Clinical
Electrocardiography

Derek J Rowlands

Consultant Cardiologist
Manchester Area Health Authority
Hon. Lecturer in Cardiology
University of Manchester

Gower Medical Publishing • London • New York
J B Lippincott Company • Philadelphia

Distributed in USA and Canada by:
J.B. Lippincott Company
East Washington Square
Philadelphia, PA 19105
USA
and
Gower Medical Publishing
101 Fifth Avenue
New York, NY 10003
USA

Distributed in Australia and New Zealand by:
Harper and Row (Australia) Pty Ltd.
P.O. Box 226
Artarmon, N.S.W. 2064
Australia

Distributed in UK, Europe and rest of the world by:
Gower Medical Publishing
Middlesex House
34-42 Cleveland Street
London W1P 5FB
UK

Distributed in Japan by:
Nankodo Co. Ltd.
42-6 Hongo 3-Chrome
Bunkyo-Ku
Tokyo 113
Japan

British Library Cataloguing in Publication Data:
Rowlands, Derek J.
Clinical Electrocardiography
1. Man. Heart. Diagnosis. Electrocardiography
1. Title
616.1207547

Library of Congress Cataloging in Publication Data
Rowlands, Derek J.
Clinical Electrocardiography/Derek Rowlands.
Includes index
1. Electrocardiography. 1. Title
[DNLM:1. Electrocardiography. 2. Heart disease — diagnosis. WG 140 R883c]
Rc683.5.E5R67 1991
616. 1'207547—dc20

ISBN: 0-397-44763-9 (Lippincott/Gower)
Printed in Singapore by Imago Productions (FE) PTE, Ltd.

Project group
Publisher: Fiona Foley
Project Editor: Sally Paviour
Designer: John Codling
Production Controller: Susan Bishop

Acknowledgements

The production of a book is always a complex business and inevitably it involves many people. It would be impossible here to list all who have contributed to this volume, but it includes those who taught me in earlier years, those who teach me today, my medical, nursing and technical colleagues, and most important of all, my students (undergraduate and postgraduate) whose own struggles to learn this difficult subject have been the driving force of this work.

On a more practical level, however, a specific mention has to be made of two names — one of a major international organisation and the other of an employee of that organisation. The organisation is ICI Pharmaceuticals Division, which supported the project over a period of years. Without its generous and enthusiastic backing this work would have been impossible. The unstinting support which it has provided has ensured the high quality of the illustrations, which is a very important aspect of the final product. Within that giant organisation one man, more than any other, has been identified with the book from its inception to its completion. That man is Roger Tittensor. It is quite impossible for me to convey the enormity of my debt to him in relation to this publication. I doubt if anyone within his firm has any real understanding of the extent of his contribution. I, of course, do and I wish to pay tribute now to that contribution. I could not have found a more reliable, committed or unselfish collaborator. To Roger, therefore, my sincerest thanks.

Finally, I would like to dedicate the book to my parents Margaret and Arthur Rowlands. From the earliest years they took a lively interest in my education and did everything within their power to support it. This is a matter which could easily be overlooked. To do so would be unforgivable. I, therefore, now dedicate this work to them.

Derek J Rowlands

Contents

Section 1: The Normal ECG

Section 2: Morphological Abnormalities

Section 3: Rhythm abnormalities

Pacemaker Electrocardiography

Preface

It is over one hundred years since the first electrocardiogram (ECG) was recorded, but electrocardiography remains an essential tool in the investigation of heart disease (the major cause of death in developed countries of the world). Despite the advent of many new investigative and diagnostic techniques, no cardiological assessment is complete without a 12-lead ECG. It has been currently estimated that one hundred million ECGs are recorded worldwide each year. Each generation of doctors has to learn afresh the difficult technique of electrocardiographic interpretation.

It is against this background that **Clinical Electrocardiography** has been produced. It assumes no prior knowledge of the subject but progresses from very basic principles to a comprehensive presentation of all clinically common electrocardiographic problems. Since it starts from first principles and progresses in a logical and disciplined manner to complex areas of electrocardiography, it is equally well suited for the beginner and also as a standard reference manual for the established practitioner. It is also well placed to serve as a manual for the teacher. Unlike other texts **Clinical Electrocardiography** has a disciplined format of presentation. Thus strict diagnostic criteria are provided rather than loose descriptions. For example, most texts will, in relation to (say) left bundle branch block, provide a list of all possible ECG changes in this condition. This is ideal if the reader's objective is to be able to write an essay on left bundle branch block but is of very limited usefulness if his objective is to decide whether or not a given ECG shows this condition. In relation to the latter objective what he needs is the *sine qua non* of the diagnosis and a separate list of the ECG features which may additionally occur in that condition. This text responds always to these dual needs. It was the author's own frustration at the inadequacies of existing books, revealed by this kind of challenge, that gave rise to the method of presentation used here.

Clinical Electrocardiography is a unique book, with a comprehensive text presented in three sections. The first of these, the Normal ECG, is an original section displaying a wide range of possible normal patterns. The second and third sections give detailed accounts of Morphological and Rhythm Abnormalities.

The text gives a frank account of the theory and practice of electrocardiography and is complemented with numerous carefully illustrated electrocardiograms. Every care has been taken to produce illustrations of the highest possible calibre and all illustrations are produced life-size. The book provides an enormous range of ECG traces, each specifically annotated. The illustrations are an extremely important feature and make the book as useful for teaching as it is for learning.

Derek J Rowlands

How to use this book

Generally, there are three approaches a reader may use to learn from this book, either as a trainee or as an established clinician re-newing his knowledge.

Approach 1. The reader wishes to have rapid access to information enabling him to discriminate among normal appearances, specific and non-specific abnormalities, and various possible rhythms without being committed to 'background reading'. To fulfill such a requirement the reader should carefully study the following pages:

Section 1: 32-33; 40-69 paying particular attention to pages 66-69. He should then work through the annotated records on pages 70-104.

Section 2: The reader should study the data contained in the blue

> "diagnostic boxes"

found on the pages which have a blue triangle in the top corner – as on this page. He should then pay particular attention to pages 265-269.

Section 3: 337-376 omitting only those paragraphs marked with a blue edge as shown here. He should also pay particular attention to pages 359-370 and 557-579. The reader should then study the data contained in the blue diagnostic boxes found on the pages which have a blue triangle in the top corner – as on this page.

Approach 2. The reader wishes to understand the basis of the normal electrocardiogram and the more important principles underlying the common morphological and rhythm abnormalities, but does not wish to concern himself with aspects which are conceptually difficult, contentious, less important or rare. In this case the reader should read through the text sequentially omitting those paragraphs marked with a blue edge as shown above.

Approach 3. The reader wishes to follow each step in the full understanding of the electrocardiogram. In this case the reader must follow the whole text sequentially.

Once you have read the book, it is likely that you will wish to dip into it from time to time, to answer questions concerning morphological or rhythm abnormalities that you come across. In such a case I suggest you work through the sections on ECG interpretation and rhythm assessment on pages 265-269 and 562-574 respectively. Readers should also benefit from working through the annotated records on pages 70-104, 270-329 and 580-609.

Derek J Rowlands

SECTION 1: **The Normal ECG**

The Normal Electrocardiogram and the Twelve Lead System

A Normal Electrocardiogram

Figure 1 shows a normal electrocardiogram (ECG). It consists of records from each of the 12 leads. The use of 12 recording leads is a convention which grew as electrocardiography developed. It has no logical or scientific basis. The two greatest obstacles to the learning of electrocardiography are:
i) the great variation in the electrocardiographic appearances of any one lead, within a population of normal subjects
and **ii)** the substantial range of different electrocardiographic appearances amongst the twelve conventional leads of a single, normal subject.

The aim of this section will be to enable the reader to overcome these twin obstacles.

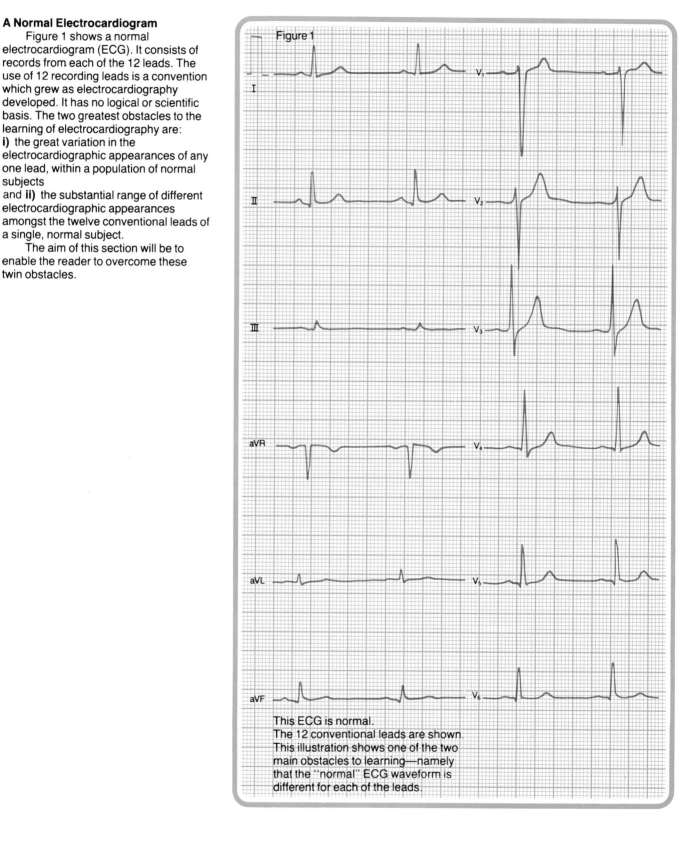

Figure 1

This ECG is normal.
The 12 conventional leads are shown.
This illustration shows one of the two main obstacles to learning—namely that the "normal" ECG waveform is different for each of the leads.

The Basic ECG Waveform

The basic ECG waveform consists of three recognisable deflections. These were termed 'P wave', 'QRS complex' and 'T wave' by Einthoven (Figure 2). He allocated sequential alphabetical lettering to the waves because he did not know their origins and did not wish to suggest any interpretation by the labelling.

In the normal 12-lead ECG all three basic waves are recorded in each lead. The P wave and T wave are relatively simple shapes. Therefore, although they vary in amplitude and in being either positive (i.e. upward deflections) or negative, they exhibit relatively few variations in shape. The QRS complexes, however, have more clearly defined shapes and they therefore exhibit readily recognisable differences in pattern in different leads within the same ECG (Figure 1).

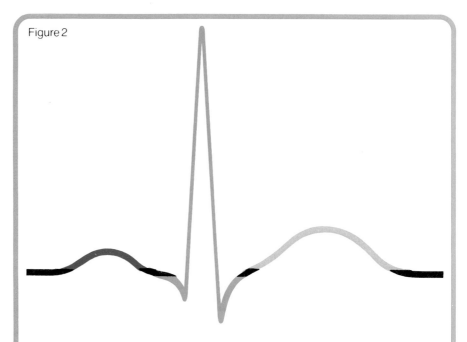

Figure 2

The **P wave** represents the spread of electrical activation through the atrial myocardium. In the normal ECG it is a small, smooth, rounded deflection preceding the QRS complex. The **QRS complex** represents the spread of electrical activation through the ventricular myocardium. It is usually, but not always, the largest deflection of the ECG. It is always 'spiky' in shape. The **T wave** represents electrical recovery of the ventricular myocardium. This must inevitably follow electrical activation and must be accomplished before any repeat electrical activation is possible. It is a broad rounded wave. A T wave follows each QRS complex and is separated from it by an interval which is constant in any given ECG.

QRS Waveform Nomenclature

All sharp, pointed deflections resulting from electrical activation of the ventricles are called "QRS complexes" whether they start with a positive (upright) deflection or a negative one, whether they finish with a positive or with a negative deflection and whether they have one, two, three or more recognisable deflections within them.

The presence and relative size of the several possible components of the QRS complex may be indicated by a convention using combinations of the letters q, r, s, Q, R, S.

The rules of the convention are as follows:-

i) The first positive (upgoing) wave is labelled r or R.

ii) Any second positive wave is labelled r' or R.'

iii) A negative wave (i.e. one descending below the base line) is labelled an s or S wave if it follows an r or R wave.

iv) A negative wave is labelled q or Q if it precedes r or R (in which case it must inevitably also be the first wave to occur).

v) Any wave which is entirely negative is labelled qs or QS.

vi) LARGE DEFLECTIONS ARE LABELLED WITH AN APPROPRIATE UPPER CASE (CAPITAL) LETTER. Small deflections are labelled with an appropriate lower case letter.

Figure 3 shows twelve of the possible variations in QRS waveform with colour-coded labelling. Note that each is. in the generic sense, a QRS complex.

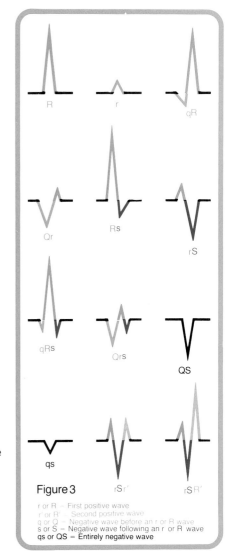

Figure 3

r or R = First positive wave
r' or R' = Second positive wave
q or Q = Negative wave before an r or R wave
s or S = Negative wave following an r or R wave
qs or QS = Entirely negative wave

Returning to Figure 1, it can now be seen that Leads I, II, aVF, V_5 and V_6 show qR-type QRS complexes, V_1 and V_2 show rS-type QRS complexes, V_3 shows Rs type, V_4 shows qRs-type, III shows r-type, aVL shows rs-type and aVR shows QS-type QRS complexes. The expression "type QRS complexes" is often abbreviated to "complexes". Thus "V_3 shows Rs-type QRS complexes" may be abbreviated to "V_3 shows Rs complexes".

Initiation and Spread of Electrical Activation in the Heart

In normal circumstances the whole process of electrical activation of the heart begins in the sino-atrial node. Spontaneous activation occurs in the sino-atrial node and activation then spreads to the adjacent atrial myocardium. Activation next spreads in all directions across the atrial myocardium. The activation process reaches the atrio-ventricular node and passes through this to the bundle of His and into the right and left bundle branches, through the Purkinje network and into the ventricular myocardium.

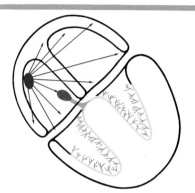

Figure 4

The common bundle (bundle of His) forms the only electrical connection between the atria and the ventricles. It arises as a continuation of the atrio-ventricular node.

The right and left bundle branches are the divisions of the common bundle. They run below the endocardial surfaces of their respective ventricles.

The sino-atrial node is situated high up in the right atrium . . . It normally initiates activation of the atrial myocardium. The atrio-ventricular node is situated low in the right atrium. It transmits activation received from the sino-atrial node (via the atrial myocardium) to the common bundle.

The Purkinje network is a fine arborisation of branches. This network spreads over the endocardial surfaces of the ventricles.

Myocardium has the ability to conduct electrical activation in **any** direction. The **actual** direction of conduction will therefore depend on the position at which activation is initiated. Conduction must necessarily occur in all directions from this starting point. The **predominant** direction of spread will be that direction in which the greatest mass of myocardium is available from the given starting point.

Activation of the atrial myocardium begins high up in the right atrium and spreads from this site in all available directions. The predominant direction of spread of atrial activation is to the left and somewhat downwards. (Large arrow Figure 5).

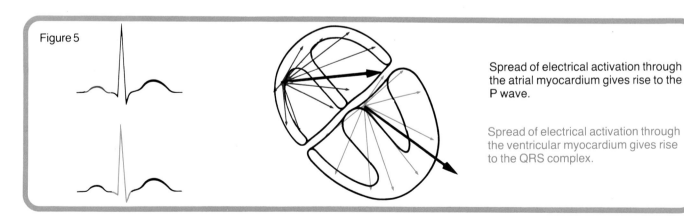

Figure 5

Spread of electrical activation through the atrial myocardium gives rise to the P wave.

Spread of electrical activation through the ventricular myocardium gives rise to the QRS complex.

The first part of the ventricular myocardium to receive the activation process is high up in the left side of the interventricular septum. Because of this, the predominant direction of ventricular activation is downwards. Since the ventricles are initially activated from the left side of the interventricular septum it might be expected that the predominant direction would also be slightly to the right. However, the mass of the left ventricle is substantially greater than that of the right ventricle and left ventricular activation dominates the production of the QRS complex in all normal and most abnormal ECG's. Because of this, ventricular activation predominantly occurs downwards and somewhat to the left. (Figure 5).

The Magnitude and Direction of the Activation Processes

Figures 4 and 5 both indicate numerous activation waves travelling over the atria and over the ventricles.

The waves occur in all available directions from their starting points. The multiple arrows over the atria and ventricles indicate the directions of the activation waves. The arrows shown are a representative group from an infinite number of actual directions.

The arrows vary, not only in direction, but also in length. The length of the arrow is determined by the extent of myocardium available for activation in any given direction. Each arrow therefore represents the activation wave in magnitude and direction. In other words, each arrow represents an activation vector.

Activation Vectors

The term 'vector' is one which often has an inhibiting effect on those seeking to learn electrocardiography. It often invokes the feeling that complexity will now increase and understanding will be left behind. There is no need for such a fear. A vector is simply something which has magnitude and direction. The activation waves so far discussed are vectors because they have these two properties. The arrows in Figure 5 are the graphical representations of these vectors. By accepted convention, arrows are used to represent vectors.
The direction in which the arrow points represents the direction of the vector. The length of the arrow represents the magnitude of the vector.

The importance of the **combination** of direction and magnitude is that **apparent** magnitude of a vector depends upon the direction in which it is sensed. This is not true of **scalar** properties which have magnitude only. The difference may be illustrated by considering two examples:
(a) George Brown weighs 75 Kgm. It does not matter whether George Brown is standing up, sitting down or standing on his head—he still weighs 75 Kgm. Weight has magnitude only it is a scalar property.
(b) A wind is blowing due East with a velocity of 10 units (Figure 6).

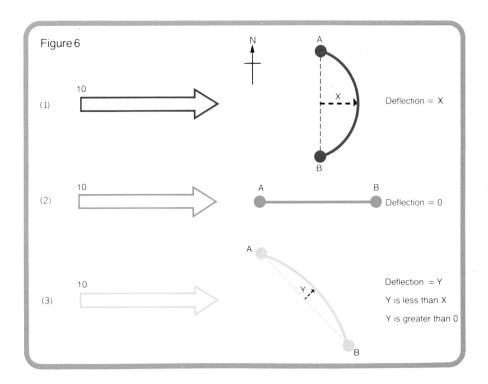

Figure 6

Figure 6 shows the vector representation of the wind as an arrow pointing due East, with a length equivalent to 10 units. To sense this wind an enterprising student of electrocardiography has erected two vertical poles (sticking up out of the ground) and has fixed a thin sheet of aluminium between them. Figure 6 shows the poles (A & B) with the aluminium sheet between them **as seen from above.** The student is anxious to discover the influence of sensing direction on the apparent magnitude of the vector, and he tries three different arrangements of his apparatus. In arrangement (1) the aluminium sheet buckles away from the wind. The maximum deflection 'x' of the aluminium

from its resting position is dependent on the magnitude of the wind vector, i.e. it is related to the velocity, 10 units (of course it is also related to the bending properties of the aluminium sheet but we need not consider this further here). In arrangement (2) no deflection of the aluminium sheet occurs. Thus, despite the fact that the **actual** magnitude and direction of the wind are unchanged, the **apparent** magnitude of the vector is zero. In arrangement (3) an intermediate orientation is used for the aluminium sheet and an intermediate deflection results. The student has demonstrated that the apparent magnitude of a vector will vary if the direction in which that vector is sensed is varied.

Essential points to note about activation wave vectors are as follows:-
(i) Activation wave vectors have magnitude and direction.

(ii) Since these two properties must be considered together, the apparent magnitude of the activation wave will depend on the direction from which it is sensed.

Using the same example as in Figure 6, the importance of the direction in which the activation wave is sensed can be illustrated as shown in Figure 7.

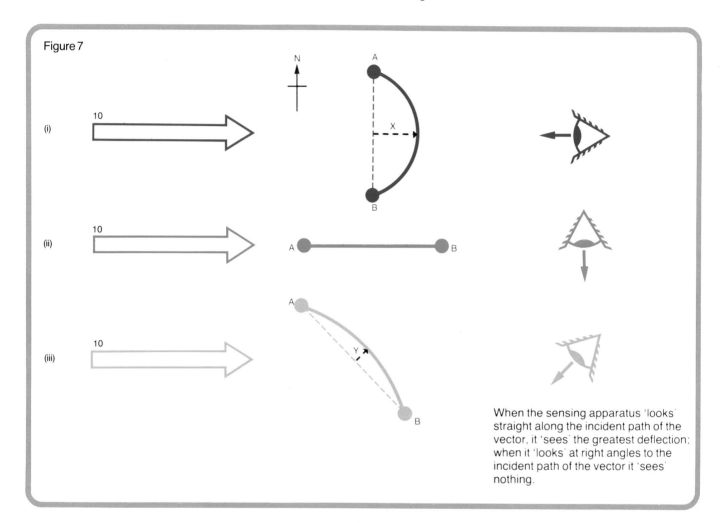

Figure 7

When the sensing apparatus 'looks' straight along the incident path of the vector, it 'sees' the greatest deflection; when it 'looks' at right angles to the incident path of the vector it 'sees' nothing.

Polarisation and Depolarisation

So far we have discussed 'activation' of areas of myocardium without specifying what this process is. 'Activation' is actually the process of depolarisation and the spontaneous spread of this process over the lining membrane of the myocardial cells.

Resting, healthy, myocardial cells are 'polarised'. That is to say, the surface membrane of each cell has an accumulation of charges - positive ones on the outside and an equal number of negative ones on the inside (Figure 8).

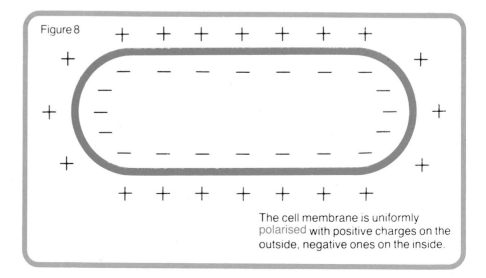

Figure 8

The cell membrane is uniformly polarised with positive charges on the outside, negative ones on the inside.

This state of affairs (ie. polarisation) persists until some external interference (eg. artificial stimulation, or the arrival of some natural activation wave) induces depolarisation. **Note that polarisation is the normal, resting state of affairs for myocardial cells. Depolarisation has to be induced.**

Depolarisation consists not simply of the abolition of the normal distribution of charges on the two sides of the surface membrane but implies a **reversal** of this normal distribution, so that **during depolarisation the outside of the membrane has negative charges and the inside positive.**

Figure 9 is a diagrammatic representation of a myocardial cell in which depolarisation has been induced in a small area of the surface membrane.

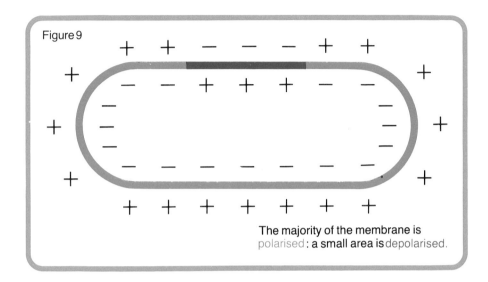

Figure 9

The majority of the membrane is polarised: a small area is depolarised.

As has already been stated, depolarisation must be induced. It does not occur spontaneously in myocardial cells. However, once depolarisation has been induced in any area of the myocardial cell membrane it will spread spontaneously over the whole of the membrane of that cell and to all other cells with which it is in electrical contact. (Figure 10).

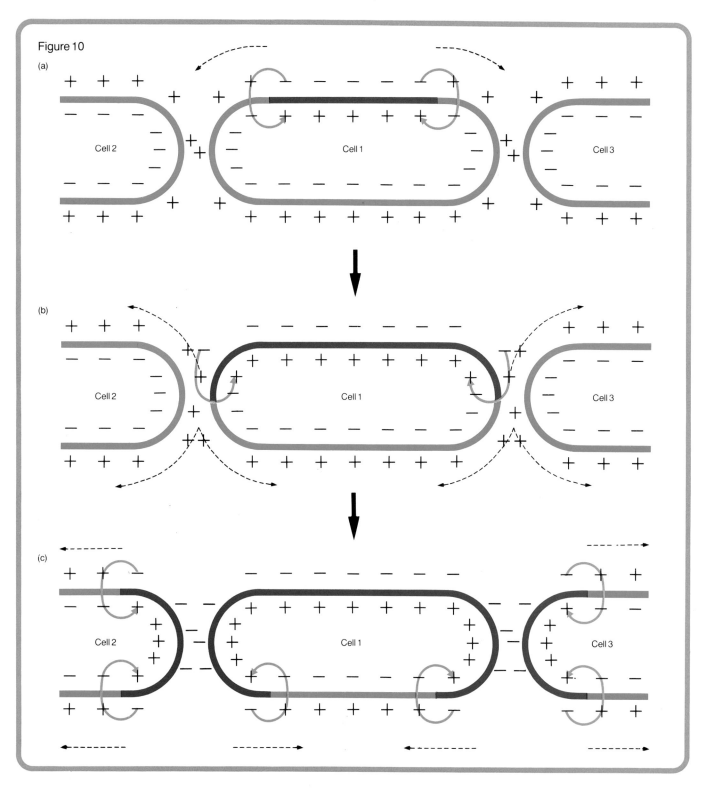

Figure 10

The self-propagation of depolarisation occurs because, at the margins between depolarised and polarised membranes, battery conditions exist with adjacent positive and negative charges giving rise to local current flow ( ) which is sufficient to induce depolarisation in the adjacent segments, and so on until the whole membrane is depolarised.

Thus, depolarisation spreads as a wave across the membranes of myocardial cells. The depolarisation (= activation) wave has vector properties, ie. it has magnitude and direction. Its magnitude depends simply on the mass of myocardium being depolarised. Its direction depends upon (a) the position on the surface membrane at which depolarisation is first induced and (b) the anatomical distribution of myocardium available for depolarisation starting from that point.

The spread of electrical activation over the ventricular myocardium gives rise to the QRS complex and we are now in a position to consider the form of the QRS complex in the conventional ECG.

The QRS Complex

To understand the appearance of the QRS complex in the leads of the ECG it is best initially to simplify matters by considering something much less complex than the arrangement of the myocardium of the right and left ventricles. Let us therefore consider a single myocardial strip with electrodes arranged around it (Figure 11).

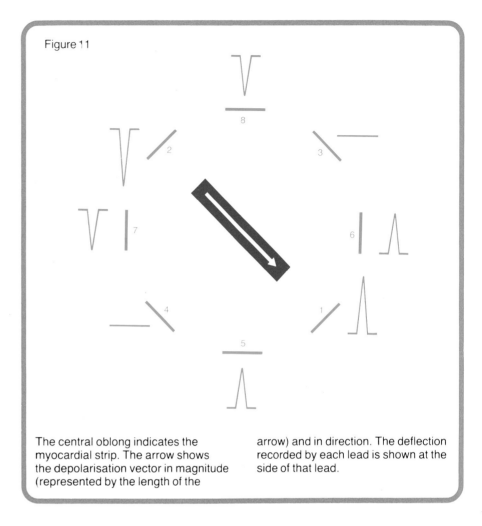

Figure 11

The central oblong indicates the myocardial strip. The arrow shows the depolarisation vector in magnitude (represented by the length of the arrow) and in direction. The deflection recorded by each lead is shown at the side of that lead.

An electrode sited in position 1 would see a large positive deflection. An electrode in position 2 would see a deflection of equal size but negative. Electrodes at position 3 or 4 would see no deflection. Electrodes at position 5 and 6 would see positive deflections of (identical) intermediate size. Electrodes at position 7 and 8 would see negative deflections of (identical) intermediate size. **Despite the fact that all eight electrodes are looking at the same wave, they see very different things because of their differing orientations.**

It is important also to realise that two electrodes each looking along a direction at the same angle to the incident wave but on different sides of it (as with 5 and 6, 3 and 4, 7 and 8) will see the same deflection.

Note that only electrodes 1 and 2 in Figure 11 above see the full magnitude of the vector.

If the left ventricle were a simple muscle strip, then eight electrodes arranged as in Figure 11 would record eight QRS complexes as shown.

If we now consider an infinite number of electrode positions arranged in a continuous circle at the centre of which is the origin of the depolarisation wave, we can predict how the appearance of the recorded deflection would be affected by the siting of the electrode (Figure 12).

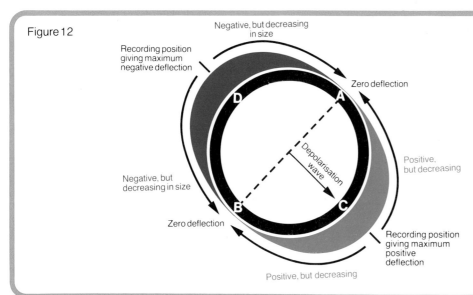

Figure 12

The thick black circle represents the infinite number of possible electrode positions occupying a circle whose centre is the origin of the depolarisation wave. Thus, leads recording from positions A or B would record no deflection. A lead in position C would give a maximum positive deflection and one in position D would give a maximum negative deflection. Any lead positioned between C and A or between C and B would show a positive deflection which would be larger or smaller depending upon whether it was nearer or farther from C. Similarly, negative deflections of varying possible size would occur using leads positioned between D and A or between D and B.

It is clear that the position of the recording electrode exerts a profound influence on the record obtained. However, before this undoubted truth can be applied to explain the form of the recordings in the twelve leads of the conventional ECG, it is necessary to consider the difference between the behaviour of a **volume** conductor and that of a **linear** conductor. The most important difference is that a linear conductor has virtually identical voltages at all points along its length, whereas the voltage may vary appreciably at different locations within a volume conductor.

The trunk behaves as a volume conductor and therefore electrode positioning on the trunk materially affects the record obtained and correct positioning of the chest electrodes is essential if a meaningful ECG is to be obtained.

The most common example of a linear conductor is a wire. An electrical waveform applied at one end of a wire is transmitted without significant change along the wire. The waveform may therefore be sensed close to or distant from its origin without appreciable differences. Within reasonable limits, the length of the wire is irrelevant. **The limbs behave like linear conductors.**

The limbs may therefore be regarded as simple extensions of the lead wire. The same record would be obtained whether the recording electrode is attached to the wrist, forearm, elbow, upper arm or shoulder. The left arm of the patient can therefore be regarded as an extension of the left arm lead of the ECG and the **left arm connection can therefore be regarded as recording from the position where the left arm meets the trunk (ie the left shoulder) no matter where on the left arm the recording electrode is placed.** Likewise the right arm lead simply records from the right shoulder and the left leg records from the left groin.

Leads R, L and F (the unipolar limb leads).

We are now in a position to understand the disposition of the unipolar limb leads, in which recordings are made from the right arm (R), the left arm (L) and the left leg ("foot", F). For convenience, the physical connections are usually made to the extremities of the limbs, ie to the wrists and left ankle. Since the limbs act as linear conductors, however, the effective locations of the recording electrodes are at the shoulders and the left groin (Figure 13,a).

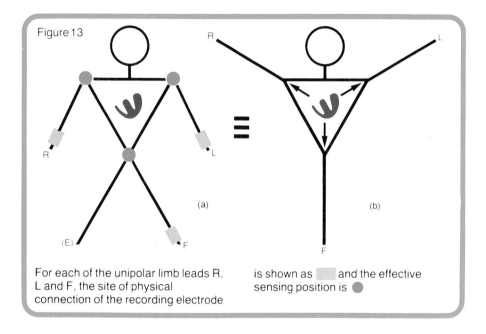

Figure 13

(a)

(b)

(E)

For each of the unipolar limb leads R, L and F, the site of physical connection of the recording electrode

is shown as ▮ and the effective sensing position is ●

The direction in which the limb electrodes sense the cardiac electrical activity is best appreciated if the limbs are rearranged as in the right hand side of the diagram (Figure 13,b).

The right leg connection (E) is simply an earth connection to minimise interference.

The Einthoven Triangle Hypothesis

Figure 13 shows the heart at the centre of an equilateral triangle. This is a diagrammatic representation of the **Einthoven Triangle Hypothesis.** This hypothesis, which was published in 1913, was an attempt to explain the principles of electrocardiography in scientific terms. It depends upon four simplifying assumptions. None of these assumptions is completely true but the error in each case is relatively small and the assumptions are sufficiently close to the truth to ensure that the hypothesis provides an adequate working base.

The assumptions of this hypothesis are as follows:-
1. **The trunk is a homogeneous volume conductor.** (It is obvious that the conductivities of the various body tissues differ from one another but the differences are surprisingly small).
2. **The sum of all the electrical forces being produced at any instant or the mean of all the electrical forces generated during the cardiac cycle can be considered as originating in a dipole located in the centre of the heart.** (A dipole is a positive charge and a negative charge of equal magnitude located so close to one another that they may be considered to be at the same point).

3. **The extremity leads (R, L and F) pick up potential changes in the frontal plane only.** (In general this is true).
4. **The attachments of the three extremities used in making the limb leads (R, L and F) form the apices of an equilateral triangle with reference to a dipole located at its centre.** (Anatomically, of course, the roots of the right arm, left arm and left leg in no sense form an equilateral triangle.) However, if the cardiac electrical field is considered as originating from a dipole the positive and negative charges are, by definition, extremely close together (ie the distance separating them is zero) and, in relative terms the distances of each of the limb roots from this dipole are great enough to be considered infinite.

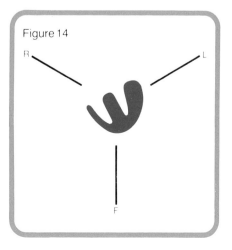

Figure 14

R

L

W

F

Thus the heart may be considered to lie at the centre of an equilateral triangle, the apices of which are the two shoulders and the left groin, which are the effective sensing points of the right arm, left arm and left leg connections (R, L and F).

Leads R, L & F are in fact looking at the heart along the directions shown in Figure 13b and in Figure 14.

We can now return to our simplified concept of the ventricles as a simple muscle strip and consider how depolarisation of this strip will give rise to deflections in R, L and F.

If the muscle is arranged as in Figure 15, L is at right angles to the direction of the depolarisation vector and therefore shows no deflection. R sees the vector retreating and gives a negative deflection and F faces the oncoming vector and gives a positive deflection. If there were some other lead, 'X', the direction of sensing of which were precisely that of the incident depolarisation wave, it would see a positive deflection larger than that seen in F.

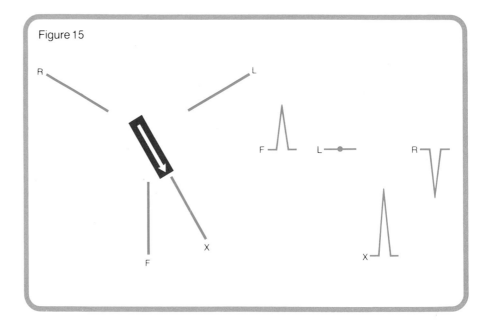

Figure 15

The limb leads so far discussed are the so-called unipolar limb leads. No voltage measurement is ever truly unipolar. Any voltage must be measured against a reference voltage. In the case of the 'unipolar' leads there is an exploring electrode (attached to the limb in question and reflecting variations in potential at that limb) and a 'reference' electrode (which is so arranged that its potential does not vary during the cardiac cycle). The reference electrode is formed by joining together leads from R, L and F. The sum total of these deflections is zero, provided the limb leads are evenly distributed around the heart. Thus in the diagram above, the "cardiac" muscle strip is at the centre of an equilateral triangle from the apices of which Leads R, L and F emerge. These leads are evenly distributed around the "heart" and it is easy to see, from inspection of the deflections at R, L and F (Figure 15),

that the sum total of their recorded deflections is close to zero. Note also that if we include Lead X, we no longer have our leads evenly distributed and the sum total of the deflections would not be zero. The proof that the sum of simultaneous deflections at R, L and F is zero will be given later (see p 19).

When this 'indifferent' connection, formed by joining R, L and F together, is used as the reference connection, the lead so formed is called a "V" lead (the "V" originally stood for voltage). Such a connection is used for the limb leads VR, VL and VF and also for the chest leads V_1 to V_6. Nowadays the limb connections are slightly modified to augment the size of the deflections obtained from R, L and F and these augmented leads are called aVR, aVL and aVF. The precordial leads are not augmented. The augmented leads will be described in detail later (pp 18, 19).

**Leads I, II and III
(the bipolar limb leads, the
'standard' limb leads)**

Before the modern unipolar leads were developed, three bipolar limb leads were used. These leads are formed by connecting one end of the recording galvanometer to one limb and the other end to a second limb. Only three limbs (right arm, left arm, left leg) are used and three combinations: known as Leads, I, II and III are achieved.

Lead I connects the galvanometer imputs to the right and left arm. Any voltage change observed could be the result of a change at either arm or at both arms, so the lead is truly bipolar.

The second connection (Lead II) is made between the right arm and the left leg and the third connection (Lead III) between the left arm and the left leg.

There was no logic in the choice of this arrangement, it was simply a matter of convenience. The right leg was used as an 'earth to minimise interference. With a bipolar system, one lead has to be connected to the positive terminal of the galvanometer and one to the negative. Again, **the way in which these connections were assigned was fortuitous, not by design.** Einthoven manipulated the connections until the ECG waveforms from all three leads were upright. It so happened then that in the case of Lead I the left arm was connected to the positive and the right arm to the negative terminals of the galvanometer, in the case of Lead II the left leg was connected to the positive and

the right arm to the negative terminals and in the case of Lead III, the left leg was connected to the positive and the left arm to the negative terminals.
This system of connection is now the accepted convention and these connections are incorporated into the lead selector switch on the ECG machine. (Had Einthoven used a different subject he may well have had to use a different arrangement of connections in order to obtain three upright deflections. In that event we would all now be using that different set of connections as our accepted convention).

From the accepted, conventional system of connections it follows that the limb leads are related to the unipolar limb leads thus:-

$$I = L - R$$
$$II = F - R$$
$$III = F - L$$

[These relationships are presented here for completeness. The student will not be required to remember these nor to use them in the process of ECG interpretation.]

Since each bipolar lead represents the result of electrical activity occurring at two sites simultaneously it becomes necessary to consider the consequences of two vectors acting simultaneously if we are to understand the effective disposition of the bipolar leads.

Summation of Vectors

If two or more vectors act simultaneously on the same object they may be added together. The result of this addition is the same as the arithmetic sum of their magnitudes only if they act in the same direction.

Consider a boat of circular outline seen from above as in Figure 16. (It is readily conceded that this shape will win no prizes for nautical design, but it is ideal for our purposes).

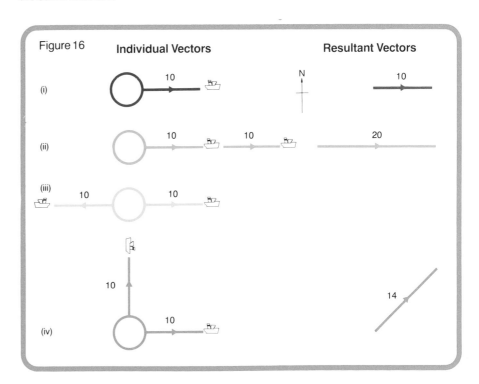

Figure 16 — Individual Vectors — Resultant Vectors

In situation (i) a single tug boat pulls our craft due east with a speed of 10 units. In (ii) the two tugs pull east each with independent speed 10 units. The total effective speed, therefore, is 20 units due east. In (iii) the two tugs pull in opposing directions and our craft does not move (though it may tear apart). In (iv) one tug pulls due north and one due east each with a velocity of 10 units. Our craft will move north east with a velocity of approximately 14 units.

The above examples show the results of vector addition in a few, very specialised, vector combinations.

In general, vectors may be added by constructing a parallelogram of vectors. (Figure 17).

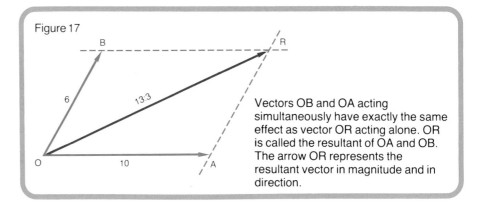

Figure 17

Vectors OB and OA acting simultaneously have exactly the same effect as vector OR acting alone. OR is called the resultant of OA and OB. The arrow OR represents the resultant vector in magnitude and in direction.

Subtraction of Vectors

Since the bipolar limb leads record the **difference** between simultaneous vectors (one end of the lead being connected to the positive and one to the negative terminal of the galvanometer) we need to understand how to subtract vectors. This requires an additional step— we have to understand a negative vector. A negative vector can be considered simply as a vector acting in the opposite direction. Thus in Figure 18, vector OC is the negative of vector OA.

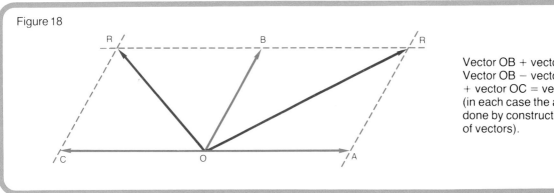

Figure 18

Vector OB + vector OA = vector OR
Vector OB − vector OA = vector OB + vector OC = vector OR′
(in each case the actual summation is done by constructing a parallelogram of vectors).

Arrangement of the Standard Limb Leads (I, II and III)

Since we now know (a) the effective arrangement of the unipolar limb leads R, L and F (b) the connections between R, L and F, used in the standard limb leads and (c) how to subtract vectors, we are now in a position to understand the **effective** arrangement of I, II and III.

Lead I is obtained by connecting L to the positive terminal of the galvanometer and R to the negative terminal.

Therefore I = L − R
we have seen that this can be manipulated to I = L + "inverse R."

Figure 19 shows how the effective position of Lead I can be visualised:-

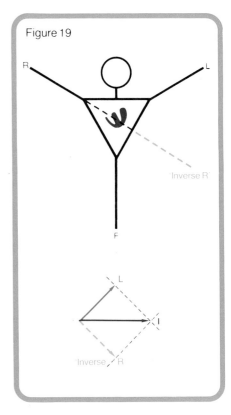

Figure 19

Thus Lead I effectively looks at the heart from the left, ie. from a position anatomically inferior to that from which the left arm lead looks.

Similarly, Lead II which records with the left leg ("foot") connected to the positive and the right arm to the negative terminal of the galvanometer, can be seen to look at the heart from a position to the left of that of the foot lead. (Figure 20).

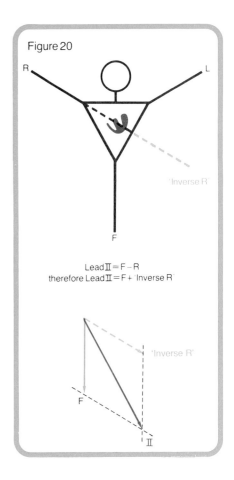

Figure 20

Lead II = F − R
therefore Lead II = F + 'Inverse R'

Similarly Lead III, in which the left leg ("foot") is connected to the positive galvanometer terminal and the left arm to the negative terminal, effectively looks at the heart from a position to the right of the foot lead. (Figure 21).

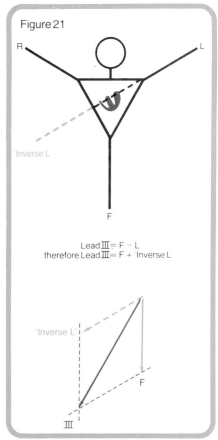

Figure 21

Lead III = F − L
therefore Lead III = F + 'Inverse L'

**The Six Limb Leads
(the frontal plane leads)**

The orientation around the heart of the six limb leads can now be understood (Figure 22).

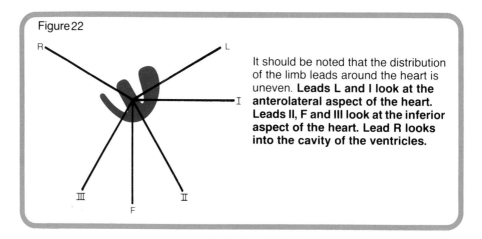

Figure 22

It should be noted that the distribution of the limb leads around the heart is uneven. **Leads L and I look at the anterolateral aspect of the heart. Leads II, F and III look at the inferior aspect of the heart. Lead R looks into the cavity of the ventricles.**

An understanding of the arrangement of the limb leads around the heart helps to make clear why it is that certain appearances are found in certain leads. For example, the changes of **inferior** infarction are seen in Leads **II, F and III** (the inferior limb leads), and those of **anterolateral** infarction are seen in **L and I** (the anterolateral leads). Lead **R** always shows appearances which are different from those of the other five limb leads for it looks into the cavity of the heart ("a cavity lead") whereas L tends to show appearances similar to I (being close to it), II tends to show similar appearances to F and F tends to show similar appearances to III.

The Augmented Limb Leads

Reference was made earlier (p.14) to the augmented limb leads. All current ECG machines use augmented limb leads, ie. they record aVL, aVF and aVR and not L, F and R. The student need not in any way concern himself with this. Everything which has been understood for L, F and R is equally applicable to aVL, aVF and aVR. Students who can accept this assurance should omit the following section. Those who require demonstration of the assertion should study the section.

The Indifferent Connection

Reference was made earlier to the 'indifferent connection' in the unipolar limb leads (p.14). It was stated that if all three connections in the frontal plane (ie. the right arm, left arm and foot connections) are joined together, the resultant deflection is zero and that this is true whatever deflections might be recorded in any single lead, provided the three leads are evenly distributed in the frontal plane. Consider leads R, L and F, with each making an angle of 120° with adjacent leads (Figure 23):-

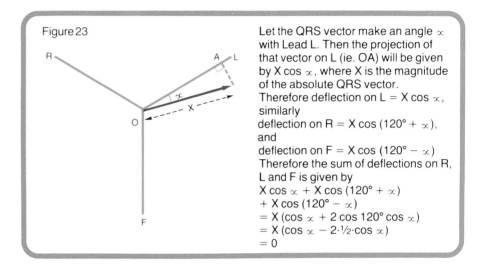

Figure 23

Let the QRS vector make an angle α with Lead L. Then the projection of that vector on L (ie. OA) will be given by $X \cos \alpha$, where X is the magnitude of the absolute QRS vector.
Therefore deflection on L = $X \cos \alpha$, similarly
deflection on R = $X \cos (120° + \alpha)$, and
deflection on F = $X \cos (120° - \alpha)$
Therefore the sum of deflections on R, L and F is given by
$X \cos \alpha + X \cos (120° + \alpha)$
$+ X \cos (120° - \alpha)$
$= X (\cos \alpha + 2 \cos 120° \cos \alpha)$
$= X (\cos \alpha - 2 \cdot \frac{1}{2} \cdot \cos \alpha)$
$= 0$

Thus the sum of the deflections on leads R, L and F is zero. We may express this as:
$$R + L + F = 0$$
Figure 24 shows how this principle is used to obtain Lead VL.

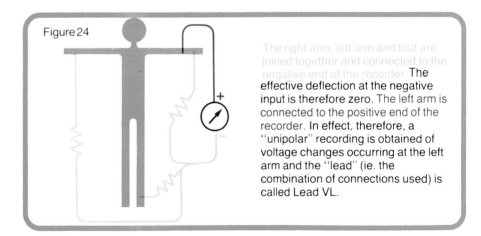

Figure 24

The right arm, left arm and foot are joined together and connected to the negative end of the recorder. The effective deflection at the negative input is therefore zero. The left arm is connected to the positive end of the recorder. In effect, therefore, a "unipolar" recording is obtained of voltage changes occurring at the left arm and the "lead" (ie. the combination of connections used) is called Lead VL.

The use of a system joining the right arm, left arm and foot together and connecting this to the negative input of the galvanometer was devised by Wilson. The joint lead is known as the Wilson central terminal. Any lead using this central terminal for the negative connection and an exploring lead for the positive connection is known as a "V lead" (The "V" originally stood for voltage).

The augmented ("aV") limb leads are obtained by omitting a limb connection from the indifferent electrode whenever that limb is connected to the exploring electrode. Figure 25 shows the connections used in recording aVL.

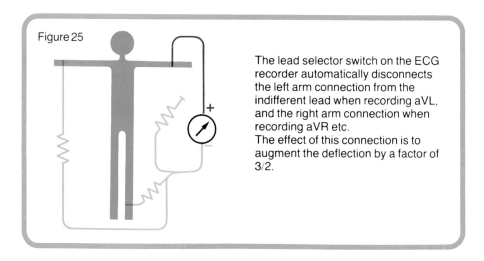

Figure 25

The lead selector switch on the ECG recorder automatically disconnects the left arm connection from the indifferent lead when recording aVL, and the right arm connection when recording aVR etc.
The effect of this connection is to augment the deflection by a factor of 3/2.

The augmentation produced can be calculated as follows:-
$R + L + F = 0$ (see p 19).
(ie. the sum of the voltage from the three limb connections is zero)
therefore $L = - (F + R) \ldots$ (i)

From the connection of aVL as shown in Figure 25 it is clear that:-
$aVL = L - (\frac{F + R}{2}) \ldots$ (ii)
(The voltage measured is the difference between that at the positive terminal (L) and that at the negative terminal $(\frac{F + R}{2})$

Substituting for L (from equation (i)) in equation (ii)
$aVL = - (F + R) - (\frac{F + R}{2})$
$\quad\quad = \frac{3}{2} (-(F + R))$
but $- (F + R) = L$ (equation (i))
therefore $aVL = \frac{3}{2} L$
Similarly $aVR = \frac{3}{2} R$
and $aVF = \frac{3}{2} F$

Augmentation of the limb leads in this way is now standard procedure in ECG recorders. It makes no difference to the **morphology** of any of the deflections. **Whenever the limb leads are shown or discussed from now on it may be taken for granted aVR, aVL and aVF are implied.**

**The General Form of the QRS
Complexes in the Six Limb Leads**

Returning once more to the strip of myocardium as a simple model for the ventricles, we can now see how the six limb leads would record their differing deflections when this strip is depolarised (Figure 26).

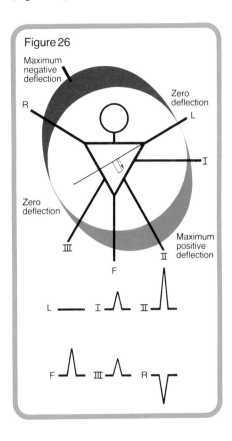

Figure 26

The myocardial strip is arranged to be parallel to Lead II. Depolarisation of the strip is arranged to be from the top right hand side (of the subject) and it therefore occurs downwards and to the left.

Depolarisation therefore spreads towards Lead II. Because of this, Lead II shows a large, positive deflection. F also 'sees' the deflection coming towards it and therefore also gives a positive deflection, but F is not placed precisely along (ie parallel to) the direction of depolarisation and therefore the size of the deflection in F is less than that in II. Similarly, I and III are orientated in front of the depolarisation waves, but less advantageously so and they see smaller positive deflections (compare Figure 12). Since the depolarisation wave approaches I and III at the same angle, these two leads show equal deflections. L is at right angles to the strip and therefore shows zero deflection but R lies behind the depolarisation wave and records a negative deflection.

We are now in a position to progress from the consideration of recordings obtained during depolarisation of a simple muscle strip to a more realistic model of the heart. The heart is a complicated arrangement of myocardial fibres organised as two atria and two ventricles with a common wall (septum) in between. The mass of the left ventricle is many times greater than that of the right, and **for a first simplification, to facilitate understanding of the genesis of the QRS complex, the effect of the right ventricular myocardium can be ignored.** It should be remembered that the QRS complex represents **depolarisation** of the **ventricular myocardium** and since, in the first instance, we are going to ignore the right ventricle we may now consider how **depolarisation of the left ventricular myocardium gives rise to the QRS complex.**

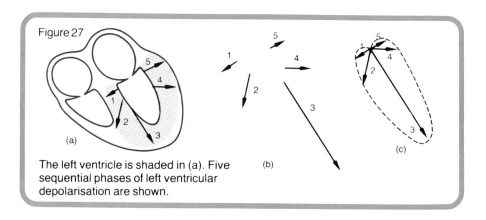

Figure 27

(a)

(b)

(c)

The left ventricle is shaded in (a). Five sequential phases of left ventricular depolarisation are shown.

Ventricular activation (depolarisation) begins high up in the inter-ventricular septum on its left side (Figure 5, p 6). The inter-ventricular septum is depolarised from left to right (phase 1, Figure 27 (a)). Depolarisation spreads down the septum, towards the apex of the heart (phase 2, Figure 27 (a)) and then progressively along the free wall of the left ventricle - but always from endocardium to pericardium (phases 3, 4, 5, Figure 27 (a)).

Figure 27 (a) shows the **direction** (only) of each phase of depolarisatioin (ie. the length of the arrows is not a scale representation of their magnitude). Figures 27 (b) and (c) show the **direction and magnitude** (ie. the vectors) of each of these five representative phases of depolarisation.

Thus, instead of the single arrow representing the depolarisation of a simple muscle strip, we have five arrows representing (a simplification of) the sequence of ventricular depolarisation (Figure 27 (b)). In fact since the direction of ventricular depolarisation is constantly changing, there are an infinite number of such **instantaneous** arrows (just as there are an infinite number of points between any two marks on a ruler) and the arrangement of this infinite series of instantaneous vectors can be visualised as in Figure 27 (c). Here the vectors are given a common origin and the interrupted line shows the position of the tips of the infinite array of arrows as one progresses counterclockwise around

the interrupted line. The five simplified arrows are shown. The interrupted line is the **vector loop.** It merely demonstrates the continuously varying **magnitude** and **direction** of the left ventricular depolarisation waves. Such a loop, including as it does the infinite number of instantaneous depolarisation vectors occurring during a single ventricular depolarisation, provides a much more realistic model of the process than the single arrow. From this model one can see how deflections more complex than those shown in Figure 26 may arise. Figure 28 shows the deflections produced in the six limb leads by a vector loop of the type shown in Figure 27.

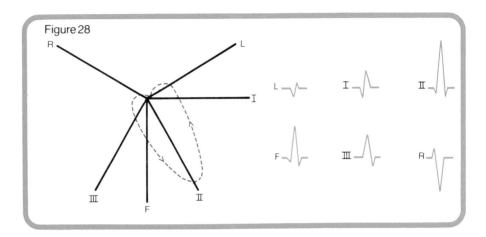

Figure 28

It may not be immediately apparent how the vector loop gives rise to QRS deflections of the form shown. It might therefore prove helpful to consider in detail how the vector loop shown in Figure 28 gives rise to the QRS morphology in two of the limb leads, for example, L (Figure 29) and II (Figure 30).

As regards the QRS appearances in L:-

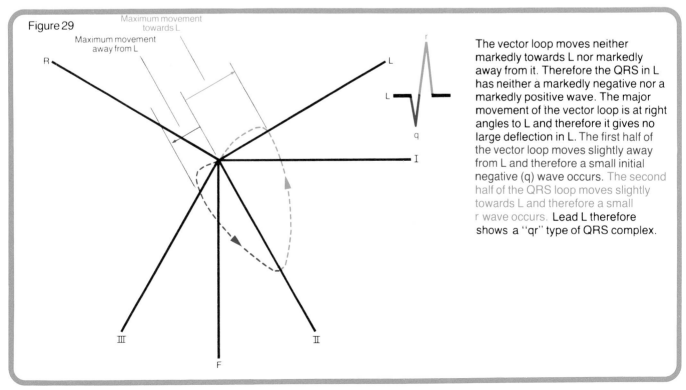

Figure 29

Maximum movement towards L

Maximum movement away from L

The vector loop moves neither markedly towards L nor markedly away from it. Therefore the QRS in L has neither a markedly negative nor a markedly positive wave. The major movement of the vector loop is at right angles to L and therefore it gives no large deflection in L. The first half of the vector loop moves slightly away from L and therefore a small initial negative (q) wave occurs. The second half of the QRS loop moves slightly towards L and therefore a small r wave occurs. Lead L therefore shows a ''qr'' type of QRS complex.

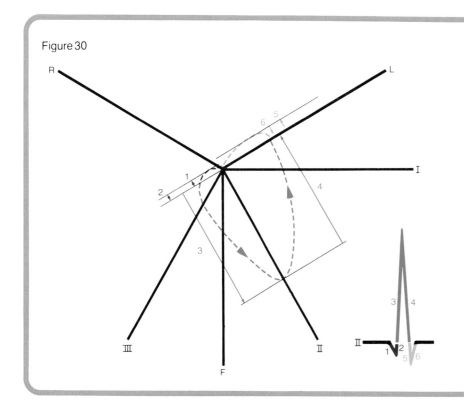

Figure 30

Note that the vector initially moves away from Lead II (phase one) and this brief trend is reversed (phase two). The loop then moves towards Lead II (phase three) until this is reversed (phase four). There is then a final movement away from II (phase five) and this, too, is finally reversed (phase six). As shown in the enlarged QRS complex, phases 1 and 2 give rise to the q wave, phases 3 and 4 to the R wave and phases 5 and 6 to the s wave. Lead II therefore shows a "qRs" type of QRS complex.

The Electrical Axis

The vector loop shown in Figures 29 and 30 is the same as that in Figure 28. It is apparent that, even though real ventricles produce a loop (compared with an **arrow** produced by a simple muscle strip), it is still possible to recognise a predominant direction in which the loop 'points'. In this example the direction is along Lead II. It is because the loop points along Lead II that a large, positive wave is seen in that lead. The direction in which the loop points is called the **electrical axis of the heart.**

The electrical axis is important for two reasons:- (a) it has clinical significance in its own right - some clinical conditions are associated with axes within certain ranges - and (b) an understanding of the axis is necessary before the variety of possible limb lead appearances among different, normal ECG's can be appreciated.

Hexaxial Reference System

Although it is quite satisfactory to describe the axis as being 'along Lead II' when the vector loop clearly points along one specific lead (as in Figure 28), such a descriptive approach would become extremely cumbersome if the axis did not conveniently point along a lead. To overcome this difficulty, the six limb leads are used in a hexaxial reference system as shown in Figure 31.

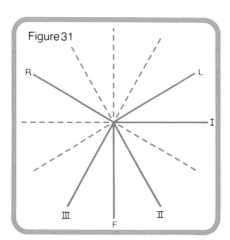

Figure 31

In this system the six leads are each produced through the origin. The resulting six lines (each line shown half continuous, half interrupted) divide the circle into twelve angles each of 30° and this reference frame is used to define the direction of the axis, as shown in Figure 32.

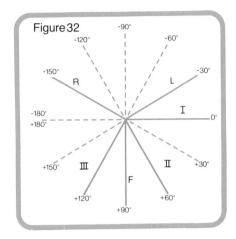

Each end of the six lines is labelled in degrees. **Lead I is arbitrarily chosen as the reference zero.** Moving clockwise from Lead I the lines are labelled in 30° increments until + 180° is reached. Moving counter-clockwise from Lead I the points are labelled − 30°, − 60° etc. This bizarre convention (for which the author disclaims all responsibility) results in the curious anomaly that + 180° and − 180° define the same point. **It should clearly be understood that the + and − signs have nothing to do with whether the QRS complex is predominantly positive or negative in any given lead. The signs in the hexaxial reference system are purely labels to identify the position of the axis. It would be just as reasonable to label the points 0°, a30°, a60°, a90° etc., passing clockwise and as 0°, b30°, b60°, b90° etc., passing anticlockwise** – but this is not the accepted convention. The use of '+' and ' −' signs in this way often gives rise to confusion because of the tendency to equate them with positivity or negativity of the QRS deflection. One or two examples may help to eliminate this possible confusion:-(Figure 33).

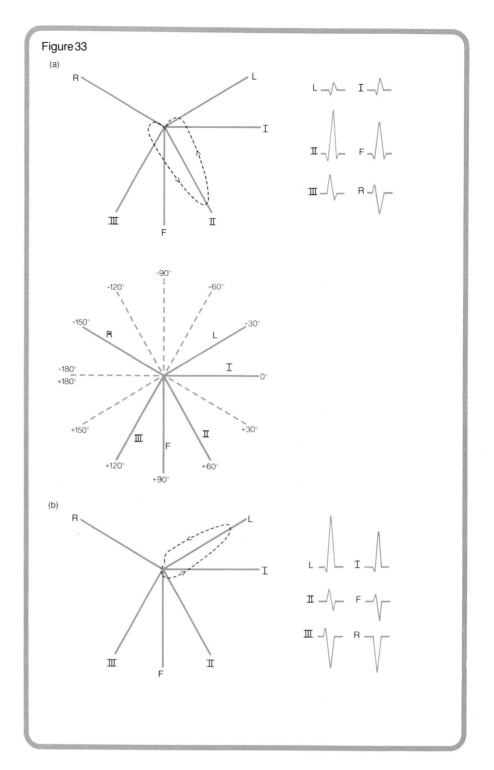

Figure 33

In Figure 33, example (a) shows a vector loop identical with that shown in Figures 27-29. The electrical axis is towards II, ie the vector loop 'points' towards Lead II. Using the hexaxial reference system we may now more precisely and more elegantly say "the electrical axis is +60°". The right hand side of Figure 33 (a) shows the appearance of the QRS complexes in the limb leads. The tallest (most positive) QRS occurs in that lead to which the axis lies closest (Lead II). In example (b) the vector loop 'points' along L and the axis

is therefore towards L. Again we may now say, 'the axis is −30°'. The right hand side of Figure 33 (b) shows the QRS appearances in the limb leads. **As is always the case, that lead to which the axis lies closest, shows the tallest (most positive) QRS complex**—in this case L. Note that the axis is—30°, ie towards L and yet QRS is positive in L. **The '+' and '−' signs of the hexaxial reference system are labels only, they do not imply positivity or negativity of the QRS complex in any lead.**

So far we have learned that the direction in which the vector loop points is the electrical axis. Strictly speaking we should refer to the **mean frontal plane QRS axis,** for we are talking about the **average** direction in which the QRS vector points as determined from the **frontal plane** leads. When the term 'axis' or 'electrical axis' is used without qualification it is deemed to refer to the mean frontal plane QRS axis. (Although it is possible to consider the horizontal and sagittal plane QRS axes, and the

P and T wave axes in all three planes, these have much less significance than the mean frontal plane QRS axes and are only used infrequently).

So far we have only learned the **meaning** of "the axis". We have not learned how to **measure** the frontal plane QRS axis from the QRS deflections in the limb leads, neither have we learned the **clinical significance** of the axis. These important matters will be dealt with on pp 46-52 and 53, respectively.

**The Precordial Leads
(the chest leads)**

In the case of each precordial lead, the positive (recording) terminal of the galvanometer is connected to an electrode at an agreed site on the chest wall. Since the connection to the negative terminal of the galvanometer is the "indifferent" one formed by joining together leads R, L and F, the chest leads are "V" leads and are designated V_1, V_2, V_3, V_4, V_5 and V_6.

A standard anatomical siting of the precordial electrodes has been agreed between the British Cardiac Society and the American Heart Association and is shown in Figure 34.

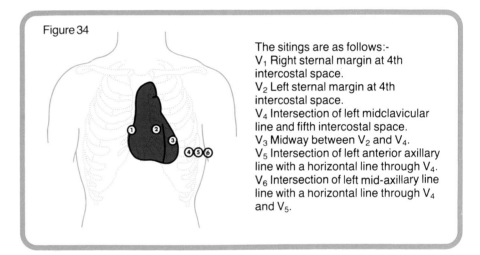

Figure 34

The sitings are as follows:-
V_1 Right sternal margin at 4th intercostal space.
V_2 Left sternal margin at 4th intercostal space.
V_4 Intersection of left midclavicular line and fifth intercostal space.
V_3 Midway between V_2 and V_4.
V_5 Intersection of left anterior axillary line with a horizontal line through V_4.
V_6 Intersection of left mid-axillary line line with a horizontal line through V_4 and V_5.

Figure 35 shows the important relationship of the precordial leads to the cardiac chambers.

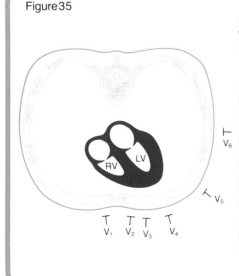

Figure 35

A horizontal cross section through the thorax at the level of the ventricles (seen from above).

Note that V_1 and V_2 face and lie close to the free wall of the right ventricle, V_3 and V_4 lie near to the interventricular septum and V_5 and V_6 face the free wall of the left ventricle but are separated from it by a substantial distance. V_4 is usually at the cardiac apex. Note, in particular **how far round in the axilla is V_6. The novice electrocardiographer places V_5 and V_6 too anteriorly and does not get a true left ventricular recording.**

The Conventional Twelve ECG Leads

We are now in a position to look at all twelve conventional electrocardiographic leads and to see how they relate to one another and to the heart (Figure 36).

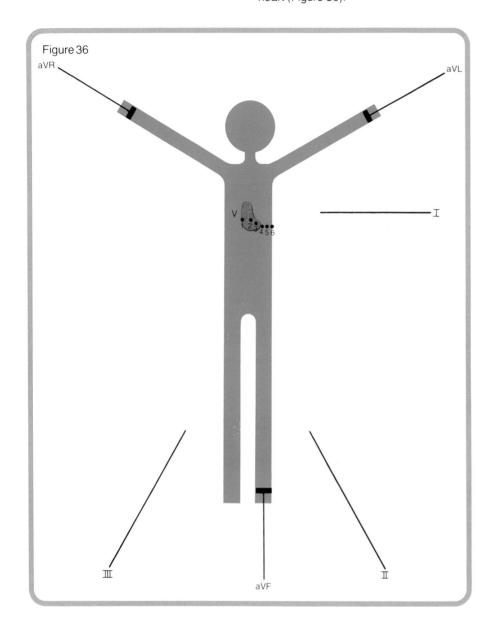

Figure 36

Note the following:-

(i) **I, II and III are bipolar leads. Their orientation with respect to the heart is not intuitively obvious. However, their effective orientation is as shown (see pp16-18 for the demonstration of this).**

(ii) **aVR, aVL, aVF and V_1-V_6 are unipolar leads and their anatomical orientation is readily apparent.**

(iii) **I, II, III, aVR, aVL and aVF are all in the frontal plane (giving information only on up and down and side-to-side movement) and are all remote from the heart. Because they are remote, they tend to give information about dominant electrical forces in the heart rather than about specific areas of the heart such as the right, or left ventricles.**

(iv) **V_1-V_6 are all in the horizontal plane. Each of these leads overlies part of the ventricular myocardium and gives detailed information about this local area.**

(v) **aVL, I, V_5 and V_6 all look at the anterolateral part of the heart and will often show similar appearances to each other.**

(vi) **II, aVF and III all look at the inferior wall of the heart, and will often show similar appearances to each other.**

Normal Electrocardiographic Appearances

We are now in a position to learn the full range of appearances possible in the normal 12-lead ECG. This is unquestionably the single most important step in the mastery of electrocardiography.

Normal Appearances in the Precordial Leads

The Morphology of the QRS Complexes

To understand the form of the normal precordial QRS complexes, we must remind ourselves of the normal sequence of depolarisation (activation) of the ventricles. The QRS complex is the electrical manifestation at the body surface of ventricular myocardial depolarisation. Since the trunk acts as a volume conductor, the siting on the trunk of the recording electrode will have a dramatic effect on the recording obtained (p 12).

Ventricular activation begins on the left side of the interventricular septum (p 6). It then spreads from left to right within the septum and later, from endocardium to epicardium in the free walls of the two ventricles.

Although the full sequence of ventricular depolarisation is an extremely complex process, it is possible to simplify it into three stages to facilitate understanding the form of the QRS complexes in the precordial leads. The three phases are (1) depolarisation of the interventricular septum, (2) depolarisation of the free wall of the right ventricle and (3) depolarisation of the free wall of the left ventricle. These three phases are represented in Figure 37. **In all future representations of this type the chest wall will be omitted, whilst the positioning of the electrodes relative to the heart is maintained—as in Figure 38.**

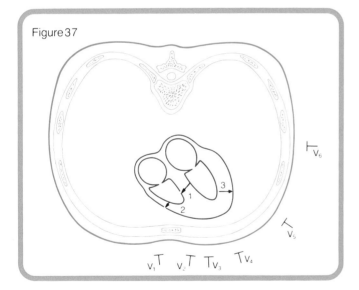

Figure 37

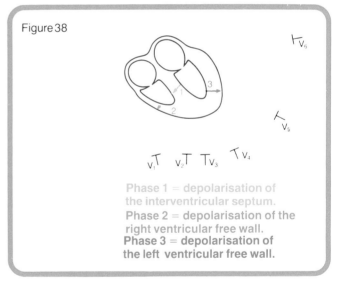

Figure 38

Phase 1 = depolarisation of the interventricular septum.
Phase 2 = depolarisation of the right ventricular free wall.
Phase 3 = depolarisation of the left ventricular free wall.

Note 1

The division into three "phases" is simply a matter of convenience to facilitate the understanding of the precordial ECG. These three phases bear no relationship to the five phases into which ventricular depolarisation was arbitrarily subdivided when considering the QRS complexes in the limb leads (p.22). Both sets of subdivisions are arbitrary and were chosen to promote understanding.

Note 2

When the generation of the QRS complex was first considered (pp 21-24) we were concerned with the limb leads. These are remote from the heart and therefore record the dominant deflection. It was therefore reasonable to ignore the influence of the right ventricle. However, since we are now considering the precordial leads, which lie close to the heart and are influenced not only by the major forces of the left ventricle but also by the activation waves from any myocardium close to the electrode. it is no longer reasonable to ignore the right ventricle and this will therefore be included in all future discussions.

The interventricular septum is depolarised first. Depolarisation of the right and left ventricular free walls then follows. Thus Phase 1 activation occurs initially, alone, and Phases 2 and 3 activation occur simultaneously after Phase 1.

Electrode V_1 'sees' Phases 1 and 2 as positive, since the depolarisation processes of these phases are carried towards V_1. However, V_1 sees Phase 3 as negative since the depolarisation process of Phase 3 is occurring away from V_1 (Figure 38). The result of these three waves of depolarisation can be assessed from Figure 39.

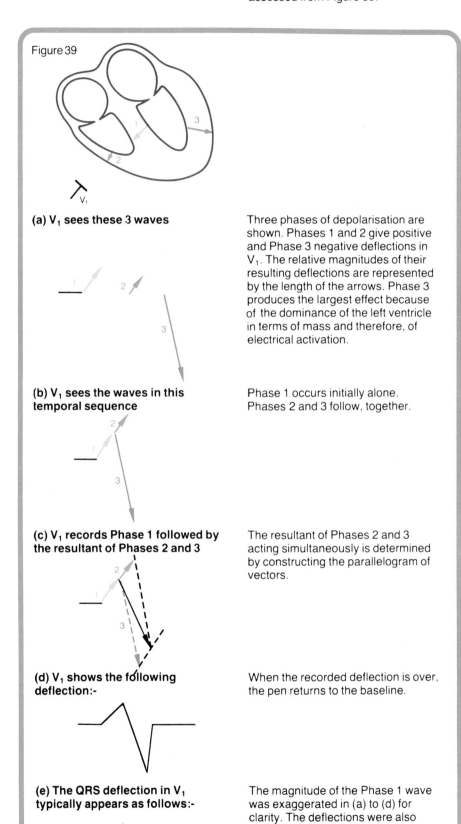

Figure 39

(a) V_1 sees these 3 waves

Three phases of depolarisation are shown. Phases 1 and 2 give positive and Phase 3 negative deflections in V_1. The relative magnitudes of their resulting deflections are represented by the length of the arrows. Phase 3 produces the largest effect because of the dominance of the left ventricle in terms of mass and therefore, of electrical activation.

(b) V_1 sees the waves in this temporal sequence

Phase 1 occurs initially alone. Phases 2 and 3 follow, together.

(c) V_1 records Phase 1 followed by the resultant of Phases 2 and 3

The resultant of Phases 2 and 3 acting simultaneously is determined by constructing the parallelogram of vectors.

(d) V_1 shows the following deflection:-

When the recorded deflection is over, the pen returns to the baseline.

(e) The QRS deflection in V_1 typically appears as follows:-

The magnitude of the Phase 1 wave was exaggerated in (a) to (d) for clarity. The deflections were also spread out for the same reason. **The typical QRS deflection in V_1 has a small initial positive wave followed by a larger negative wave.**

Using the same approach, the typical QRS deflection in V_6 can be predicted (Figure 40).

Figure 40

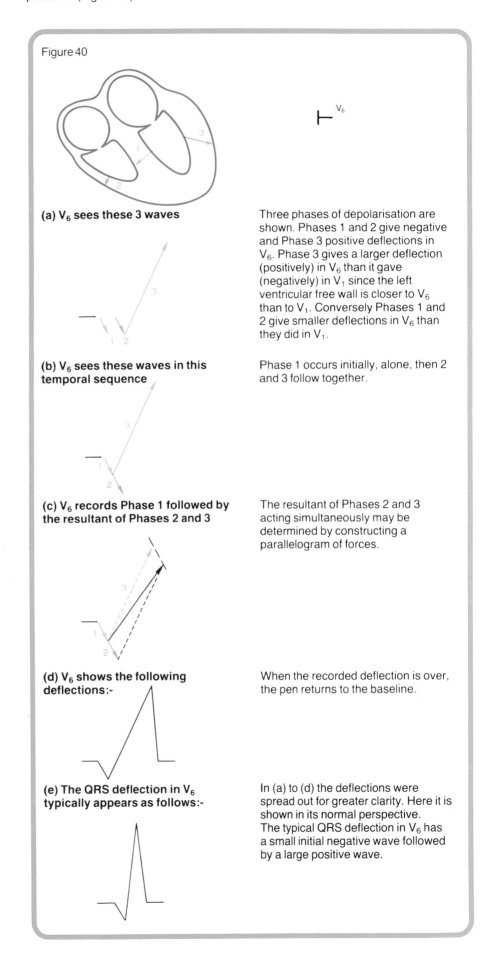

(a) V_6 sees these 3 waves

Three phases of depolarisation are shown. Phases 1 and 2 give negative and Phase 3 positive deflections in V_6. Phase 3 gives a larger deflection (positively) in V_6 than it gave (negatively) in V_1 since the left ventricular free wall is closer to V_6 than to V_1. Conversely Phases 1 and 2 give smaller deflections in V_6 than they did in V_1.

(b) V_6 sees these waves in this temporal sequence

Phase 1 occurs initially, alone, then 2 and 3 follow together.

(c) V_6 records Phase 1 followed by the resultant of Phases 2 and 3

The resultant of Phases 2 and 3 acting simultaneously may be determined by constructing a parallelogram of forces.

(d) V_6 shows the following deflections:-

When the recorded deflection is over, the pen returns to the baseline.

(e) The QRS deflection in V_6 typically appears as follows:-

In (a) to (d) the deflections were spread out for greater clarity. Here it is shown in its normal perspective. The typical QRS deflection in V_6 has a small initial negative wave followed by a large positive wave.

We have now learned the basic QRS morphology for a lead facing the right ventricle (eg V_1) and for one facing the left ventricle (eg V_6). This information is absolutely fundamental to the understanding of the ECG, and it is therefore worth repeating.

The criteria for normality of the morphology of the precordial QRS complexes are as follows:-

The QRS complex in V_1, typically shows a small initial positive wave followed by a larger negative wave. The QRS complex in V_6 typically shows a small initial negative wave followed by a large positive wave. Using the QRS waveform nomenclature (page 5):-

V_1 typically shows an rS pattern of QRS complex:-

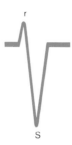

V_6 typically shows a qR pattern of QRS complex:-

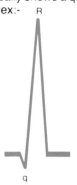

We may now consider the form of the QRS complexes in the remaining precordial leads. Typical normal appearances are shown in Figure 41.

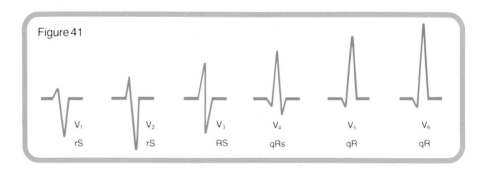

Figure 41

The salient features of these waveforms are as follows:-

1. In general, the size of the initial positive wave (r (or R) wave) increases progressively from V_1 to V_6. However, it is quite normal for the R wave in V_6 to be smaller than that in V_5. It is also normal for the R wave in V_5 to be smaller than that in V_4, provided that the R wave in V_6 is also smaller than the R wave in V_5.

2. The size of the negative wave following the r wave (ie the s (or S) wave) may or may not increase from V_1 to V_2 but it steadily decreases thereafter.

3. The direction of the **initial** part of the QRS is upward (ie positive) in V_1, V_2 and V_3 but downward (ie negative) in V_4-V_6. That is, V_1-V_3 show initial r waves and V_4-V_6 initial q waves. (We shall learn later that this is modified by rotation of the heart – pages 34-37).

These concepts are illustrated in Figure 42.

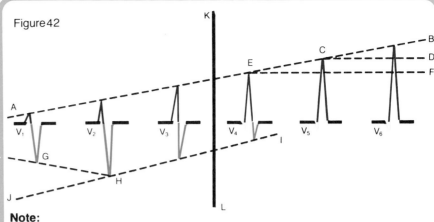

Figure 42

Note:

    Line AB. This illustrates that the **R wave** in each precordial lead is larger than in the lead preceding it in the series from V_1 to V_6.

    Line CD. However, it is quite normal for the **R wave** in V_6 to be smaller than that in V_5.

    Line EF. It is also normal for the **R wave** in V_5 to be smaller than that in V_4, provided that the **R wave** in V_6 is also smaller than that in V_5.

    Line JI. The size of the S wave diminishes progressively across the precordial leads and may ultimately disappear altogether.

    Line GH. The size of the S wave in V_2 is often greater than that in V_1.

    Leads before line KL have an initial deflection which is positive (an r wave).

    Leads after line KL have an initial negative deflection (a   ).

    Three important features should be noted:-

1. The progressive increase in the size of the r wave from V_1 to V_6 occurs because the myocardium underlying the electrodes becomes progressively thicker in the same sequence and because myocardial depolarisation is always from endocardium to epicardium, thus reflecting myocardial thickness. The voltage change resulting from local myocardial depolarisation necessarily increases from V_1 to V_6.

2. However, since V_6, and to a lesser extent V_5, are further from the heart than the other precordial electrodes, the recorded R wave voltage may be less in V_6 than in V_5. For the same reason it may be less in V_5 than in V_4, but in this situation it will always also be less in V_6 than in V_5.

3. The tall positive waves in the left precordial leads are generated by depolarisation of the left ventricular free wall (Phase 3, Figure 40). The same process gives rise to the deep S waves in the right precordial leads (Phase 3, Figure 39). Therefore, just as the R wave height increases (in general) from V_1 to V_6 so the S wave depth diminishes.

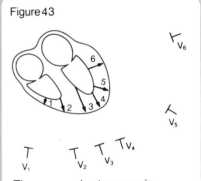

Figure 43

The progressive increase in myocardial thickness underlying electrodes V_1 to V_6 gives rise to a progressive increase in the positive deflection.

**Clockwise and Counterclockwise
Cardiac Rotation.**

We have considered the normal shape and the common, normal variations in the relative size of the various waves within the precordial QRS complexes. We must now consider an important variation in the morphology of the complexes. This variation, called **clockwise or counterclockwise rotation, is important not because it has major clinical significance but because apparently striking differences in the QRS waveform may appear between one individual and the next without clinical significance.** Cardiac 'rotation' is not something which **develops** in any given person between one recording and the next—it is something which describes normal differences between individuals—in the same manner as colour of eyes and size of nose describe normal differences between individuals. The degree of rotation may **occasionally** be so extreme as to constitute an abnormality (just as the colour of the eyes or size of the nose may occasionally be so extreme as to constitute an abnormality) but this is not usually the case.

"Rotation" actually refers to the relative **electrical** positions of the two ventricles but it is convenient to conceive of it in terms of their relative **anatomical** positions. The axis around which the heart is considered to be rotated runs from a position anteriorly, inferiorly and to the left (ie above left hip anteriorly) to one posteriorly, superiorly and to the right (ie above the right shoulder posteriorly).

(NB THIS 'AXIS' HAS NOTHING WHATSOEVER TO DO WITH THE 'ELECTRICAL AXIS' OF THE HEART. IT IS MERELY A CONVENIENT WAY OF LOOKING AT THE HEART TO DESCRIBE VARIATIONS IN THE RELATIVE POSITIONS OF THE TWO VENTRICLES.) Rotation is 'viewed' from the proximal end of the arrow representing the axis of rotation. Clockwise rotation is then seen to be as illustrated in Figure 45

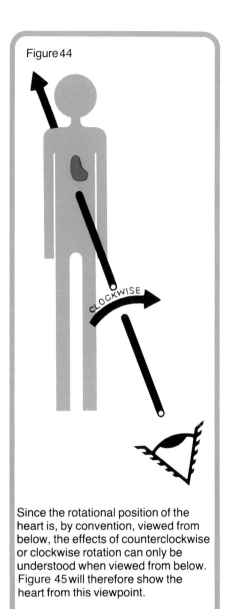

Figure 44

Since the rotational position of the heart is, by convention, viewed from below, the effects of counterclockwise or clockwise rotation can only be understood when viewed from below. Figure 45 will therefore show the heart from this viewpoint.

In the normal, intermediate position of the heart, V_1, V_2 and V_3 overly the right ventricle and V_4, V_5 and V_6 overly the left ventricle (Figure 45). The direction of depolarisation of the interventricular septum is from left to right and therefore towards V_1, V_2 and V_3 and away from V_4, V_5 and V_6 [Figures 39(a), 40(a) and 45(a)]. The first three leads therefore show **initial positive** (r) waves and the second three, **initial negative** (q) waves. Also, the initial three leads show **dominant negative** (S) waves and the second three **dominant positive** (R) waves. The zone of change between these two types (ie in this case between V_3 and V_4) is called the **transition zone.** The transition zone marks the line of the ventricular septum (line AB Figure 45a). **Moving across the precordial leads from V_1 to V_6 its position may be recognised either by the change from a dominant negative to a dominant** **positive deflection or by the change from an initial positive to an initial negative deflection.** These two definitions do not always indicate identical transitional points, but there is usually close agreement and precise identification is meaningless since transition actually occurs at a zone, not at a point. When the two definitions do differ the QRS usually becomes dominantly positive before (reading from V_1 to V_6) the initial deflection changes from positive to negative. It should also be noted that the q wave in the left precordial leads is, not infrequently, so small as to be difficult to see. If this wave is not visible, the transition zone can **only** be determined from the position of change from dominantly negative (in the right precordial leads) to dominantly positive deflections (in the left precordial leads).

The normal, intermediate position of the heart is shown in Figure 45 (a), with the heart shown in a horizontal cross section of the thorax **viewed from below.** The line AB, which indicates the transitional zone, lies along the interventricular septum. The axis around which rotation is possible passes from below to above and therefore passes down 'into' the plane of the paper of the illustration of Figure 45. Thus clockwise rotation is ↘ and counterclockwise is ↙ in this presentation.

With clockwise cardiac rotation more of the right ventricle comes to underly the precordial leads and the transition zone is moved from the intermediate position between V_3 and V_4) to a position further to the left of the chest–in Figure 45(b) actually to V_5/V_6.

Conversely, with counterclockwise rotation the transition zone moves further to the right of the chest–in Figure 45 (c) actually to V_1/V_2.

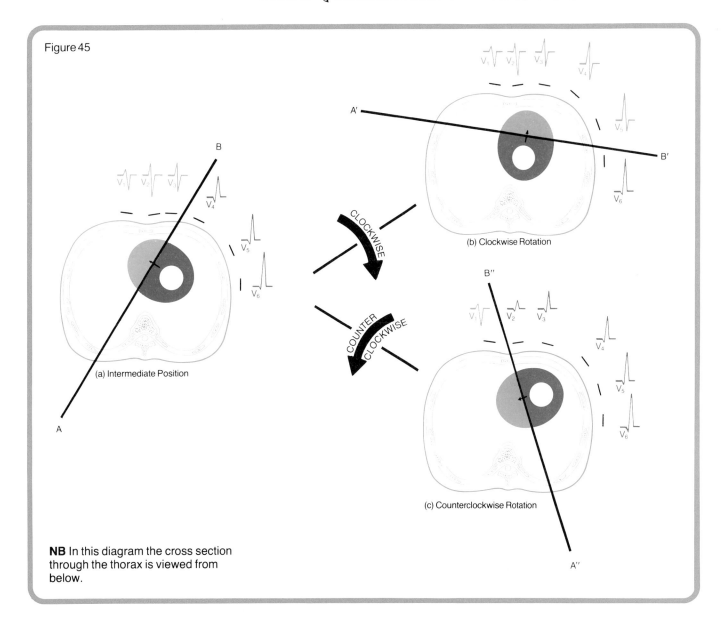

Figure 45

(a) Intermediate Position

CLOCKWISE

COUNTER CLOCKWISE

(b) Clockwise Rotation

(c) Counterclockwise Rotation

NB In this diagram the cross section through the thorax is viewed from below.

The typical precordial QRS complexes
of the intermediate position and of
clockwise and counterclockwise rotation
are shown in Figure 46.

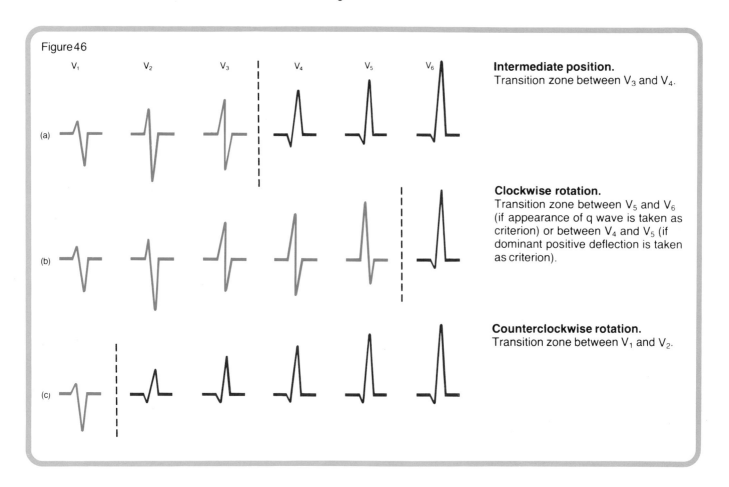

Figure 46

Intermediate position.
Transition zone between V_3 and V_4.

Clockwise rotation.
Transition zone between V_5 and V_6
(if appearance of q wave is taken as
criterion) or between V_4 and V_5 (if
dominant positive deflection is taken
as criterion).

Counterclockwise rotation.
Transition zone between V_1 and V_2.

Note:
(i) Figure 46 demonstrates only the
precordial leads and only the **QRS
complexes.** The terms clockwise and
counterclockwise cardiac rotation refer
only to variation in the form of the
precordial QRS complexes.
(ii) The appearances in Figure 46 (a),
46 (b), and 46 (c) are normal. **The first
two salient features of the normal
precordial QRS morphology given on
p32 still obtain, ie:-**
a) the size of the initial positive wave
increases progressively from V_1 to V_6
(except that it may get smaller between
V_5 and V_6 or between V_4 and V_5 **and**
between V_5 and V_6).
b) the size of the negative wave following
the r wave may or may not increase from
V_1 to V_2 but continuously decreases
thereafter from V_2 to V_6).

**However, the third feature (p32)
of the typical normal precordial QRS
morphology is altered by rotation:-**
c) the direction of the initial part of the
QRS is positive only in V_1 in
counterclockwise rotation but from V_1 to
V_5 in clockwise rotation. Similarly, an
initial negative wave is permissible from
V_2 to V_6 in counterclockwise rotation but
is only present in V_6 in clockwise rotation.
The third salient feature must therefore
be amended to read 'the direction of the
initial deflection in the QRS complex is
upright in the right precordial lead(s) and
downward in the left precordial lead(s).'

(iii) Occasionally, rotation may be so
extreme that all the leads may record
from one side of the interventricular
septum only (Figure 47).

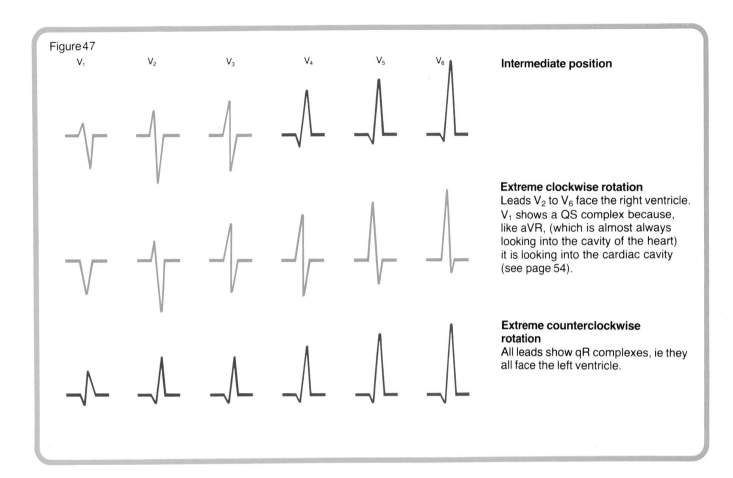

Figure 47

Intermediate position

Extreme clockwise rotation
Leads V_2 to V_6 face the right ventricle.
V_1 shows a QS complex because,
like aVR, (which is almost always
looking into the cavity of the heart)
it is looking into the cardiac cavity
(see page 54).

**Extreme counterclockwise
rotation**
All leads show qR complexes, ie they
all face the left ventricle.

Note that in the presence of extreme
clockwise rotation, an entirely negative
wave (a QS complex) is permissible in V_1.
Similarly, in the presence of extreme
counterclockwise rotation there may be
no initial q wave in V_6.

The Dimensions of the QRS Complexes

Having ascertained the essential features of the configuration of the QRS complexes in the precordial leads, it is now necessary to establish the criteria for the height (or depth) and duration of each component wave within these QRS complexes. The ECG deflections are recorded on a graticule which facilitates measurement. This graticule is shown diagrammatically and magnified in Figure 48 (a) and a natural sized graticule is shown in Figure 48 (b).

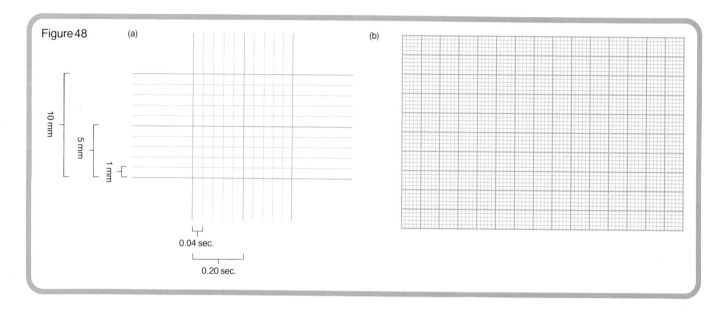

Figure 48

(a)

10 mm

5 mm

1 mm

0.04 sec.

0.20 sec.

(b)

Each electrocardiogram should include a calibration signal of 1 millivolt. The gain on the recorder is adjusted until this calibration signal occupies 10mm vertical distance on the graticule. All normal values for voltage on the ECG are dependent upon a normal gain calibration. All normal values for time measurements are dependent upon the recording having been made at a standard recording speed of 25mm per second.

The graticule is used (provided the voltage calibration and paper speed are standard) to measure the voltages and duration of various parts of the QRS complexes. The following measurements are made (Figure 49).

Figure 49

R wave height. Height in mm of the first positive wave above the base line.

Q wave depth. Depth in mm of any initial (ie. preceding an R wave) negative wave below the base line.

S wave depth. Depth in mm below the base line of any negative wave which follows an R wave.

q wave duration. Time in seconds from the onset of the q wave to the point where the upstroke of the R wave re-crosses the base line.

Total QRS duration. Time in seconds from the onset of the QRS complex (whether the initial wave be negative or positive) to the end of the QRS complex (whether the final wave be negative or positive).

Ventricular Activation Time. Time in seconds from the beginning of the q wave to the peak of the R wave. It can only be measured in leads showing a qR type of QRS complex.

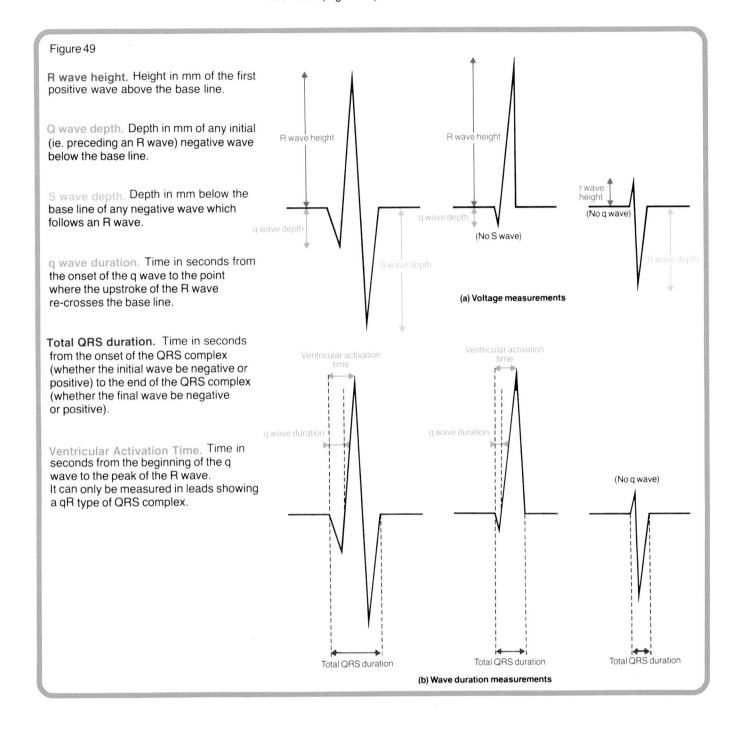

(a) Voltage measurements

(b) Wave duration measurements

The criteria for normality of dimensions in the precordial QRS complexes are as follows:-

(i) Minimum voltage: at least one R wave in the precordial leads must exceed 8mm in height.

(ii) Maximum voltage: (a) the tallest R wave in the left precordial leads must not exceed 27mm. (b) the deepest S wave in the right precordial leads must not exceed 30mm. (c) the sum of the tallest R wave in the left precordial leads and the deepest S wave in the right precordial leads must not exceed 40mm.

(iii) Maximum duration:-the total QRS duration in any one precordial lead must not exceed 0.10 sec. (2½ small squares).

(iv) q wave criteria:-(a) precordial q waves must not equal or exceed 0.04 sec. in duration (one small square). (b) precordial q waves must not have a depth greater than ¼ of the height of the R wave in the same lead.

(v) Ventricular activation time:-in leads facing the left ventricle (ie. showing qR complexes) must not exceed 0.04 sec. (one small square).

The Precordial T waves

The reader will be delighted to learn that, from every point of view, the T wave is simpler than the QRS complex and the range of normal is therefore much easier to understand.

The criteria for normality of T waves in the precordial leads of adults are as follows:-

V_1. 80% of normal adults have upright T waves, 20% have flat or inverted T waves. Therefore the finding of an inverted T wave in V_1 cannot be considered an abnormality (unless it was upright in a previous ECG in that same person).

V_2. 95% of normal adults show upright T waves and 5% have flat or inverted T waves in V_2. Therefore there is a 1/20 possibility of inverted T waves in V_2 occurring by chance and not indicating an abnormality. However, if the T wave in V_2 is inverted when it was formerly upright in a record from the same subject, it is abnormal. Further. if there is T wave inversion in V_2 with an upright T wave in V_1 (which more often has T wave inversion in normal subjects than V_2) then this is an abnormality.

$V_3 - V_6$. The T wave is normally upright in these leads. T wave inversion in V_4, V_5 or V_6 is **always** abnormal. T wave inversion in V_3, as well as in V_1 and V_2 may sometimes (though rarely) be found in healthy young adults.

There are no strict criteria for T wave size. In general the tallest precordial T wave is found in V_3 or V_4 and the smallest in V_1 and V_2 and, as a general rule, the T wave should not be less than ⅛ and not more than ⅔ of the height of the preceding R wave in each of the leads V_3-V_6.

Three normal and two abnormal
precordial series of QRS complexes and
T wave from normal adults are shown in
Figure 50.

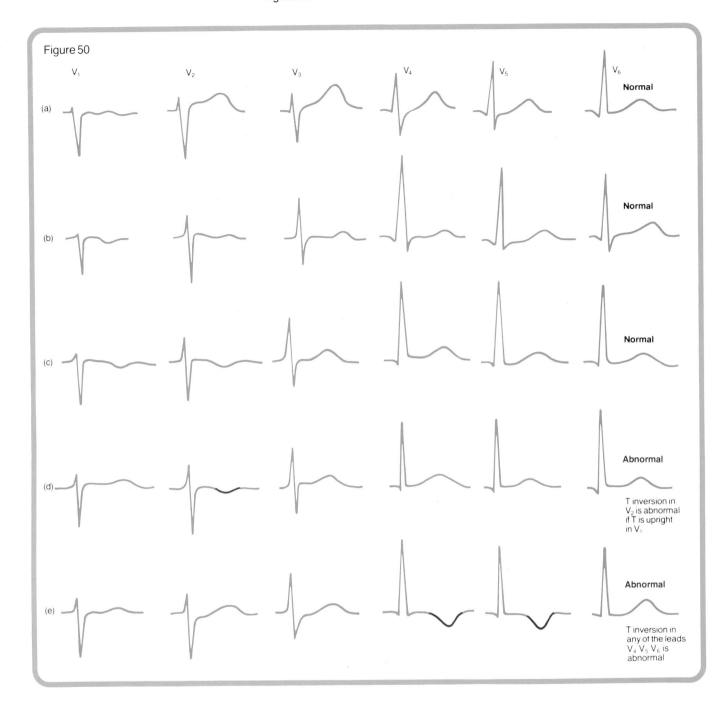

Figure 50

The S-T Segment

Any reader who was relieved (and probably a little surprised) to discover that the author's promise of simplicity in explaining the T wave was adhered to in the subsequent text can now give his or her joy full reign, for the S-T segment is even simpler than the T wave.

There is one single rule for normality of the S-T segment. The S-T segment must not deviate by more than 1mm above or below the iso-electric line in any precordial lead. This is a simple rule. The only problem lies in defining (i) the iso-electric line and (ii) the S-T segment.

(i) The iso-electric line is the horizontal level of the recording at a time when there is no cardiac activity, ie. in the T-P interval (Figure 51).

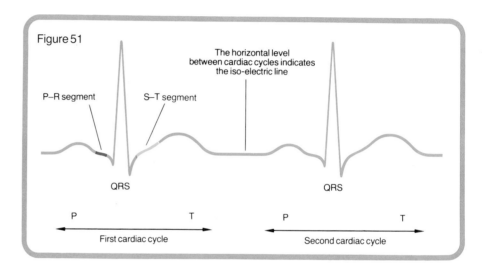

Figure 51

The horizontal level between cardiac cycles indicates the iso-electric line

P–R segment

S–T segment

QRS

QRS

P

T

P

T

First cardiac cycle

Second cardiac cycle

In Figure 51 the T-P interval is clearly visible and the horizontal position of the T-P interval marks the iso-electric line. In this case it is easily recognisable and is on the same level as the P-R segment and the S-T interval. However, the T-P interval cannot always be recognised and when it is recognisable it is not always on the same level as the P-R segment or the S-T interval. When the heart rate is rapid, the P wave may begin before the T wave of the preceding complex has been completed and there will be no T-P interval. (Figure 52). In this event the position of the S-T segment relative to the true iso-electric line cannot be determined with confidence and conclusions that the S-T segment is elevated or depressed must only be made if the changes are striking (Figure 52).

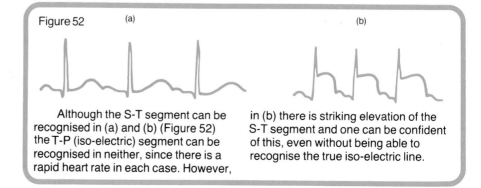

Figure 52   (a)   (b)

Although the S-T segment can be recognised in (a) and (b) (Figure 52) the T-P (iso-electric) segment can be recognised in neither, since there is a rapid heart rate in each case. However, in (b) there is striking elevation of the S-T segment and one can be confident of this, even without being able to recognise the true iso-electric line.

(ii) Recognising the **S-T segment itself** is not always easy. It is defined as the interval between the end of the QRS complex and the beginning of the T wave. This interval is easier to see in some leads than in others. If one looks at a normal precordial series it is clear that the S-T segment is more clearly defined in the left precordial leads than in the right precordial leads and one should exercise caution in concluding that minor degrees of S-T segment elevation in the right precordial leads are abormal, for in these leads the QRS may pass straight into the take-off for the T wave without a discrete S-T interval (Figure 53).

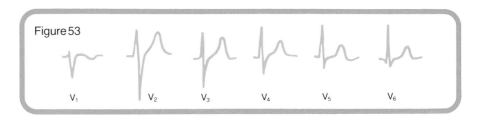

Figure 53

V_1 V_2 V_3 V_4 V_5 V_6

The S-T segment is well defined in V_4, V_5 and V_6 but poorly defined in V_2 and V_3. The appearances are normal.

The P Waves

We have not discussed the P waves since page 5 when it was established that they represent depolarisation of the atrial myocardium. We may now consider the form of the P waves in the precordial leads (Figure 54).

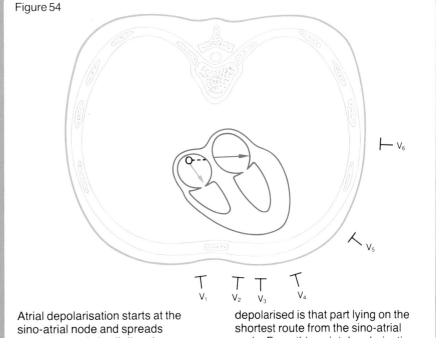

Figure 54

Atrial depolarisation starts at the sino-atrial node and spreads simultaneously in all directions through the myocardium of the right atrium. That direction of spread of depolarisation within the right atrium which produces the longest available pathway is the effective, predominant direction of depolarisation of the right atrium and this determines the direction of the right atrial P wave vector (blue arrow, Figure 54). The first part of the left atrium to be depolarised is that part lying on the shortest route from the sino-atrial node. From this point depolarisation spreads in all directions through the left atrial myocardium. That direction of spread of depolarisation within the left atrium which provides the longest available pathway is the effective, predominant direction of depolarisation of the left atrium and this determines the direction of the left atrial P wave vector (red arrow, Figure 54).

Leads V_1 and V_2 "see" the right atrial vector coming towards them and therefore exhibit a positive wave in response to right atrial depolarisation. The left atrial vector moves away from these leads which therefore "see" a negative deflection when the left atrium depolarises. Left atrial depolarisation occurs later than right atrial depolarisation. The P wave in V_1 and V_2 is therefore often biphasic (Figure 55).

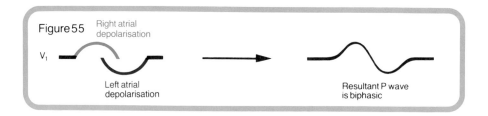

Figure 55   Right atrial depolarisation

V_1

Left atrial depolarisation

Resultant P wave is biphasic

Leads V_3 to V_6 "see" both right and left atrial depolarisation coming towards them and therefore the normal P wave is entirely upright in these leads.

Therefore **the normal P wave in the precordial leads is a small, rounded deflection. It is always upright in V_3-V_6 but may be upright or biphasic in V_1 and V_2. When it is biphasic in these leads the area of the** (second) **negative component must not exceed the area of the** (first) **positive component.** (see later under "atrial hypertrophy").

We are now in a position to summarise the important criteria for normality of all the waves of the precordial leads. These criteria must be memorised.

Summary: Normal appearances in precordial leads

(NB ensure calibration is 10mm and paper speed is 25mm per second)

P waves

Upright in V_4-V_6. Upright or biphasic in V_1, V_2. If biphasic, then negative component must have smaller area than positive component.

S-T segments

Must not deviate above or below the iso-electric line by more than 1mm. Caution must be exercised in diagnosing abnormal S-T segment elevation in the right precordial leads unless it is striking.

T waves

Upright in V_4-V_6. Often inverted in V_1. May be inverted in V_2 provided they are also inverted in V_1 and have not previously been upright in V_2. In general, the T wave height should be not more than $\frac{2}{3}$ and not less than $\frac{1}{8}$ of the height of the preceding R wave in any of the leads V_3-V_6.

QRS Complexes

(a) Morphology

V_1 shows an rS pattern and V_6 shows a qR pattern. The size of the r wave increases progressively from V_1 to V_6, although it may fall off slightly between V_5 and V_6 or between V_4 and V_5 and again between V_5 and V_6. [Occasionally the r wave in V_2, V_3 or V_4 may be smaller than that in the lead immediately to its right in the precordial series. This is also acceptable as being within normal limits provided it occurs in the transition zone. When this is a normal finding, the adjacent r waves are usually small]. The S wave in V_2 may be deeper than that in V_1 but from V_2 onwards the S wave depth decreases. The initial part of the QRS deflection is positive in the right precordial leads. There comes a point in progression from V_1 to V_6 where the initial deflection ceases to be positive and becomes negative. When this point is reached it indicates that the transition zone has been crossed. To the left of this point of transition the dominant deflection is positive, to the right it is negative. Many people define the transition zone as the point at which the deflection becomes dominantly positive. These two definitions do not always locate the same point but they usually agree approximately. When the transition zone is in the region of V_3/V_4 the heart is neither clockwise nor counterclockwise rotated but is intermediate in position. When the transition zone is between V_2 and V_3 or between V_1 and V_2 there is counterclockwise cardiac rotation. When the transition zone is between V_4 and V_5 or V_5 and V_6 there is clockwise rotation. Both are normal variations. In the presence of pronounced clockwise cardiac rotation a QS complex may be found in V_1.

(b) Dimensions

At least one R wave in the precordial leads must exceed 8mm. The tallest R wave in the precordial leads must not exceed 27mm. The deepest S wave in the precordial leads must not exceed 30mm. The sum of the tallest R wave in the left precordial leads and the deepest S wave in the right precordial leads must not exceed 40mm. The total QRS duration in any lead must not exceed 0.10 sec. Precordial q waves must not equal or exceed 0.04 sec in duration. Precordial q waves must never have a depth greater than one quarter of the height of the R wave which follows them. The ventricular activation time must not exceed 0.04 sec.

The summary above contains **all** the criteria essential to establish the normality or otherwise of the precordial ECG.

We may now return to consider the normal appearances in the limb leads.

Normal Appearances in the Limb Leads

Only three criteria need to be applied to the limb leads to determine normality or otherwise of the QRS complexes. These criteria concern:

i) The size of any q waves in aVL, I, II or aVF.

ii) The size of the R waves in aVL and aVF.

iii) The electrical axis of the heart.

Of these, the third is the most difficult and we will tackle this first. The general consideration of the morphology and dimensions of the QRS complexes in the limbs will be resumed after the explanation of the electrical axis (p 53).

The **meaning** of the term "mean frontal plain QRS axis" (usually abbreviated to "electrical axis") was explained on pages 24-27. We must now learn to **measure** the axis from the QRS appearances in the six limb leads.

The Assessment of the Electrical Axis

The electrical axis can be determined by simple inspection of the six frontal plane leads. This gives the axis to an accuracy of ± 15°. It is not possible **by any technique** to obtain a greater accuracy than this for the assumptions of the Einthoven hypothesis (pp13, 14) on which the hexaxial reference system is based are only approximately true and to attempt to resolve the axis to a greater level of accuracy than 15° is, therefore, to pretend to an accuracy which cannot exist.

The axis is measured by reference to the hexaxial reference system (Figure 56).

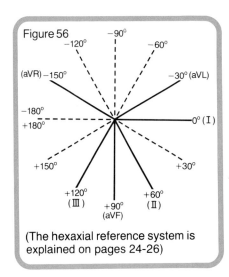

Figure 56

(The hexaxial reference system is explained on pages 24-26)

To calculate the axis it is necessary to determine the algebraic sum of the QRS deflections in each limb lead. This is done by adding all the positive deflections and subtracting all the negative deflections of the QRS complex in any given lead (Figure 57).

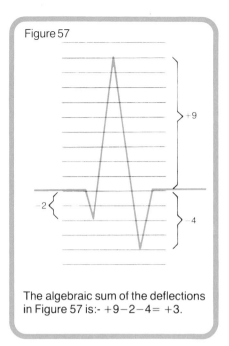

Figure 57

The algebraic sum of the deflections in Figure 57 is:- $+9-2-4= +3$.

To determine the axis, proceed as follows:-
1. Decide, by inspection, in which frontal-plane lead the algebraic sum of QRS-complex deflections most closely approximates to zero. (This is not necessarily the smallest QRS complex. A small but entirely positive QRS complex has a greater algebraic sum than a large one in which the positive and negative waves are equal). **The axis is approximately at right angles to this lead and must therefore lie in one of two approximate directions.** For example, using the hexaxial system in Figure 56 suppose that the algebraic sum of QRS− complex deflections is most nearly equal to zero in Lead I. Then the axis must lie at approximately $+90°$ or $-90°$ which are the two directions at right angles to Lead I. Since each of the six frontal-plane leads has another lead at right angles to it, one of these two choices necessarily lies on another lead (which in this case is Lead aVF).
2. Examine the form of the QRS complex in that limb lead which occupies a position at right angles to the limb lead in which the algebraic sum of QRS complexes was closest to zero. The QRS complex in this second lead must have a dominantly positive form or a dominantly negative form. If the form is dominantly positive the axis must point towards this second lead (and be $+90°$ in this example), if dominantly negative it must point away from this lead (in this example $-90°$).

This procedure gives the axis to the nearest 30°. To improve resolution to the nearest 15° a further step must be taken as follows:-
3. Return to the first lead chosen (Lead I in this example). The algebraic sum of QRS complex deflections is close to zero. Is it actually zero or is it slightly positive or slightly negative?
(i) If the sum is slightly positive, the axis must point slightly towards this first lead. Therefore the initial estimate of its position must be altered by 15°* in a direction taking it towards the position of the first lead (in this example, from $+90°$ to $+75°$ or from $-90°$ to $-75°$ depending on whether the initial estimate of the axis was $+90°$ or $-90°$. Note, by inspection of Figure 56 that in both cases this adjustment of the calculated axis moves it slightly towards the first lead, in this example Lead I).
(ii) If the sum is slightly negative the axis must point slightly away from the first lead and the initial estimate of its position must be altered by 15°* in a direction taking it away from the position of the first lead. (In this example from $+90°$ to $+105°$ or from $-90°$ to $-105°$ depending on whether the initial estimate of the axis was $+90°$ or $-90°$. Note, by inspection of the Figure 56 that in both cases this adjustment of the calculated axis moves slightly away from the first lead, which in this example is Lead I.
(iii) If the sum is actually zero the initial estimate of the axis need not be altered. This estimate is now correct to the nearest 15°.

*Adjustments of 15° are made because this angle is half of that of the measuring reference system (the hexaxial system). It is accepted scientific convention that one cannot claim a greater accuracy than half of the smallest directly obtainable measurement, eg. using a ruler calibrated in mms the limit of accuracy is ½ mm.

An example may help to clarify the technique. Consider the ECG in Figure 58 (the hexaxial reference system is reproduced beside the ECG).

Figure 58

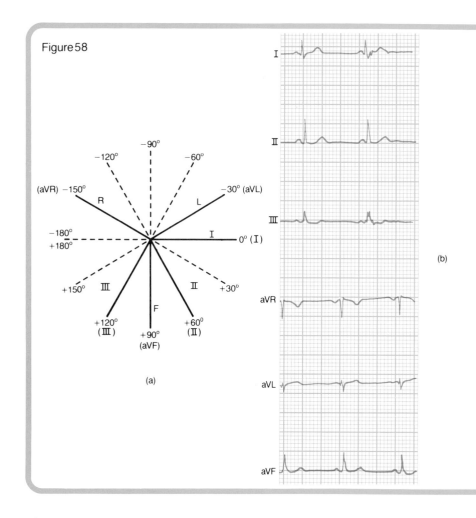

(a)

(b)

The limb leads only are shown since the precordial leads are not relevant to the analysis of the frontal plane axis. Inspection of the six limb leads indicates that the algebraic sum of QRS deflections is most nearly equal to zero in aVL. The QRS axis must therefore be approximately at right angles to this lead. Figure 58(a) reveals two possible directions for the axis, namely + 60° and − 120°, both of which are right angles to Lead aVL. One of these possible directions, + 60°, lies on another lead (Lead II). In Figure 58(b) Lead II shows a clearly positive dominant deflection of the QRS complex. Of the two possible directions, therefore, the axis must be along Lead II, that is at + 60°. This gives the axis to the nearest 30°. Further inspection of the QRS complex in Lead aVL reveals that the algebraic sum of QRS-complex deflections in this lead while being closer to zero than in any other lead, is in fact slightly negative. It is thus necessary to make an adjustment to the first estimate for the axis (+ 60°) and to move the axis 15° further away from Lead aVL (since the QRS is slightly negative in Lead aVL). Thus the final estimate of the axis is + 75° and this is correct to the nearest 15°.

Several points should be noted about this technique for axis determination.

1. The plus and minus signs on the hexaxial reference system (Figure 58a) have nothing to do with the polarity of the QRS complexes in any lead. The description of axes as 0° to + 180° or 0° to − 180° is an arbitrary convention (page 25).

2. It is not acceptable merely to look for the lead with the largest positive QRS-complex deflection. It is true that this is the lead closest to the axial direction, but the degree of accuracy achieved by estimating the axis in this way will vary with the actual value of the axis. If the axis is between + 60° and + 120°, where three limb leads are close together, the estimate will be correct to 30°. However, if the axis lies between − 30° and − 150° the calculation will be considerably less reliable (note the distribution of the frontal-plane leads in Figure 58a).

3. When there are two leads in which the algebraic sum of QRS-complex deflections is close to zero these will either be at 30° or at 150° to one another and the same answer (to 15° accuracy) will be given whichever is first chosen.

4. If all six frontal-plane leads have QRS complexes with algebraic sums close to zero, the axis is indeterminate (by any technique) since the QRS-complex vector is directed predominantly forwards or backwards and, either way, subtends only a small angle on the frontal plane.

5. Slight variations in QRS complex morphology may take place with the changes in anatomical heart position that occur in association with respiration-induced variations in the axis.

Two of these points are illustrated in Figure 59.

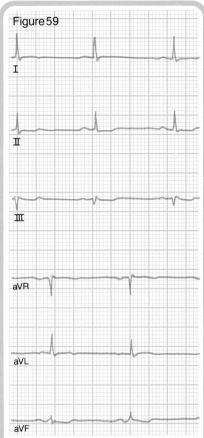

Figure 59

I

II

III

aVR

aVL

aVF

Figure 59 illustrates points 3 and 5 above. Respiratory variation in QRS-complex size occurs and is best seen where the QRS complex is small as in Leads III and aVF (point 5). Also, either of these leads could be chosen as the one in which the algebraic sum of deflections is closest to zero (point 3). If Lead III is picked the initial estimated axis becomes + 30° or −150°. Since Lead aVR (−150°) shows a negative QRS complex the initial axial estimate must be +30°. Reinspection of Lead III reveals a slightly negative QRS complex, so the revised estimate of the axis becomes +15° (as a result of moving the axial estimate 15° away from Lead III). If Lead aVF is chosen as the one in which the QRS-complex algebraic sum is closest to zero, initial axial estimates of 0° or 180° are possible. Since Lead I has a positive QRS complex 0° is the true initial axial estimate. Re-inspection of Lead aVF shows the algebraic sum of QRS-complex deflections to be both truly zero for the first complex and positive for the second, giving revised axial estimates of 0° (now to 15° accuracy) and +15° respectively. Each of these agrees (to 15° with that made if Lead III is first selected).

Figure 60 provides four sets of limb leads on which the reader may practice determining the axis. Use the diagram of the hexaxial reference system provided. The answers are given on page 52.

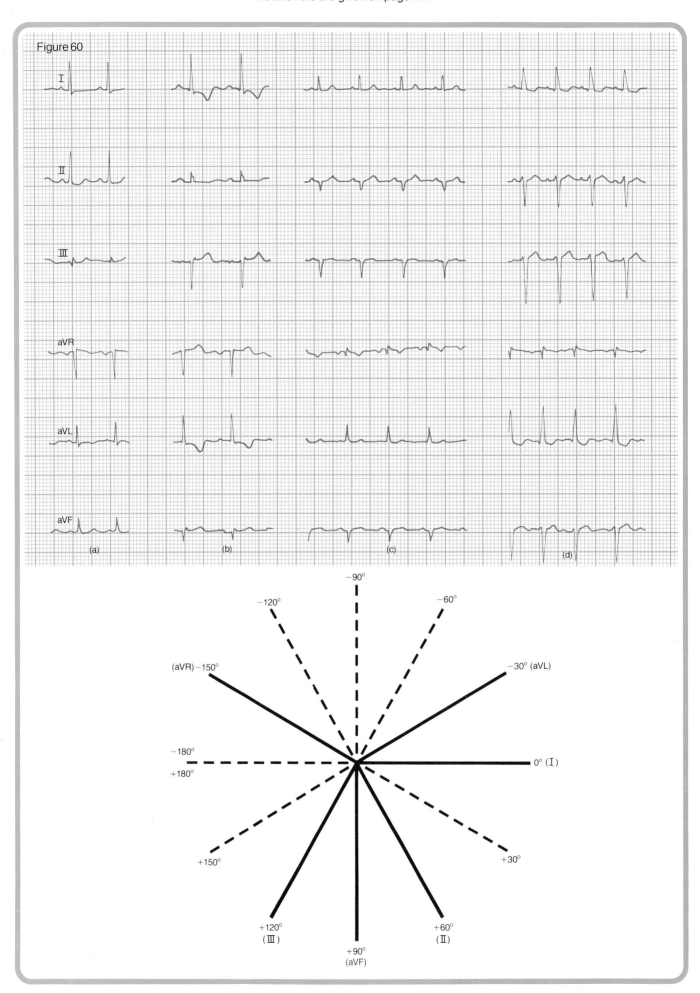

Answers to axis determination from Figure 60

Answers:-
(a) +30°; (b) −15°; (c) −60°; (d) −45°.

Technique of obtaining these answers:-

(a) (i) QRS algebraic sum closest to zero in III. Therefore axis is either +30° or −150°.
(ii) −150° lies on aVR. The QRS is negative in aVR thus the axis points away from aVR, therefore of the two alternatives the correct one must be +30°.
(This gives the axis to the nearest 30°).
(iii) Re-inspection of III shows algebraic sum of QRS is effectively zero, therefore no adjustment is necessary, therefore to the nearest 15° the axis is +30°.

(b) (i) QRS algebraic sum closest to zero in aVF. Therefore axis is either zero degrees or 180°.
(ii) Zero degrees lies on I. The QRS is positive in I thus the axis points towards I. Therefore of the two alternatives the axis is 0°. This is accurate to 30°.
(iii) Re-inspection of aVF shows that the QRS is not exactly zero, but is slightly negative. The QRS axis must thus be slightly away from aVF, therefore we must make a 15° adjustment of our first assessment to move this assessment 15° away from aVF. We must therefore alter our assessment from 0° to −15°.

(c) (i) QRS algebraic sum is most closely equal to zero in aVR. Therefore the axis is either −60° or +120°.
(ii) Of these two possibilities, +120° lies on III. The QRS is negative in III therefore the axis points away from III and of the two possibilities the axis must be −60°. This is correct to 30°.
(iii) Re-inspection of aVR shows that the algebraic sum of QRS deflections is indistinguishable from zero and the first assessment therefore requires no adjustment. The answer −60° is thus accurate to 15°.

(d) (i) The QRS algebraic sum is closest to zero in aVR. Therefore the axis is either −60° or +120°.
(ii) Of these two possibilities, +120° lies on III. The QRS is predominantly negative in III and the axis therefore points away from III and of the two possibilities the axis must be −60°. This is accurate to 30°.
(iii) Re-inspection of aVR shows that the QRS algebraic sum is slightly negative. The initial estimate of the axis must therefore be adjusted by 15° to move it away from aVR slightly. The axis estimate thus becomes −45°, which is correct to 15°.

The Significance of the Electrical Axis

In the normal adult the mean frontal plane QRS axis lies between −30° and +90° (Figure 61).

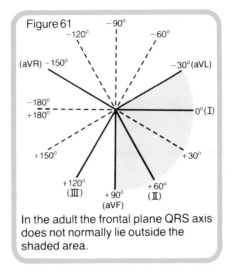

Figure 61

In the adult the frontal plane QRS axis does not normally lie outside the shaded area.

As explained on page 24 the axis is important for two reasons:-

(i) It is an index for normality or abnormality in its own right. Thus if the ECG from an adult shows an axis of +120° or of −45° it is definitely abnormal in either case.

(ii) The large normal range of the frontal plane axis explains the tremendous variation of normal appearances in the limb leads.

It should be remembered that the left ventricle dominates the electrical activity of the heart and determines the position of the mean QRS vector. Thus when the QRS axis is zero degrees, Lead I will show a left ventricular type of complex (ie a qR complex such as is normally found in V_6). Therefore when the axis is 0° appearances like those in V_6 will be seen in Lead I. When it is −30° those appearances will be seen in aVL, when it is +90° those appearances will be seen in aVF etc. Because of this enormous range of possible variations in the QRS in the limb leads it is not possible to describe the QRS morphology in the limb leads in the same way as for the precordial leads.

Instead one determines the axis.

The Horizontal Heart and the Vertical Heart

When the mean frontal plane QRS axis is in the approximate region of 0° to −30°, the heart is said to be horizontal. When the axis lies approximately in the region of +60° to +90° the heart is said to be vertical.

The Morphology and Dimensions of the QRS Complexes

We may now elaborate on the points listed on page 46, where it was stated that only three criteria need be applied to the limb leads to determine whether the QRS appearances are normal or not:-

(i) The size of any q waves present in aVL, I, II, or aVF

Any q wave present in aVL , I, II or aVF must not have a depth exceeding one quarter the height of the ensuing R wave and must not equal or exceed 0.04 sec in duration. (The same criteria which were applied in the precordial leads). **Any q wave present in aVR or III should be ignored.** If the reader is prepared to accept this advice without requiring demonstration of its validity, he should omit the following section.

see ＊ page 54

Lead aVR looks into the cavity of the heart and therefore 'sees' the endocardial surface of the ventricles. Since ventricular depolarisation occurs from endocardium to epicardium at all parts of the ventricular free walls, it follows that ventricular depolarisation travels away from aVR and, therefore, that aVR shows an entirely negative QRS complex, ie a QS complex. **Deep Q waves and QS complexes are therefore never abnormal in Lead aVR.**

Lead III is a bipolar lead. It measures the voltage difference between two unipolar limb connections:-
III = F − L (page 15)

It is perfectly possible in the normal ECG for the QRS deflections to be dominantly positive both in F and in L and for the size of the positive wave in L to exceed that in F. When L has a larger positive deflection than F, (F-L) will be negative and a dominant Q wave may be produced. This Q wave is the result of subtracting one normal voltage (in L) from another normal voltage (in F). In this situation, the Q wave in III is normal, no matter what its dimensions. **It follows that deep Q waves and QS complexes in III may be completely normal.** Unfortunately, abnormal Q waves or QS complexes may also be found in III. However, whenever this occurs, abnormal Q waves or QS complexes are also found in aVF. This is not surprising since aVF is close to III in orientation but cannot be subject to the same risk of producing an "abnormal" appearance by the subtraction of one normal appearance from another for the simple reason that it is a unipolar lead. There is no situation in which prominent Q waves or QS complexes in III reliably indicate abnormality in the absence of similar appearances in aVF. **The simplest and safest approach therefore is to ignore Lead III when looking for abnormal Q waves.**

It should be noted that the same problems do not arise with the other two bipolar leads, I and II. This is because the subtracted lead is R in each case:-
I = L − R (page 15)
II = F − R (page 15)

Since R is always negative in the normal ECG I and II will not show more negativity than L and F respectively. When abnormal Q waves are seen in I they will usually be present (and larger) in L. Similarly abnormal Q waves in II will be present and larger in F.

Q waves of greater duration than 0·04 sec or of depth in excess of one quarter the height of the ensuing R wave are permissible in aVL if the mean frontal plane QRS axis is in the region of 75° to +90° (normal axis) or further to the right (abnormal axis) — ie when the heart is vertical. The reason for this is that when the heart is vertical aVL "looks" into the cavity of the heart. Leads which look into the cavity of the heart ("cavity leads") show QS complexes because in all parts of the ventricular myocardium depolarisation travels from endocardium to epicardium and the depolarisation process necessarily travels away from any cavity leads.
Figure 62 demonstrates this.

Figure 62

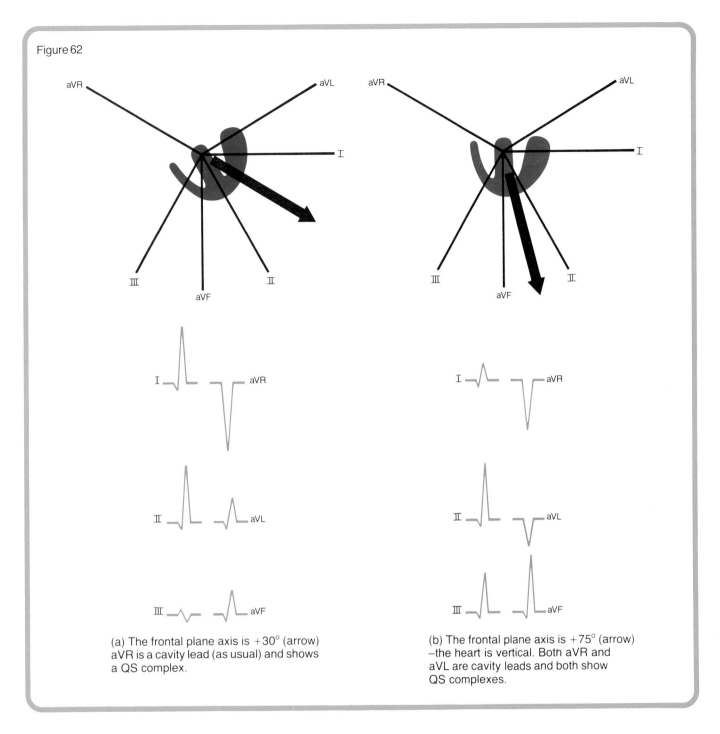

(a) The frontal plane axis is +30° (arrow)
aVR is a cavity lead (as usual) and shows
a QS complex.

(b) The frontal plane axis is +75° (arrow)
–the heart is vertical. Both aVR and
aVL are cavity leads and both show
QS complexes.

Thus QS complexes or dominant
Q waves may occur normally in aVL if
(but only if) the heart is vertical.

**(ii) The size of the R waves in aVL and
aVF**
The R wave in aVL must not exceed
13mm and that in aVF must not exceed
20mm.
(iii) The electrical axis of the heart
The mean frontal plane QRS axis must
not lie outside the limits −30° to +90°.

The above ((i), (ii) and (iii)) are the only
criteria needed to establish whether the
QRS complexes in the limb leads are
normal or not.

The S-T Segments

The rule for normality is the same as that applied in the case of the precordial leads, namely, that the S-T segments must not deviate above or below the iso-electric line by more than 1mm.

The T Waves

In general, the T waves and QRS complexes in the limb leads are concordant, ie when the QRS complexes are upright, the T waves are upright and when the QRS complexes are negative the T waves are negative. This means that the normal T wave will always be negative in aVR and will always be positive in I and II. Unfortunately the normal T wave can be positive or negative in aVL, aVF and III without indicating abnormality.

A **rough** guide by which to assess normality or otherwise of the T waves in the limb leads is the following:-

In any lead in which the QRS is predominantly upright the T wave must be clearly upright. In any lead in which the QRS is predominantly negative the T wave should be clearly negative. In any lead in which the algebraic sum of QRS deflections is close to zero the T wave may be positive or negative (though small in either case) or iso-electric (flat). The normal T wave is always upright in Leads I and II.

The only way, however, **definitively** to determine whether the T waves are normal or abnormal in the limb leads is to determine the angle between the mean frontal plane QRS axis and the mean frontal plane T axis.

We have learned to measure the mean frontal plane QRS axis. The mean frontal plane T axis is measured in exactly the same way except that one looks for T deflections instead of QRS deflections. (Also the phrase "algebraic sum of" is unnecessary with the T waves because, unlike the QRS complexes, they are usually uniphasic). The normal T wave axis does not differ from the frontal plane axis by more than +45° (Figure 63). Apart from one specific situation (p 58) this is the only criterion which must be applied to determine whether the T waves in the limb leads are normal or not.

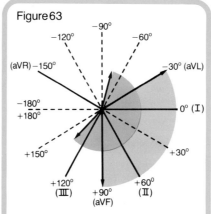

Figure 63

Figure 63 shows the normal range of QRS axes from −30° to +90°. It is possible for T wave axes to be normal from −75° to +135° but the T axis cannot be decreed normal or abnormal without reference to the QRS axis. The T wave axis is abnormal if it differs from the QRS axis by more than 45° in either direction.

Thus if the T wave axis is −75° and the QRS axis −30° they are both within normal limits, the QRS being at the limit of normal and the T wave being separated from the QRS by the maximum permissible (ie normal) angle. However, if the T wave axis is −15° and the QRS axis is +60°, the T waves are abnormal for the angle between the T axis and the QRS axis is then 75°.

Examples may help (Figure 64).

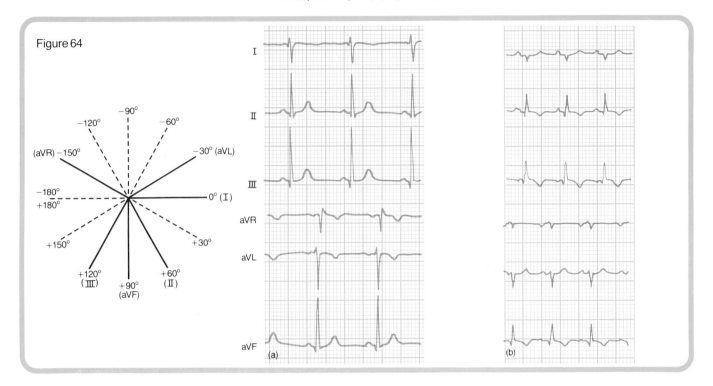

Figure 64

I

II

III

aVR

aVL

aVF

(a)

(b)

Consider Figure 64(a).
First determine the QRS axis:-
(i) The lead with the algebraic sum of QRS deflections most nearly zero is Lead I. Therefore the axis is either +90° or −90°. Of these two options, +90° lies on aVF therefore:-
(ii) inspect aVF. The QRS is positive therefore the axis is towards this lead. Thus, of the two options, the correct axis (to the nearest 30°) is +90°.
(iii) Re-inspection of Lead I shows that the QRS is actually slightly negative in this lead. Therefore our estimate of the axis must be adjusted 15° away from Lead I. It therefore becomes +105°. (The QRS axis is abnormal).
Next determine the T axis:-
(i) The lead with the T wave most nearly equal to zero is Lead I. Therefore the T axis is either −90° or +90°. +90° lies on aVF therefore:-
(ii) inspect the T waves in aVF. They are positive, therefore the T axis is towards aVF. Therefore of the two possible T wave axes (−90° and +90°) +90° must be correct.
(iii) Re-inspection of Lead I shows that the T wave size is indistinguishable from zero and therefore no further adjustment is necessary. The T axis is therefore +90°.

Thus, we know (a) the QRS axis is +105° and (b) the T axis is +90°. We can conclude that the QRS axis is abnormal because it falls outside the normal range (−30 to +90°). The only criterion for the T axis is its relationship to the QRS. The difference between the QRS and T axes is 15°. This is within normal limits and the T waves are normal.

Consider Figure 64(b).
First determine the QRS axis:-
(i) The algebraic sum of QRS deflections is most closely equal to zero in Lead I (if aVR be chosen, the answer will work out the same (see page 48). The QRS axis is therefore either +90° or −90°,
(ii) The QRS in aVF is positive therefore the QRS axis is +90° (to 30° accuracy).
(iii) The QRS is slightly negative in Lead I therefore the estimated QRS axis must be moved 15° away from Lead I giving a frontal plane QRS axis of +105°.
Next determine the T axis:-
(i) The T wave is closest to zero in aVR. The T axis is therefore either −60° or +120°. Of these, +120° lies on Lead III.
(ii) The T wave in Lead III is negative, therefore the T axis is not +120° and must be −60°.
(iii)Re-inspection of aVR shows the T wave is indistinguishable from zero and therefore the T axis does not need to be adjusted. It is therefore −60°.
Thus we know (a) the QRS is +105° (b) the T axis is −60°.

The QRS axis is definitely abnormal. The T axis differs from the QRS by +165° and the T waves are therefore abnormal.

Note

1. Where the limb leads are concerned one is only asking the question "are the T waves normal?" - one is not asking the question of individual leads. In this respect the limb leads differ strikingly from the precordial leads. The reason for the difference is that the precordial leads look at local areas of the heart and give preferential information concerning these areas. It is therefore reasonable to ask if repolarisation (the event which gives rise to the T waves) is normal or otherwise in a given lead. However, the limb leads are remote from the heart and give an overall impression only. One may therefore only ask if repolarisation of the ventricles is normally or abnormally related to their polarisation. One cannot use the limb leads to ask questions about local areas of the heart.

2. In one specific instance, T waves in the limb leads are considered abnormal despite having an axis identical with or very close to (and certainly within 45° of) that of the QRS complex. This situation occurs when there are abnormal Q waves (of myocardial infarction) in the inferior limb leads. This single exception will be dealt with in the section on ischaemic heart disease. An example is shown in record 26, page 97.

3. If the QRS axis is determinate and the T axis indeterminate, or vice versa, then the T waves in the limb leads are abnormal.

We may now summarise the two features which indicate the normality or otherwise of T waves in the limb leads:-

1 (a) Using soft criteria.

When the QRS is upright, T should be upright.

When the QRS is negative, T should be negative.

When the QRS is close to zero, T should be small but may be positive or negative.

(b) Using reliable criteria.

The angle between the mean frontal plane QRS axis and the mean frontal plane T axis must not exceed 45°.

2. In the presence of QS complexes or abnormal Q waves in II, III, and aVF, negative T waves in these leads are abnormal despite failure to fulfil the soft or reliable criteria in 1 above.

The P Waves

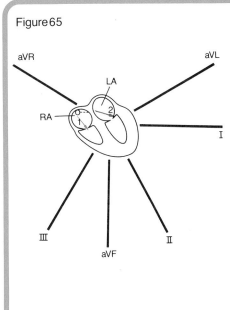

Figure 65

Atrial depolarisation begins in the sino-atrial node and spreads in all directions across the right atrial myocardium. The longest available direction determines the direction in which most right atrial myocardium is available for depolarisation and therefore the direction in which the right atrial component of the P wave (blue arrow, Figure 65) is best seen. Left atrial depolarisation begins at that point which is on the shortest depolarisation route from the sino-atrial node. The longest available direction within the left atrium then determines the predominant left atrial depolarisation pathway (purple arrow, Figure 65).. The right and left atrial depolarisation waves are therefore both positive in Lead II, the right atrial wave beginning before but overlapping with the left (Figure 66).

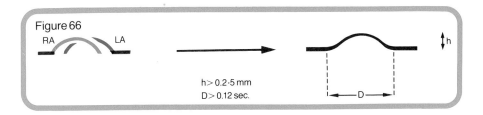

Figure 66

h > 0.2-5 mm
D > 0.12 sec.

The P wave seen as a result of overlapping right and left atrial depolarisation is a smooth, rounded wave (Figure 66). Its total duration does not normally exceed 0·12 sec (three small squares) and its height does not normally exceed 2·5mm (these readings are true for any limb lead but the readings will normally be greatest in Lead II)

We are now in a position to summarise the important criteria for normality of all the waves in the limb leads. These criteria must be memorised.

Summary:
Normal appearances
in limb leads

(NB ensure calibration is 10mm and
paper speed is 25mm/sec)

P waves

(Best seen in II) These should be
small rounded waves. The height should
not exceed 2·5mm. Duration should not
exceed 0·12 sec.

S-T segments

Must not deviate above or below the
iso-electric line by more than 1mm in any
lead.

QRS Complexes

R wave in aVL must not exceed 13mm.
R wave in aVF must not exceed 20mm.
Mean frontal plane QRS axis must not lie
outside the limits −30° to +90°.

Any q wave present in aVL *, I, II aVF
must not have a depth greater than one
quarter the height of the ensuing R wave
and must not have a duration equal to or
in excess of 0.04 sec (1 small square).

* When the frontal plane QRS axis is
further to the right than +60° (ie. from
+75° on to abnormal right axis deviation)
q waves exceeding these criteria, and
even QS complexes may be found in aVL
without constituting an abnormality.

T waves

The angle between the mean frontal
plane QRS axis and the mean frontal
plane T axis must be 45° or less. * *

* * If QS complexes or abnormal
Q waves are present in II, III and aVF, .
negative T waves in these leads are also
to be considered abnormal even though
the angle between the frontal plane QRS
and T axes may be less than 45° (See
record 26, page 97)

The Normal Rhythm of the Heart

We have now covered the important features of the normal P waves, QRS complexes, S-T segments and T waves in the precordial leads and in the limb leads. All that remains is to examine the **frequency** and **relationship in time** of atrial and ventricular depolarisation, ie. the cardiac rhythm. The rhythm of the heart is the ordered sequence of depolarisation of the myocardium. Since this definition refers only to depolarisation it concerns only P waves and QRS complexes. **The S-T segments and T waves have no relevance to the question of the cardiac rhythm. The rhythm can be determined from any ECG lead provided that the QRS complexes and P waves can each be recognised in that lead.**

The normal rhythm of the heart is sinus rhythm. This term implies that depolarisation begins in the sino-atrial node, spreads through the atrial myocardium, reaches the A-V node and spreads to the ventricles through the bundle of His, the right and left bundle branches and the Purkinje network, finally giving rise to ventricular depolarisation.

Figure 67 shows an example of sinus rhythm. The rhythm is said to be normal when it is sinus rhythm and when the heart rate is not less than 60 and not more than 100 beats per minute.

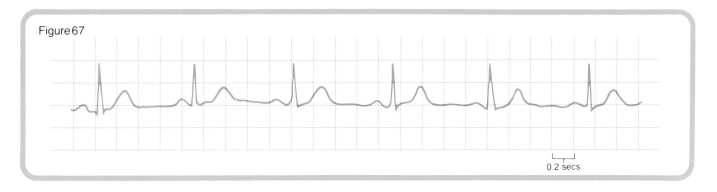

Figure 67

0.2 secs

A surprisingly large number of ECG criteria must be fulfilled before one can confidently state that the rhythm is sinus:-
P waves must be present.
The P waves must be regular.
The P waves must be the usual form for that patient.
The P wave frequency must not be outside the range 60-100 per minute.
There must be one P wave to each QRS complex.
The P wave must precede each QRS complex.
The P-R interval must be normal.
The P-R interval must be constant.
The QRS complex must be the usual form for that patient.

For example a patient may have left atrial hypertrophy and left ventricular hypertrophy. In this event the P waves and QRS complexes will be abnormal, but their morphology will be constant for that patient. If a P wave occurs different in form from the one recognised to be usual for that patient, it will not be of sinus origin.

An arrhythmia is any cardiac rhythm other than "sinus rhythm with rates between 60 and 100 per minute".

A Systematic Approach to the Interpretation of the ECG

If the reader has followed the text so far, he can be confident that all the basic groundwork has been covered. He may feel a little anxious that, despite spending so much time and effort, he has only learned about the normal ECG. He should accept the assurance that this is the most difficult aspect to learn in the whole of electrocardiography. The rest is "downhill'.

It is now necessary to develop a systematic approach to the examination of a standard, 12-lead ECG. This should consist of three sequential phases:

   1. **Documentation**
   2. **Recording quality**
   3. **Interpretation**

1. Documentation

Any record which does not include the **name** of the person from whom it was taken and the **date** on which it was recorded, is potentially misleading. It is important to establish the habit of writing the subject's name and the recording date on the record immediately it is taken. Equally, it is important to establish the habit of looking for the name and date whenever a record is to be interpreted. The learner is also urged to label each lead on the recording immediately the record is completed. This will save time and difficulty later (although an expert electrocardiographer can usually tell which lead is which without the labelling).

2. Recording Quality

It is futile to try to make sophisticated judgements on a record of inferior quality. All records should be taken with care. Lack of attention to detail during the recording will lead to serious imperfections in the tracing which may make interpretation difficult or impossible. Before interpretation of a record is attempted, four precautions must be observed:-

a. Baseline drift must be looked for. If present this renders interpretation of S-T segment changes impossible and seriously interferes with T wave interpretation (Figure 68).

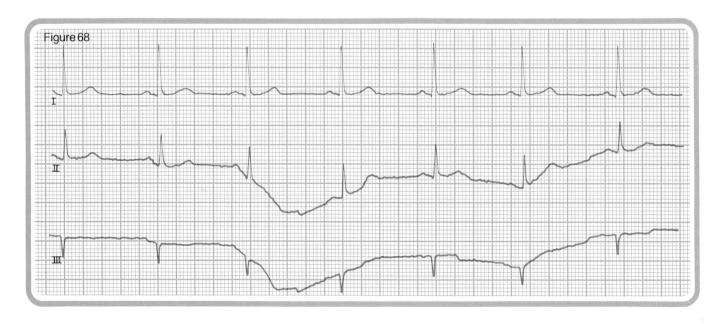

Figure 68

In Figure 68 the baseline is steady in Lead I, but drifts seriously in Leads II and III. Note how this appears to flatten the T waves following the third QRS complex in Lead II.

b. The record should be inspected for skeletal muscle interference (Figure 69)

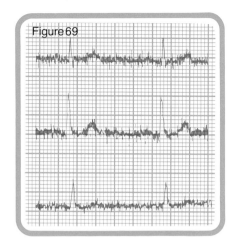

Figure 69

Figure 69 shows irregular, sharp, spiky waves throughout the record. These waves are produced by depolarisation of small groups of skeletal muscle fibres. This type of interference most commonly occurs when the patient is shivering or is moving his limbs or trunk. It may also occur if skeletal muscle tremor is present, eg in patients with Parkinson's disease. When present, it precludes adequate assessment of the baseline and interferes with the assessment of all low voltage deflections.

c. The record should be examined for mains frequency interference. This consists of regular sine wave oscillation (with a frequency of 50Hz in UK and 60 Hz in USA). This interferes with the assessment of all low voltage deflections (Figure 70).

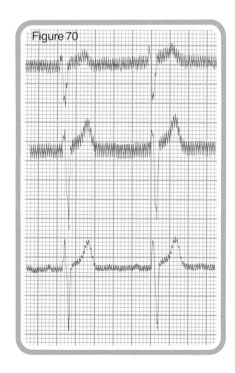

Figure 70

Baseline drift, skeletal muscle interference and mains frequency interference all result from faulty recording technique.

d. Finally, **the calibration signal must be checked.** All ECG machines have a calibration button which, when pressed, puts a 1 millivolt signal through the ECG amplifier. The amplifier gain is normally adjusted so that the resulting deflection is 10mm (2 large ECG squares). All voltage measurements made on the ECG are entirely dependent on the accuracy of the calibration signal (Figure 71).

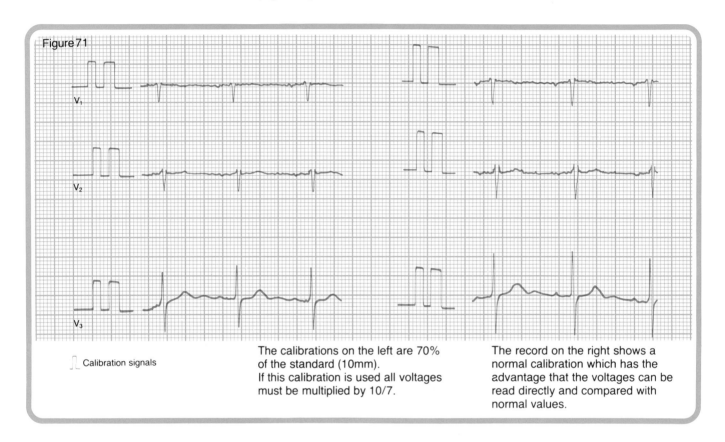

Figure 71

⌐ Calibration signals

The calibrations on the left are 70% of the standard (10mm).
If this calibration is used all voltages must be multiplied by 10/7.

The record on the right shows a normal calibration which has the advantage that the voltages can be read directly and compared with normal values.

Sometimes a deliberate reduction in standardisation is made in order to fit the deflections on the recording paper. This is most often necessary when there is left ventricular hypertrophy and sometimes when there is left bundle branch block. It is customary then to adjust the gain so that the usual 1mV pulse now gives a 5mm deflection. When this is done, the vertical deflections merely require to be doubled before they can be assessed against the normal voltage criteria. On most occasions when this "half standardisation" is necessary it is only the precordial leads which require this modification. It is then of greatest importance to record a calibration signal for the limb leads at full standardisation and at the precordial leads at half standardisation. An example is shown in Figure 72.

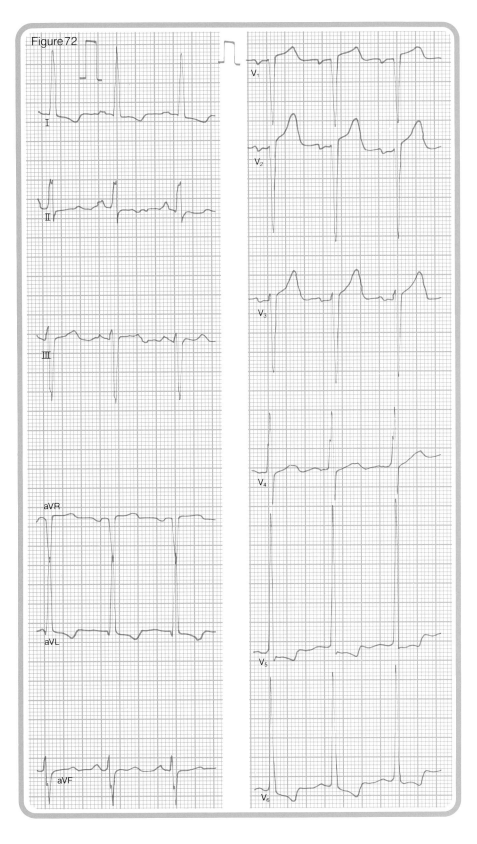

Figure 72

Figure 72 shows a 12-lead ECG with the limb leads fully standardised (10mm per mV) and the chest leads half standardised (5mm per mV). The R wave height in the left precordial leads and the S wave depth in the right precordial leads are clearly greater than normal. The R waves and S waves are actually even more impressive than they look for they must be doubled to give the true deflection.

3. Interpretation

Once the appropriate precautions listed under 1 and 2 above have been observed it is possible to proceed with interpretation.

The 12-lead ECG contains two discrete areas of information:-

(a) information about the rhythm of the heart

(b) morphological information

(a) The rhythm. As discussed on page 61, the rhythm of the heart describes the ordered sequence of depolarisation of the myocardium. It is concerned with the timing and sequence of atrial depolarisation, the timing and sequence of ventricular depolarisation and the relationship between the two. In practice this means the **timing** and **frequency** of **P waves** and of **QRS complexes** and **their inter-relationships.** As far as rhythm analysis is concerned, the **size** and **shape** of the P wave and of the QRS complexes are only important in so far as they have a bearing on the site of initiation of depolarisation and the direction of spread of that depolarisation over the atria and ventricles respectively The S-T segment and T waves have no relevance to rhythm analysis.

(b) Morphological information. "Morphological information" is information concerning the physical condition of the heart. Such information is contained in P waves, QRS complexes, S-T segments and T waves, but not in the relationship between P waves and QRS complexes (except by clinical inference).

As will become clear during subsequent discussion of the abnormal ECG, there is a narrow field of overlap and, therefore, of possible confusion between these otherwise discrete areas. For example, sustained atrial arrhythmias (atrial tachycardia, atrial flutter, atrial fibrillation) preclude the assessment of P wave morphology and sustained ventricular arrhythmias (ventricular tachycardia, ventricular pre-excitation) preclude the assessment of QRS morphology. These matters will be dealt with in detail in the sections on the abnormal ECG.

Any systematic approach to electrocardiographic interpretation must take the rhythm and arrhythmias into account. For the present, however, until the main morphological and rhythm abnormalities are described, we must make the scheme for systematic interpretation dependent upon the presence of normal (sinus) rhythm.

Systematic Interpretation

Preliminary Checks

Check the patient identification and the date.

Check the recording quality noting any baseline drift, skeletal muscle interference and mains frequency.

Check the calibration.

1. Inspect the record to determine the cardiac rhythm.

Assuming there is normal sinus rhythm throughout the recording:-

2. Assess the Qrs morphology in the precordial leads.

V₁ should have an rS complex

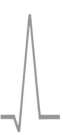

V₆ should have a qR complex

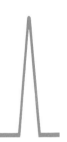

(Sometimes the q wave is not visible in V₆, ie the QRS waveform is an R complex).

Occasionally an S wave may also be found in V₆, so that the waveform may be qRs

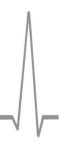

or Rs.

V_1-V_6 (Figure 73) The r wave voltage should increase progressively from V_1 to V_6, although it will often fall off (a) between V_5 and V_6 or (b) between V_4 and V_5 and again between V_5 and V_6. The **S wave** is usually deeper in V_2 than in V_1, it then becomes progressively smaller across the precordial leads. As indicated above, it may occasionally still be visible in V_6.

The initial deflection of the QRS complex should be positive (ie an r wave) in the right precordial leads, but there will usually come a point, in progression across the precordial leads, when the initial positive deflection will give way to an initial negative deflection (ie a q wave). (If no initial q wave is present in the left precordial leads one may be seen in leads further to the left than V_6, ie in I or aVL).

Figure 73

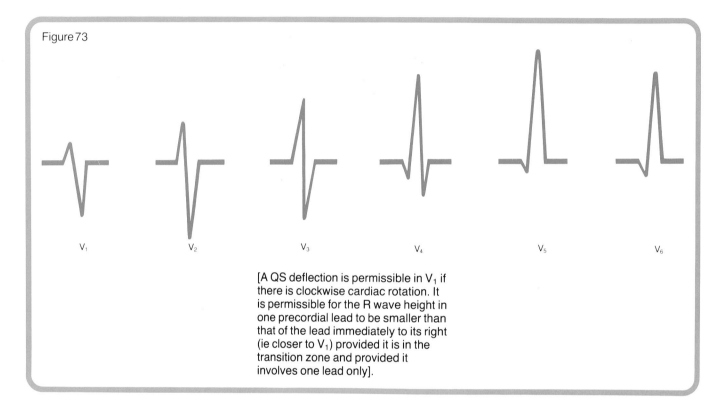

V_1 V_2 V_3 V_4 V_5 V_6

[A QS deflection is permissible in V_1 if there is clockwise cardiac rotation. It is permissible for the R wave height in one precordial lead to be smaller than that of the lead immediately to its right (ie closer to V_1) provided it is in the transition zone and provided it involves one lead only].

3. Assess the QRS dimensions in the precordial leads
(a) The total QRS duration in any lead should not exceed 0.10 sec (2½ small squares).
(b) At least one R wave should exceed 8mm in height.
(c) The tallest R wave should not exceed 27mm.
(d) The deepest S wave should not exceed 30mm.
(e) The sum of the deepest S wave and the tallest R wave should not exceed 40mm.
(f) The ventricular activation time (time from the onset of QRS to peak of the R wave in a lead showing a qR complex) should not exceed 0.04sec (1 small square).
(g) Any q waves seen should not have a depth exceeding one quarter the height of the ensuing R wave.
(h) Any q waves seen should not equal or exceed 0.04 sec (one small square) in duration.

4. Assess the precordial T waves

V_1 The T wave may be upright, inverted, biphasic or flat (**unless** it was formerly upright in the same subject, in which case it should still be upright).

V_2 The T wave may be upright, inverted, biphasic or flat (**unless** (a) it was formerly upright in the same subject or (b) the T wave is upright in V_1 in the same subject — either of which cases the T wave should be upright in V_2.) It is **usual** for the T wave to be upright in V_2.

V_3-V_6 The T wave should be upright. In general, in V_3-V_6 the T wave height should be more than $1/8$ — but less than $2/3$ of the height of the R wave in the same lead.

5. Assess the precordial S-T segments

These should not deviate by more than 1mm above or below the iso-electric (T-P) line in any lead. **This rule should not be rigidly interpreted in V_1 and V_2 where the QRS complex may merge imperceptibly into the S-T segment and the latter may likewise merge into the T wave.**

6. Assess the QRS complexes in the limb leads

(a) q waves. Any q waves present in aVL , I, II or aVF should not have a depth in excess of one quarter the height of the ensuing R wave.

Any q wave present in aVL , I, II or aVF should not equal or exceed 0.04 sec (one small square) in duration.

(If the frontal plane QRS axis is $+75°$ or further to the right, aVL will, like aVR, be a "cavity lead" and q waves in this lead should then be ignored, whatever their size).

(b) R waves. The R wave in aVL should not exceed 13mm and that in aVF should not exceed 20mm.

(c) The frontal plane QRS axis. This should lie within the range $-30°$ to $+90°$, inclusive.

7. Assess the T waves in the limb leads

The mean frontal plane T wave axis should not differ from the mean frontal plane QRS axis by more than $\pm 45°$.

In the presence of abnormal q waves in II and aVF, inverted T waves in these leads are abnormal even if the angle between the mean frontal plane QRS and T wave axes does not exceed $45°$.

8. Assess the S-T segments in the limb leads

These should not deviate from the iso-electric (T-P) line by more than ± 1mm.

9. Assess the P waves

These should not exceed 0.12 sec in duration or 2.5mm in height in II. Any negative component visible in V_1, should not have a greater area than that of the positive component.

The 12-Lead ECG: Annotated Records

This final section will review a series of thirty 12-lead ECG's. For each of the first seven records each detailed step of the systematic interpretation detailed on pages 66-69 will be followed and described using the same numbering for the paragraphs. Abnormalities will be shown in **heavy type.** Records 8 to 30 then appear without any supporting text. On page 102 each of the records 8 to 30 will be defined as being normal or abnormal. For those records which are abnormal a list of the abnormal features will appear on pages 103-104. These lists will use the paragraph headings corresponding to the systematic approach described on pages 66-69. The student may therefore use this section either for further systematic tuition or for self-evaluation.

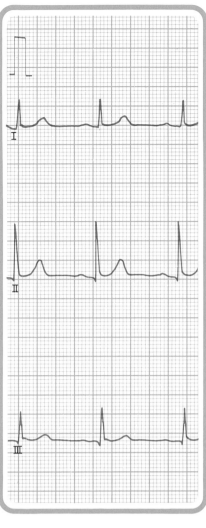

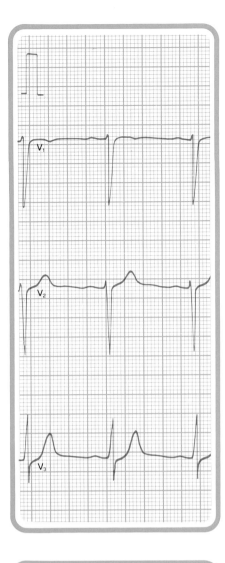

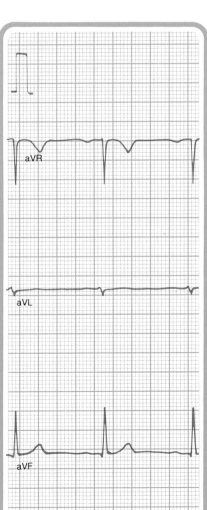

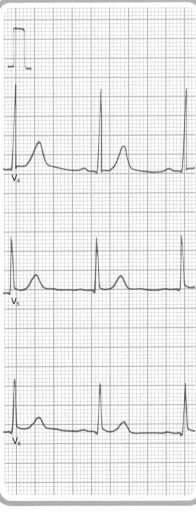

Record 1

Normal record

1. Sinus rhythm

2. V_1 — has an rS complex
V_6 — has a qR complex
V_1-V_6 — normal wave progression from V_1 to V_4 with slight fall-off between V_4 and V_5 and again between V_5 and V_6.

3. (a) Total QRS duration = 0·08 sec.
  (b) R waves in V_3, V_4, V_5, V_6 all exceed 8mm.
  (c) Tallest precordial R wave (V_4) = 22mm.
  (d) Deepest precordial S wave (V_2) = 18mm.
  (e) $S_{V_2} + R_{V_4}$ = 40mm.
  (f) Ventricular activation time = 0·04 sec.
  (g) q waves in $V_{4,\,5,\,6}$ are not deeper than one quarter the height of the R waves in the same lead.
  (h) q waves in V_4, V_5; V_6 are less than 0·04 sec in duration.

4. T waves in V_1 are inverted (normal).
T waves in V_2, V_3, V_4, V_5, V_6 are upright.

5. The precordial S-T segments are iso-electric. Note that it is easier to see a discrete S-T segment in V_6 than in V_2. This is usually the case.

6. (a) Small q waves are seen in I, II and aVF. They are less than 0·04 sec in duration and do not have a depth more than one quarter the height of the R wave in the same lead. (q waves present in aVR and III should be ignored).
  (b) R wave in aVL does not exceed 13mm (is actually only 1mm).
R wave in aVF does not exceed 20mm.
  (c) Mean frontal plane QRS axis = +60°.

7. Mean frontal plane T wave axis = +60° (Difference from QRS axis is 0°).

8. The S-T segments in the limb leads are iso-electric.

9. The P wave duration is 0.10 sec.
The P wave height in II is 1mm.

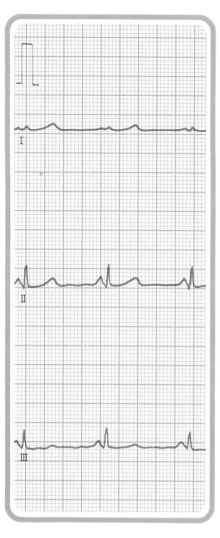

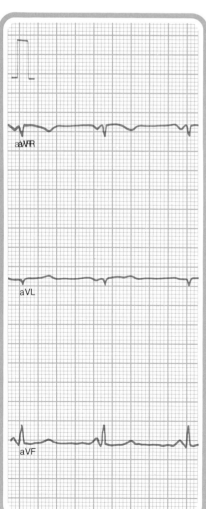

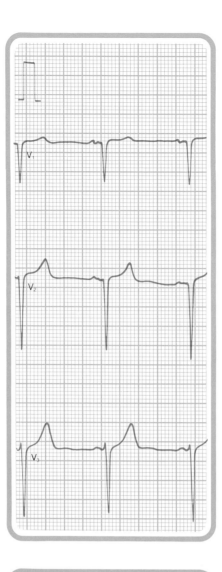

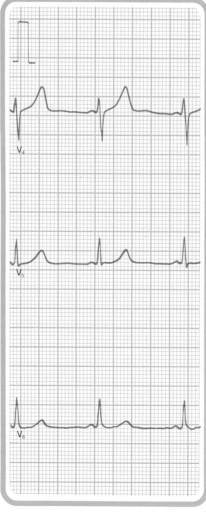

Record 2

Normal record

1. Sinus rhythm

2. V_1 — has an rS complex [r wave is very small. If there is no r wave at all in V_1 (ie if the complex is QS) it does not constitute an abnormality provided there is obvious clockwise rotation*. This requires that the transition zone must be towards the left side of the precordial leads. There **must** be an r wave in V_2 otherwise the record is definitely abnormal].

V_6—has an R wave (No initial q wave is visible).

V_1-V_6—normal R wave progression from V_2 to V_6. Since no q wave is visible in V_6, the transition zone can only be assessed by the position in which the precordial lead becomes dominantly positive. In this record this is between V_4 and V_5, ie there is some degree of clockwise cardiac rotation.*

3. (a) total QRS duration is 0·08 sec.

(b) R wave in V_6 is 8mm (borderline abnormal—tallest R wave in precordial leads should exceed 8mm)

(c) Tallest precordial R wave (V_6) = 8mm (ie does not exceed 27mm).

(d) Deepest precordial S wave (V_2) = 22mm (ie does not exceed 30mm).

(e) $S_{V_2} + R_{V_6} = 30$mm (ie does not exceed 40).

(f) Ventricular activation time cannot be measured since there is no qR complex in the precordial leads.

(g) and (h) No q waves are seen in the chest leads.

4. The T waves are upright in all the precordial leads.

5. The S-T segments are iso-electric. Note that it is easier to distinguish the S-T segment from the T wave in the left than in the right precordial leads. The gentle, rising S-T segment passing straight into the T wave is normal in the right precordial leads (V_1-V_3).

6. (a) q waves, in this case QS complexes (which are one specific example of q waves), are seen in aVL. This is normal because the axis is +75°**

(b) There is no R wave in aVL. The R wave in aVF is 5mm (ie does not exceed 20mm).

(c) The mean frontal plane QRS axis is +75°**

7. The mean frontal plane T wave axis is +45°. The difference between the frontal plane T axis and QRS axis is therefore within normal limits at 30°.

8. The S-T segments in the limb leads are normal.

9. The P wave duration is 0.10 sec. The P wave height in II is 2.5mm.

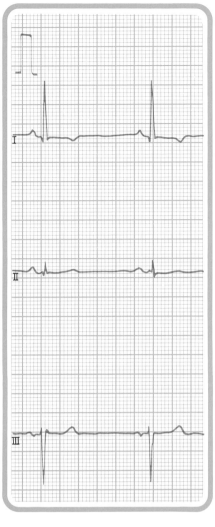

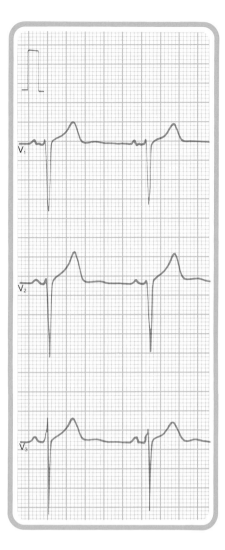

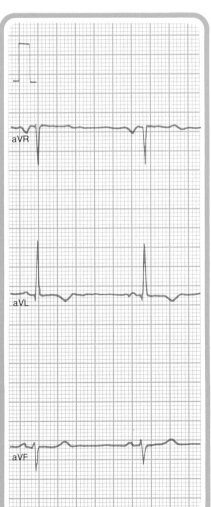

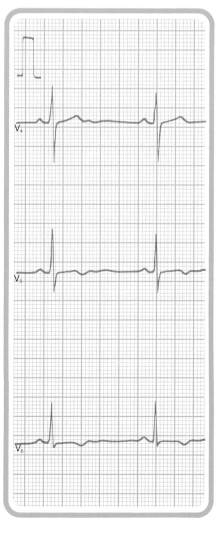

Record 3

Abnormal record

1. Sinus rhythm

2. V_1 — has an rS complex
V_6 — has an Rs complex [whenever V_6 does not have a q wave one should inspect other leads which "look at" the left ventricle. Most commonly these other leads are I and aVL, but if the axis is in the range $+60°$ to $+120°$ then it is II and aVF which show left ventricular type QRS complexes. In this case I and aVL show qR complexes. The significance of finding a normal q wave in at least one lead facing the left ventricle will become clear when left bundle branch block is discussed in the section on morphological abnormalities of the ECG. At this point, refer back to Record 2. In this record no R wave was seen in V_6. Since the heart was vertical (axis $+75°$) the normal, left ventricular q waves were seen in II and aVF.
V_1-V_6—normal R wave progression from V_1 to V_6.

3. (a) total QRS duration = 0·06 sec.
(b) R wave in V_5 exceeds 8mm (actually = 12mm).
(c) Tallest precordial R wave (V_5) = 12mm.
(d) Deepest precordial S wave (V_2) = 20mm.
(e) $S_{V_2} + R_{V_5} = 32mm$.
(f) Ventricular activation time cannot be measured since there is no precordial lead showing a qR complex.
(g) and (h) No q waves are seen in the precordial leads.

4. The T waves are normal in V_1-V_4. **There is T wave inversion in V_5 and V_6. This is abnormal.**

5. The S-T segments are normal in the precordial lead.

6. (a) q waves are present in I and aVL. They are less than 0·04 sec. in duration and do not exceed one quarter of their corresponding R wave height.
(b) R wave in aVL is 14mm. **(This just exceeds the voltage criterion of 13mm in aVL).**
R wave in aVF is less than 20mm.
(c) Frontal plane QRS axis is $-15°$.

7. Mean frontal plane T axis is $+120°$. **The difference between the frontal plane QRS and T wave axes is $135°$. This is abnormal.**

8. The S-T segments in the limb leads are normal.

9. The P wave duration is 0·08 sec. The P wave height in II is 2mm.

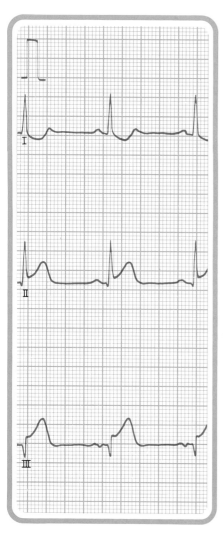

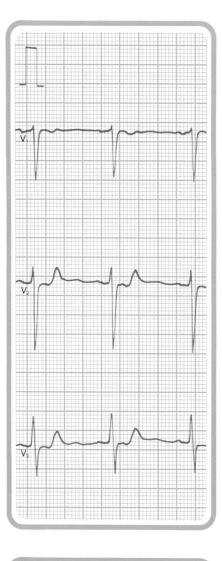

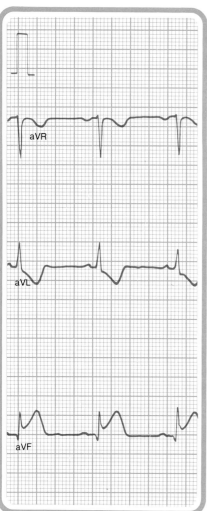

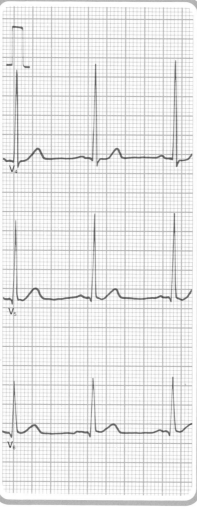

Record 4

Abnormal record

1. Sinus rhythm

2. V_1 — has an rS complex
V_6 — has a qR complex
V_1-V_6—normal R wave progression
(maximal in V_4).

3. (a) QRS duration 0·09 sec.
   (b) R wave in V_4, V_5, V_6 all exceed
8mm.
   (c) Tallest precordial R wave (V_4)
= 26mm.
   (d) Deepest precordial S wave (V_2)
= 18mm.
   (e) $S_{V_2} + R_{V_4} = 44$ **(This is abnormal,
this sum should not exceed 40mm).**
   (f) **Ventricular activation time (best
seen in V_5) is 0·05 sec. This is
abnormal.**
   (g) q waves are seen in V_5 and V_6.
They do not have a depth exceeding one
quarter the height of the ensuing R wave.
   (h) the q waves in V_5 and V_6 are less
than 0·04 sec in duration – they are
actually 0·02 sec.

4. The precordial T waves are normal.

**5. The precordial S-T segments are
depressed in V_2 and V_3. This is
abnormal** (Note the depression must be
assessed against the T-P segment).

6. (a) q waves are seen in I, II and aVF.
In none of these cases does their depth
exceed one quarter the height of the
ensuing R wave nor does their duration
equal or exceed 0·04 sec. (Remember to
ignore the QRS complex in III).
   (b) The R waves in aVL and aVF do
not exceed 13 and 20mm respectively.
   (c) The mean frontal plane QRS axis
is +30°.

7. The mean frontal plane T wave axis is
+90°. This is not too easy to assess
since the S-T segment tends to merge
gradually into the T waves).
**The angle between the mean frontal
plane QRS and T wave axes is
therefore 60°. This is abnormal.**

**8. The S-T segments are elevated in II,
III and aVF and are depressed in I and
aVL. These features are abnormal.**

9. The P wave duration is 0·10 sec. The
P wave height in II is 1mm, **The P wave
in V_1 has a dominant terminal
negative phase. This is abnormal.**

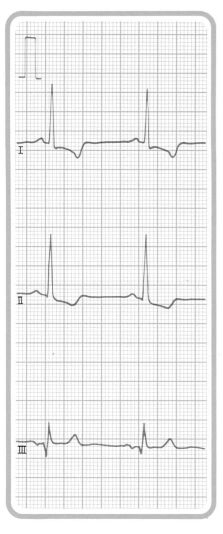

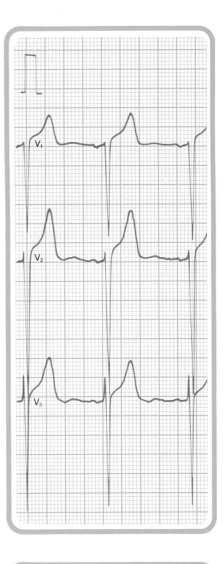

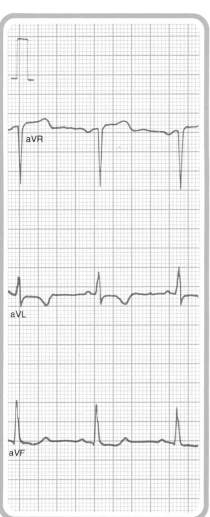

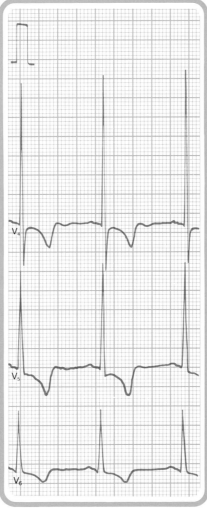

Record 5

Abnormal record

1. Sinus rhythm

2. V_1 – has an rS complex
V_6 – has a qR complex
V_1-V_6 – normal R wave progression to maximum voltage in V_4.

3. (a) Total QRS duration is 0·09 sec.
   (b) R waves in V_4, V_5 and V_6 all exceed 8mm.
   (c) **Tallest precordial R wave exceeds 27mm.** (V_4 is tallest R wave – 40mm). **This is abnormal.**
   (d) **Deepest precordial S wave exceeds 30mm. This is abnormal.** (Deepest S wave is V_2 - 37mm).
   (e) **Deepest S + tallest R wave exceeds 40mm. This is abnormal.** ($S_{V_2} + R_{V_4} = 77$mm).
   (f) Ventricular activation time is 0·03 sec.
   (g) q wave depths do not exceed one quarter the height of ensuing R wave.
   (h) q wave duration is less than 0·04 sec.

4. There is T wave inversion in V_4, V_5 and V_6. This is abnormal.

5. There is S-T depression in V_4, V_5 and V_6. This is abnormal.

6. (a) q waves are present in aVF. They are less than 0·04 sec. in duration and do not have a depth exceeding one quarter the height of the ensuing R wave.
   (b) The R wave in aVL does not exceed 13mm and that in aVF does not exceed 20mm.
   (c) The mean frontal plane QRS axis is +45°.

7. The mean frontal plane T axis is +135°. This is not easy to assess because the S-T segment merges into the T wave. **The angle between the frontal plane QRS and T axes is 90°. This is abnormal.**

8. There is S-T segment depression in I, II and aVF. This is abnormal.

9. The P wave duration is 0.10 sec. The P wave height in II is 1·5mm. **There is a terminal negative component to the P wave in V_1 which is larger than the initial positive component. This is abnormal.**

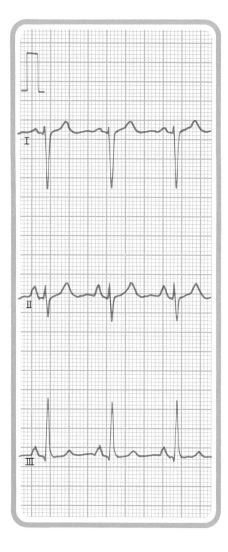

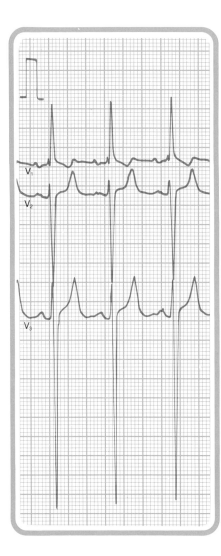

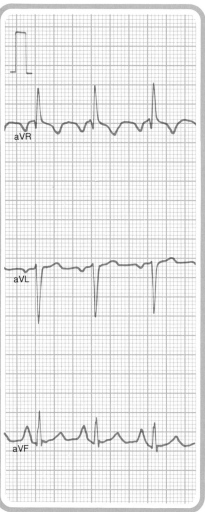

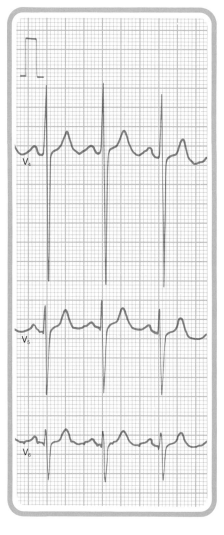

Record 6

Abnormal record

1. Sinus rhythm

2. V_1 – **has R wave (or rR′). This is abnormal.** (It should be rS).
V_6 – **has qrS complex. It is abnormal for the S waves to be larger than the r in V_6.** (On page 67 it was explained that V_6 can normally have a qRs complex. In each case the R wave is dominant. A qrS or an rS complex is abnormal for V_6)
V_1 - V_6 – **The r wave progression is quite abnormal.** R in V_1 is larger than that in V_2.

3. (a) Total QRS duration is 0·10 sec.
(b) One precordial R wave exceeds 8mm (R in V_1 is 21mm).
(c) Tallest R does not exceed 27mm.
(d) **Deepest S wave exceeds 30mm. This is abnormal.** (S in V_3 is 51mm).
(e) **Sum of deepest S and tallest R exceeds 40mm. This is abnormal.**
(f) Ventricular activation time is 0·03 sec.
(g) q waves in V_5 and V_6 do not have a depth exceeding one quarter the height of ensuing R wave.
(h) q waves in V_5 and V_6 have a duration less than 0·04 sec.

4. Precordial T waves are normal.

5. Precordial S-T segments are normal.

6. (a) q waves present in aVF are not more than one quarter the height of the ensuing R wave and are less than 0·04 sec. in duration.
(b) R waves in aVL do not exceed 13mm and those in aVF do not exceed 20mm.
(c) **The mean frontal plane QRS axis is +165°. This is abnormal.**

7. The mean frontal plane T axis is +45°. **The angle between the frontal plane QRS and T axes is 120°. This is abnormal.**
[Note that it is possible to have (i) a normal QRS axis with an abnormal angle between the QRS and T axes (eg. records 3, 4 and 5), (ii) an abnormal QRS axis with an abnormal angle between the QRS and T axes (example 6), (iii) an abnormal QRS axis with a normal angle between QRS and T axes (no example yet shown - see example 26)].

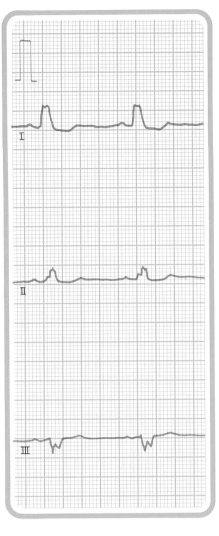

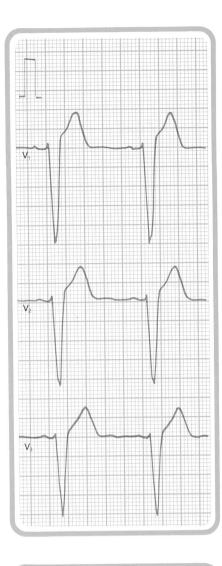

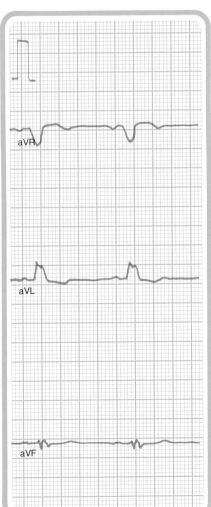

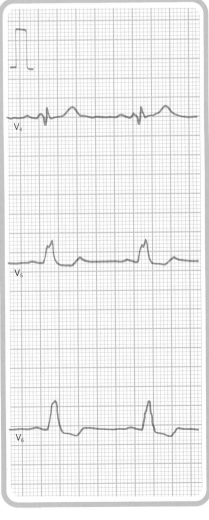

Record 7

The record is abnormal

1. Sinus rhythm

2. V_1 – has an rS complex
V_6 – has an R wave (no q wave). This finding should prompt the reader to inspect I and aVL for q waves. No q wave is seen in these leads either. (I and aVL are chosen in preference to II and aVF since the heart is horizontal - axis 0° see 6(c), below. I and aVL are therefore the most likely of the limb leads to show q waves - other than aVR and III where q waves are never significant). **V_1 - V_6 – R wave progression is abnormal.** (There is very little increase in the r wave from V_1 to V_4 with a sudden increase between V_4 and V_5.)

3. (a) **The total QRS duration is 0·16 sec. This is abnormal.**
(b) The tallest R wave (in V_6) is only 8mm in height. This is on the borderline of abnormality.
(c) The tallest R wave does not exceed 27mm.
(d) The deepest S wave does not exceed 30mm.
(e) The deepest S plus tallest R wave does not exceed 40mm.
(f) The ventricular activation time cannot be measured since no qR complex is seen in the precordial leads.
(g) and (h) No q waves are seen in the precordial leads.

4. There is T wave inversion in V_6. This is abnormal.

5. The S-T segments are depressed in V_5 and V_6. This is abnormal.

6. (a) There are no q waves seen in aVL, I, II or aVF.
The fact that there are no q waves in V_4, V_5, V_6, I, II or aVF is abnormal.
(b) The R wave in aVL does not exceed 13mm and that in aVF does not exceed 20mm.
(c) The frontal plane QRS axis is 0°.

7. The mean frontal plane T wave axis is indeterminate (see page 48) One cannot, therefore, estimate the difference between the frontal plane QRS and T axes. **However, since the QRS axis is determinate, the fact that the T wave axis is not determinate is significant and constitutes an abnormality.**

8. The S-T segments in I, II, aVL are depressed. This is abnormal.

9. The P wave duration is 0·10 sec. The P wave height in II is 1mm.

Further examples now follow. No description is given with the record. At the end of the examples (page 102) the records 8 - 30 are documented as being normal or abnormal and, if abnormal, the specific features which constitute the deviation from normal are listed - again using the paragraph numbering system of pages 66-69.

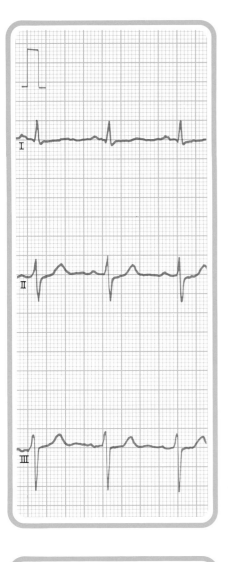

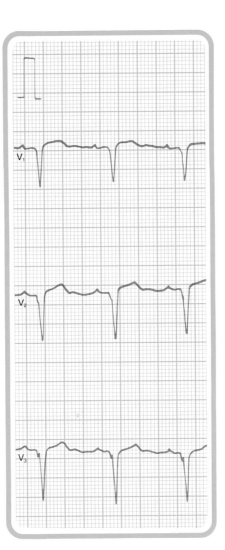

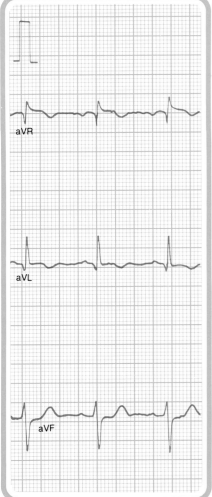

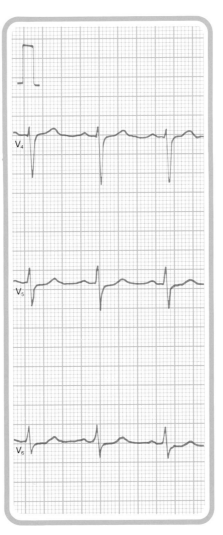

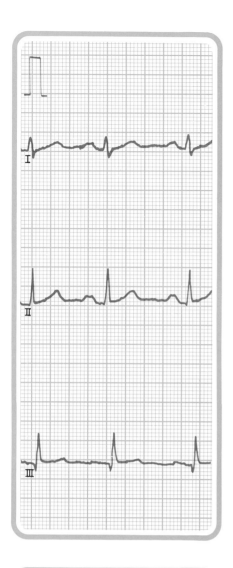

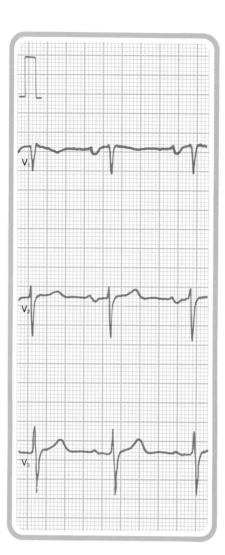

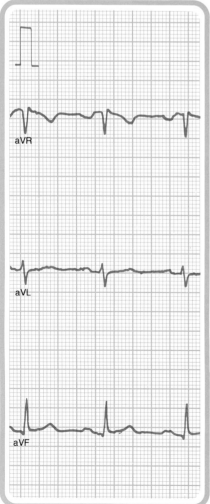

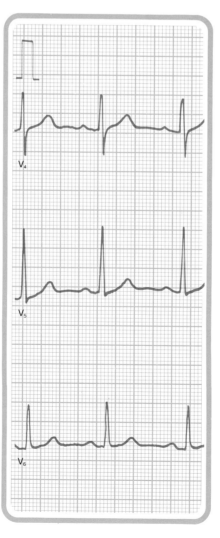

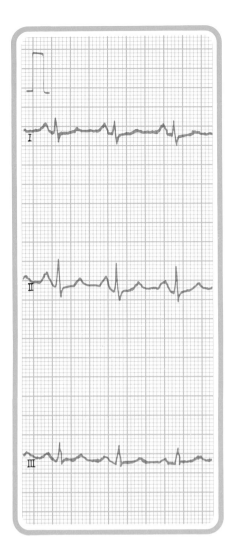

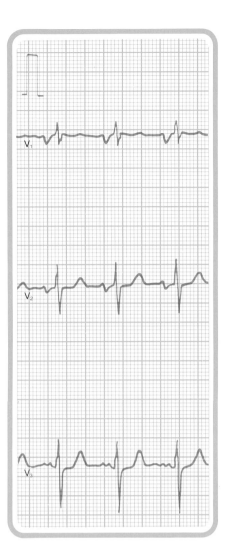

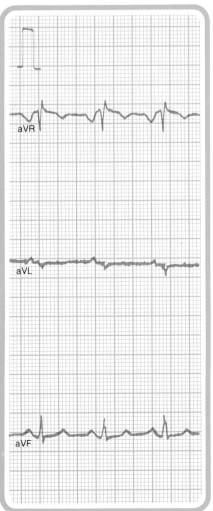

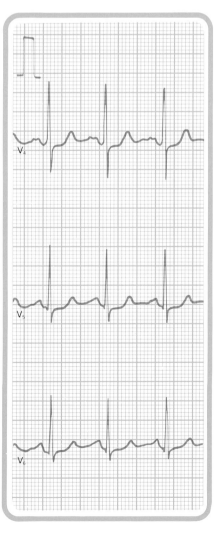

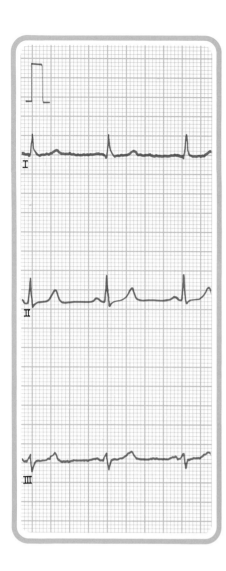
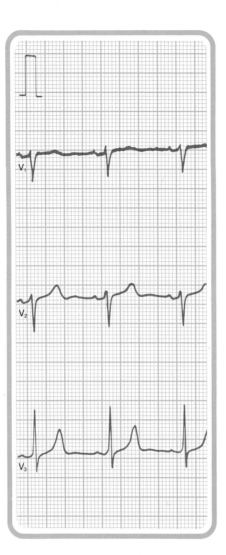
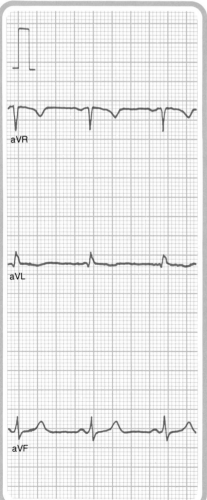
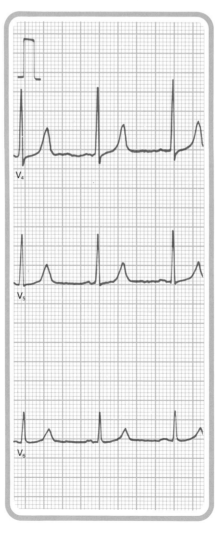

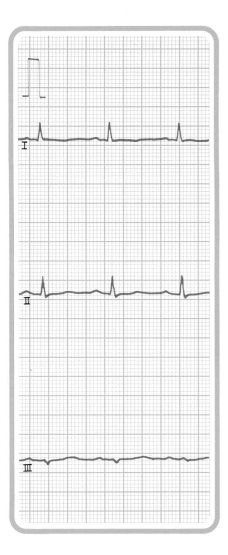

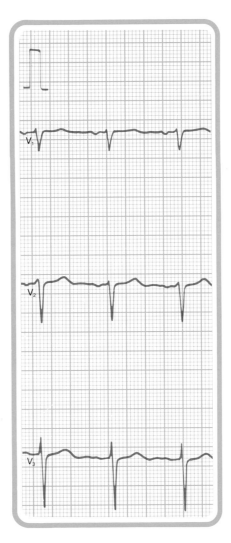

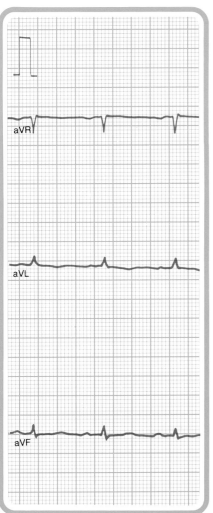

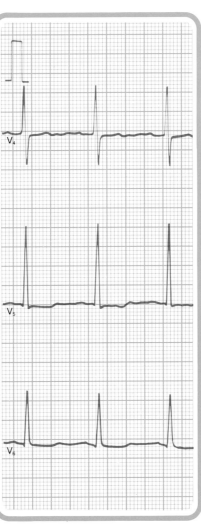

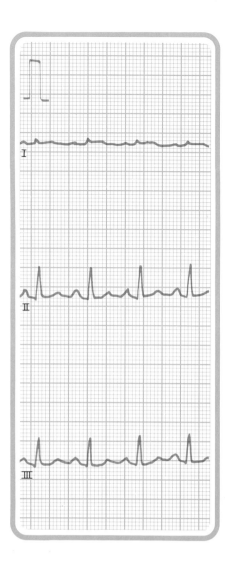
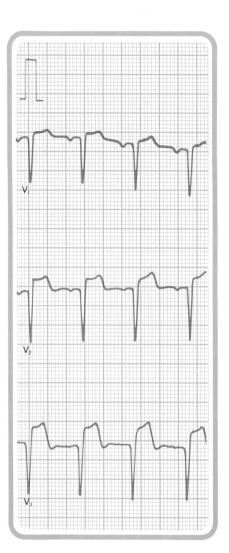
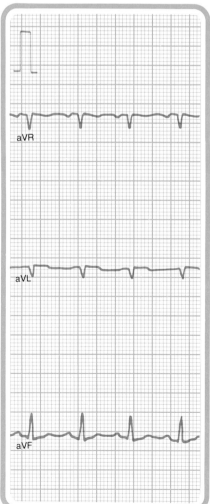
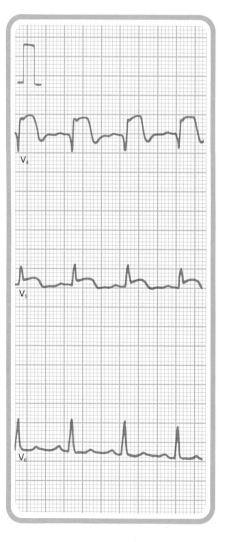

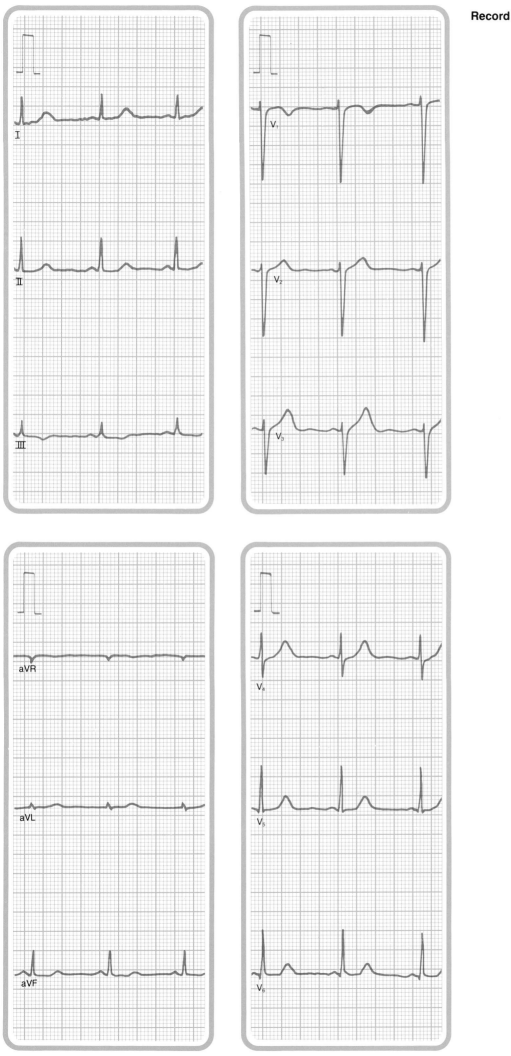

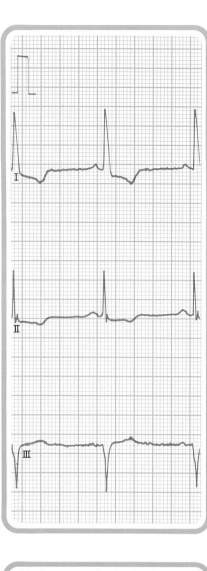

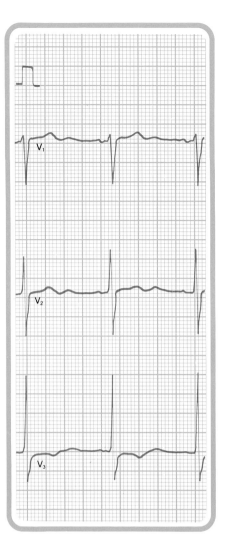

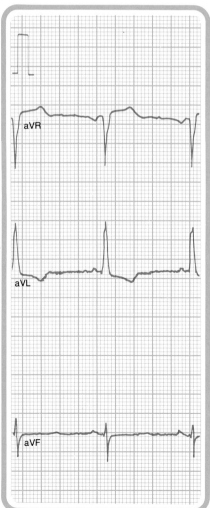

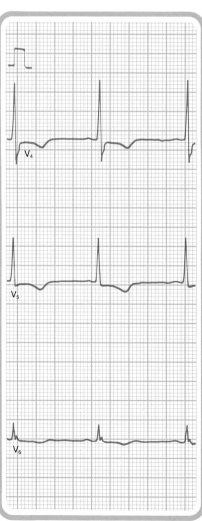

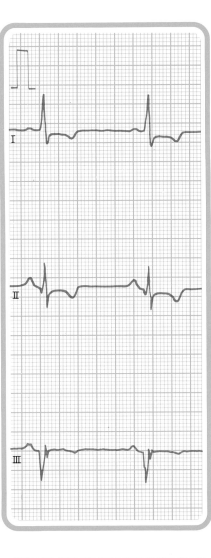

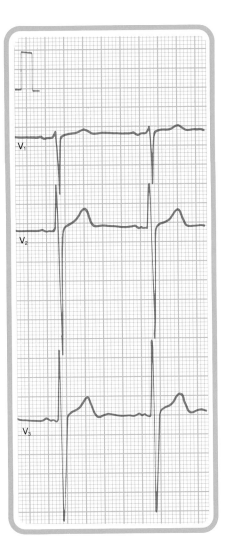

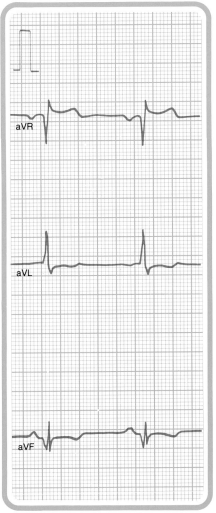

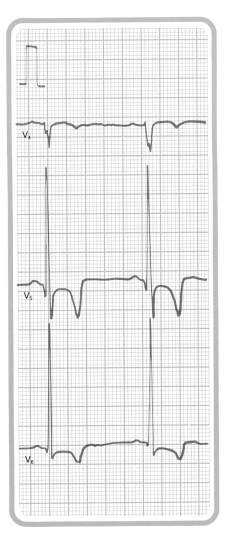

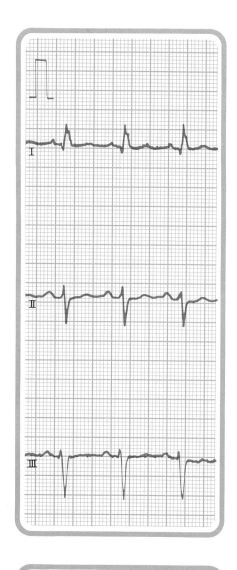

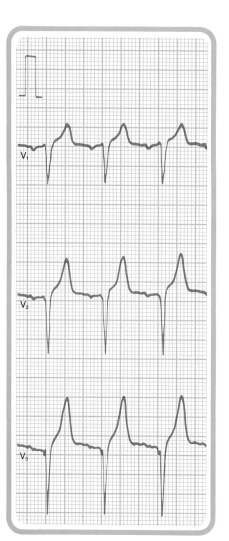

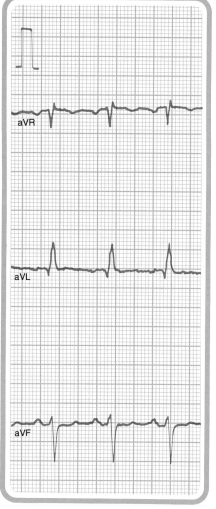

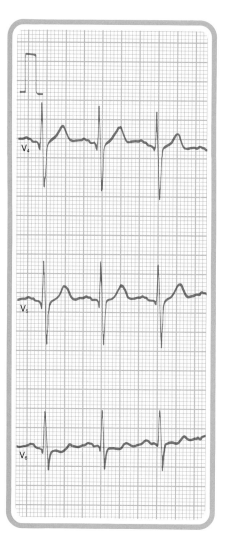

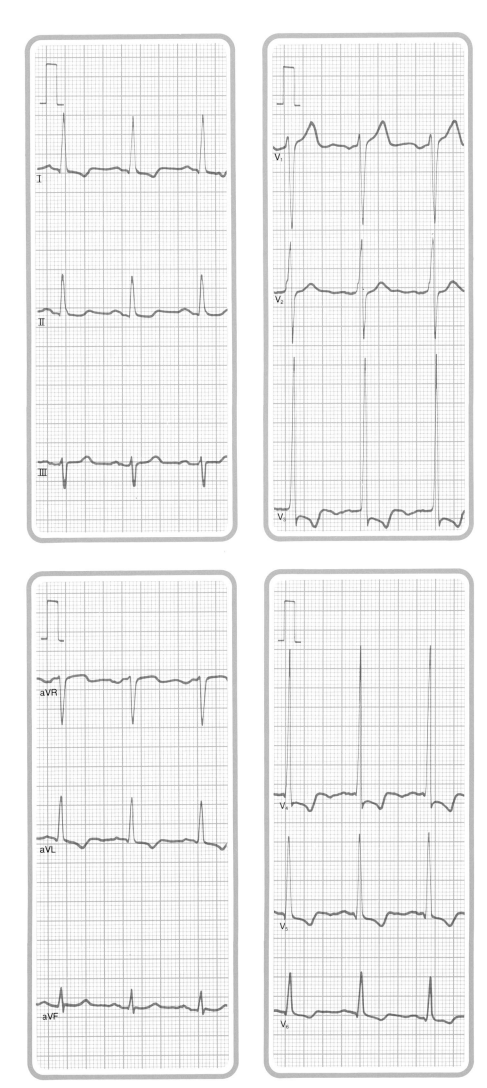

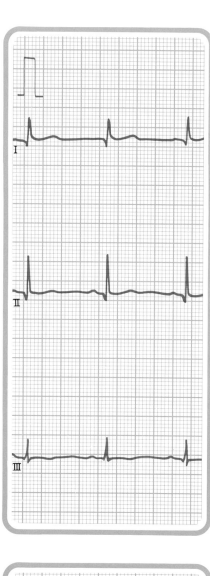

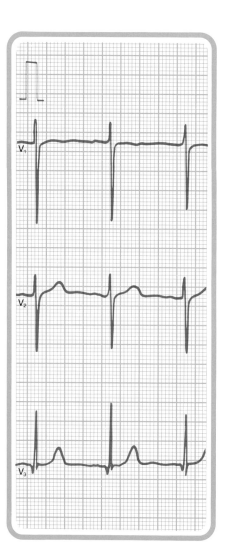

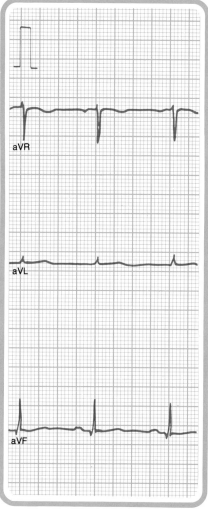

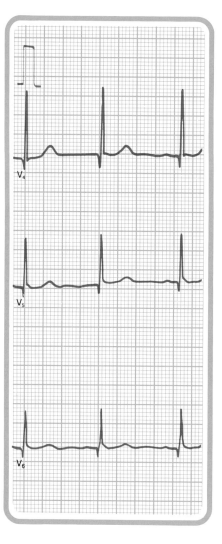

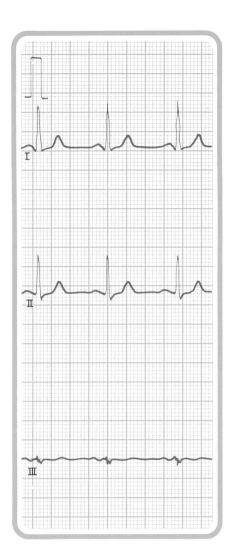

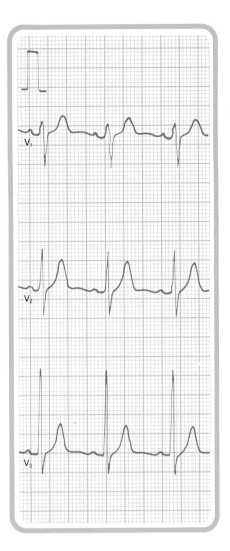

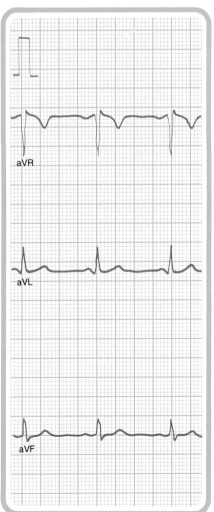

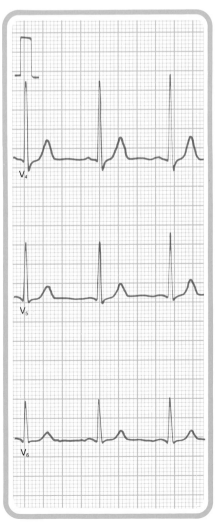

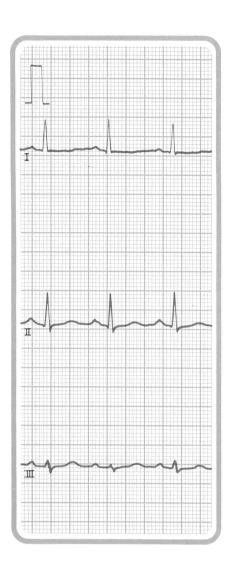
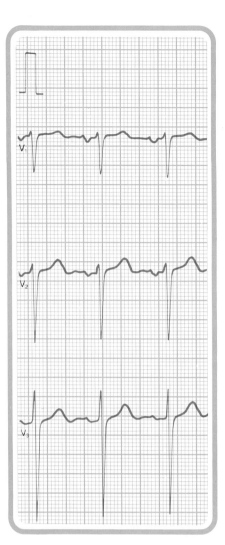
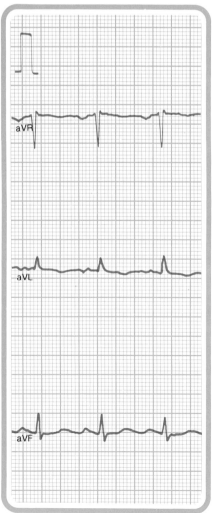
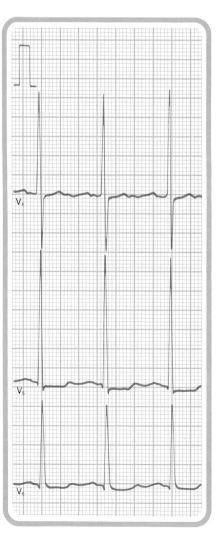

Record 21

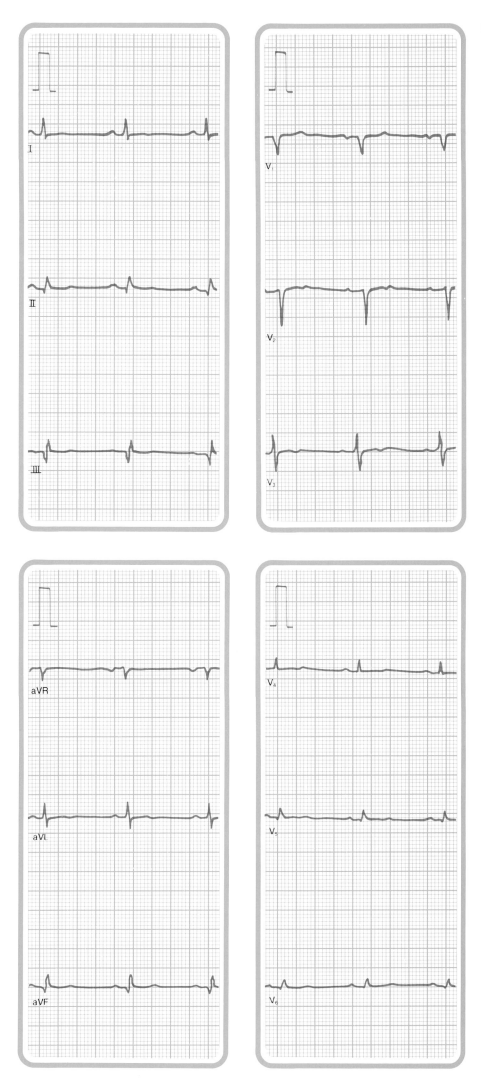

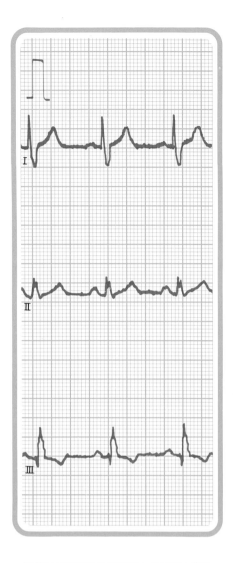

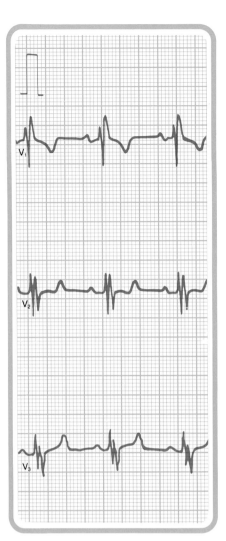

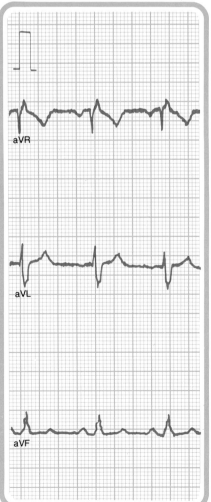

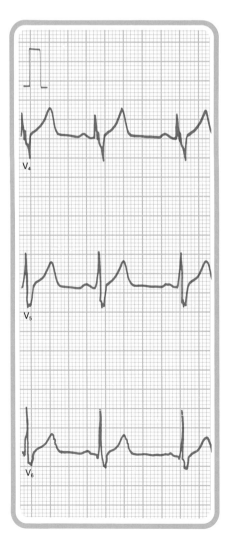

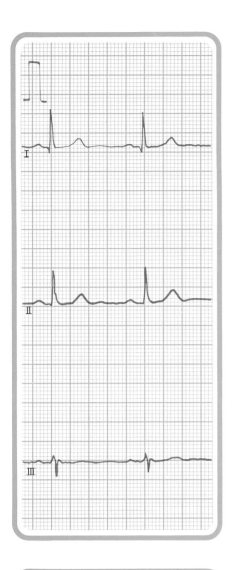
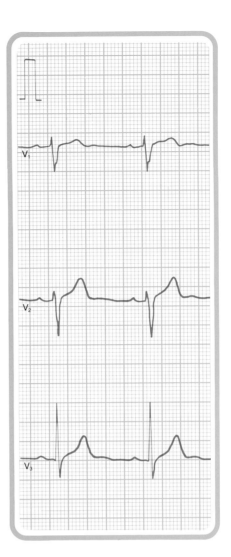
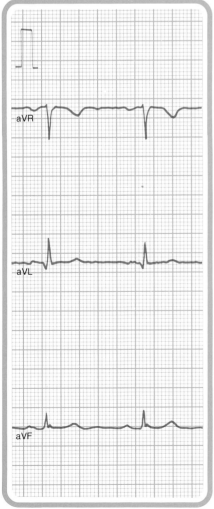
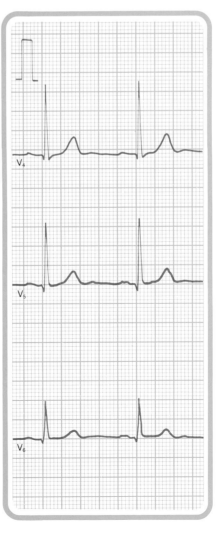

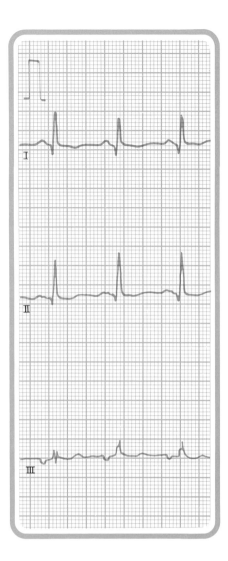

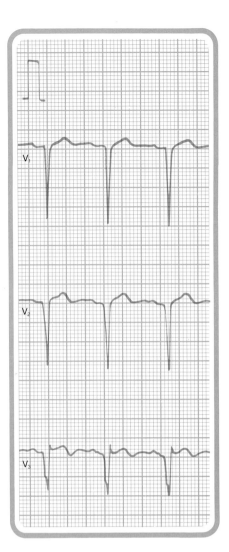

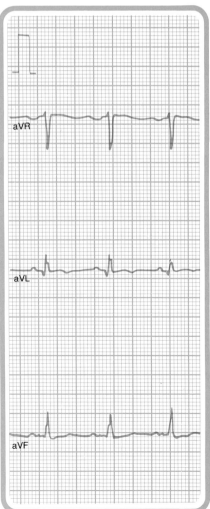

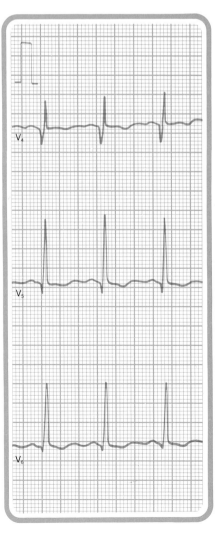

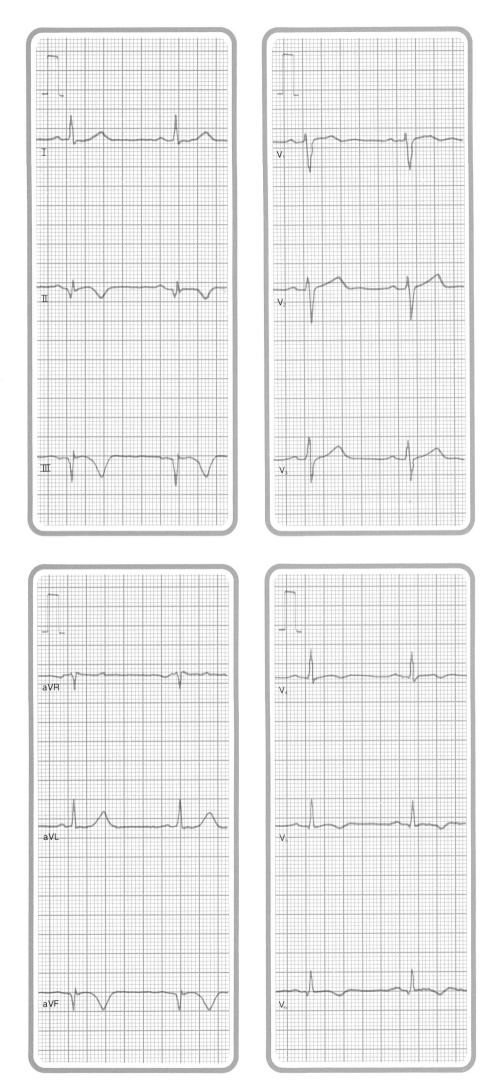

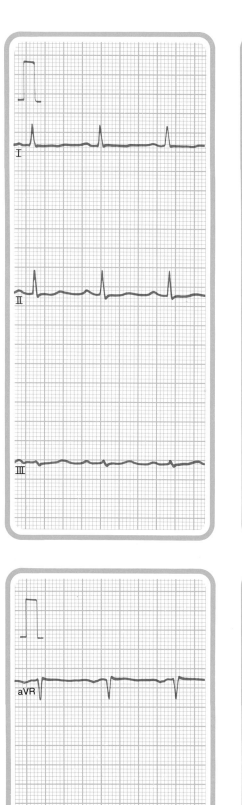

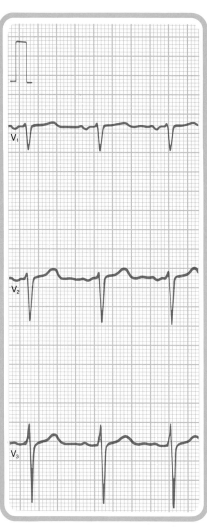

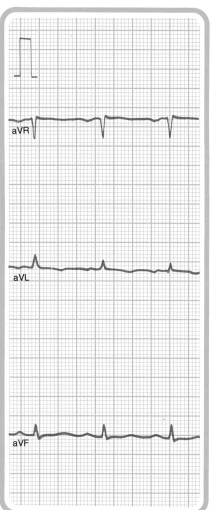

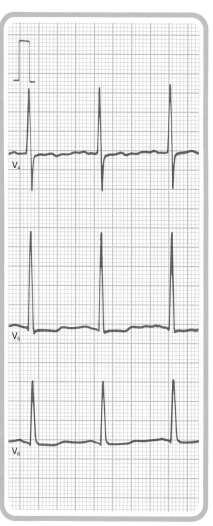

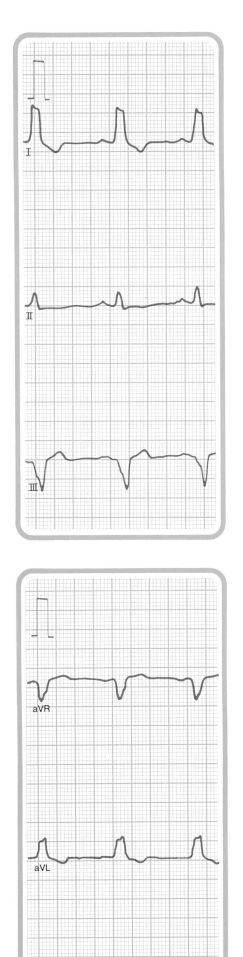
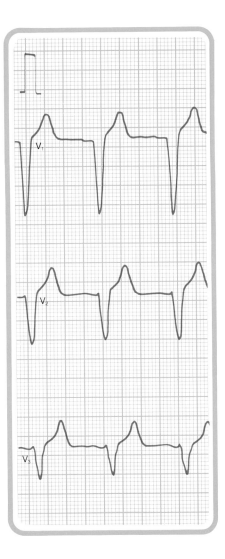
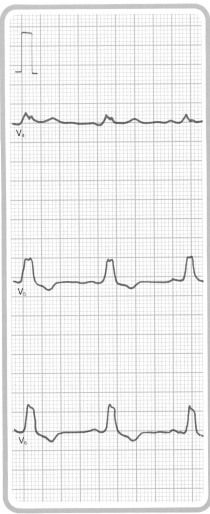

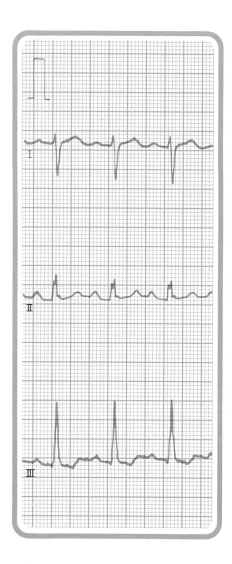

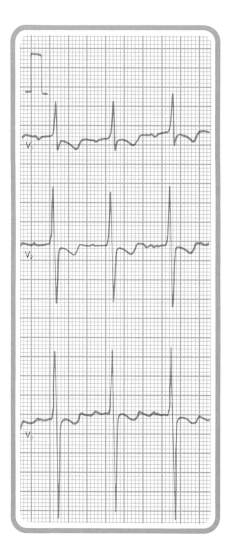

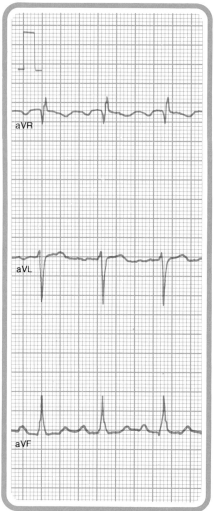

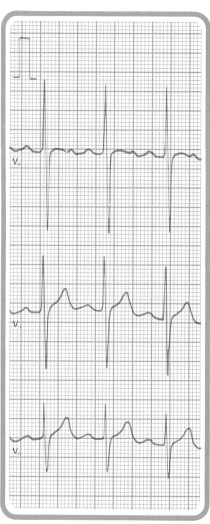

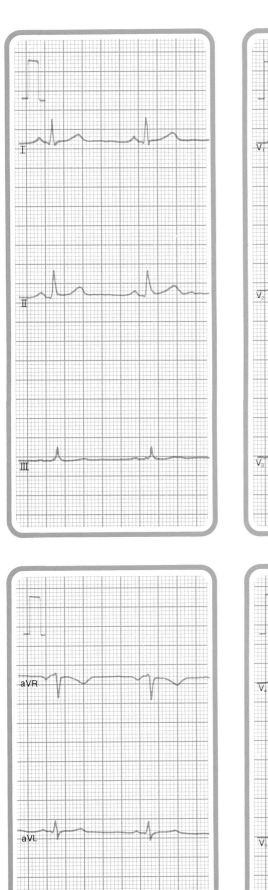
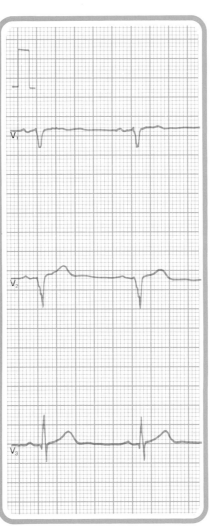
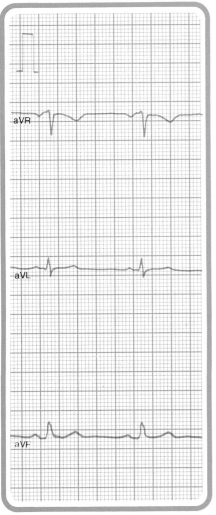
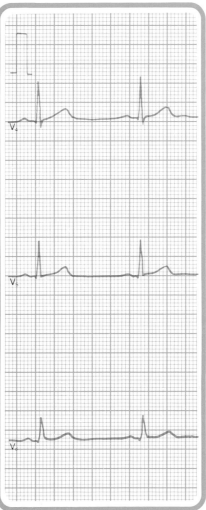

Records 8 - 30

Within normal limits	Abnormal
	8
	9
	10
11	
	12
	13
14	
	15
	16
	17
	18
19	
20	
	21
	22
	23
24	
	25
	26
	27
	28
	29
30*	30*

*This record is probably abnormal, but appearances of this type are occasionally seen normally - see details under abnormal record 30.

Listing of abnormalities in record examples 8 - 30

(The numbers refer to the paragraph numbers of "systematic interpretation" on pages 66-69)

Record 8

2. V_1 shows QS complex in V_1. In the presence of clockwise rotation this can be a normal finding, but even then there must be an rS complex in V_2. The presence of a QS in V_2 is definitely abnormal and in this record there is also a QS in V_3. (The **only** precordial lead in which a QS complex can be found in the normal ECG is V_1).
V_6 does not have a qR complex but has an Rs wave. This is related to the extreme degree of clockwise cardiac rotation here (transition zone is even further to the left than V_6). Normal septal q waves **are** seen in this record but only in leads further round the left ventricle than V_6 – in this case I and aVL.
$V_1 - V_6$ r wave progression is slight.
3. (b) No precordial R wave exceeds 8mm.
5. There is slight but probably significant S-T segment elevation in V_2 and V_3.
6. (a) The q waves in aVL are 0·05 sec in duration and are, therefore, abnormal.
   (c) The mean frontal plane QRS axis is abnormal at $-45°$.
7. The mean frontal plane T wave axis is $+75°$. Therefore, the angle between the frontal plane QRS and T axes is $120°$ –which is abnormal.

Record 9

9. The P wave duration is 0·14 sec. This is abnormal. The P waves are bifid in II and biphasic in V_1. The negative component in V_1 is much larger in area than the initial positive component. This is abnormal.

Record 10

2. V_1 has RS complex and the size of the R and S waves are equal. This is abnormal. The r wave should be smaller than the S wave.
5. It appears that there is S-T segment depression in V_4, V_5 and V_6 but closer inspection reveals that the segment before the QRS is also depressed and that the QRS is "sitting in" a zone of depression:-
This is abnormal. It is an exaggerated atrial T wave.
9. The P wave in V_1 has a negative component greater in area than the positive component (it is virtually all negative).

Record 12

4. The T waves are iso-electric in V_4, V_5 and V_6.
5. There is S-T segment depression in V_5 and V_6.
7. The T wave axis is indeterminate. The QRS axis is determinate $(+15°)$. Therefore, the T waves are abnormal in the frontal plane leads.

Record 13

2. No initial r wave is seen in V_1 and V_2, V_3, V_4—all have Q waves rather than initial r waves. This is abnormal.
3. (g) the q waves in V_1, V_2, V_3 and V_4 all exceed one quarter of their ensuing R wave.
   (h) the q waves in V_1, V_2, V_3 and V_4 all exceed 0·04 sec in duration.
4. There is inversion of the terminal part of the T wave in V_3 and V_4.
5. There is S-T elevation in V_1, V_2, V_3, V_4 and V_5.

Record 15

3. (c) R wave in V_3 = 42mm
(NOTE HALF STANDARDISATION)
   (e) $S_{V_2} + R_{V_3}$ = 64mm
(NOTE HALF STANDARDISATION)
4. There is T wave inversion in V_3, V_4, V_5 and V_6.
5. There is S-T depression in V_4, V_5 and V_6.
7. The frontal plane T wave axis is $180°$. Since the frontal plane QRS axis is $-15°$ the angle between the two is abnormal (ie more than $45°$).
8. There is S-T depression in I, II, aVL.
9. The P waves in V_1 have a dominant negative deflection.

Record 16

2. The r wave voltage does not increase progressively across the chest—it increases from V_1 to V_3, falls off at V_4 and increases again in V_5 and V_6. Although it was stated on p 45 that the R wave voltage in one of the leads V_2, V_3 or V_4 may be smaller than that in the lead to its immediate right (in the precordial series) this is only likely to be a normal finding where the adjacent r waves are small. In this case, the R waves in V_3 and V_5 are large and the difference in R wave size in these leads compared with that in V_4 is very substantial. This is an abnormality.
3. (c) R_{V_5} = 30mm.
   (d) S_{V_2} = 33mm.
   (e) $S_{V_2} + R_{V_5}$ = 63mm.
   (f) Ventricular activation time = 0·06 sec.
4. There is T inversion in V_4, V_5 and V_6.
6. (a) The q in aVF exceeds one quarter the length of the ensuing R wave and is longer than 0·04 sec in duration.
7. The T wave axis is $-135°$. Since the QRS axis is $0°$, the angle between the two $(135°)$ is abnormal.
8. There is S-T depression in I, II, III, aVL and aVF.

Record 17

2. The r wave progression is abnormal. A small r wave (normal) is seen in V_1. V_2 and V_3 have QS complexes (they should have taller r waves than V_1).
3. (g) The Q wave in V_2 and V_3 exceeds one quarter the height of the ensuing r wave, since there is no ensuing r wave!
   (h) The Q waves (actually QS complexes) in V_2 and V_3 exceed 0·04 sec in duration.
5. There is S-T depression in V_6.
6. (c) The mean frontal plane QRS axis is $-45°$.
7. The mean T wave axis is $+60°$. Since this is $105°$ from the QRS axis the limb lead T waves are abnormal.
9. The P waves in V_1 have a dominant negative component.

   (Note, the T waves in V_3 look unusually tall. No **specific** criteria are available to enable us to determine whether these are normal or not but these T waves are abnormal according to the **general** guidelines given on page 44).

Record 18

3. (c) R_{V_3} = 40
   (e) $S_{V_1} + R_{V_3}$ = 60
   (f) ventricular activation time = 0·07 sec. (best seen in V_4).
4. The T waves are inverted in V_3, V_4, V_5 and V_6.
5. There is S-T depression in V_3, V_4, V_5 and V_6.
7. The frontal plane T axis is $+135°$. Since the QRS axis is $+15°$ the angle between the two $(120°)$ is abnormal.
8. There is S-T depression in I, II and aVL.
9. The P waves have a dominant negative component in V_1.

Record 21

3. (c) R_{V_5} = 34
   (e) $S_{V_3} + R_{V_5}$ = 60
4. The T waves are flat in V_4, V_5, V_6.
5. There is S-T depression in V_5, V_6.
7. The frontal plane T axis is $+90°$. Since the QRS axis is $+30°$ the angle between the two is abnormal, $(60°)$.
9. The P waves in V_1 have a dominant negative component.

Record 22

3. (b) No precordial R wave exceeds 8mm.
4. The precordial T waves are inverted in V_3 and flat in V_4, V_5 and V_6.
6. (a) The q waves present in II and aVF are greater in depth than one quarter the height of the ensuing R wave.
The q waves in aVF are more than 0·04 sec. in duration.

Record 23

2. V_1 has an rSR complex.

3. (a) The total QRS duration is 0·14 sec. (best seen in V_5).

7. The frontal plane T axis is +30°. Since the frontal plane QRS axis is +90° the frontal plane T waves are marginally abnormal.

Record 25

2. V_1 has no r wave — it has an initial Q wave and initial Q waves are also seen in V_2, V_3, V_4. The r wave does not begin until V_3 (which has Qr). The r wave progression is, therefore, abnormal.

3. (f) The ventricular activation time is 0·05 sec. (best seen in V_5).

   (g) The q waves in V_1, V_2, V_3 and V_4 all have depths in excess of one quarter the height of the ensuing r wave.

   (h) The q waves in V_1, V_2, V_3 and V_4 exceed 0·04 sec. in duration.

4. The T waves are inverted in V_3 and V_4, and are flat in V_5 and V_6.

5. There is S-T elevation in V_2 and V_3.

6. The q waves in I have a depth exceeding one quarter the height of the ensuing r wave.

7. The frontal plane T axis is indeterminate. Since the frontal plane QRS axis is determinate the T waves are abnormal in the frontal plane leads.

Record 26

4. The T waves are flat in V_4 and inverted in V_5 and V_6.

6. The q waves in II and aVF exceed one quarter the height of the ensuing R waves and are more than 0·04 sec. in duration.

7. The T waves in II, III and aVF are abnormal even though the angle between the QRS axis (−30°) and the T axis (−60°) is within normal limits (30°). This is an example of the exception to the general rule. This exception was described on page 58.

Record 27

4. The T waves are flat (iso-electric) in V_4, V_5 and V_6.

5. There is S-T segment depression in V_5 and V_6.

7. The mean frontal plane T wave axis is +90. Since the frontal plane QRS axis is +30° the angle between the frontal plane QRS and T wave axes is abnormal.

Record 28

2. There is no r wave in V_1. The complex is a QS one.

3. (a) The total QRS duration is 0.14 sec.

4. There is T wave inversion in V_5 and V_6.

5. There is S-T segment depression in V_5 and V_6.

6. There are abnormal q waves in aVF. (They are QS complexes and, therefore, the Q wave has a depth greater than one quarter the height of the ensuing R wave —which is in fact zero).
The Q waves in aVF are also abnormally wide.

7. The mean frontal plane T wave axis is +150°. Since the frontal plane QRS axis is −15° the angle between the two axes (165°) is abnormal.

8. There is S-T segment depression in I and aVL.

Record 29

2. V_1 has an Rs complex. It should have an rS complex. It is abnormal for the initial positive wave in V_1 to be larger than the subsequent negative wave. V_6 has an RS complex. The positive wave should be clearly dominant in V_6 (ie. Rs, qR or qRs).

4. The T waves are flat or inverted in V_3.

5. There is S-T segment depression in V_1, V_2 and V_3.

6. The mean frontal plane QRS axis is +120°.

7. The mean frontal plane T wave axis is +30°. It is therefore differs by more than 45° from the QRS axis.

8. There is S-T segment depression in III and aVF.

Record 30

2. The R wave progression is not typical of normal. The R wave in V_2 is smaller than that in V_1. This is usually abnormal but if the deviation from the normal precordial R wave progression only occurs in a single precordial lead and if that lead lies in the region of the interventricular septum (as here) then it is not necessarily abnormal (page 45). Since it is always better to under-report rather than over-report abnormalities on the ECG this record should be regarded as normal. Note that the transition zone very clearly lies between V_2 and V_3. Sometimes an abnormality of R wave progression like this can indicate an old antero-septal myocardial infarction. (See the section on morphological abnormalities of the ECG).

SECTION 2: **Morphological Abnormalities**

Introduction

Inter-relationships between Morphological and Rhythm Information

The electrocardiogram provides greater or lesser degrees of information about the structure, shape, orientation, size and state of health of the atrial and ventricular myocardium (**"morphological" information**) and on the direction, timing and sequence of the depolarisation of myocardium and the relationship between atrial and ventricular depolarisation (**"rhythm" information**). In the majority of electrocardiograms the morphological information and the rhythm information are mutually discrete. Occasionally, however, a disturbance of the cardiac rhythm may interfere with morphological analysis (as when ventricular tachycardia precludes the recognition of ventricular hypertrophy, bundle branch block or myocardial infarction) and sometimes a morphological abnormality may interfere with the determination of cardiac rhythm (as when bundle branch block occurring in association with a supraventricular tachycardia may lead to an incorrect diagnosis of ventricular tachycardia). In most electrocardiograms it is possible both to determine the cardiac rhythm and to assess the morphological state. Reports of electrocardiograms should always give both items of information, wherever possible.

Simple electrocardiographic reports therefore often take one of the general forms illustrated below:-
1. "Sinus rhythm. The record is within normal limits."
2. "Sinus rhythm. Left bundle branch block."
3. "Sinus bradycardia. Acute myocardial infarction."
4. "Ventricular tachycardia. This precludes morphological evaluation of the electrocardiogram."

This whole section (Section 2) will be concerned entirely with morphological abnormalities of the electrocardiograms. **Unless otherwise stated, normal sinus rhythm will be assumed.** The criteria for normality of the QRS complexes, S-T segments and T waves given in Section 1 depend upon the normal sequence of depolarisation and of repolarisation of the ventricular myocardium. This normal sequence is only possible if the activation (depolarisation) wave reaches the ventricles via the normal route, i.e. through the A-V node from a more proximal, primary initiating site. The criteria for QRS complexes, S-T segments and T waves (i.e. the ventricular part of the ECG) therefore apply to all rhythms initiated from a **supraventricular** site, i.e. sinus rhythm, sinus arrhythmia, sinus tachycardia, sinus bradycardia, atrial ectopic beats, atrial tachycardia, atrial flutter, atrial fibrillation, nodal ectopic beats, nodal rhythm and nodal tachycardia.

The only exception to this rule arises from the fact that the right and left bundle branches have different refractory periods (normally the refractory period of the right bundle is longer than that of the left bundle). Because of this, when the supraventricular rate is rapid it is possible for the depolarisation wave to emerge from the distal end of the atrio-ventricular node at a time when one bundle (usually the left) has recovered and the other has not. In this event the depolarisation wave spreads through the ventricular myocardium by pathways preferentially served by that bundle which has recovered and the QRS complexes, S-T segments and T waves are all altered. This rate-dependent conduction down one bundle only is known as **functional bundle branch block** or as **aberrant intraventricular conduction.** If the bundle which, in these circumstances, fails to conduct is the right bundle no disease of the bundle is implied. If the bundle which fails to conduct is the left bundle it is likely that the left bundle is abnormal (simply because in normal circumstances its refractory period is less than that of the right bundle).

Rate-related (functional) bundle branch block most commonly occurs in association with atrial tachycardia in which case usually each QRS complex, S-T segment and T wave is affected. It also occurs intermittently in atrial fibrillation – usually only being present in those cardiac cycles which follow closely on the preceding cycle (i.e. where the ventricular rate is transiently rapid). Sinus tachycardia is never rapid enough to give rise to "normal" functional bundle branch block, though it may give rise to bundle branch block on a rate-dependent basis by unmasking disease in one or other bundles, i.e. the occurrence of bundle branch block in association with sinus tachycardia implies disease in the appropriate bundle.

Beats which are initiated within the ventricle (ventricular ectopic beats, ventricular tachycardia) cannot possibly follow the normal pathway since they actually start in the wrong place! Such beats therefore necessarily produce abnormal QRS complexes and this primary abnormality of the QRS complex inevitably gives rise to secondary abnormalities of the S-T segments and T waves.

Sensitivity and Specificity

Electrocardiographic interpretation is an empirical process. An abnormality of the electrocardiogram is **defined** as such only because the "abnormal" feature is not generally (if ever) found in electrocardiograms taken from normal, healthy subjects. The **recognition** of any given electrocardiographic abnormality depends upon the satisfaction of the appropriate criteria. Most electrocardiographic abnormalities depend upon the presence of more than one criterion. The criteria themselves are the result of the accumulated experience of empirical interpretation of electrocardiograms and each criterion will have a greater or lesser degree of **sensitivity** and **specificity.**

A 100% sensitive criterion for any abnormality is one which guarantees that whenever it is applied to a community, every case of that abnormality within the community will be detected.

Sensitivity is defined as follows:-

$$\text{Sensitivity} = \frac{\text{Number of true positive detections}}{\text{Number of positives in the group tested}}$$

Sensitivity thus gives an index of the capability of a test to detect an abnormality.

A 100% specific criterion for any abnormality is one which guarantees that whenever it is applied to a community every case in which the test indicates that the given abnormality is present will actually have that abnormality.

Specificity is defined as follows:-

$$\text{Specificity} = \frac{\text{Number of true normals detected}}{\text{Total number of normals in the group tested}}$$

Specificity thus indicates the ability of a test to recognise a normal subject.

In practice no electrocardiographic criterion is 100% specific or 100% sensitive and when several different criteria are applicable to a given diagnosis the greater the number of criteria fulfilled the more confident can one be of the diagnosis.

Diagnostic Criteria and Associated Findings

Most electrocardiographic diagnoses require the presence of certain minimal, essential criteria. These are the *sine qua non* of the diagnosis. In addition, it may be possible to recognise certain changes which are frequently found in association with the condition in question, but which are not **essential** to the diagnosis. The presence or absence of these associated findings may be the result of matters independent of the condition in question (e.g. may depend upon the degree of cardiac rotation or the overall body build). Whenever possible, criteria subsequently given will be divided into **"diagnostic criteria"** and **"associated findings".** Unless otherwise indicated, **all** the diagnostic criteria must be fulfilled for the ECG diagnosis to be made.

In addition, it is sometimes important to note certain **negative** points in the diagnostic process, i.e. that certain features are not actually part of the diagnostic process (are neither "diagnostic criteria" nor "associated findings") and their presence indicates some additional abnormality. Such features (of which there are a very large number of possibilities) will only be mentioned if they are frequently but wrongly considered to be part of the primary diagnosis.

There is general but not absolute agreement among cardiologists on the criteria of normal and most abnormal electrocardiographic appearances. However, since agreement is not absolute, some variation in criteria amongst authors is to be expected. Wherever possible, in this presentation, reasonable criteria are given with which most would agree.

Primary and Secondary Interpretation of the Electrocardiogram

The view is widely held and frequently expressed that the electrocardiogram should never be interpreted without prior knowledge of the relevant clinical data. In fact, this viewpoint is virtually unchallenged. It is a view with which the author completely disagrees. In the author's view the electrocardiogram should be "read" and interpreted in the **absence** of clinical data ("primary interpretation"). Both this primary interpretation and the electrocardiogram on which it is based should then be re-appraised in the light of relevant clinical data ("secondary interpretation"). It is a fallacy to believe that the two processes can take place concurrently. The danger when primary and secondary interpretation are not undertaken **consecutively** is that the criteria for making a given electrocardiographic diagnosis may be modified by clinical knowledge and the modified criteria used to support the clinical conclusion. This is scientifically indefensible. When a blood sample is sent to the biochemistry laboratory with a request for estimation of the blood urea level, the chemist makes the assessment independently of the clinical data. The urea level is, or is not, raised as the case may be, irrespective of whether there is clinical evidence of renal damage ("primary interpretation" of the urea level). The clinician must then use secondary interpretation of the chemist's result in the light of the clinical data. If the chemist finds that the urea level is at the upper extreme of the normal range he says just that. He does not say it is abnormal if he knows that there is previous clinical evidence of renal damage nor does he say that it is normal if there is no such evidence. If the interpretation of an independent test is modified by prior clinical judgement, the test cannot subsequently be said to support or prove the clinical judgement. For example, if an ECG shows non-specific S-T, T changes in the left precordial leads, the report should state that fact. The clinical knowledge that the patient takes digitalis clearly means that digitalis is a possible cause of the S-T, T changes. However, it is not certain that digitalis is the cause, it could be ischaemia, electrolyte disturbances, inflammation, injury,etc. If the patient has never taken digitalis, clearly that cannot be the cause.

Primary interpretation is a definitive statement of the electrocardiographic diagnosis – an indication of whether the record is within normal limits or whether specific or non-specific abnormalities are recognisable. Secondary interpretation is an assessment of the significance of normal or abnormal appearances in the light of the full clinical picture. The author absolutely agrees that the latter process must **always** take place but it should not be allowed to interfere with a very disciplined approach to the former. A few examples may help to clarify this concept.

Example 1
A man of 45 presents with chest pain. The electrocardiogram is entirely normal.
Primary interpretation
The ECG is within normal limits.
Secondary interpretation
The electrocardiogram could still be that of a patient with myocardial ischaemia.

Secondary interpretation is essential for primary interpretation alone might result in inappropriate management.

Example 2
A fit 25-year-old man who plays squash regularly has a routine ECG for insurance purposes. The record shows abnormally tall R waves in V_5 and V_6 and abnormally deep S waves in V_1 and V_2. In other respects the record is normal.
Primary interpretation
The voltage criteria for left ventricular hypertrophy are fulfilled.
Secondary interpretation
This man is thin and athletic. The voltage criteria have high sensitivity and low specificity in the diagnosis of left ventricular hypertrophy. Although the electrocardiographic appearances suggest the possibility of left ventricular hypertrophy, in this situation they do not prove it and it is perfectly possible that the heart is completely normal.

Example 3
A grossly overweight man of 50 has a systolic murmur suggestive of aortic stenosis. His electrocardiogram is identical with that of the man in Example 2.
Primary interpretation
The voltage criteria for left ventricular hypertrophy are fulfilled.
Secondary interpretation
Obesity reduces the QRS voltages of surface electrocardiographic recordings. In the light of this fact, the abnormal R wave in V_5 and V_6 and the abnormal S waves in V_1 and V_2 more strongly point to true left ventricular hypertrophy. The presence of systolic murmur of aortic stenosis provides a possible explanation for the left ventricular hypertrophy but does not itself add to the evidence that left ventricular hypertrophy is actually present.

Perhaps a final illustration outside electrocardiography might help to highlight the pitfalls associated with interpreting a clinical test initially in full conjunction with clinical data. A clinician suspects that a patient has a mitral diastolic murmur but is not sure of this. He requests a chest X-ray. If he provides no clinical information about his suspicion on the X-ray request card and the radiologist thinks that the left atrium is slightly enlarged, the radiological opinion legitimately re-enforces the possibility of mitral stenosis. If, however, the clinician writes "? mitral stenosis" on the X-ray request card, there is the danger that the radiologist might, despite seeing appearances which he would otherwise regard as normal, be tempted by the clinical information on the card to write some such report as "Normal appearances. There is perhaps minimal left atrial enlargement". Should this happen the clinician might then, quite unjustifiably, use this dubious information as supportive evidence of his own doubtful opinion. The radiologist should just have said "Normal appearances" if the criteria for abnormality were not fulfilled. In that situation, the clinician would still be able to entertain his initial diagnosis but this would no longer be falsely reinforced via an interpretation of a test distorted by the initial clinical suspicion.

Intraventricular Conduction Disturbances

The Pacemaker and Conducting Tissue

The three waves most easily recognisable in the normal electrocardiogram are the result of electrical activity in **myocardium,** i.e. not in the cardiac conducting tissue. The P wave, QRS complex and T wave are the surface electrocardiographic manifestations of atrial myocardial depolarisation, ventricular myocardial depolarisation and ventricular myocardial repolarisation respectively. (Atrial myocardial repolarisation gives rise to the Ta wave on the surface ECG, but this is completely obscured in most records by the QRS complex which is much larger and which occurs at about the same time). Myocardium cannot **initiate** depolarisation but it has the ability to **conduct** a depolarisation wave once it has been initiated and myocardial depolarisation is followed by **myocardial contraction.**

The pacemaker and conducting tissue of the heart is histologically different from myocardium and can be seen to consist of modified myocardium with very few contractile elements. It, too, has the ability to **conduct** any depolarisation process already initiated, but it differs from myocardium in that (a) **it can initiate such depolarisation,** and (b) **depolarisation** (whether conducted or initiated) **does not result in contraction** (Table 1).

Table 1

	Properties		
Tissue	Conduction of depolarisation	Contraction in response to depolarisation	Initiation of depolarisation
Myocardium	+	+	−
Pacemaker and conducting tissue	+	−	+

The pacemaker and conducting tissue of the heart are arranged as shown in Figure 74. It consists of the sino-atrial node, the atrio-ventricular node, the common bundle (bundle of His) the right bundle branch, the left bundle branch (which has antero-superior and postero-inferior divisions) and the Purkinje network emanating from the bundle branches.

The **sinus node** (sino-atrial node, SA node) is located in the right atrium at the mouth of the superior vena cava. It is approximately 15mm in length, 5 to 7mm wide and 1.5 to 2mm thick. It is the primary cardiac pacemaker. The **atrio-ventricular node** (AV node) lies on the right side of the lower part of the interatrial septum. It is about 5-6mm long, 2-3mm wide and 0.5 to 1mm thick. The **common bundle** (bundle of His, AV Bundle) is continuous with the AV node. It penetrates the central fibrous body of

the heart to reach the crest of the interventricular septum. It is 10-20mm in length and 1-4mm in diameter. The **right bundle branch** runs directly down from the common bundle, on the subendocardial surface of the right ventricle. After a "bare" initial portion, fine branches of the **Purkinje tissue** (Purkinje network, Purkinje arborisation) arise from the remainder of its length to spread over the endocardial surface of the right ventricle. The **left bundle branch** is a less discrete structure than the right bundle. It has two major subdivisions, the antero-superior and the postero-inferior divisions. Each division forms a fan, rather than a fasciculus, of fibres, spreads on the endocardial surface of the left ventricle and gives rise to Purkinje tissue in the same way as the right bundle. Purkinje branches arise earlier (i.e. more proximally) from the left than from the right bundle.

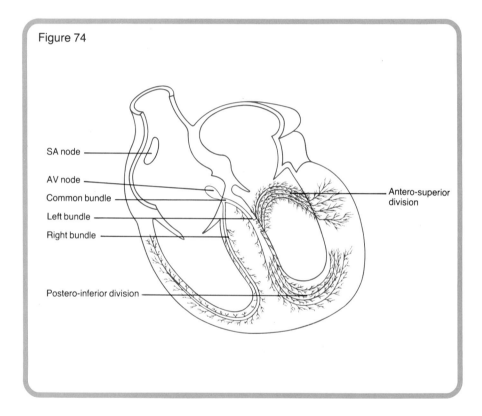

Figure 74

SA node

AV node

Common bundle

Left bundle

Right bundle

Postero-inferior division

Antero-superior division

Normal Atrio-ventricular and Intraventricular Conduction

The sino-atrial node, all parts of the right and left atrial myocardium and the AV node are in electrical continuity (i.e. a depolarisation arising in any part is normally conducted to all other parts). This whole supraventricular system maintains electrical continuity with the ventricular system only via the common atrio-ventricular bundle (bundle of His). In normal circumstances, no electrical conduction is possible directly from atrial myocardium to ventricular myocardium, because of the interposition of the non-conducting, fibrous atrio-ventricular ring (which is electrically bridged by the His bundle). It follows that the depolarisation wave (which, if the rhythm is sinus, originates from the sino-atrial node) reaches ventricular myocardium only after its passage through the bundle of His and the beginnings of the right and left bundle branch systems. Thus the first part of the intraventricular myocardium to be depolarised is the superior part of the

interventricular septum adjacent to the mitral and tricuspid valves. The main stem of the left branch (before it bifurcates into its two divisions), is very short and the left bundle branch gives off fine Purkinje fibres more proximally than the right bundle branch. Because of this **the first (superior) part of the interventricular septum is depolarised from left to right.** Sequential depolarisation of the left and right ventricles then occurs, the sequence being dependent upon (a) the site of initiation of septal depolarisation and (b) the distribution of the fast conducting pacemaker tissue. The rate of conduction through the common bundle, bundle branches and Purkinje system is rapid (4000mm/sec) compared with that through the ventricular myocardium (400mm/sec). The AV node ("AV" junction) conducts most slowly of all at 200mm/sec.

The excitation wave arising at the AV node (having been conducted through atrial myocardium after initiation at the SA node) thus passes down the common bundle and simultaneously down both bundle branches. Because of the earlier origin of Purkinje fibres on the left, the superior part of the interventricular septum is depolarised from left to right. Lower down, the septum is depolarised simultaneously from both sides and subsequently the free walls of the ventricles are depolarised from endocardium to epicardium. Because of the relatively great speed of conduction down the bundle branches and Purkinje cells, the entire endocardial surface of both ventricles becomes depolarised at about the same time. Conduction then spreads more slowly transmurally from endocardium to epicardium.

It is therefore possible to simplify the sequence of depolarisation of the ventricular myocardium into three phases (as discussed on page 29). Phase 1 (Figure 75) represents depolarisation of the superior portion of the interventricular septum. This occurs initially and on its own. Phase 2 represents depolarisation of the free wall of the right ventricle and Phase 3 that of the free wall of the left ventricle – in both cases from endocardium to epicardium. Phases 2 and 3 are effectively simultaneous.

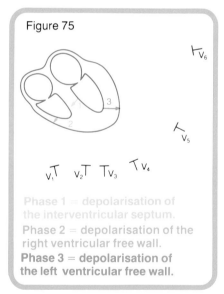

Figure 75

Phase 1 = depolarisation of the interventricular septum.
Phase 2 = depolarisation of the right ventricular free wall.
Phase 3 = depolarisation of the left ventricular free wall.

This sequence of ventricular myocardial depolarisation gives rise to the typical normal QRS wave forms in V_1 and V_6 (Figures 76, 77).

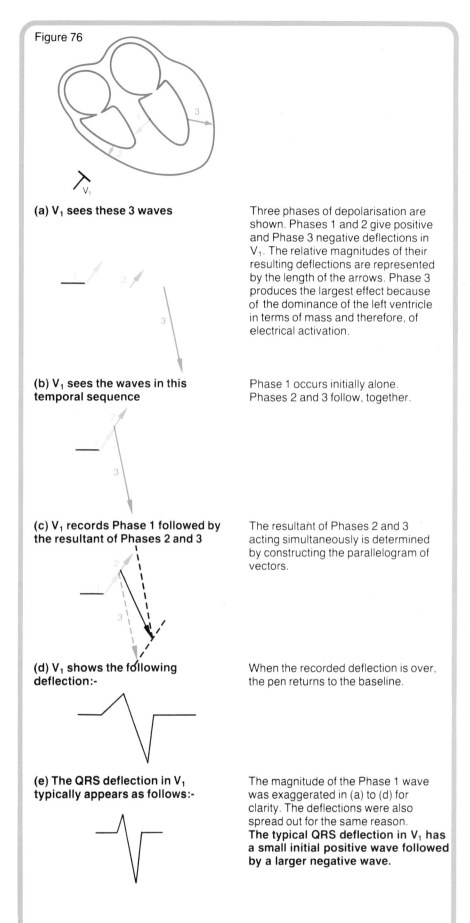

Figure 76

(a) V_1 sees these 3 waves

Three phases of depolarisation are shown. Phases 1 and 2 give positive and Phase 3 negative deflections in V_1. The relative magnitudes of their resulting deflections are represented by the length of the arrows. Phase 3 produces the largest effect because of the dominance of the left ventricle in terms of mass and therefore, of electrical activation.

(b) V_1 sees the waves in this temporal sequence

Phase 1 occurs initially alone. Phases 2 and 3 follow, together.

(c) V_1 records Phase 1 followed by the resultant of Phases 2 and 3

The resultant of Phases 2 and 3 acting simultaneously is determined by constructing the parallelogram of vectors.

(d) V_1 shows the following deflection:-

When the recorded deflection is over, the pen returns to the baseline.

(e) The QRS deflection in V_1 typically appears as follows:-

The magnitude of the Phase 1 wave was exaggerated in (a) to (d) for clarity. The deflections were also spread out for the same reason. **The typical QRS deflection in V_1 has a small initial positive wave followed by a larger negative wave.**

Figure 77

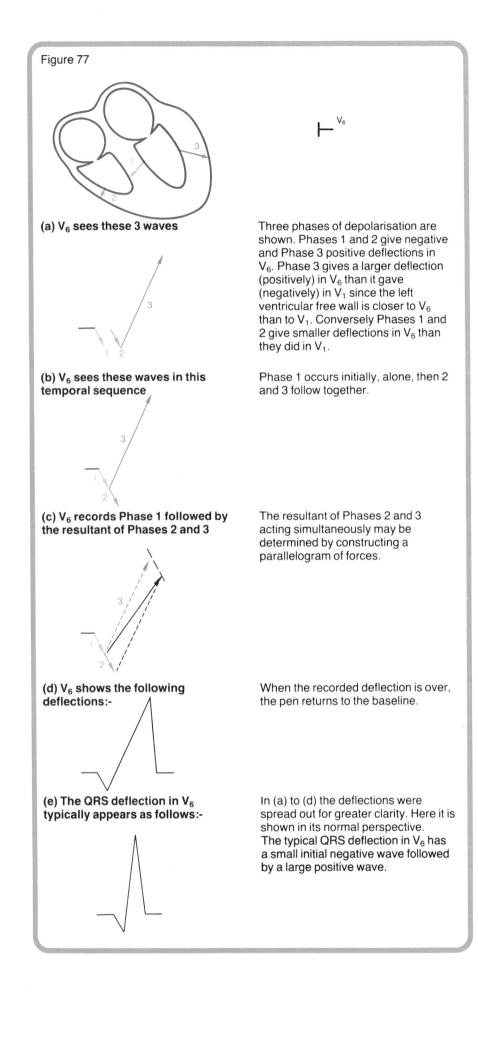

(a) V₆ sees these 3 waves

Three phases of depolarisation are shown. Phases 1 and 2 give negative and Phase 3 positive deflections in V_6. Phase 3 gives a larger deflection (positively) in V_6 than it gave (negatively) in V_1 since the left ventricular free wall is closer to V_6 than to V_1. Conversely Phases 1 and 2 give smaller deflections in V_6 than they did in V_1.

(b) V₆ sees these waves in this temporal sequence

Phase 1 occurs initially, alone, then 2 and 3 follow together.

(c) V₆ records Phase 1 followed by the resultant of Phases 2 and 3

The resultant of Phases 2 and 3 acting simultaneously may be determined by constructing a parallelogram of forces.

(d) V₆ shows the following deflections:-

When the recorded deflection is over, the pen returns to the baseline.

(e) The QRS deflection in V₆ typically appears as follows:-

In (a) to (d) the deflections were spread out for greater clarity. Here it is shown in its normal perspective. The typical QRS deflection in V_6 has a small initial negative wave followed by a large positive wave.

Ventricular Pre-excitation

Ventricular pre-excitation is a relatively rare condition in which an abnormal (additional or "accessory") atrio-ventricular conduction pathway exists between the atrial and ventricular myocardium. The accessory pathway usually conducts the depolarisation wave more quickly than does the normal atrio-ventricular conducting tissue. The accessory pathway makes electrical contact with the ventricular myocardium at a location other than that which is the usual starting point for ventricular myocardial depolarisation. It follows that, in the presence of ventricular pre-excitation, myocardial depolarisation commences at an "abnormal" location and the whole sequence of ventricular myocardial depolarisation must therefore follow an abnormal pathway. This results in the development of an abnormal QRS complex in association with the short P-R interval which is indicative of the accelerated atrio-ventricular conduction.

The concept of ventricular pre-excitation and the changes induced by it on the electrocardiogram are fully discussed in the section on "Miscellaneous Abnormalities" (pages 212 to 249). However, it is necessary at this stage to be aware of its existence for the discussion which follows and the scheme for analysis of normal and abnormal electrocardiograms will both subsequently require modification in the light of the possibility of ventricular pre-excitation. All discussion prior to the formal consideration of pre-excitation will involve the assumption that atrio-ventricular conduction is normal.

Abnormal Intraventricular Conduction

When the normal sequence of conduction of a depolarisation wave is disturbed after it has descended through the AV node an intraventricular conduction disturbance is said to have occurred. The following intraventricular conduction disturbances are recognisable (with greater or lesser degrees of facility) on the 12-lead ECG:

Right bundle branch block (RBBB – partial or complete, permanent or intermittent)

Left bundle branch block (LBBB – partial or complete, permanent or intermittent)

Left anterior hemiblock (LAH – also known as left superior intraventricular block)

Left posterior hemiblock (LPH – also known as left inferior intraventricular block)

RBBB+LAH
RBBB+LPH
Diffuse intraventricular block

Right Bundle Branch Block (RBBB)

When there is total failure of conduction in the right bundle branch system (Figure 78), there is no change in the direction of depolarisation of the interventricular septum (Phase 1) and no change in the timing or direction of depolarisation of the free wall of the left ventricle (Phase 3), but depolarisation of the free wall of the right ventricle (Phase 2) is delayed and prolonged since the depolarisation wave reaches the right ventricular myocardium after slow conduction through the myocardium of the septum. Phase 2 depolarisation starts later than normal and takes longer to reach its peak and these features give rise to typical changes in the precordial electrocardiogram (Figures 79 and 80).

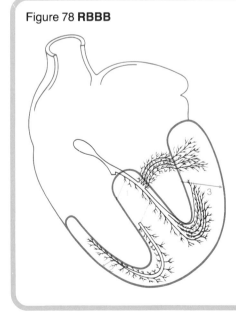

Figure 78 **RBBB**

There is failure of conduction in the right bundle branch proximally. Septal depolarisation (Phase 1) is unaffected since it is initiated via Purkinje fibres which arise proximally from the left bundle before its division into two fasciculi. Left ventricular depolarisation takes place at the normal time and at normal rate. Right ventricular depolarisation is delayed because of the slow conduction through myocardium which forms the only electrical continuity between the nearest Purkinje fibres arising from the left bundle and the distal, functioning part of the right bundle (interrupted arrow). The extent of the defect in the right bundle determines the extent of the delay in initiating and in completing right ventricular depolarisation.

Both in V$_1$ and V$_6$ the QRS complex differs from normal in its terminal portion only. The overall QRS duration is prolonged (since Phase 2 depolarisation starts late and takes longer than normal), a secondary slurred R wave occurs in V$_1$ and a secondary slurred S wave occurs in V$_6$.

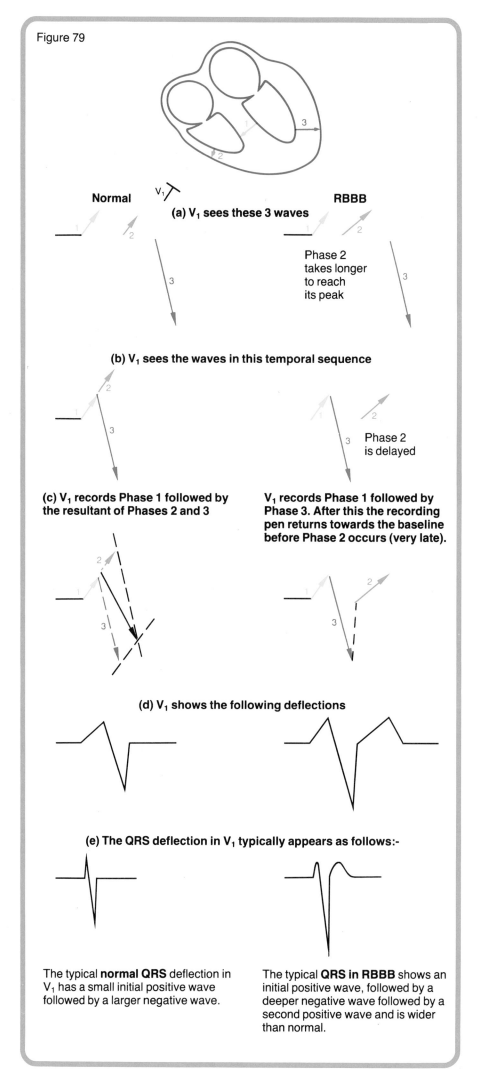

Figure 79

Normal   V$_1$ **(a) V$_1$ sees these 3 waves**   **RBBB**

Phase 2 takes longer to reach its peak

(b) V$_1$ sees the waves in this temporal sequence

Phase 2 is delayed

(c) V$_1$ records Phase 1 followed by the resultant of Phases 2 and 3

V$_1$ records Phase 1 followed by Phase 3. After this the recording pen returns towards the baseline before Phase 2 occurs (very late).

(d) V$_1$ shows the following deflections

(e) The QRS deflection in V$_1$ typically appears as follows:-

The typical **normal QRS** deflection in V$_1$ has a small initial positive wave followed by a larger negative wave.

The typical **QRS in RBBB** shows an initial positive wave, followed by a deeper negative wave followed by a second positive wave and is wider than normal.

Figure 80

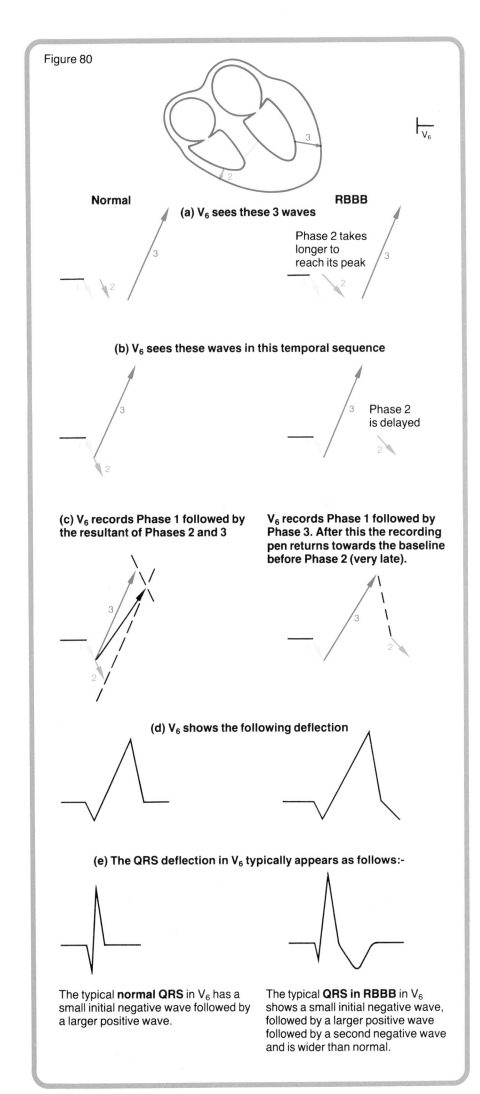

Normal   **RBBB**

(a) V$_6$ sees these 3 waves

Phase 2 takes longer to reach its peak

(b) V$_6$ sees these waves in this temporal sequence

Phase 2 is delayed

(c) V$_6$ records Phase 1 followed by the resultant of Phases 2 and 3

V$_6$ records Phase 1 followed by Phase 3. After this the recording pen returns towards the baseline before Phase 2 (very late).

(d) V$_6$ shows the following deflection

(e) The QRS deflection in V$_6$ typically appears as follows:-

The typical **normal QRS** in V$_6$ has a small initial negative wave followed by a larger positive wave.

The typical **QRS in RBBB** in V$_6$ shows a small initial negative wave, followed by a larger positive wave followed by a second negative wave and is wider than normal.

The changes in ventricular depolarisation (which are represented by the QRS changes) inevitably give rise to secondary changes in ventricular repolarisation (i.e. changes in the S-T segment and T waves). In consequence, there is often S-T segment depression and T wave inversion in the right precordial leads. Leads I and aVL tend to show appearances similar to those in V_6. The mean frontal plane QRS axis is not abnormal in uncomplicated right bundle branch block, although it may not infrequently be indeterminate. These features are all illustrated in Figure 81. This ECG would be reported as follows: "Sinus rhythm. The mean frontal plane QRS axis is indeterminate. There is complete right bundle branch block."

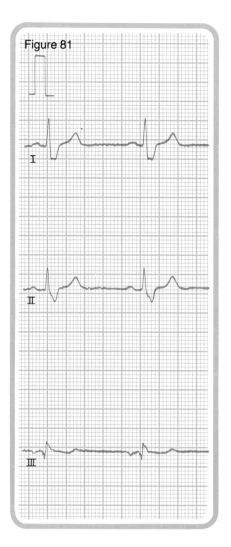

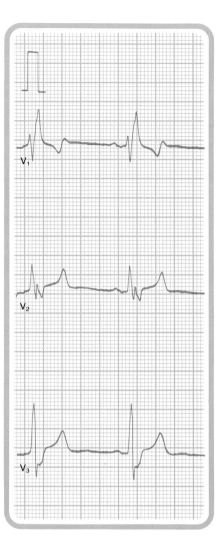

Figure 81

The rhythm is sinus. The total QRS duration is abnormally long (0.16 sec – most easily seen in the first QRS in V_1 or the second QRS in I). V_1 has a large secondary R wave (i.e. it has an rSR′ complex). The combination of prolongation of the total QRS duration with a secondary R wave in V_1 is diagnostic of right bundle branch block. As is usually the case there is a broad, slurred S wave in V_6 (the equivalent of the broad, slurred R wave in V_1). The mean frontal plane QRS axis is indeterminate but, as is often the case, the QRS appearances in V_6 are transmitted to I and aVL. There is secondary S-T segment depression in V_1 (often is present in V_2 and V_3 as well).

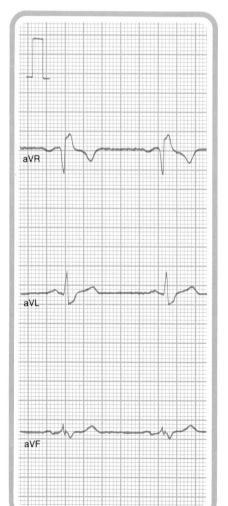

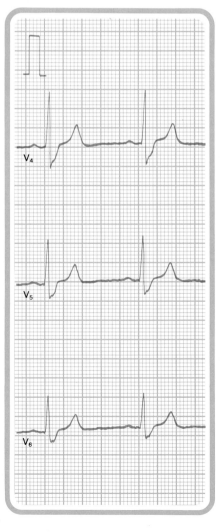

Diagnostic criteria for right bundle branch block

(Assuming the rhythm to be supraventricular)

1. Total QRS duration is 0.12 sec or greater.
2. A secondary R wave is seen in V_1. The secondary wave is usually broad and slurred, (the complex in V_1 may be rsr', rSr', RSr', RSR', or M-shaped).

Additional features frequently present in right bundle branch block

1. Deep, slurred S waves are seen in the left precordial leads (typically V_4, V_5 and V_6), though they may also be seen in V_3 and even V_2 if there is counterclockwise rotation, or they may be seen only in V_6 if there is clockwise rotation).
2. Deep slurred S waves are usually seen also in I and aVL.
3. S-T segment depression and T wave inversion are seen in the right precordial leads (typically $V_1 - V_3$, but only in V_1 in counterclockwise rotation and possibly from $V_1 - V_5$ in clockwise rotation).

Important negative points in right bundle branch block

1. The mean frontal plane QRS axis is usually within the normal range in uncomplicated complete right bundle branch block. The axis may move 15–30° towards the right when right bundle branch block develops but **abnormal** right axis deviation is **not** a routine feature of right bundle branch block. The axis is often indeterminate (page 48). This is not in itself an abnormality. When right bundle branch block is combined with a clearly abnormal axis, bifascicular block (i.e. RBBB+LAH if there is abnormal left axis deviation or RBBB+LPH if there is abnormal right axis deviation) is considered to be present (pages 139 to 142).
2. The initial part of the QRS complex is normal in every lead. In fact, each lead only differs from the normal QRS because of the presence of a late, slurred "addition" to the basic waveform (Figure 82).

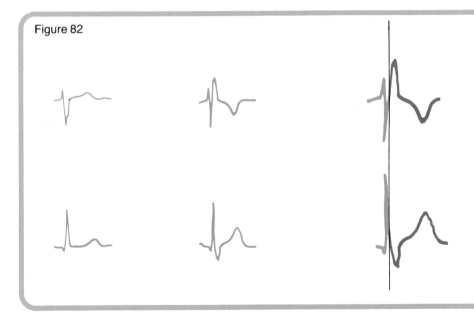

Figure 82

The left-hand column shows typical normal QRS configurations, S-T segments and T waves in V_1 and V_6. The central column shows typical appearances in right bundle branch block. The right-hand column shows the same appearances as the central column, enlarged by a factor of 2 to emphasise that in both these leads (and in fact in all 12 leads) both the initial and the dominant deflections of the QRS complexes in right bundle branch block are almost identical with those in the presence of normal intraventricular conduction. (The parts of the QRS deflections to the left of the vertical line are virtually the same as those in the normal QRS complexes).

The main reasons that all but the terminal part of the QRS is normal are because:
1. The direction of septal depolarisation (the earliest part of ventricular depolarisation) is normal and therefore the initial direction of the QRS in every lead remains unchanged, and
2. The depolarisation of the left ventricular free wall (which is the influence dominating QRS deflections in all leads in most circumstances) is unaltered.

Because the most important diagnostic parts of the QRS complexes are unaltered in right bundle branch block, the criteria for normality or abnormality of voltage, R wave progression and q waves can be applied (e.g. it is still possible to diagnose left ventricular hypertrophy or myocardial infarction).

Incomplete Right Bundle Branch Block

Incomplete right bundle branch block is diagnosed when:

1. A secondary R wave is seen in V_1 (which therefore has an rsr', rSr', rSR', Rsr', RSr', RSR' or M-shaped complex), and

2. The total QRS duration is 0.11 sec or less. An example is shown in Figure 83.

The ECG in Figure 83 would be reported as follows:
"Sinus tachycardia. The mean frontal plane QRS axis is +45°. There is incomplete right bundle branch block".

When the term "right bundle branch block" is used without qualification, it is deemed to refer to complete right bundle branch block.

Although incomplete right bundle branch block can occur in disease states (listed below) it is usually of no clinical significance, being found in 2–3% normals.

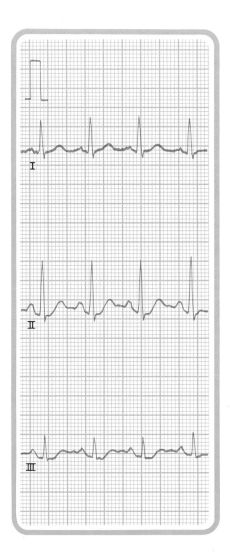

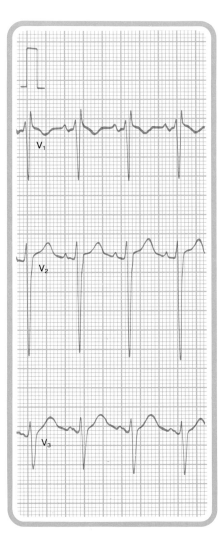

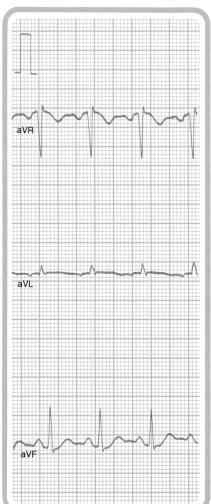

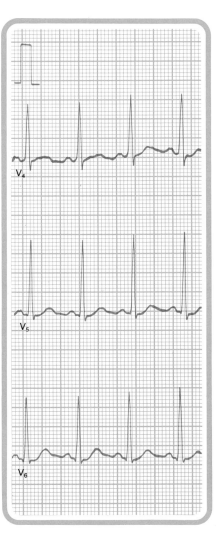

Figure 83

The rhythm is sinus. There is an rSr' configuration to the QRS complex in V_1. However, the total QRS duration is within normal limits at 0.09 sec (best seen in V_1). There is therefore incomplete right bundle branch block.

Intermittent Right Bundle Branch Block

Right bundle branch block may develop secondary to myocardial infarction or ischaemia, may develop in the pulmonary embolism and may appear as a functional disturbance whenever the supraventricular rate exceeds a critical value. In all of these situations, the right bundle branch block may disappear and normal intraventricular conduction may return when the underlying abnormality improves. Rarely, right bundle branch block, unassociated with any overt cardiac abnormality may be present intermittently.

Clinical Significance

Complete right bundle branch block may occur congenitally in hearts which are in all respects completely normal. When it is the sole "abnormal" finding it must not be taken to be conclusive of the presence of cardiac disease.

It can, however, develop in a variety of cardiac diseases including ischaemic heart disease, hypertension, pulmonary embolism, cardiomyopathy, myocarditis, rheumatic heart disease, pericarditis, Chagas disease, and can be found congenitally in atrial septal defect (in which condition it is always found – complete or incomplete) and Fallot's Tetralogy.

Left Bundle Branch Block (LBBB)

When there is total failure of conduction in the left bundle branch system (Figure 84) there is delay in the initiation and in the velocity of depolarisation of the free wall of the left ventricle – Phase 3. (This is the precise corollary of the delay in depolarisation of the free wall of the right ventricle in the right bundle branch block). However, in LBBB there is a very important additional change – complete reversal of the direction of depolarisation of the interventricular septum (Phase 1). This latter feature produces dramatic changes in the electrocardiogram for it alters the initial direction of the QRS complex in every lead – all those leads which formerly showed an initial r wave will now have an initial q wave, and the leads with initial q waves will now have initial r waves.

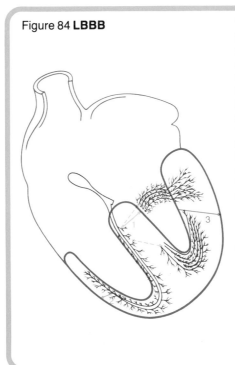

Figure 84 **LBBB**

There is failure of conduction in the left bundle branch system. Septal depolarisation arrow (1) is reversed (since it must take place from the earliest Purkinje fibres arising from the right bundle). In addition to this reversal of the direction of septal depolarisation, the depolarisation of the myocardium of the left ventricle starts later than normal and takes longer than normal because of the slow conduction through myocardium which forms the only electrical continuity between the nearest Purkinje fibres arising from the right bundle and the distal, functioning parts of the left bundle. Each of the two major divisions of the left bundle will receive the depolarisation wave (2 interrupted arrows) in the same way. The extent of the defect in the left bundle determines the extent of the delay in initiating and in completing left ventricular depolarisation.

The two changes from normal produce typical changes in the precordial QRS complexes (Figures 85 and 86). Both in V_1 and V_6 the QRS complex differs radically from normal in its configuration. The overall QRS duration is prolonged (since Phase 3 starts late and takes longer than usual). The cardinal features are absence of the (normal) septal q wave in V_6 and prolongation of the total QRS duration.

Figure 85

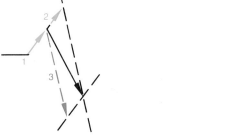

Normal   **LBBB**

(a) V₁ sees these 3 waves

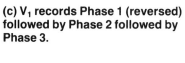

(b) V₁ sees these waves in this temporal sequence

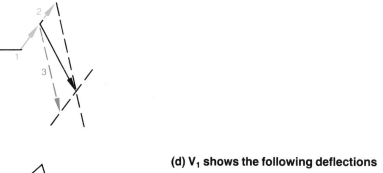

(c) V₁ records Phase 1 followed by resultant of Phases 2 and 3

(c) V₁ records Phase 1 (reversed) followed by Phase 2 followed by Phase 3.

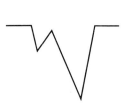

(d) V₁ shows the following deflections

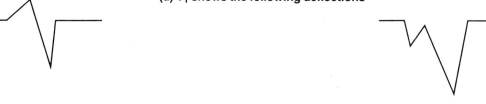

(e) The QRS deflection in V₁ typically appears as follows:-

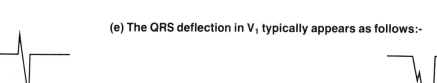

The typical **normal QRS** deflection in V₁ has a small initial positive wave followed by a larger negative wave

The typical **QRS in LBBB** in V₁ shows no initial positive wave, a deep negative wave and is wider than normal.

121

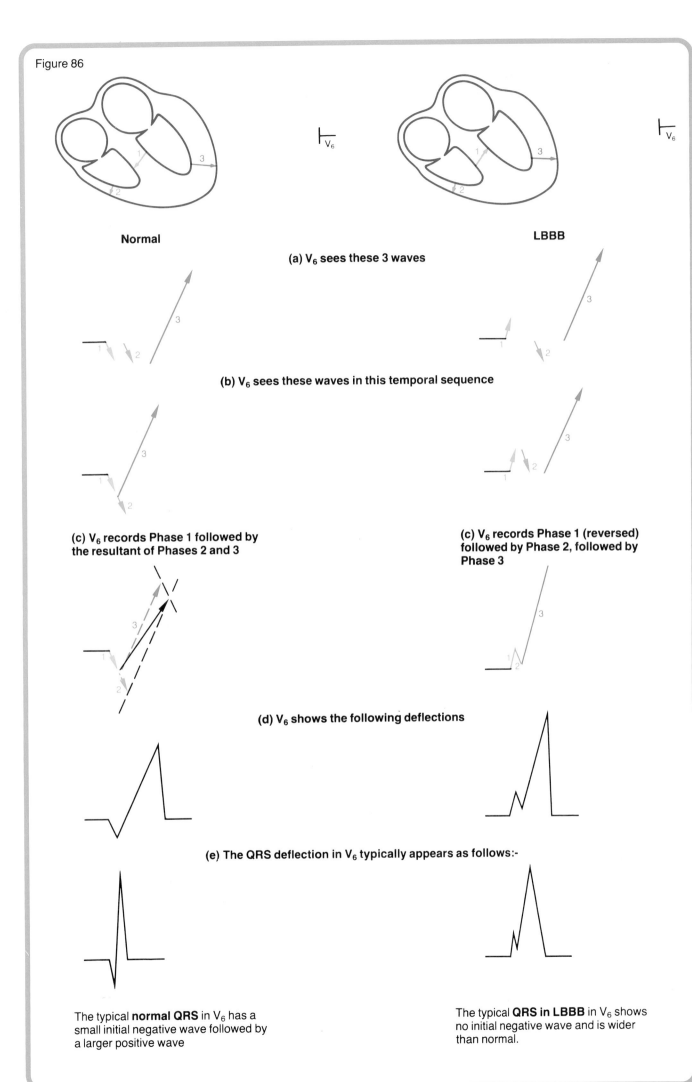

Figure 86

Normal

LBBB

(a) V$_6$ sees these 3 waves

(b) V$_6$ sees these waves in this temporal sequence

(c) V$_6$ records Phase 1 followed by the resultant of Phases 2 and 3

(c) V$_6$ records Phase 1 (reversed) followed by Phase 2, followed by Phase 3

(d) V$_6$ shows the following deflections

(e) The QRS deflection in V$_6$ typically appears as follows:-

The typical **normal QRS** in V$_6$ has a small initial negative wave followed by a larger positive wave

The typical **QRS in LBBB** in V$_6$ shows no initial negative wave and is wider than normal.

122

The changes in ventricular depolarisation (which are represented by the QRS changes) inevitably give rise to secondary changes in ventricular repolarisation (i.e. changes in the S-T segment and T waves). There is therefore often S-T segment depression and T wave inversion in the left precordial leads and S-T segment elevation with tall T waves in the right precordial leads. Leads I and aVL tend to show appearances similar to those in V_6. The mean frontal plane QRS axis is not abnormal in uncomplicated left bundle branch block, although it may be indeterminate. These features are illustrated in Figure 87. This ECG would be reported as follows: "Sinus rhythm. The mean frontal plane QRS axis is $+15°$. There is complete left bundle branch block".

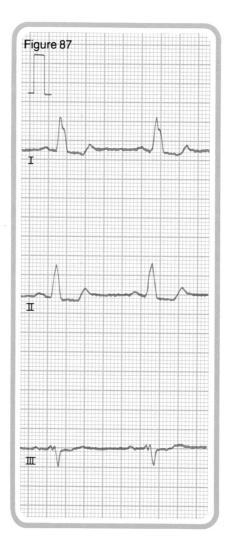

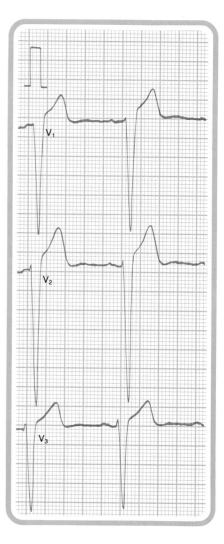

Figure 87

The rhythm is sinus. The total QRS duration is abnormally long (0.14 sec – most easily seen in the first QRS complex in V_6). Deep S waves (in this case with a small initial r wave) are seen in V_1. There is no secondary R wave in V_1 to indicate right bundle branch block. There is no initial (septal) q wave in V_6 or in leads further to the left than V_6 (i.e. I and aVL). In the absence of right bundle branch block this combination of absent left-sided q waves and abnormally long total QRS duration is indicative of left bundle branch block. S-T segment depression (which is secondary to the QRS abnormality) is seen in V_6, I, II and aVL. The frontal plane QRS axis is within the normal range of $+15°$. The heart is horizontal (page 53) and because of this the appearances in left ventricular leads (typically V_6) are transmitted to Leads I and aVL (i.e. to those frontal plane leads which lie closest to the direction of the frontal plane axis).

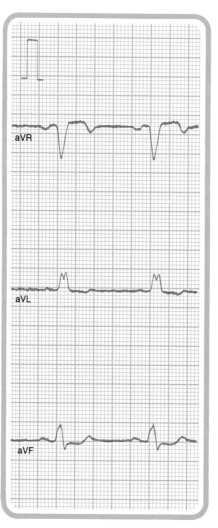

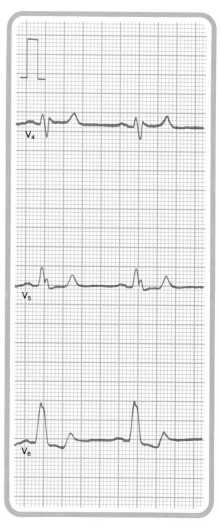

Diagnostic criteria for left bundle branch block

(Assuming that the rhythm is supraventricular and that there is no ventricular pre-excitation[†]).

1. Total QRS duration is 0.12 sec or greater.
2. There is no secondary R wave in V_1, to indicate RBBB[*].
3. There is no septal q wave in V_5, V_6 or in leads further to the left (in the case of horizontal hearts, I and aVL).

Additional features frequently present in left bundle branch block

1. The QRS complexes in some leads may be notched (e.g. Leads I, aVL, V_5 and V_6 in Figure 87).
2. The QRS complexes in V_5, V_6, I and aVL tend to have rsR', "M" pattern or broad monophasic R waves. If the heart is clockwise-rotated V_5, V_6, I and aVL tend to show RS complexes.
3. Secondary S-T segment depression and possibly T wave inversion may be present in left precordial leads and also in I and aVL.
4. The S-T segments are often elevated and the T waves abnormally tall in the right precordial leads.
5. The S waves in the right precordial leads are often abnormally deep.
6. The initial r waves in the right precordial leads may be very small or absent. If absent the QRS complexes, by definition, have deep Q waves not deep S waves.
7. In the precordial leads the dominant direction of the T waves and the S-T segments tends to be opposite to the dominant direction of the QRS complexes in any given lead.
8. In the limb leads there is an abnormal angle between the mean frontal plane QRS and T wave axes – or the QRS axis is highly determinate and the T wave axis indeterminate (which is equally abnormal (page 58)).

Note

[*] It is necessary to include this criterion since it is possible for no initial q wave to be visible in V_6 normally (page 67). If right bundle branch block develops on top of this normal variation the combination of (1) prolongation of the total QRS duration, and (2) absence of septal q waves in V_6 would lead to an incorrect diagnosis of LBBB. (The criteria for the recognition of RBBB would not be affected by this possibility (Figure 88)).
See pages 212 to 220 and 266.

Important negative points in left bundle branch block

1. The mean frontal plane QRS axis is usually within the normal range in uncomplicated cases. The axis may move 15–30° towards the left (Figures 90 and 91) when left bundle branch block develops but **abnormal left axis deviation is not a routine feature of left bundle branch block.** Sometimes the axis may be indeterminate. This is not in itself an abnormality (page 48). When LBBB is combined with abnormal left axis deviation, extensive disease of the left ventricular conducting tissue is likely to be present involving the peripheral part of the antero-superior division of the left bundle branch system as well as the proximal part of the main left bundle. When LBBB is combined with right axis deviation, the possibility of co-existing right ventricular hypertrophy should be considered.

2. The initial part of the QRS complex in every lead takes place in a direction opposite from normal. Therefore, **once the diagnosis of left bundle branch block has been established, no further diagnostic processes utilising criteria for QRS complexes, S-T segments or T waves should be used - except for the measurement of the frontal plane QRS axis.**

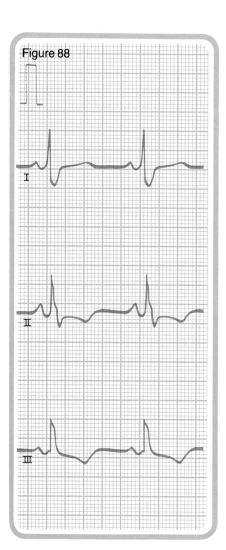

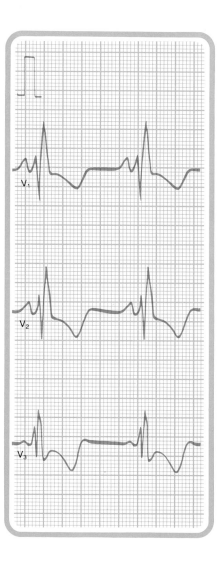

Figure 88

The rhythm is sinus. There is an rSR′ configuration of the QRS complex in V_1 and the total QRS duration is prolonged to 0.12 sec (best seen in V_1). There is therefore complete right bundle branch block. (No septal q wave is seen in V_6 or I. This is not in itself, abnormal. Had there been no septal q wave in V_6 and a prolongation of the total QRS duration **without a secondary r wave in V_1,** there would have been **left** bundle branch block. In that event one would have expected deep S (or Q) waves in V_1). There is S-T segment depression with T wave inversion from V_1 to V_4. These are changes commonly associated with right bundle branch block and no additional abnormality need be invoked.

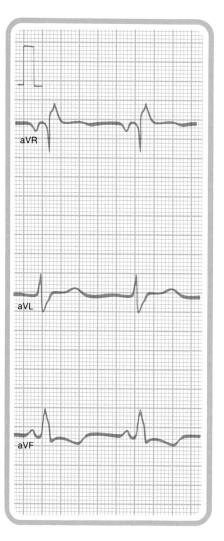

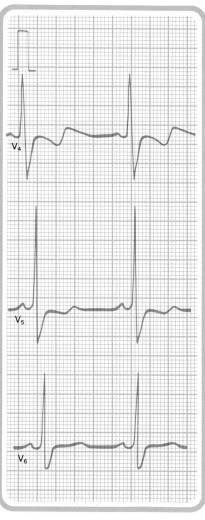

Incomplete Left Bundle Branch Block

Incomplete left bundle branch block is diagnosed when there is no septal q wave in left-sided precordial leads or in Lead I or aVL and when the total QRS duration is 0.10 or 0.11 sec. Thus the only difference between complete and incomplete LBBB is the duration of the QRS complex. An example is shown in Figure 89. This record would be reported as follows:

"Sinus tachycardia. Incomplete left bundle branch block. There are non-specific S-T, T changes throughout the limb leads and in the left precordial leads. These may well be secondary to the intraventricular conduction disturbance. Left atrial hypertrophy."

When the term "left bundle branch block" is used without qualification, it is deemed to refer to complete left bundle branch block. When the total QRS duration is 0.10 sec (i.e. still acceptable as "normal") and there is no septal q wave in V_5, V_6, I or aVL it does not necessarily indicate disease* (even though it is technically incomplete left bundle branch block) since the q wave can sometimes be absent in these leads under normal circumstances (page 67).

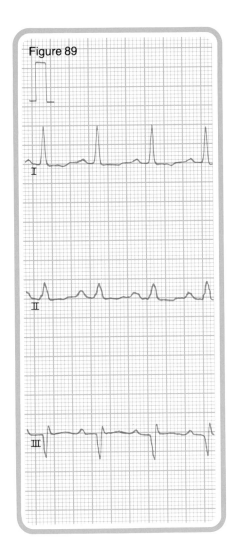

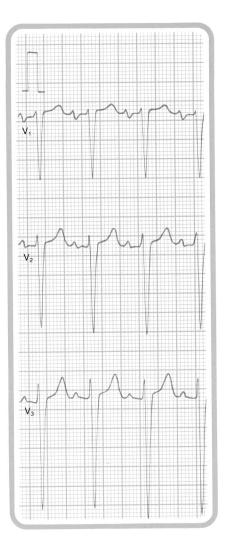

Figure 89

The rhythm is sinus but the rate is more rapid than 100 per minute, therefore the rhythm is actually sinus tachycardia. The S waves in the right precordial leads are deeper than normal, the R waves in the left precordial leads are taller than normal, but the important point to note is that there is no evidence of any normal septal q wave in V_5, V_6, Lead I or aVL. The septum is therefore depolarising from right to left and not from left to right as is the normal situation.

This suggests a defect of conduction in the left bundle branch system. Total QRS duration is only 0.11 sec (best seen in the first QRS complex in V_2) and there is therefore incomplete left bundle branch block. The T waves are of low voltage throughout the limb leads and there is T wave inversion and S-T segment depression in the left precordial leads. These are non-specific changes which may well be secondary to the intraventricular conduction disturbance. The P waves are also abnormal (page 163).

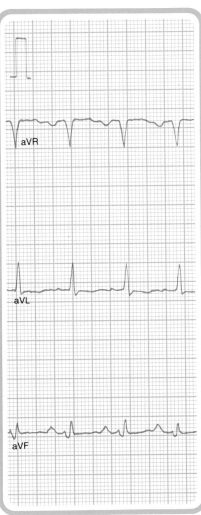

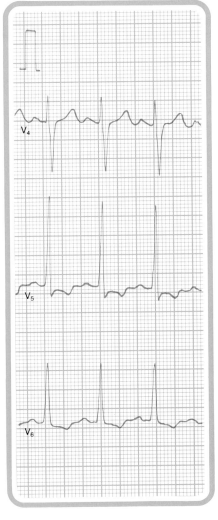

Intermittent Left Bundle Branch Block

Left bundle branch block may be intermittently present in relation to varying pathology, such as myocardial ischaemia. It can sometimes appear as a functional disturbance when the ventricular rate exceeds a certain value, but is less likely to do so than is right bundle branch block. In all of these situations, the left bundle branch block may disappear and normal intraventricular conduction may return when the underlying abnormality improves.

Figures 90 and 91 are taken from a patient with intermittent left bundle branch block.

Figure 90 shows the electrocardiogram of a patient with hypertrophic cardiomyopathy. The rhythm is sinus, there is normal intraventricular conduction. The record is within normal limits. Note that the frontal plane QRS axis is +15°.

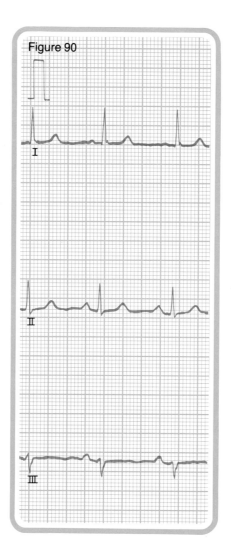

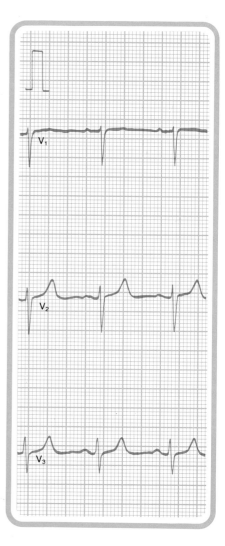

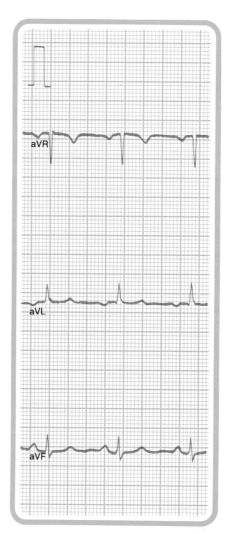

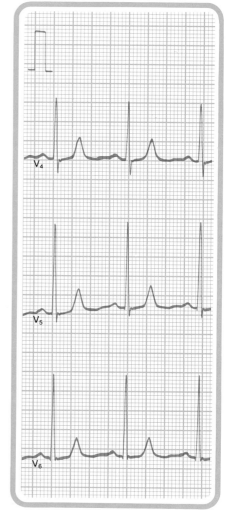

Figure 90

A normal ECG from a patient with hypertrophic cardiomyopathy.

Figure 91 shows an ECG taken from the same patient as that in Figure 90 and about 2 weeks later. Complete LBBB has developed. (The record is recognisably that of the same patient as Figure 90 since the P wave configuration in each lead is identical in the two records). Note that with the development of LBBB the frontal plane QRS axis has moved from +15° (Figure 90) to −15°. This degree of left-axis shift on developing LBBB is typical.

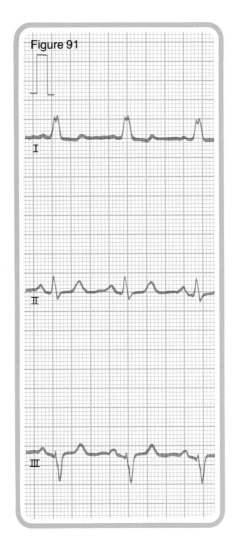

Figure 91

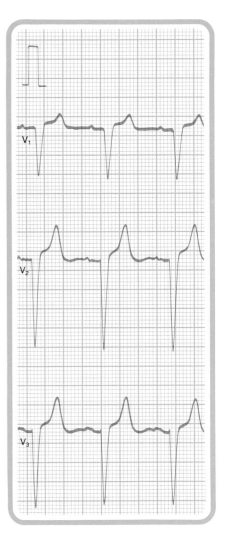

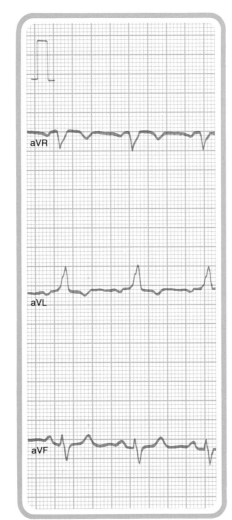

Figure 91

A record taken from the same patient as that in Figure 90, about 2 weeks later. Left bundle branch block has developed. The axis has moved minimally to the left but is still within the normal range. This patient developed and lost LBBB intermittently over many months. Cardiac catheterisation confirmed the (clinical) diagnosis of hypertrophic cardiomyopathy and coronary angiography showed normal coronary vessels.

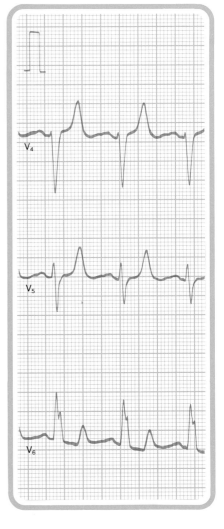

Clinical Significance

Left bundle branch block always indicates the presence of significant cardiac disease. It occurs most commonly in ischaemic heart disease, hypertension, aortic stenosis and fibrous degeneration within the conducting tissue. It may also occur in congestive and in hypertrophic cardiomyopathy, myocarditis, acute rheumatic fever, syphilis, cardiac tumours, following cardiac surgery and in congenital heart disease.

Fascicular Blocks

The concept of "fascicular blocks" has caused much confusion, partly because there is some genuine disagreement about the meaning of the terms used, but mainly because of loose application of the terms. According to this concept there are three fascicles of conduction, those of the right bundle branch, the anterior division of the left bundle and the posterior division of the left bundle.

Unifascicular block thus includes (1) RBBB, (2) LAH and (3) LPH,

Bifascicular block includes (1) LBBB (2) LAH + RBBB and (3) LPH + RBBB

Trifascicular block corresponds to complete AV block where uni- or bifascicular block has been known to be present previously. Complete heart block can, of course, also arise because of complete failure of conduction through the AV node or through the common bundle.

(It should be noted that LBBB can arise either from a discrete lesion proximally in the left bundle branch or from simultaneous LAH and LPH).

The Hemiblocks

It is possible to recognise blocks which involve either of the two divisions of the left bundle branch system.

When we first considered a simplified system describing the sequence of depolarisation of the ventricular myocardium, we divided myocardium depolarisation up into three phases (page 29). These were:

Phase 1 – Depolarisation of the interventricular septum.

Phase 2 – Depolarisation of the free wall of the right ventricle, and

Phase 3 – Depolarisation of the free wall of the left ventricle.

As long as the two divisions of the left bundle branch system are either both conducting normally or are both failing to conduct, this simplified scheme still explains the basic form of the QRS complex in the various leads. However, when we come to consider the hemiblocks it is necessary to consider Phase 3 depolarisation as having two separate parts (Figure 92).

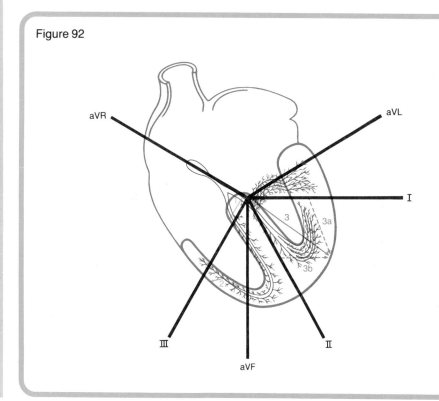

Figure 92

Phases 1, 2 and 3 represent depolarisation **(in the frontal plane)** of the interventricular septum, of the free wall of the right ventricle and of the free wall of the left ventricle respectively. Phase 3 is a result of depolarisation of the left ventricle simultaneously from two directions – a depolarisation wave spreading from below upwards and to the left as a result of transmission through the posterior (inferior) division (3b) and a depolarisation wave spreading from above downwards and to the left as a result of transmission down the anterior (superior) division (3a). In both cases the depolarisation wave also spreads from endocardium to epicardium. The phases of depolarisation can then be simplified as in Figure 93. Phase 1 occurs first, then Phases 2, 3a and 3b occur simultaneously, 3a and 3b add together to give 3 and Phases 3 and 2 add together to produce a resultant deflection which follows Phase I (Figure 93).

Normally the two parts of Phase 3 occur simultaneously with each other and with Phase 2 and they both follow Phase 1. The sequence of ventricular depolarisation in the frontal plane is therefore as outlined in Figure 93, with initial (septal) depolarisation downwards and to the right of the heart (towards Lead III) and subsequently a greater voltage depolarisation downwards and to the left of the heart. It is in this way that the normal counterclockwise direction of the vector loop in the frontal plane is inscribed and the resultant normal frontal plane axis (in the case shown in Figure 93 approximately +45°) is achieved.

The hemiblocks refer to failure of normal Phase 3a (anterior hemiblock) or of Phase 3b (posterior hemiblock) conduction.

The important functional disturbance produced by a hemiblock is a dramatic shift in the mean frontal plane QRS axis without any change in the initial direction of ventricular (septal) depolarisation.

Figure 93

Phase 1 occurs initially, alone. This is followed by Phases 2, 3a and 3b, all occurring simultaneously. Phases 2, 3a and 3b can be considered as acting from the point in time and in space at which Phase 1 ends.

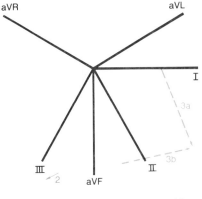

Starting from this point, Phases 3a and 3b can be seen to give rise to Phase 3:-

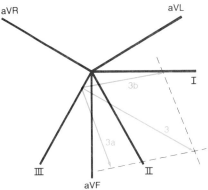

Phases 2 and 3 acting from this same point in time and space can be seen to give rise to R (which is the resultant of 2, 3a and 3b, all acting simultaneously).

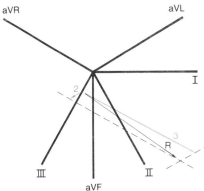

Thus the frontal plane representation of ventricular depolarisation has two sequential phases (1 and R).

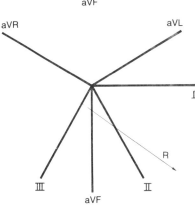

This gives rise to the normal frontal plane loop (in this case with an axis of 45°). (The axis is the direction in which the frontal plane loop "points").

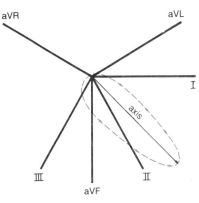

Left Anterior Hemiblock (LAH)

In left anterior hemiblock the antero-superior part of the left ventricle is not activated through the fast-conducting antero-superior division of the left bundle branch. Instead, it is activated only by the transmission of the depolarisation wave after it emerges from the postero-inferior part of the left ventricular myocardium which receives the depolarisation wave in normal manner through the postero-inferior division of the left bundle (Figure 94).

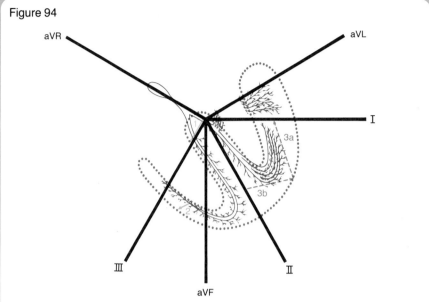

Figure 94

The antero-superior division of the left bundle totally fails to conduct. Septal depolarisation (Phase 1) and depolarisation of the free wall of the right ventricle (Phase 2) take place normally. Depolarisation of the inferior portion of the left ventricle (Phase 3b) also takes place normally. As usual Phase 1 occurs first, alone. Phases 2 and 3b then occur simultaneously. Depolarisation of the superior part of the left ventricle can only occur when a depolarisation wave reaches it from the postero-inferior division (i.e. after Phase 3b). However, since the impulse travels rapidly down the fast-conducting posterior division, Phase 3a is only minimally delayed. Since depolarisation of the superior part of the ventricle starts from the lower end rather than (as normal) from the upper end, the direction of Phase 3a is reversed.

The two basic changes, therefore, are:-
1. Delay in the initiation of, and
2. Reversal of the direction of Phase 3a

The depolarisation delay is much less than that in bundle branch block since there is rapid travel down the inferior bundle to the mid-portion of the left ventricle. The total QRS duration is therefore not abnormal, though it does tend to be at the upper end of the normal range.

The effects of these changes are shown in Figure 95.

Figure 95

Left anterior hemiblock.
The antero-superior division of the left
bundle totally fails to conduct.

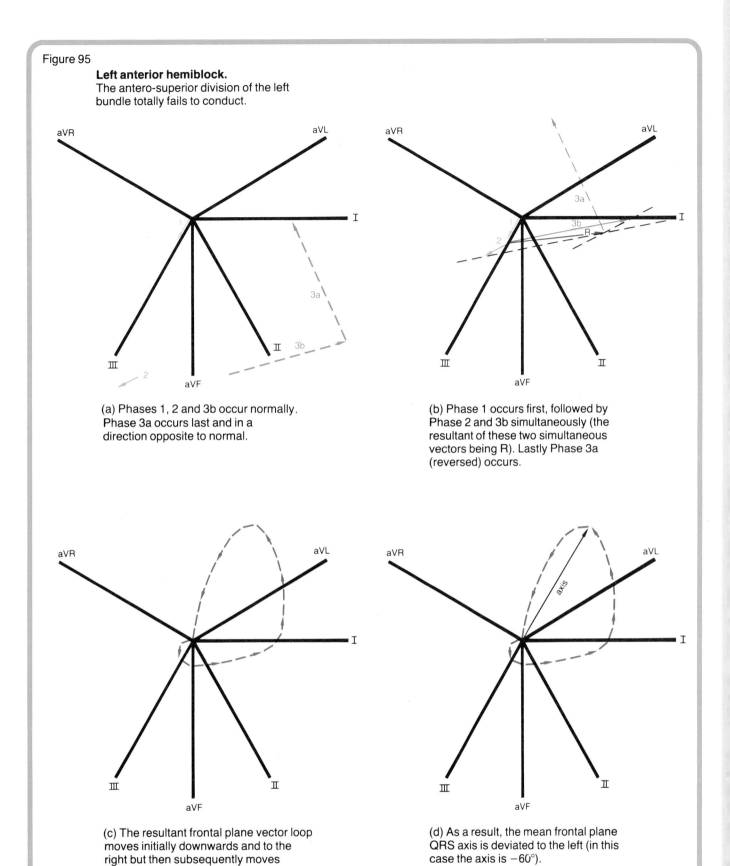

(a) Phases 1, 2 and 3b occur normally.
Phase 3a occurs last and in a
direction opposite to normal.

(b) Phase 1 occurs first, followed by
Phase 2 and 3b simultaneously (the
resultant of these two simultaneous
vectors being R). Lastly Phase 3a
(reversed) occurs.

(c) The resultant frontal plane vector loop
moves initially downwards and to the
right but then subsequently moves
powerfully upwards and to the left.

(d) As a result, the mean frontal plane
QRS axis is deviated to the left (in this
case the axis is −60°).

The cardinal features of left anterior
hemiblock are thus an abnormal degree
of left axis deviation with an initial
movement of depolarisation directed
inferiorly (i.e. left axis deviation but with
initial r waves in II, III and aVF).

Diagnostic criteria for left anterior hemiblock

1. A mean frontal plane QRS axis more negative than −30°.
2. Initial r waves in all inferior limb leads (II, III, aVF).
3. Other recognised causes of left axis deviation must be absent.

Other causes of abnormal left axis deviation

Other recognised causes of left axis deviation include some types of ventricular pre-excitation (the electrocardiographic features of the Wolff-Parkinson-White Syndrome), hyperkalaemia, tricuspid atresia, ostium primum atrial-septal defect. The only one of these easily missed is the Wolff-Parkinson-White Syndrome (see page 212). Artificial cardiac pacing from the apex of the right or left ventricle and injection of contrast in the left coronary artery are even more obviously recognisable alternative causes of left axis deviation.

Inferior myocardial infarction is an important, common cause of abnormal left axis deviation but does not come into the differential diagnosis if the diagnostic criteria (above) are fulfilled, since there is loss of the initial r waves in the inferior limb leads (II, III and aVF) in inferior infarction (see page 197).

Associated feature frequently present in left anterior hemiblock

The total QRS duration is usually at the upper end of the normal range (0.09 or 0.10 sec).

Important negative point in left anterior hemiblock

The total QRS duration is not prolonged beyond normal limits.

An example of left anterior hemiblock is shown in Figure 96.

This record would be reported as follows:-

"Sinus rhythm. The mean frontal plane QRS axis is −45°.
Left anterior hemiblock. Clockwise cardiac rotation".

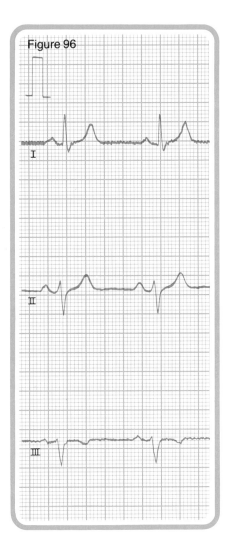

Figure 96

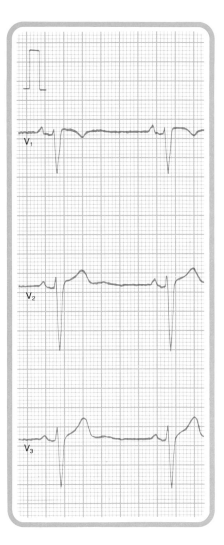

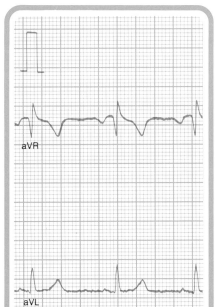

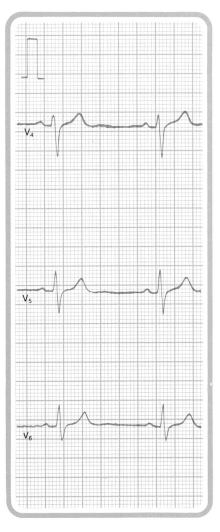

Figure 96

The rhythm is sinus. The mean frontal plane QRS axis is $-45°$. Normal initial r waves are seen in the inferior leads (II, III and aVF) and the abnormal degree of left axis deviation therefore indicates the presence of left anterior hemiblock (also known as left superior intraventricular block). The total QRS duration is 0.10 sec (best seen in the first QRS complex in Lead II). There is pronounced clockwise cardiac rotation (see pages 34–37). This accounts for the fact that no septal q waves are seen in the V_6. They are absent also from Lead 1 but are present in aVL and because of the latter, incomplete left bundle branch block cannot be said to be present.

Intermittent Left Anterior Hemiblock

Just as left and right bundle branch block can be intermittent if the pathological condition giving rise to the conduction problem varies, so left anterior hemiblock can be intermittent.

Clinical Significance

Chronic left anterior hemiblock is most commonly found in elderly people without other evidence of heart disease. In this situation it probably reflects fibrous degeneration in the anterior division of the left bundle branch. It may also be present in chronic ischaemic heart disease (e.g. in patients with chronic stable angina) in acute ischaemic heart disease (e.g. after acute ischaemia or infarction involving the appropriate division of the left bundle), in hypertension, in congestive cardiomyopathy, in hypertrophic cardiomyopathy, in calcific aortic stenosis (the calcium may extend into the conducting tissue), in myocarditis and as a result of surgical trauma (e.g. after aortic valve replacement).

Important differential diagnoses of left anterior hemiblock

The most striking feature of left anterior hemiblock is abnormal left axis deviation. The second commonest cause of abnormal left axis deviation is inferior myocardial infarction. The vital difference in the electrocardiogram between left anterior hemiblock and left axis deviation due to inferior myocardial infarction is the presence of initial r waves in the inferior leads (II, III and aVF) in left anterior hemiblock, compared with the abnormal Q wave in the inferior leads in inferior infarction (page 205). The third most common cause of left axis deviation is Wolff-Parkinson-White syndrome. This is easily missed unless looked for early in the assessment of the ECG (page 266). Other causes of left axis deviation are usually obvious and are listed on page 133.

Left Posterior Hemiblock (LPH)

Left posterior hemiblock occurs less frequently than left anterior hemiblock but as in anterior hemiblock the most dramatic change it produces is in the frontal plane QRS axis.

In left posterior hemiblock the postero-inferior part of the left ventricle is not activated through the fast-conducting postero-inferior division of the left bundle branch. Instead it is activated only by the transmission of the depolarisation wave after it emerges from the antero-superior part of the left ventricular myocardium which receives the depolarisation wave in the normal manner through the antero-superior division of the left bundle (Figure 97).

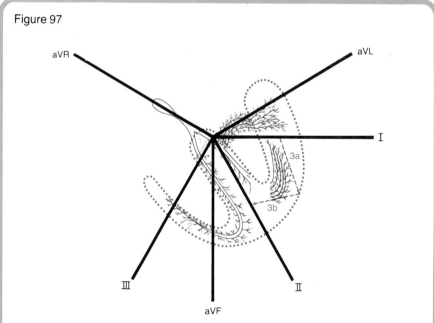

Figure 97

The postero-inferior division of the left bundle totally fails to conduct. Septal depolarisation (Phase 1) and depolarisation of the free wall of the right ventricle (Phase 2) take place normally. Depolarisation of the superior portion of the left ventricle (Phase 3a) also takes place normally. As usual, Phase 1 occurs first, alone. Phases 2 and 3a then occur simultaneously. Depolarisation of the inferior part of the left ventricle can only occur when the depolarisation wave reaches it from the antero-superior division. However, since the impulse travels rapidly down the fast-conducting anterior division, Phase 3b is only minimally delayed. Since depolarisation of the inferior part of the ventricle starts from the upper end, the direction of Phase 3b is reversed.

The two basic changes, therefore, are:-
1. **Delay in the initiation of, and**
2. **Reversal in the direction of, Phase 3b**

The depolarisation delay is much less than that in bundle branch block since there is rapid travel down the superior bundle to the mid-portion of the left ventricle. The total QRS duration is therefore not abnormal, though it does tend to be at the upper end of the normal range.

The effect of these changes is seen in Figure 98.

Figure 98

Left posterior hemiblock.
The postero-inferior division of the left bundle totally fails to conduct.

Phases 1, 2 and 3a occur normally. Phase 3b occurs last and in a direction opposite to normal.

Phase 1 occurs first, followed by Phase 2 and 3a simultaneously (the resultant of these two simultaneous vectors being R). Lastly Phase 3b (reversed) occurs.

The resultant frontal plane vector loop moves initially downwards and to the right. It then moves more definitively downwards. Finally it moves markedly to the right before returning to the origin.

As a result, the mean frontal plane QRS axis is deviated to the right (in this case the axis is +110°).

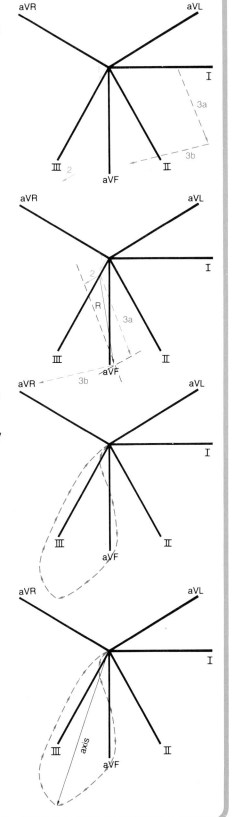

Cardinal feature of left posterior hemiblock

Unfortunately, it is not possible to be totally dogmatic about the presence of this lesion. One cannot, therefore, legitimately talk of "diagnostic criteria" but only of the "cardinal feature".

Its only electrocardiographic feature is a mild degree of right axis deviation (between $+90°$ and $+120°$). The total QRS duration is usually at the upper end of the normal range at 0.09 to 0.10 sec.

Such relatively subtle alterations as slight right axis deviation and a total QRS duration at the upper end of the normal range make it impossible to be totally confident of the diagnosis from the electrocardiogram alone. Other possible causes of right axis deviation must be excluded (on clinical or investigative grounds), before it can reasonably be concluded that left posterior hemiblock is present. These alternative causes include:- a vertical heart in a tall thin subject, emphysema, right ventricular hypertrophy, atrial-septal defect and extensive antero-lateral myocardial infarction.

An example of left posterior hemiblock is shown in Figure 99.

The ECG of Figure 99 would be reported as follows:- "Sinus rhythm. The mean frontal plane QRS axis is $+105°$. This is an abnormal degree of right axis deviation. There is no evidence of right ventricular hypertrophy and the appearance could be indicative of left posterior hemiblock. The frontal plane T waves are minimally abnormal".

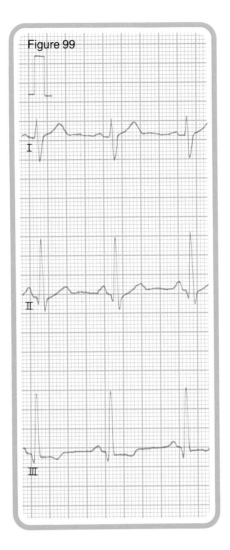

Figure 99

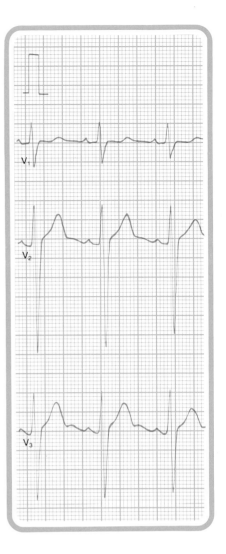

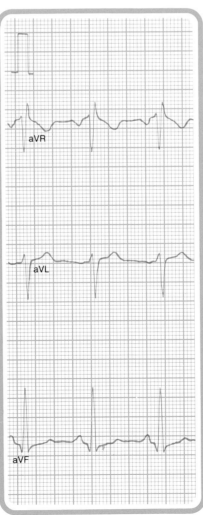

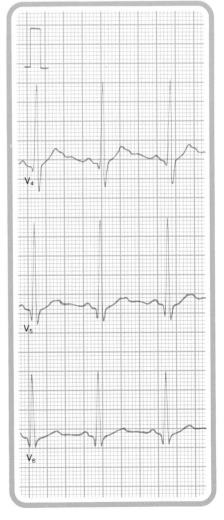

Figure 99

The rhythm is sinus, the mean frontal plane QRS axis is slightly deviated towards the right at +105°. The mean frontal plane T wave axis is +30°. The angle between this and the mean frontal plane QRS axis (75°) is thus abnormal (pages 56 and 57).

The T waves in the frontal plane are therefore minimally abnormal. There is no evidence in the precordial leads of right ventricular hypertrophy to account for the right axis deviation. There is no clockwise cardiac rotation such as might be found in the presence of chronic lung disease. Left posterior hemiblock is therefore a real possibility, but one cannot be totally dogmatic about this. If one had been able to see an earlier electro-cardiogram in the same subject which was similar in all respects but showed an axis within the normal range, then it would have been reasonable to conclude that left posterior hemiblock had developed.

Bifascicular Blocks

The term "Bifascicular block" is used when two fascicles are blocked simultaneously. The more common combination is right bundle branch block and left anterior hemiblock, and the less common combination is right bundle branch block and left posterior hemiblock. (The combination of left anterior hemiblock and left posterior hemiblock is indistinguishable from left bundle branch block).

Right Bundle Branch Block with Left Anterior Hemiblock

This combination is relatively easy to recognize. The criteria for right bundle branch block are fulfilled and there is an abnormal degree of left axis deviation (i.e. more negative than −30°).

Criteria for right bundle branch block with left anterior hemiblock

1. Total QRS duration is 0.12 sec or greater.
2. A secondary R wave is seen in V_1 (see page 118).
3. The mean frontal plane QRS axis is more negative than −30°.
4. An initial r wave is seen in the inferior limb leads (II, III and aVF).

An example is shown in Figure 100. The ECG in Figure 100 would be reported as follows:- "Sinus rhythm. There is complete right bundle branch block. There is left anterior hemiblock giving rise to a mean frontal plane QRS axis of −75°. There is left atrial hypertrophy and pronounced clockwise cardiac rotation and the r waves are of abnormally low voltage in the left precordial leads".

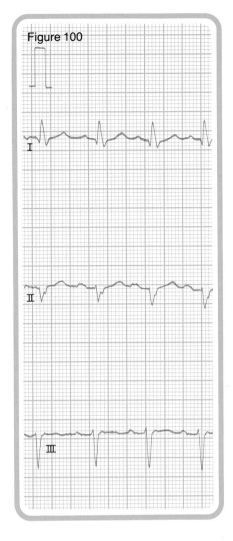

Figure 100

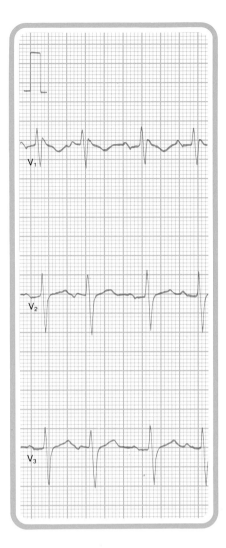

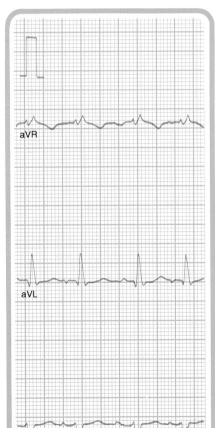

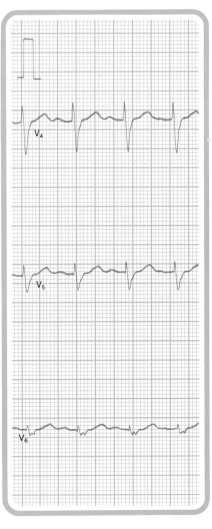

Figure 100

The rhythm is sinus. There is a secondary r wave in V_1. The total QRS duration is 0.13 sec (best seen in the first QRS complex in I). There is therefore right bundle branch block. The mean frontal plane QRS axis is $-75°$ and there are small initial r waves in II, III and aVF. There is therefore also left anterior hemiblock. (The bifid P waves in II and biphasic P waves in V_1 suggest left atrial hypertrophy – see later). There is clockwise cardiac rotation with very poor R wave progression across the precordial leads (such changes can occur in obesity and in anterolateral infarction – see later).

Right Bundle Branch Block with Left Posterior Hemiblock

Just as it is impossible from the ECG alone to be certain that there is left posterior hemiblock, so it is impossible to be **certain** of the combination of right bundle branch block and left posterior hemiblock. The criteria required are those for right bundle branch block and, in addition, an abnormal degree of right axis deviation. However, as is also true with regard to the diagnosis of right posterior hemiblock alone, other recognisable causes of right axis deviation must be included before the diagnosis of the combination can be made.

Cardinal features of right bundle branch block with left posterior hemiblock

1. Total QRS duration of 0.12 sec or greater.
2. A secondary R wave in V_1.
3. A mean frontal plane QRS axis more positive than $+90°$.

The first two criteria are those for right bundle branch block. The third criterion is that for left posterior hemiblock but is not specific, therefore other causes of right axis deviation need to be eliminated before the diagnosis can be made with confidence.

An example of the combination is shown in Figure 101. The ECG in Figure 101 would be reported as follows:-
"Sinus rhythm. Complete right bundle branch block. Abnormal right axis deviation ($+120°$) consistent with right posterior hemiblock. Clockwise cardiac rotation."

Figure 101

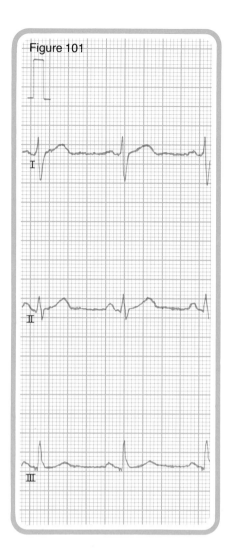
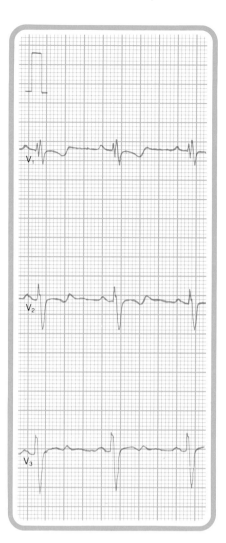
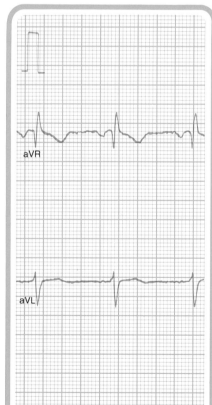
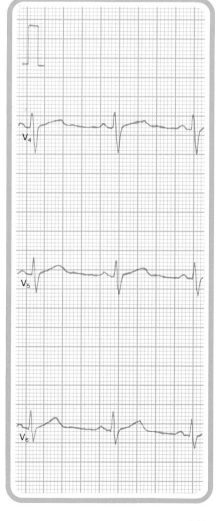

Figure 101

The rhythm is sinus. There is an
rsR'S' pattern in V₁. The total QRS
duration is prolonged, at 0.12 sec
(best seen in the first QRS complex
in V₁). There is therefore complete
right bundle branch block. There is an
abnormal degree of right axis
deviation (+120°). Since no other
clinical or investigative cause for right
axis deviation was apparent, right
posterior hemiblock is a possible
explanation. There is also clockwise
cardiac rotation.

Clinical Significance of Bifascicular Blocks

The combination of right bundle branch block and left anterior hemiblock is relatively common. It is most frequently found in asymptomatic elderly patients with fibrotic degeneration in the conducting tissues, and only rarely does it proceed to complete heart block. It may also be seen in atherosclerotic heart disease, calcific aortic stenosis, hypertrophic cardiomyopathy, congestive cardiomyopathy and congenital endocardial cushion defects. When it occurs in the context of acute myocardial infarction some 25–50% may progress to complete heart block, but when found in other situations only 5–15% of the patients progressed to complete block.

Right bundle branch block with left posterior hemiblock is a much less frequent combination, but may occur in any of the conditions listed for combination of right bundle branch block and left anterior hemiblock (above). However, when it does occur it is much more likely to progress to complete heart block and this happens in 60–70% of the patients in whom the combination is found.

The main reason that left posterior hemiblock is much less common than left anterior hemiblock is because the posterior division is thicker and shorter and has a much better blood supply than the anterior division. Higher vulnerability of the anterior division explains why right bundle branch block and left anterior hemiblock is more common than right bundle branch block and left posterior hemiblock and also why the combination of right bundle branch block and left posterior hemiblock is more likely to progress to complete heart block.

Other Forms of Intraventricular Block

The terms "parietal block" and "peri-infarction block" have been used for many years, but are poorly defined and are often used by different authorities to mean different things. These terms are therefore best abandoned and will not be discussed further.

The term "diffuse intraventricular block" refers to a rare but defined condition in which the delay occurs in the myofibrils rather than in the conducting tissue. The **diagnostic criteria** are the presence of abnormally wide (0.11 sec or longer) QRS complexes with a normal frontal plane QRS axis and with a QRS configuration which is either similar to normal or to that of left bundle branch block. This rare condition is most commonly seen in severe cardiomyopathy or myocarditis. It may also occur in infiltrative myocardial disease, occasionally in severe rheumatic disease, in ischaemic heart disease (especially in the presence of ventricular aneurysms), in hyperkalaemia, severe hypoxia, hypothermia and sometimes following over-dosage with quinidine or procainamide.

Ventricular Hypertrophy

Appreciable hypertrophy of the right or left ventricle produces characteristic changes in the electrocardiogram. Lesser degrees of hypertrophy may be present without ECG changes or with only non-specific changes. This is more often true in the case of right than of left ventricular hypertrophy. In general, the limb leads are of less diagnostic value than the precordial leads in detecting these conditions. Once again, this is particularly true with respect to right ventricular hypertrophy and, indeed, there is no certain way of diagnosing right ventricular hypertrophy from the limb leads alone – however severe the changes.

In normal circumstances the thickness of the left ventricular free wall is about three times greater than that of the right ventricular free wall. The mass of the left ventricular myocardium is therefore many times greater than that of the right ventricle (page 22). The voltages generated by left ventricular depolarisation are of the order of ten times greater than those generated by right ventricular depolarisation and, for this reason, in normal circumstances (and in most abnormal circumstances) left ventricular depolarisation is the dominant influence in determining the appearances of the QRS complexes and the resultant S–T segment and T waves. As would be expected, therefore, left ventricular hypertrophy produces, in effect, an exaggeration of the normal QRS pattern whereas right ventricular hypertrophy alters the QRS pattern in the various leads. In both cases secondary S–T segment and T wave changes follow the primary changes in QRS complexes.

Left Ventricular Hypertrophy (LVH)

The increased myocardial bulk associated with hypertrophy of the left ventricle results in an increase in the voltage contribution of Phase 3 depolarisation (Figure 102 and 103). This gives **taller R waves in the left precordial leads** and **deeper S waves in the right precordial leads**. The increased bulk also gives rise to prolongation in the time taken to travel from endocardium to the (now more distant) epicardium. This time, known as the "ventricular activation time" or the "intrinsicoid deflection time" is measured from the onset of the QRS complex to the peak of the R wave (page 39). It is measured only in left precordial leads showing a qR complex.

With the development of LVH the total QRS duration may increase minimally compared with its volume before the development of LVH. It usually still remains within the normal range but may sometimes reach 0.10 or 0.11 sec. It does not reach 0.12 sec. The primary depolarisation (QRS) abnormality gives rise to secondary repolarisation changes in the form of S–T segment depression and T wave inversion in leads facing the left ventricle. The precordial leads which face the left ventricle are, of course, the left precordial leads. The limb leads which face the left ventricle are Leads I and aVL (when the heart is horizontal) or II and aVF (when the heart is vertical). In the presence of left ventricular hypertrophy, the heart is usually but not always horizontal.

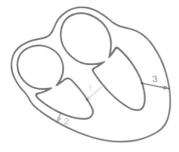

Normal

(a) The timing, sequence and relative voltages of the three phases of ventricular depolarisation are as shown:-

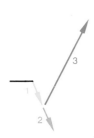

(b) The normal QRS complex in V₆ is of the qR pattern:-

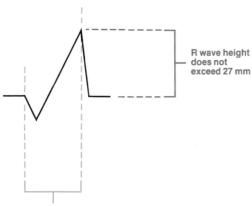

R wave height does not exceed 27 mm

Ventricular activation time does not exceed 0.04 sec

(c) The normal qR complex is followed by an iso-electric S-T segment and upright T wave

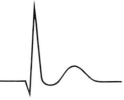

Left Ventricular Hypertrophy

(a) The timing and sequence of the three phases of ventricular depolarisation are normal. The voltage resulting from Phase 3 is substantially increased. That resulting from Phase 1 may also be slightly increased.

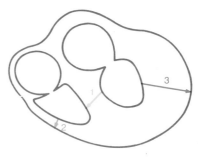

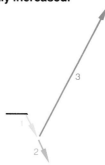

(b) The qR configuration of the QRS complex in V₆ is unchanged, but the R wave height and the ventricular activation time are increased.

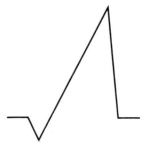

R wave height may exceed 27 mm

Ventricular activation time may exceed 0.04 sec

(c) The abnormal QRS complex is followed by a depressed S-T segment and an inverted T wave.

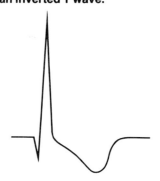

Figure 103

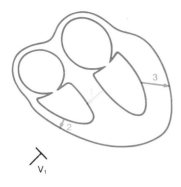

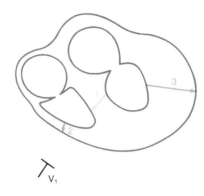

Normal

Left Ventricular Hypertrophy

(a) The timing, sequence and relative voltages of the three phases of ventricular depolarisation are as shown:-

(a) The timing and sequence of the three phases of ventricular depolarisation are normal. The voltage resulting from Phase 3 is substantially increased. That resulting from Phase 1 may also be slightly increased.

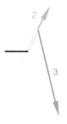

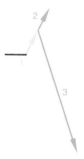

(b) The normal QRS complex in V_1 is of the rS pattern:-

(b) The normal rS configuration of the QRS complex in V_1 is unchanged but the S wave depth is increased.

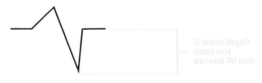

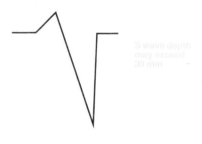

S wave depth does not exceed 30 mm

S wave depth may exceed 30 mm

(c) The normal rS complex is followed by an iso-electric S-T segment. The T waves may be upright, flat or inverted.

(c) No definitive changes in the S-T segment or T wave occur in this lead.

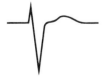

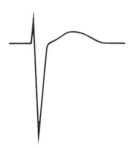

An example of severe left ventricular hypertrophy is shown in Figure 104. This ECG would be reported as follows:- "Sinus rhythm. The mean frontal plane QRS axis is −15°. There are pronounced changes of left ventricular hypertrophy. There is evidence of left atrial hypertrophy". (Left atrial hypertrophy is described in the next chapter. It is usually present when there is left ventricular hypertrophy).

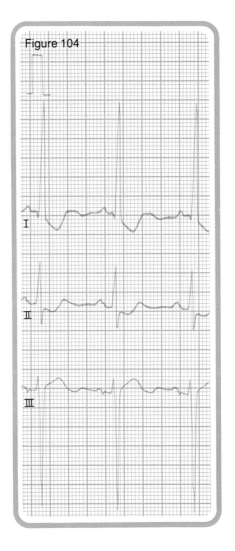

Figure 104

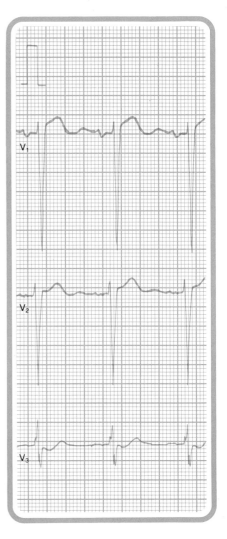

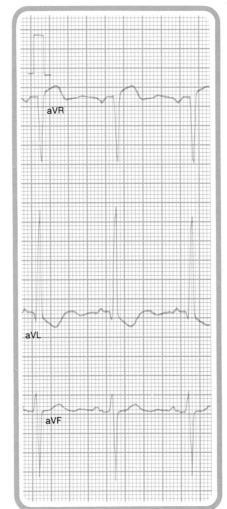

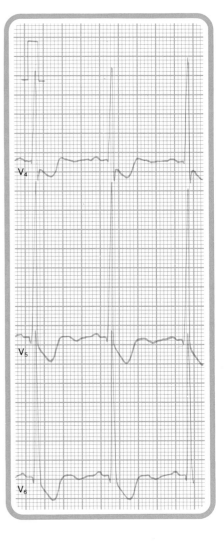

Figure 104

The rhythm is sinus. The axis is towards the left end of the normal range (−15°) i.e. the heart is horizontal. R wave height in V_5 and V_6 is abnormal (the peak R wave height in V_5 is 41mm). The S wave depth in V_1 is abnormal (31mm). The ventricular activation time in V_5 and V_6 is prolonged (0.06 sec). There is S–T segment depression and T wave inversion in the left precordial leads. Since the heart is horizontal the changes seen in the left precordial leads are also shown in I and aVL. There is also evidence of left atrial hypertrophy (page 165).

Criteria for left ventricular hypertrophy*

(Normal calibration assumed (pages 64 and 65))

1. The R waves in any one or more of the Leads, V_4, V_5 or V_6 exceeds 27mm.

2. The tallest R waves in any of the Leads V_4, V_5 or V_6 plus the deepest S waves in any of the Leads V_1, V_2 or V_3 exceeds 40mm.

3. The S waves in one or more of the Leads V_1, V_2 or V_3 exceeds 30mm.

4. R wave in aVL exceeds 13mm.

5. R in aVL exceeds 20mm.

6. The ventricular activation time (intrinsicoid deflection time) exceeds 0.04 sec (i.e. equals or exceeds 0.05 sec)**.

7. Abnormal S-T segment depression (i.e. more than 1mm below the iso-electric line (page 42)) in any lead facing the left ventricle (i.e. in V_4, V_5 or V_6, and in Lead I and aVL when heart is horizontal or in II and aVF when the heart is vertical).

8. T wave inversion in leads facing the left ventricle (as outlined in (7) above).

Unfortunately, there are no internationally agreed criteria for left ventricular hypertrophy. The above criteria would meet general but not universal acceptance. The voltage criteria (1–5 above) are generally sensitive criteria. As such they are frequently fulfilled in the absence of definitive, clinical or pathological evidence of left ventricular hypertrophy. **R waves beyond the normally accepted height or S waves beyond the normally accepted depth are often found in thin-chested persons (especially if they indulge in regular physical activity which may induce "physiological" hypertrophy). If the voltage criteria only are fulfilled it is better to report the ECG as "the voltage criteria for left ventricular hypertrophy are fulfilled" rather than "left ventricular hypertrophy" for the former can be normal in thin-chested persons.** This is a good example of "secondary" interpretation of the electrocardiogram in the light of clinical data (page 109).

Prolongation of the ventricular activation time is a more specific criterion but is considerably less sensitive than the voltage criteria.

Note

* Left ventricular hypertrophy is a **graded** abnormality (not an all-or-none abnormality like complete bundle branch block). Because of this there are no "diagnostic" criteria. A whole range of criteria may point towards left ventricular hypertrophy. Some are more sensitive than specific (page 108) and some more specific and sensitive. In general the greater the number of criteria fulfilled, the more likely the diagnosis becomes.

** The small squares on the ECG graticule indicate 0.04 sec and it is not considered possible to distinguish differences less than 0.01 sec. If this is accepted, "exceeds 0.04 sec" is the same as "equals or exceeds 0.05 sec".

Systolic overload, diastolic overload, "strain"

Hypertrophy of the left ventricle can be produced by conditions giving rise to additional load in the ventricle during systole (e.g. aortic stenosis) or during diastole (e.g. aortic incompetence). The so-called "Systolic overload pattern" is one in which the S–T segment and T wave changes are **relatively** more prominent than the QRS changes. The so-called "Diastolic overload pattern", conversely, is one in which the QRS changes are **relatively** more pronounced than the S–T segment and T wave changes. However, it should be stressed that these are "soft" (i.e. ill-defined) concepts and are not reliable indicators of the cause of the hypertrophy.

The term "strain" is even less well-defined (and carries physical, physiological and prognostic overtones which it cannot possibly justify). Like "systolic overload" it refers to the pronounced S–T segment and T wave changes **thought to have arisen on the basis of ventricular hypertrophy**. The term is not significantly different in concept from "systolic overload". For this reason (and also because the terms imply pathophysiological consequences which cannot possibly be predicted from the ECG) the terms "strain" and "strain pattern" are best avoided. The terms "systolic overload pattern" and "diastolic overload pattern" do have some minor discriminatory power but are not of major usefulness.

Associated features in left ventricular hypertrophy

1. Since the physical size of the left ventricle is increased in left ventricular hypertrophy, there is more left ventricle underlying the chest leads. Because of this, left ventricular (i.e. qR) complexes may appear further to the right in the precordial leads than the usual V_4 to V_6 – i.e. **there is often counterclockwise cardiac rotation** (pages 34 to 37).
2. Usually the development of left ventricular hypertrophy results in a **slight** shift of the mean frontal plane QRS axis towards the left. However, the axis usually remains within the normal range and typically it is between $+30°$ and $-30°$. This means that the heart is **horizontal** (page 53). In this event the changes in QRS complexes, S–T segments and T waves induced in the left precordial leads will be seen also in I and aVL.

Occasionally, left ventricular hypertrophy can occur with a mean frontal plane QRS axis of $+60°$ to $+90°$ – i.e. the heart is vertical (page 53). In this situation the changes in the QRS complexes, S–T segments and T waves induced in the left precordial leads are seen also in II and aVF.

Figure 104 shows a typical example of left ventricular hypertrophy in a horizontal heart. Leads I and aVL show appearances similar to those found in V_5 and V_6. Figure 105 shows an example of left ventricular hypertrophy in a vertical heart (the mean frontal plane QRS axis is $+60°$). Leads II and aVF show appearances similar to those found in V_5 and V_6.

The ECG of Figure 105 would be reported as follows:–
"Sinus rhythm. The mean frontal plane QRS axis is $+60°$. The precordial QRS complexes satisfy the voltage criteria for left ventricular hypertrophy".

3. Electrocardiographic evidence of left atrial hypertrophy usually accompanies that of left ventricular hypertrophy. Electrocardiographic evidence of atrial hypertrophy can only be recognised if the rhythm is sinus.
4. Prominent U waves are often seen in the right and mid-precordial leads of patients with left ventricular hypertrophy.

The U Wave

The U wave is a small, rounded, upright wave occurring immediately at the end of the T wave. It is part of the repolarisation process. It is visible in many normal electrocardiograms. It becomes more prominent in left ventricular hypertrophy, myocardial ischaemia, hypokalaemia and following exercise. It is thus a non-specific change. A U wave is deemed to be definitively abnormal if it is taller than the T wave preceding it (in the same lead). Prominent, but not abnormal, U waves are seen in V_1–V_3 of Figure 105. In this figure small U waves are also visible in V_4.

The normal U wave is described in more detail on page 195. Conditions giving rise to abnormally tall U waves are listed on page 263.

Important negative points in left ventricular hypertrophy

Left ventricular hypertrophy does not give rise to an abnormal degree of left axis deviation. The presence of an axis more negative than −30° in an electrocardiogram showing left ventricular hypertrophy suggests the presence of left anterior hemiblock (provided initial r waves are visible in the inferior limb leads).

Clinical Significance

The main causes of recognisable left ventricular hypertrophy on the electrocardiogram are systemic hypertension, aortic stenosis, coarctation of the aorta, mitral incompetence, aortic incompetence and hypertrophic cardiomyopathy. Of these, systemic hypertension almost certainly represents the commonest cause. Aortic and mitral incompetence both cause diastolic loads on the left ventricle and patent ductus arteriosus may do the same if the shunt is very large. The other causes listed result in systolic overload of the ventricle.

It is partly because left ventricular hypertrophy is associated with a **slight** shift of the frontal plane axis towards the left (though usually still within the normal range) and partly because those conditions most commonly giving rise to left ventricular hypertrophy tend to present in the middle and later age groups (when the axis normally lies towards the left end of the normal range) that left ventricular hypertrophy is usually associated with a horizontal heart. If appreciable left ventricular hypertrophy develops in a child, the heart may well be vertical, for the normal frontal plane QRS axis is at the extreme right hand end of the normal range in infancy and progresses gradually towards the left hand end of the range with increasing age. Left ventricular hypertrophy with a vertical heart is thus most commonly seen in childhood in association with valvar or subvalvar aortic stenosis or coarctation of the aorta.

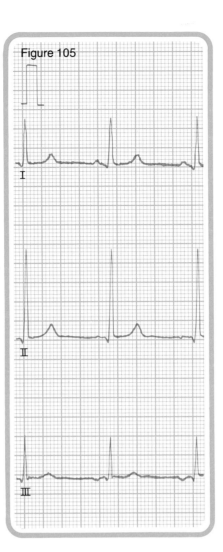

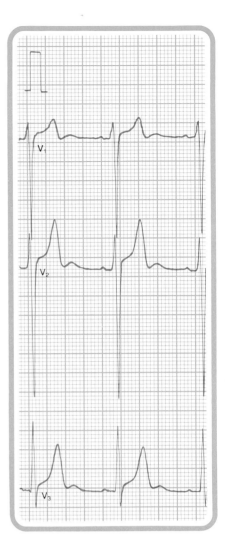

Figure 105

The rhythm is sinus. The frontal plane QRS axis is +60° and the heart is therefore vertical. The precordial QRS complexes satisfy the voltage criteria for left ventricular hypertrophy. In other respects the record is within normal limits. Since the heart is vertical, the form of the QRS complexes in II and aVF is similar to that in V_6. Contrast this with Figure 104, where the heart is horizontal (frontal plane axis −15°). In this situation, Leads aVL and I show QRS appearances similar to those in V_6.

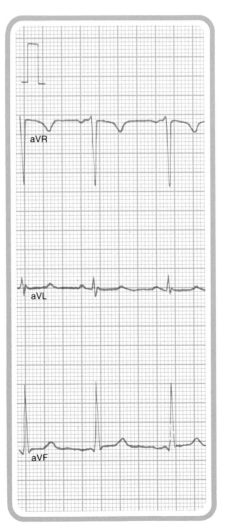

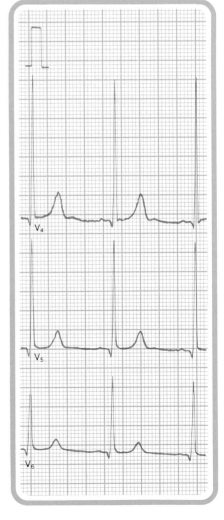

Right Ventricular Hypertrophy (RVH)

In all normal and in most abnormal electrocardiograms, the voltages generated by left ventricular depolarisation dominate the electrocardiographic appearances in every lead. Minor degrees of right ventricular enlargement have no appreciable effect on the appearances. However, the increased bulk of the right ventricle in more pronounced right ventricular hypertrophy results in a major increase in the voltage contribution of Phase 2 of ventricular depolarisation and this may become the dominant influence in many ECG leads.

The most obvious consequence of RVH is an increase in the voltage of the R wave in the right precordial leads (Figure 106). The most diagnostic feature is a dominant R wave in V_1[†] (the term "dominant R wave" implies that whatever the configuration of the QRS complex in V_1 the largest wave in that QRS complex is an R wave). The most readily understood configuration of the QRS complex in V_1 is an Rs complex (Figures 106 and 107). However, not uncommonly a small q wave may be present in V_1 in right ventricular hypertrophy (giving rise to a qR or a qRs complex – i.e. the QRS morphology may be different but the R wave is still dominant). An example is shown in Figure 108. The explanation for the presence of a q wave in V_1 is not fully understood. It may be that right ventricular hypertrophy involves the upper part of the interventricular septum and as a result of this the depolarisation of the interventricular septum initially passes upwards and backwards instead of forwards and downwards (Figure 109). This gives rise to an initial movement of the QRS vector away from V_1 and results in an initial negative wave (i.e. a q wave).

[†] A dominant R' wave may be seen in V_1 in the presence of RBBB. It is important to exclude RBBB (by the fact that the total QRS duration is less than 0.12 sec) before RVH is diagnosed.

Figure 106

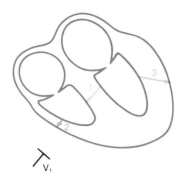

Normal

(a) The timing, sequence and relative voltages of the three phases of ventricular depolarisation are as shown:-

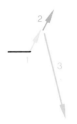

(b) The normal QRS complex in V₁ is of the rS pattern:-

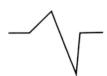

(c) The normal rS complex is followed by an iso-electric S-T segment. The T waves may be upright, flat or inverted.

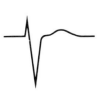

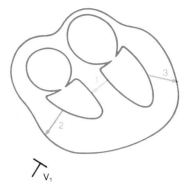

Right Ventricular Hypertrophy

(a) The timing and sequence of the three phases of ventricular depolarisation are normal. The voltage resulting from Phase 2 is substantially increased. That resulting from Phase 1 may also be slightly increased.

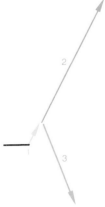

(b) The normal rS configuration in V₁ is radically altered to produce a dominant R wave.

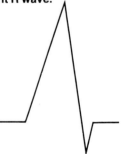

(c) The abnormal Rs complex in V₁ is followed by a depressed S-T segment and an inverted T wave.

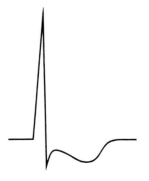

152

The ECG in Figure 107 would be
reported as follows:–
"Sinus rhythm. The mean frontal plane
QRS axis is +135°. There is a dominant
R wave in V_1. There is clockwise cardiac
rotation. The appearances are indicative
of right ventricular hypertrophy. The form
of the P waves in II suggests the
possibility of right atrial hypertrophy".

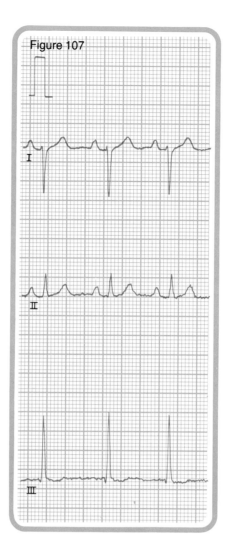

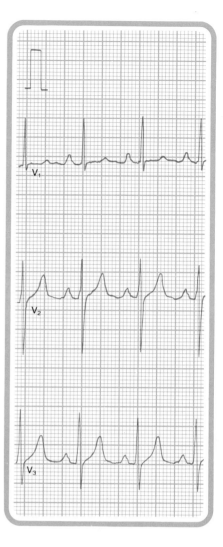

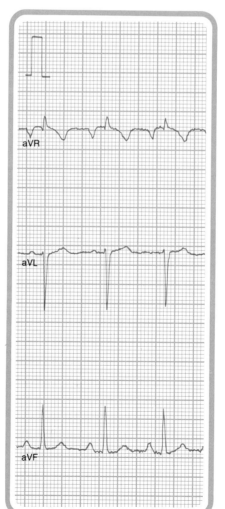

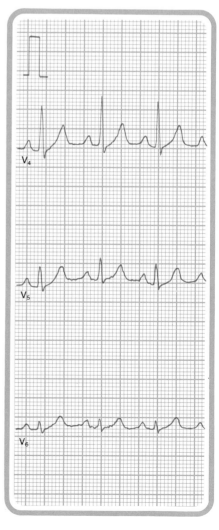

Figure 107

The rhythm is sinus. There is
abnormal right axis deviation (+135°).
There is a dominant R wave (an Rs
complex) in V_1. There is therefore
right ventricular hypertrophy. There is
clockwise cardiac rotation. There are
no S–T,T changes of right ventricular
hypertrophy (see below). The P waves
are tall and pointed in Lead II suggesting
right atrial hypertrophy (see next
section).

153

The ECG of Figure 108 would be reported as follows:–
"Sinus rhythm. The mean frontal plane QRS axis is +135°. There is a dominant R wave in V_1. There is pronounced clockwise cardiac rotation. There are non-specific S-T, T changes from V_1 to V_5. The appearances are those of right ventricular hypertrophy. There is evidence also of right atrial hypertrophy.

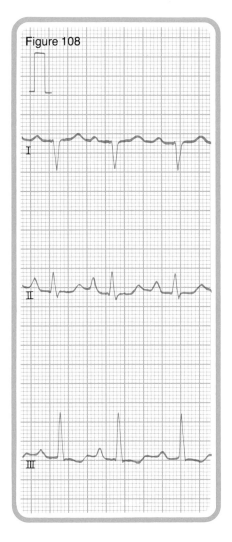

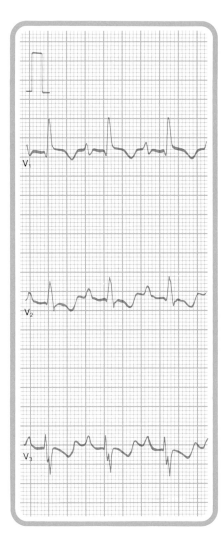

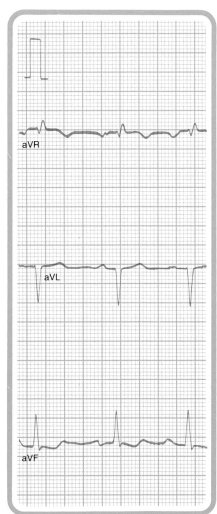

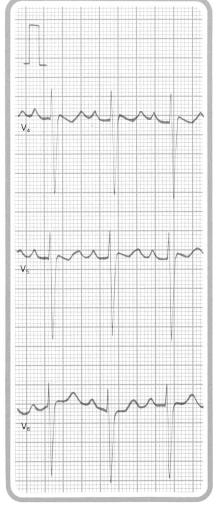

Figure 108

The rhythm is sinus. There is abnormal right axis deviation (+ 135°). There is a dominant R wave (qR complex) in V_1. There is therefore right ventricular hypertrophy. There is clockwise cardiac rotation and a deep S wave in V_6. There is S–T segment depression from V_1 to V_4. The P waves are tall and pointed in Lead II, indicating right atrial hypertrophy (see pages 159 to 161). The P-R interval is prolonged 0.22 sec.

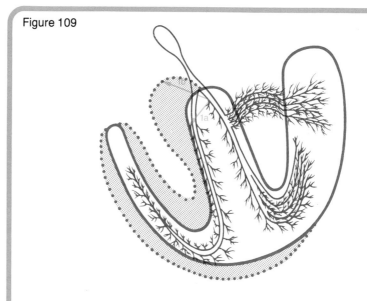

Figure 109

T_{V_1}

In the normal heart septal depolarisation passes forwards, downwards and to the right (arrow 1a). In the presence of right ventricular hypertrophy it can pass backwards, upwards and to the right (arrow 1b) to produce an initial part of the QRS complex moving away from V_1, i.e. an initial q wave.

The primary depolarisation (QRS) abnormality gives rise to secondary repolarisation changes in the form of S–T segment depression and T wave inversion in leads facing the right ventricle. These changes involve the right and mid-precordial leads.

Unlike left ventricular hypertrophy, right ventricular hypertrophy is accompanied by deviation of the axis beyond the normal range. Right ventricular hypertrophy is associated with right axis deviation. In addition, since the right ventricle is larger than normal, more of the right ventricular myocardium than usual underlies the precordial leads. The transition zone therefore moves further towards the left in the precordial series, i.e. there is usually pronounced clockwise cardiac rotation (pages 34 to 37). As a result of this the R wave size in the left precordial leads is reduced and as a result of the increased voltage of Phase 2 depolarisation the S wave in the left precordial leads is increased.

Diagnostic criteria for right ventricular hypertrophy

1. A frontal plane QRS axis more positive than +90°.
2. Dominant R wave in V_1 (Rs, R, RR', qR or qRS).
3. Absence of evidence of anterolateral infarction* (see page 197).
4. QRS duration must be less than 0.12 sec†.

Note

*Anterolateral infarction is one cause of right axis deviation (page 197 and Table 2, page 156). In the presence of both anterolateral infarction and true posterior infarction the combination of abnormal right axis deviation and a dominant R wave in V_1 may occur and this may wrongly suggest right ventricular hypertrophy. However, the true diagnosis is indicated by the evidence of anterolateral infarction.

†If the QRS duration is 0.12 sec or longer there is bundle branch block which, in the presence of a dominant R wave in V_1, would be right bundle branch block. The diagnosis of right ventricular hypertrophy in the presence of right bundle branch block is difficult and unreliable.

Additional features frequently present in right ventricular hypertrophy

1. S–T segment depression and T wave inversion in some of the Leads V_1 to V_4.
2. Deep S waves in V_5, V_6 and also in I and aVL.
3. Evidence of right atrial hypertrophy (see page 159).

Problems in the differential diagnosis of right ventricular hypertrophy

As indicated earlier, right ventricular hypertrophy may be well advanced before any ECG changes become apparent.

The earliest change is usually a shift of the axis to the right. However, a mean frontal plane QRS axis more positive than +90° occurs in a large number of conditions (see Table 2).

Table 2

Causes of mean frontal plane QRS axis more positive than +90°

Normal finding in infants and children
Occasional normal finding in tall, slim adults
Occasional finding in chronic lung disease
   (even in the absence of pulmonary hypertension)
Anterolateral myocardial infarction
Left posterior hemiblock
Right ventricular hypertrophy
Pulmonary embolism
Atrial septal defect

The second of the diagnostic criteria for right ventricular hypertrophy (the presence of a dominant R wave in V_1) also has several possible causes (see Table 3).

Table 3

Causes of increased R wave amplitude in V_1

Normal finding in children
True posterior myocardial infarction
Ventricular pre-excitation
Duchenne type muscular dystrophy
Right bundle branch block (occasionally)
Right ventricular hypertrophy

The **combination** of abnormal right axis deviation and a dominant R wave in V_1 makes it very highly likely that there is right ventricular hypertrophy. The likelihood is further increased by the presence of S-T segment depression and T wave inversion in the right precordial leads and by the presence of right atrial hypertrophy (see page 159).

Clinical Significance

The majority of conditions giving rise to right ventricular hypertrophy are conditions which produce systolic overload of the right ventricle – pulmonary stenosis, pulmonary hypertension (primary, or secondary to left ventricular insufficiency or to mitral valve disease) and Fallot's tetralogy. Only relatively rarely does chronic cor pulmonale give rise to right ventricular hypertrophy.

Diastolic overload of the right ventricle occurs in atrial septal defect, anomalous pulmonary venous return and tricuspid incompetence. The electrocardiographic appearances in diastolic overload of the right ventricle are indistinguishable from those in complete or incomplete right bundle branch block.

Bi-ventricular Hypertrophy

Bi-ventricular hypertrophy may be difficult or impossible to recognise from the electrocardiogram. The increased electrical forces of both Phases 2 and 3 ventricular depolarisation may cancel themselves out so that the precordial QRS complexes may appear completely normal. If both ventricles are enlarged, one more markedly so than the other, the pattern will be that of hypertrophy of the dominant ventricle. When both ventricles are hypertrophied to a similar degree many of the changes will cancel each other out. However, because of the increased ventricular wall thickness the time taken for depolarisation to spread from endocardium to epicardium within the ventricles will be increased and the total duration may be prolonged to 0.10 or 0.11 sec but not beyond this. In addition, T wave inversion may be apparent in any of the chest leads. Sometimes **the combination of signs of left ventricular hypertrophy with right axis deviation** (i.e. more positive than +90°) **will present and this combination, if chronically present, suggests bi-ventricular hypertrophy. Less frequently, combined ventricular hypertrophy may give rise to signs of right ventricular hypertrophy and an axis more negative than −30°.**

The essential points to note about bi-ventricular hypertrophy are as follows:-

1. It may exist without diagnostic ECG changes.

2. The total QRS duration may be prolonged to 0.10 or 0.11 sec.

3. T wave inversion may be present in the precordial leads.

4. The combination of signs of left ventricular hypertrophy and an axis more positive than +90° is suggestive of bi-ventricular hypertrophy.

5. Occasionally the combination of signs of right ventricular hypertrophy with an axis more negative than −30° is found.

Clinical Significance

Bi-ventricular hypertrophy is found in severe rheumatic valve disease (aortic valve disease with pulmonary hypertension or mitral incompetence with pulmonary hypertension) cardiomyopathy and occasionally in congenital heart disease.

Atrial Hypertrophy

Just as ventricular hypertrophy produces recognisable changes in ventricular depolarisation (i.e. in the QRS complexes) and repolarisation (i.e. in the T waves), so atrial hypertrophy produces changes in the atrial depolarisation (P) wave. Since the atrial repolarisation (Ta) wave is not usually visible in the electrocardiogram, it is not surprising that recognisable changes in its form are not usually visible in atrial hypertrophy. Enlargement of the left or right atrium gives rise to an increase in the voltage and duration of the respective component of the P wave.

The Normal P Wave

It will be recalled (pages 43, 44 and 59) that right atrial depolarisation starts before left atrial depolarisation starts and finishes before left atrial depolarisation finishes. In normal circumstances atrial depolarisation begins as soon as depolarisation of the sino-atrial node spreads to activate the adjacent right atrial myocardium. Depolarisation then spreads simultaneously in all available directions through right atrial myocardium. The direction in which the greatest amount of atrial myocardium is available determines the direction in which the right atrial component of the P wave is best seen (Figure 110). This is usually towards Lead II in the limb leads and towards V_1 in the precordial leads. The first part of the left atrial myocardium to be depolarised is that point which is on the **shortest** route of depolarisation from the sino-atrial node (Figure 110). From this point, depolarisation spreads in all available directions through the left atrial myocardium. The direction in which the greatest amount of atrial myocardium is available determines the direction in which the left atrial component of the P wave is best seen. This is usually also towards Lead II in the limb leads but is away from V_1 in the precordial leads.

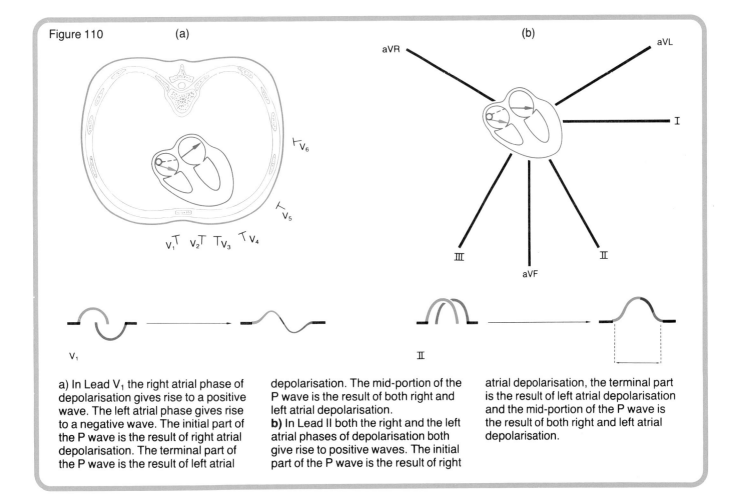

Figure 110   (a)   (b)

a) In Lead V_1 the right atrial phase of depolarisation gives rise to a positive wave. The left atrial phase gives rise to a negative wave. The initial part of the P wave is the result of right atrial depolarisation. The terminal part of the P wave is the result of left atrial depolarisation. The mid-portion of the P wave is the result of both right and left atrial depolarisation.
b) In Lead II both the right and the left atrial phases of depolarisation both give rise to positive waves. The initial part of the P wave is the result of right atrial depolarisation, the terminal part is the result of left atrial depolarisation and the mid-portion of the P wave is the result of both right and left atrial depolarisation.

Lead II therefore normally shows a uniphasic upright P wave which consists of overlapping right and left atrial components (Figure 110b), whereas V_1 normally shows a biphasic P wave with an initial positive and a subsequent negative component (Figure 110a).

In Lead II the normal P wave does not exceed 2.5mm in height or 0.12 sec in duration. In the normal P wave in V_1 the area of the negative component does not exceed the area of the positive component which precedes it.

Atrial Abnormality

The P wave is a much less well-defined wave-form than the QRS complex. Abnormalities of the P wave therefore tend to be less specific than those of the QRS complexes. Thus, while it is customary to speak of abnormal P waves as showing "hypertrophy" of the right or left atrium, there is, in fact, no means of distinguishing hypertrophy of a given atrium from ischaemia, infarction or inflammation of that atrium or from a conduction defect within the atrium. It may be therefore that the term "atrial abnormality" might be preferable to "atrial hypertrophy", but the latter term is widely used and will not easily be displaced. The important point to realise is that when there is evidence of (for example) left atrial hypertrophy, the only legitimate conclusion from the electrocardiogram is that the left atrium is in some way abnormal ("primary" interpretation). In the light of clinical data indicating the presence of mitral stenosis or of left ventricular hypertrophy, the presence of true left atrial hypertrophy might be inferred ("secondary" interpretation). In the absence of such data no assessment of the cause of the atrial abnormality can be made.

Right Atrial Hypertrophy

In right atrial hypertrophy the right atrial component of the P wave is increased in voltage and in duration. Since the right atrial component of the P wave is normally seen as a positive deflection both in Lead II and in V_1, the P wave height is increased in both of these leads. Since right atrial depolarisation is normally complete well before left atrial depolarisation is completed, the delay in the completion of right atrial depolarisation is not sufficient to prolong right atrial depolarisation beyond the end of left atrial depolarisation. Because of this the P wave duration is not increased (Figure 111a).

Figure 111

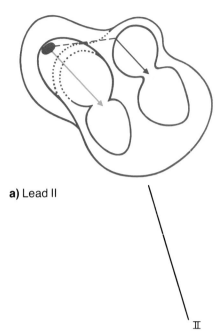

a) Lead II

In right atrial hypertrophy the (initial) right atrial component of the P wave is increased in magnitude and in duration. The resultant effect on the P wave is an increase in the P wave height but not in its duration.
a) The resultant P wave in Lead II is abnormally tall and is pointed.
b) The resultant P wave in Lead V₁ has an abnormally tall (initial) positive component.

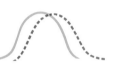

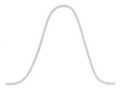

Normal P wave in II – right and left atrial components.

The P wave in II in right atrial hypertrophy – right and left atrial components. The right atrial component is increased.

The P wave in II in right atrial hypertrophy is abnormally tall.

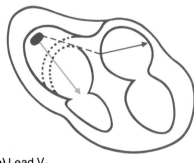

b) Lead V₁

T_{V_1}

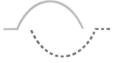

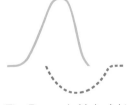

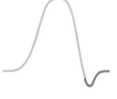

Normal P wave in V₁– right and left atrial components.

The P wave in V₁ in right atrial hypertrophy – right and left atrial components. The right atrial component is increased.

The P wave in V₁ in right atrial hypertrophy has a tall initial positive component.

The primary electrocardiographic change in right atrial hypertrophy is therefore an increase in the voltage of the P wave in Lead II and an increase in the voltage of the initial positive part of the P wave in V_1. There is a good deal of variation in the dominant direction of right atrial depolarisation in the horizontal plane and as a result of this changes in the P wave height in V_1 do not reliably occur in right atrial hypertrophy. The diagnosis of right atrial hypertrophy can therefore only safely be made from the P waves in the frontal plane leads. Lead II usually shows the changes best. An example is shown in Figure 112. The ECG in Figure 112 would be reported as follows:-

"Sinus rhythm. The mean frontal plane QRS axis is +165°. There is right ventricular hypertrophy, right atrial hypertrophy and clockwise cardiac rotation".

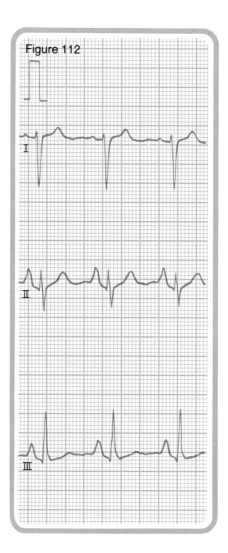

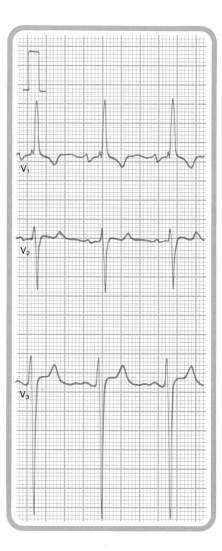

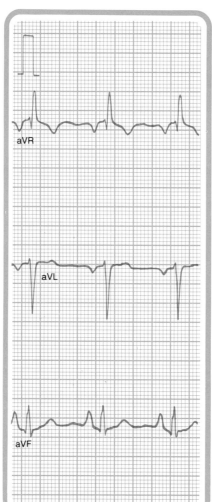

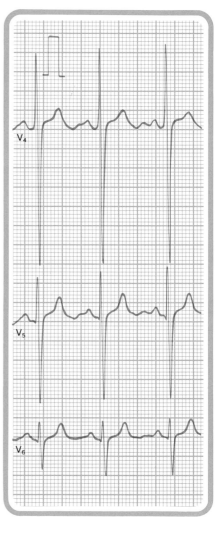

Figure 112

There is an abnormal degree of right axis deviation (+165°) and a dominant R wave in V_1. There is thus right ventricular hypertrophy. The P waves are tall and pointed in Lead II and are in excess of 3mm. There is thus right atrial hypertrophy. Right atrial hypertrophy very frequently accompanies right ventricular hypertrophy. The pronounced clockwise cardiac rotation is part of the right ventricular hypertrophy.

Criterion for right atrial hypertrophy

The P wave height is 3mm or more in Leads II, III or aVF (Leads III and aVF are included because the P wave vector is sometimes directed more closely towards either of these leads than along Lead II, i.e. the P wave axis is often +75° or more positive than this).

Associated findings

In association with right atrial hypertrophy, the positive part of the P wave in V_1 is often greater than 1.5mm tall. There is usually evidence of right ventricular hypertrophy. There is often also a prominent atrial repolarisation wave (see pages 166 and 167).

Clinical Significance

As indicated earlier, the electrocardiographic finding of "right atrial hypertrophy" strictly speaking only defines the presence of right atrial abnormality. Changes similar to those in hypertrophy also occur in ischaemia or infarction of the right atrium although the latter two are rare clinical events. The presence of associated right ventricular hypertrophy makes it much more likely that the right atrial hypertrophy pattern on the electrocardiogram does indicate true hypertrophy of the right atrium. Right atrial hypertrophy occurs in all conditions which give rise to right ventricular hypertrophy and in addition it occurs in tricuspid stenosis.

Left Atrial Hypertrophy

The electrocardiographic changes produced by left atrial hypertrophy are those changes produced by an increase in the voltage and duration of the left atrial depolarisation wave. Since the terminal part of the normal P wave is produced by left atrial depolarisation, it follows that the total P wave duration is prolonged in left atrial hypertrophy.

In addition, the P wave tends to be bifid in Lead II and biphasic in V_1 (Figure 113). In V_1 the area of the (terminal) negative component exceeds the area of the (initial) positive component. An example of left atrial hypertrophy is shown in Figure 114.

Figure 113

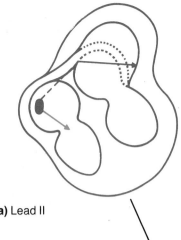

a) Lead II

In left atrial hypertrophy the left atrial (terminal) component of the P wave is increased in magnitude and in duration. The resultant effect on the P wave is to increase the size of the terminal portion and also to increase the total P wave duration.

a) The resultant P wave in Lead II is broadened (more than 0.12 sec) and bifid with a tall second component.

b) The resultant P wave in Lead V₁ is broadened and biphasic. The area of the (terminal) negative component is larger than the area of the (initial) positive component.

II

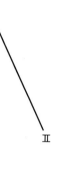

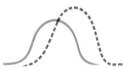

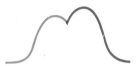

Normal P wave in II – right and left atrial components.

The P wave in II in left atrial hypertrophy – right and left atrial components. The left atrial component is increased.

The P wave in II in left atrial hypertrophy is notched and broad. The second component may be tall.

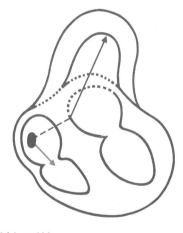

b) Lead V₁

T_{V_1}

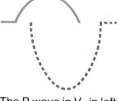

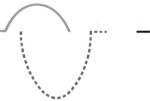

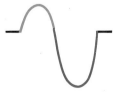

Normal P wave in V₁ – right and left atrial components.

The P wave in V₁ in left atrial hypertrophy – right and left atrial components. The left atrial component is increased.

The P wave in Lead V₁ in left atrial hypertrophy has a dominant negative (terminal) component.

The ECG in Figure 114 would be reported as follows:- "Sinus rhythm. The mean frontal plane QRS axis is +75°. The P waves are broad and bifid in Lead II and there is a dominant negative component to the P wave in V_1. The changes are indicative of left atrial hypertrophy (strictly "left atrial abnormality"). In other respects the record is within normal limits".

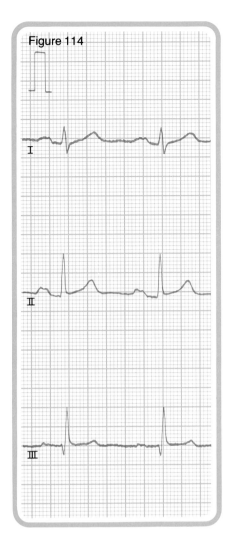

Figure 114

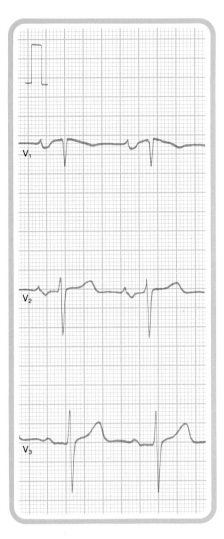

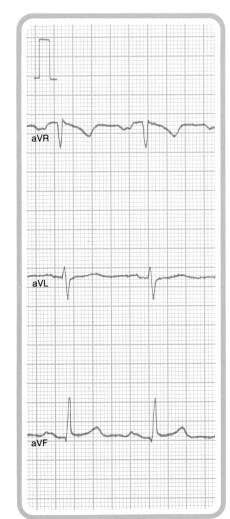

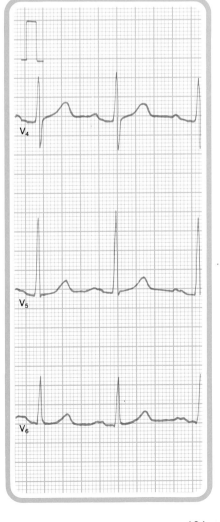

Figure 114

The rhythm is sinus. P waves are bifid in Lead II. The P wave duration in Lead II is prolonged at 0.15 sec (best seen in the second T wave in Lead II). The P waves in V_1 are clearly biphasic. In this lead there is a small, brief (and rather sharp looking) initial positive component followed by a deeper and very much broader negative component. The area of the negative component clearly exceeds that of the positive component.

164

Criteria for left atrial hypertrophy

1. The P wave is notched and exceeds 0.12 sec in duration in Leads I, II, aVF or aVL.

2. The P wave in V_1 has a dominant negative component (i.e. either it is entirely negative or alternatively the area of the (terminal) negative component exceeds that of the (initial) positive component).

(Either criterion suggests the diagnosis. If both are satisfied the diagnosis is more likely still).

Features commonly associated with left atrial hypertrophy

Just as right atrial hypertrophy is frequently found in association with right ventricular hypertrophy, so left atrial hypertrophy is frequently found in association with left ventricular hypertrophy. In patients with pure mitral stenosis, left atrial hypertrophy may occur in association with **right** ventricular hypertrophy.

Clinical Significance

Left atrial hypertrophy occurs in any condition associated with left ventricular hypertrophy and it also occurs in mitral stenosis. It is frequently found in association with systemic hypertension even when there is no electrocardiographic evidence of left ventricular hypertrophy in that condition. It may also be found in association with aortic stenosis, aortic incompetence, mitral incompetence, hypertrophic cardiomyopathy and chronic ischaemic heart disease.

As discussed earlier (under the heading of right atrial hypertrophy) the term "atrial hypertrophy" is less justifiable than "atrial abnormality". The primary electrocardiographic interpretation of the presence of broad bifid P waves in Lead II or a dominant negative component to the P wave in V_1 is that there is some *abnormality* of the left atrium. If it is known that there is mitral stenosis or left ventricular hypertrophy then true left atrial hypertrophy might well be inferred ("secondary" interpretation). The electrocardiogram itself merely provides evidence of abnormality of the left atrium and cannot distinguish between atrial hypertrophy, atrial ischaemia and atrial infarction. When electrocardiographic evidence of left atrial hypertrophy is found in a person with ischaemic heart disease it is likely that the common explanation is ischaemia or infarction of the atrium.

Bi-atrial Hypertrophy

The diagnosis of bi-atrial hypertrophy is not as difficult as the diagnosis of bi-ventricular hypertrophy since the hypertrophy of each individual atrium affects predominantly a different part of the P wave whereas hypertrophy of each individual ventricle affects the same part of the QRS complex. Bi-atrial hypertrophy may therefore be diagnosed whenever the criteria for both left and right atrial hypertrophy are fulfilled.

Diagnostic criteria for bi-atrial hypertrophy

1. P waves in the limb leads which are **both** 3mm or greater in height, and **also** in excess of 0.12 sec in duration.

2. The presence of a large biphasic P wave in V_1 with an (initial) upright portion of 2mm or more in height, and a (terminal) negative portion at least 1mm deep and 0.04 sec in duration.

3. The presence of a tall peaked P wave 2mm or more in height in V_1 in combination with wide (i.e. more than 0.12 sec in duration) notched P waves in the limb leads or in the left precordial leads.

(Any one criterion suggests the diagnosis. The more criteria are fulfilled the more likely the diagnosis becomes).

Clinical Significance

Bi-atrial enlargement is found in conditions giving rise to bi-ventricular enlargement. This includes congenital heart disease, hypertrophic cardiomyopathy and pulmonary hypertension occurring either with aortic valve disease or with mitral incompetence. The reservations expressed about the use of the term "atrial hypertrophy" with reference to hypertrophy of individual atria apply equally well with reference to hypertrophy of both atria.

Atrial Repolarisation Wave

It was pointed out (page 5) that electrical recovery of myocardium must occur following depolarisation of that myocardium before any subsequent repeat depolarisation is possible. In the case of the ventricular myocardium, depolarisation and repolarisation are both recognisable from the surface electrocardiogram. The **QRS complex is, in fact, the surface electrocardiographic manifestation of ventricular myocardial depolarisation** and **the T wave is the surface electrocardiographic manifestation of ventricular myocardial repolarisation** (though it should be noted that ventricular myocardial repolarisation is actually taking place during the S-T segment and, in some parts of the heart, even before the QRS complex is completed). **The P wave is the surface electrocardiographic manifestation of atrial myocardial depolarisation.** The process of repolarisation of the atrial myocardium does not give rise to a recognisable wave on the surface electrocardiogram (i.e. it has no surface electrocardiographic manifestation) even though repolarisation must necessarily occur before any subsequent, repeat depolarisation of the atrial myocardium is possible. The atrial repolarisation wave is called the "atrial T wave" or "Ta" wave. It is normally a shallow, smooth negative wave which, since it occurs at the same time as the much larger QRS complex, is normally totally obscured by the latter. It becomes apparent on the surface electrocardiogram only when it is increased in size. When the Ta wave becomes prominent it increases both in depth and in duration (Figure 115). It may then be apparent as a dip in the trace, seen both **before** and **after** the QRS complex. It is easily confused with a depressed S-T segment but recognition that the depression starts **before** the QRS complex should prevent this misunderstanding. Its appearance may be likened to a QRS complex standing slightly left of centre in a shallow saucer.

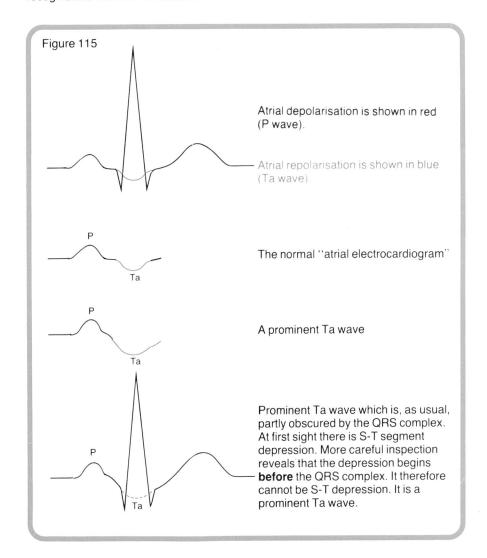

Figure 115

Atrial depolarisation is shown in red (P wave).

Atrial repolarisation is shown in blue (Ta wave).

The normal "atrial electrocardiogram"

A prominent Ta wave

Prominent Ta wave which is, as usual, partly obscured by the QRS complex. At first sight there is S-T segment depression. More careful inspection reveals that the depression begins **before** the QRS complex. It therefore cannot be S-T depression. It is a prominent Ta wave.

Causes of Prominent Atrial Repolarisation Waves

By far the commonest cause of an exaggerated Ta wave is **sinus tachycardia.** An example is shown in Figure 116. The ECG of Figure 116 would be reported as follows:-
"Sinus tachycardia. Rate 165/min. Prominent atrial repolarisation wave simulating S-T depression in some leads. Allowing for the heart rate, the record is within normal limits".

Prominent Ta waves may also occur in **right atrial hypertrophy.** Close inspection of Figure 112 shows a prominent Ta wave well seen in Leads II and aVF. Prominent Ta waves also occur in atrial infarction (see page 199).

Rarely a normal Ta wave can be seen in cases of complete heart block when the QRS complex does not obscure the wave.

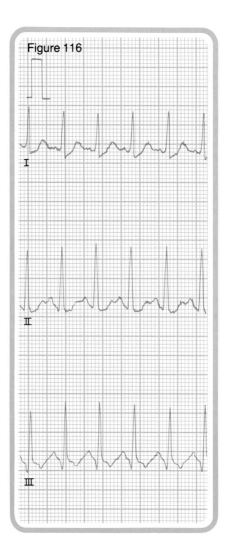

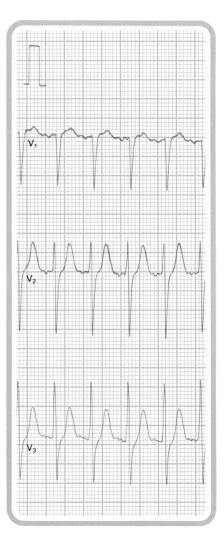

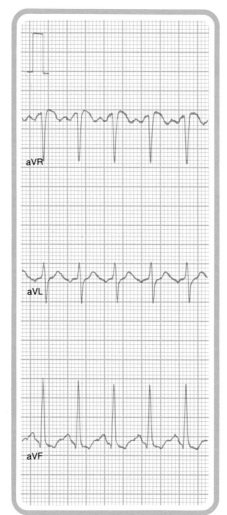

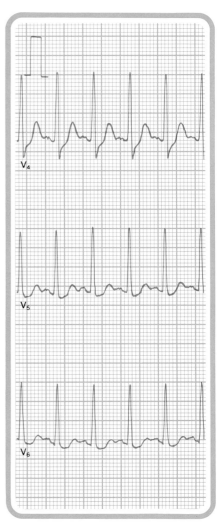

Figure 116

A 12-lead electrocardiogram taken just after the completion of an exercise test. The rhythm is sinus tachycardia and the heart rate is 165/min. There is apparent S-T depression in I, II, aVF and V_4-V_6, but closer inspection (especially in II where the T and Ta vectors are usually best seen) reveals that the negativity begins **before** the QRS complexes. It is a prominent Ta wave. There is no significant S-T abnormality and the exercise test is negative.

Ischaemic Heart Disease

The electrocardiogram is used more often in the investigation of suspected ischaemic heart disease than in that of any other condition. Since the viability of every part of the myocardium and of the conducting tissue is dependent upon the adequacy of perfusion of the tissue, it follows that coronary atheroma can induce ischaemic damage in any part of the myocardium or conducting tissue. **Ischaemia of the myocardium** may give rise to changes in the P waves, QRS complexes, S-T segments or T waves in any lead of the electrocardiogram and **ischaemia of the conducting tissue** can cause any conceivable arrhythmia. The range of cardiographic abnormalities which can occur in ischaemic heart disease is therefore vast. However, **it is perfectly possible to have severe, extensive, stenosing atheroma of the coronary arteries without there being any recognisable abnormality in the 12-lead electrocardiogram.** It must be remembered that the electrocardiogram provides information only about the **myocardium** (via the configuration and dimensions of P waves, QRS complexes, S-T segments and T waves) and about the **specialised conducting tissue** (via the electrocardiographic evidence of the cardiac rhythm). Electrocardiographic evidence of ischaemic heart disease is always **inferential.** If no ischaemic damage to the myocardium or conducting tissue has occurred (either permanently or transiently) the electrocardiogram can play no part in confirming or refuting a clinical impression of ischaemic heart disease. **For example, 50-75% of patients with unequivocal angina pectoris have normal resting 12-lead electrocardiograms when first seen.**

These two facts – namely that **almost any** ECG abnormality may occur in ischaemic heart disease and that even in the presence of severe ischaemic heart disease there may be **no abnormality** – bedevil attempts to acquire a balanced understanding of the electrocardiogram as a diagnostic tool in ischaemic heart disease. Nevertheless, it is possible to recognise the more important and the common electrocardiographic manifestation of ischaemic heart disease and these manifestations will be dealt with in this chapter.

The Electrocardiogram in Acute Myocardial Infarction

Changes in QRS complexes, in S-T segments or in T waves may occur in acute myocardial infarction and many of these changes may persist.

However, the only definitive, diagnostic changes of myocardial infarction (whether recent or old) are changes in the QRS complexes.

The QRS Complexes in Infarction

Two QRS abnormalities may be indicative of myocardial infarction. These are:-
1. Inappropriately low R wave voltage in a local area.
2. Abnormal Q waves.

Whilst these two changes may seem very dissimilar, they are actually part of the same process. The **development of a negative wave** (Q wave) and **the reduction in size of the positive wave** each result from loss of positivity which, in turn, is the result of necrosis of myocardium. This is so, simply because QRS changes of infarction are related to the reduction in the amount of, or to the total absence of, living myocardium underneath the exploring electrode. The size of the positive wave in each precordial lead is, both in normal and in abnormal circumstances, related to the thickness of viable myocardium underneath the electrode. In normal circumstances this thickness increases progressively from right to left in the precordial series (Figure 117).

Note

Figures in this chapter depicting the horizontal cross-section of the heart in the approximate level of the precordial leads omit the atria for the sake of simplicity. They show cross-sections through the ventricles below the level of the atrio-ventricular valves. (In this plane the right ventricular cavity is seen to be crescent-shaped and to be "wrapped round" the left ventricle). This simplification of the diagram is necessary to demonstrate the importance of depolarisation of the posterior wall of the heart on the appearances in the precordial leads when there is anterior infarction.

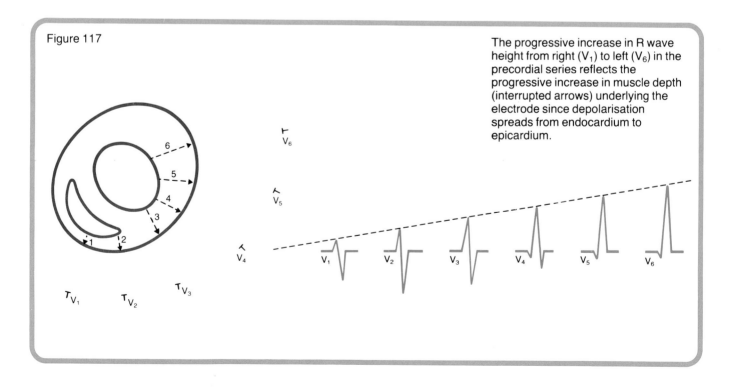

Figure 117

The progressive increase in R wave height from right (V_1) to left (V_6) in the precordial series reflects the progressive increase in muscle depth (interrupted arrows) underlying the electrode since depolarisation spreads from endocardium to epicardium.

Loss of R wave voltage

If infarction (i.e. total loss of viability) of part of the thickness of the left ventricular myocardium occurs in that part of the left ventricle underlying electrodes V_3 to V_5, the result will be a reduction in the R wave voltage under these electrodes (Figure 118).

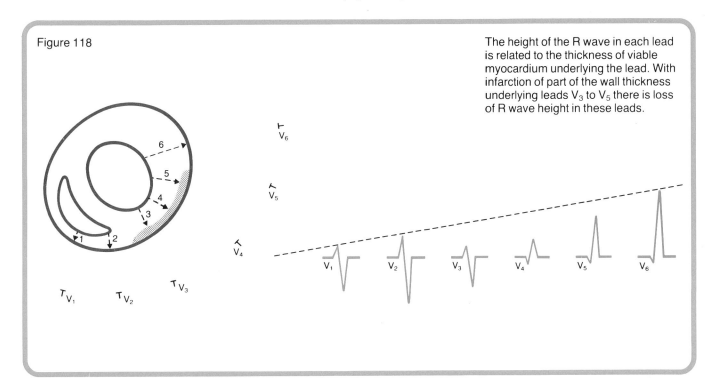

Figure 118

The height of the R wave in each lead is related to the thickness of viable myocardium underlying the lead. With infarction of part of the wall thickness underlying leads V_3 to V_5 there is loss of R wave height in these leads.

Loss of R wave height can only be judged to be present if **either** a previous record is available showing a significantly greater R wave height in the appropriate leads before the infarction occurred **or** the leads involved are two or more of the leads V_2-V_5. The criteria cannot be applied to V_1 or to V_6 since it is necessary to interpolate between these leads in order to estimate what the true R wave height should be (dotted line, Figure 117). At least two leads within the group V_2-V_5 must show evidence of R wave reduction for this criterion to be used to indicate myocardial infarction since (as noted on page 45) occasionally in a normal precordial series one R wave may be smaller in V_2, V_3 or V_4 than in the lead to its immediate right in the precordial series (i.e. V_1, V_2 or V_3 respectively). Theoretically it is possible to have reduction in R wave height in V_5 alone in myocardial infarction, but in most cases infarction involves myocardium underlying at least two leads.

Note

Infarction must **not** be diagnosed on the basis of an R wave height in V_5 or V_6 less than that in V_4 for this is a common normal variation related to the greater depth of lung lying between V_5 and V_6, on the one hand, and the heart, on the other hand, compared with that lying between V_4 and the heart (Figure 42, page 33). However, infarction may be diagnosed from reduced R wave voltage in V_5 and V_6 if a record prior to infarction is available to indicate the true initial R wave height.

Abnormal Q waves and QS complexes

When infarction involves the full thickness of the myocardium ("transmural" infarction – i.e. from endocardium to epicardium) there will be **total** loss of R waves in leads overlying the infarcted zone (Figure 119).

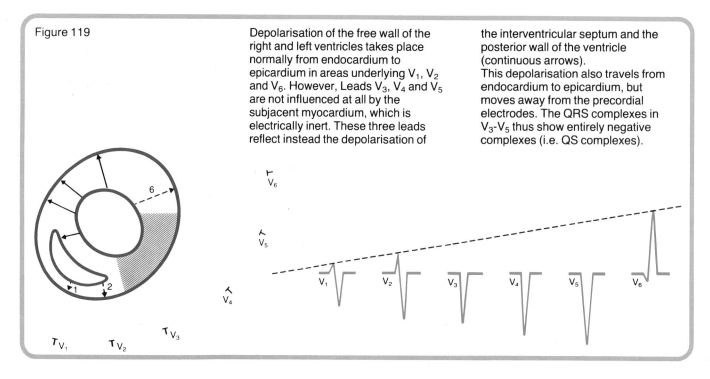

Figure 119

Depolarisation of the free wall of the right and left ventricles takes place normally from endocardium to epicardium in areas underlying V_1, V_2 and V_6. However, Leads V_3, V_4 and V_5 are not influenced at all by the subjacent myocardium, which is electrically inert. These three leads reflect instead the depolarisation of the interventricular septum and the posterior wall of the ventricle (continuous arrows).

This depolarisation also travels from endocardium to epicardium, but moves away from the precordial electrodes. The QRS complexes in V_3-V_5 thus show entirely negative complexes (i.e. QS complexes).

Total loss of R waves in the precordial leads gives rise to entirely negative waves, i.e. by definition (page 5) to QS complexes. These negative waves are the result of depolarisation of the posterior wall of the ventricle travelling from endocardium to epicardium (and therefore away from the anterior leads). These depolarisation waves from the posterior wall of the heart are, in normal circumstances, obscured by the dominant depolarisation of the anterior wall of the ventricles which lie much closer to the precordial leads.

When infarction involves less than the full thickness of the myocardium but still involves a major part of the wall thickness, less severe changes occur in which the R waves, whilst appreciably reduced in size, are still present and there are abnormal Q waves (see later, page 174) but, since there are residual R waves, no actual QS complexes (Figure 120). The finding of abnormal Q waves and reduced R wave voltage is the commonest electrocardiographic appearance in established infarction.

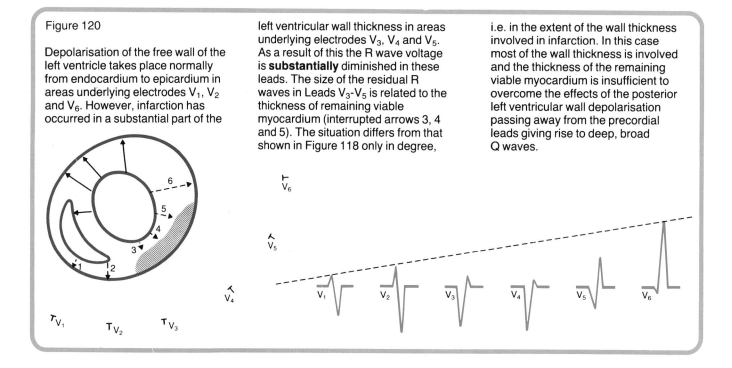

Figure 120

Depolarisation of the free wall of the left ventricle takes place normally from endocardium to epicardium in areas underlying electrodes V_1, V_2 and V_6. However, infarction has occurred in a substantial part of the left ventricular wall thickness in areas underlying electrodes V_3, V_4 and V_5. As a result of this the R wave voltage is **substantially** diminished in these leads. The size of the residual R waves in Leads V_3-V_5 is related to the thickness of remaining viable myocardium (interrupted arrows 3, 4 and 5). The situation differs from that shown in Figure 118 only in degree, i.e. in the extent of the wall thickness involved in infarction. In this case most of the wall thickness is involved and the thickness of the remaining viable myocardium is insufficient to overcome the effects of the posterior left ventricular wall depolarisation passing away from the precordial leads giving rise to deep, broad Q waves.

The reduction in R wave voltage is the result of reduction in the thickness of viable myocardium underlying the recording electrode. This reduction in viable myocardial thickness in the anterior wall of the ventricle permits the influence of the posterior wall depolarisation to dominate and abnormal Q waves develop in the relevant precordial leads (produced by depolarisation of the posterior wall travelling from endocardium to epicardium away from the anterior leads).

The reduction in R wave voltage can only be recognised if **either** a previous record is available showing a significantly greater R wave height in the appropriate leads before the infarction occurred, **or** the leads involved are two or more of the leads V_2 to V_5 (see page 170).

We therefore have four possible QRS changes indicative of infarction:-
1. Reduced R wave voltage (where this can confidently be ascertained)
2. Abnormal Q waves without any conclusive evidence of R wave reduction
3. Reduced R wave voltage in association with abnormal Q waves and,
4. QS complexes

These four changes are part of a common process and represent increasing thickness of infarction. With a non-uniform thickness of infarction, combinations of these findings may occur (Figure 121).

Figure 121

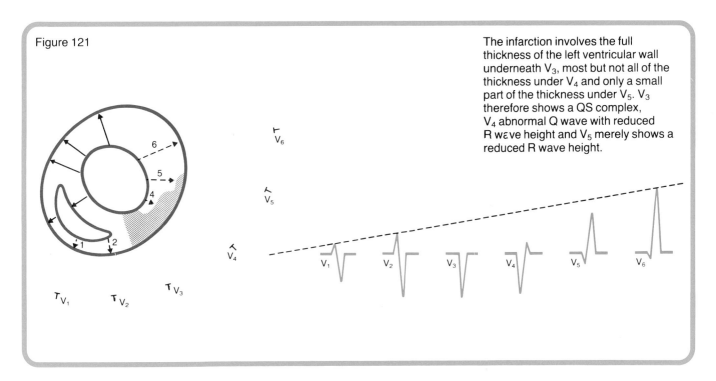

The infarction involves the full thickness of the left ventricular wall underneath V_3, most but not all of the thickness under V_4 and only a small part of the thickness under V_5. V_3 therefore shows a QS complex, V_4 abnormal Q wave with reduced R wave height and V_5 merely shows a reduced R wave height.

At this stage it is important to redefine the situations in which Q waves and QRS complexes are normal or abnormal.

Normal Q waves

In the precordial leads the normal q wave is found only to the left of the interventricular septum (since it is produced by septal depolarisation) passing from left to right (page 32)). When the heart position is indeterminate (pages 34–37) these normal q waves will be seen in V_4, V_5 and V_6 (Figure 46). With pronounced clockwise cardiac rotation they may appear in V_6 only or possibly only in leads even further to the left (Lead I and aVL) (Figures 46 and 47). In the presence of counter-clockwise cardiac rotation they may be seen from V_2 to V_6 (Figure 46), or with extreme counter-clockwise cardiac rotation from V_1 to V_6 (Figure 47).

In the limb leads the normal septal q waves will be seen in those leads which show a left ventricular configuration. The leads involved will depend upon the axis of the heart. When the heart is horizontal, i.e. the axis is in the region of zero to $-30°$ (page 53), the normal qR complex of the left precordial leads will be transmitted to Leads I and aVL and these leads will show normal q waves. When the heart is vertical (i.e. the axis is in the region of $+60°$ to $+90°$ (page 53)), the normal qR complex of the left precordial leads will be transmitted to Leads II and aVF and these leads will show normal q waves. With an axis in the region of $0°$ to $+60°$ Leads I and II will show normal q waves.

Normal QS complexes

QS complexes indicate that the whole process of depolarisation of viable ventricular myocardium takes places away from the lead in question. Since in all parts of the ventricles depolarisation is from endocardium to epicardium, it follows that **any lead which "looks into" the cavity of the heart will see QS complexes.** This is the usual, normal situation in the case of aVR and, depending on the axis of the heart, can also be normal for III or for aVL (Figure 122).

Figure 122

The arrow indicates the direction of the mean frontal plane QRS axis in each case.

Note in this figure that the heart is shown to be **physically** vertical or horizontal, this is intended to facilitate understanding of what is an **electrical** rather than a physical concept. For example the horizontal heart is one in which the main (left ventricular) electrical forces are directed horizontally and to the left.

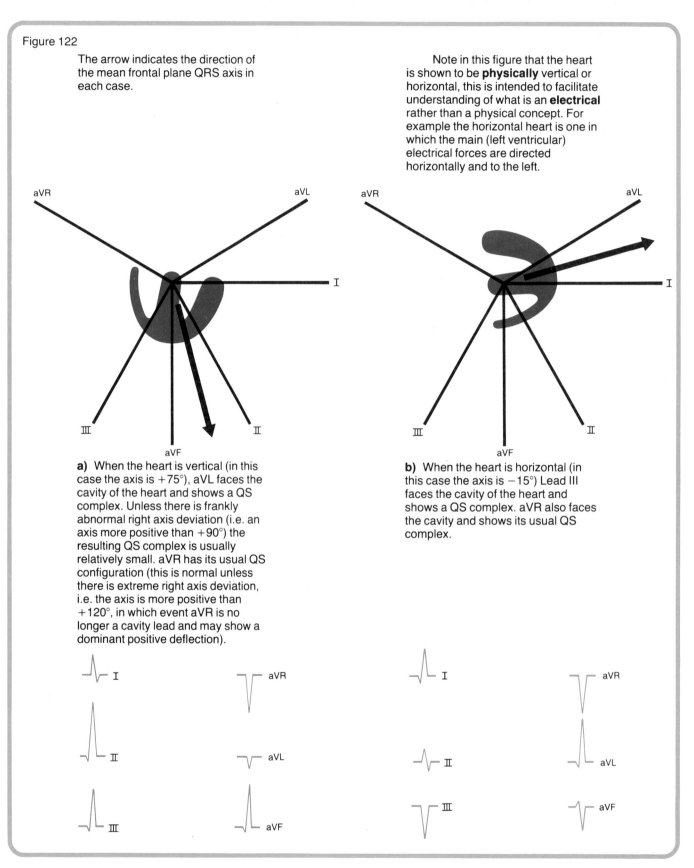

a) When the heart is vertical (in this case the axis is +75°), aVL faces the cavity of the heart and shows a QS complex. Unless there is frankly abnormal right axis deviation (i.e. an axis more positive than +90°) the resulting QS complex is usually relatively small. aVR has its usual QS configuration (this is normal unless there is extreme right axis deviation, i.e. the axis is more positive than +120°, in which event aVR is no longer a cavity lead and may show a dominant positive deflection).

b) When the heart is horizontal (in this case the axis is −15°) Lead III faces the cavity of the heart and shows a QS complex. aVR also faces the cavity and shows its usual QS complex.

Thus when the heart is vertical (Figure 122 (a)) Leads II, III and aVF show **normal septal q** waves (qR complexes), and aVL shows a **normal QS complex.** (aVR shows a QS complex as usual).

When the heart is horizontal (Figure 122 (b)) Leads I and aVL show normal **septal q waves,** and III shows a **normal QS complex** (aVR shows a QS complex as usual).

In pronounced clockwise cardiac rotation V_1 (and very occasionally V_2) may also show QS complexes (Figure 47).

Abnormal QS complexes

QS complexes in leads other than those looking into the cavity of the heart are abnormal.

Abnormal q waves

Q waves may be recognised to be abnormal because of:-
1. Abnormal width (duration)
    or
2. Abnormal depth (relative to the following R wave).

Q waves of 0.04 sec or longer duration **are abnormal** (provided they are not normal QS complexes – *vide supra*).

Q waves with a depth which is more than 25% of the height of the ensuing R wave are abnormal (Figure 123).

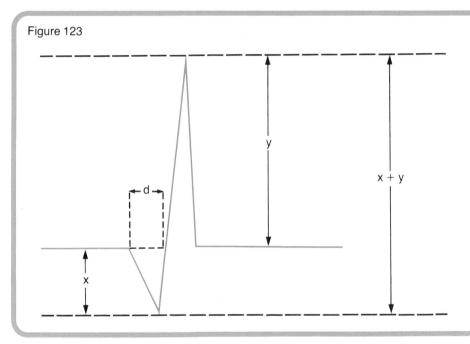

Figure 123

A qR type of QRS complex is shown diagrammatically. The q wave duration (d) is measured from the onset of the q wave to the point where the upstroke of the R wave crosses the horizontal line. The q wave depth is x. The criterion for abnormality is that $x > y/4$ (i.e. for normality $x \leqslant y/4$). Note that the height of the r waves (y) is not the same as the total QRS height (x+y). The criterion for abnormality could also be stated as $x > \frac{x+y}{5}$, and this is exactly the same criterion.

The essential electro-cardiographic criteria for the diagnosis of myocardial infarction from the QRS complexes are therefore as follows:-
1. Reduction in r wave height (from a normal level assessed either by a previous record antidating infarction or by interpolation in the precordial leads)*
    or
2. The occurrence of QS complexes in V_1*, V_2, V_3, V_4, V_5, V_6, I, II, aVF, aVL[+]
    or
3. Abnormally deep or abnormally wide q waves in V_1*, V_2, V_3, V_4, V_5, V_6, I, II, aVF, aVL[+]. q waves are abnormal if **either** they equal or exceed 0.04 sec in duration **or** if their depth exceeds one quarter of the height of the ensuing R wave.

Notes
1.* Reduction in r wave height cannot be used as a criterion in the limb leads for r wave height in the limb leads is dependent upon the mean frontal plane QRS axis and the range of possible positions for the normal axis is appreciable.
2.* In the presence of pronounced clockwise rotation QS complexes may appear normally in V_1 and occasionally in V_2.
3.[+] In the presence of a vertical heart QS complexes may be present normally in aVL.
4. Lead III is omitted from these considerations. This is because Lead III can have a deep Q wave even when the ECG is completely normal (when the heart is horizontal (above) or whenever the positive wave in aVL exceeds that in aVF (page 54)).
5. In the presence of left bundle branch block or ventricular pre-excitation none of the above criteria may be used.

Examples of electrocardiograms showing abnormal q waves are shown in Figures 124 and 125.

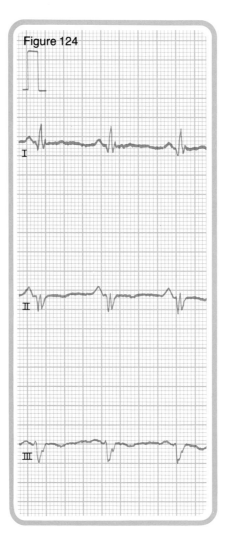

Figure 124

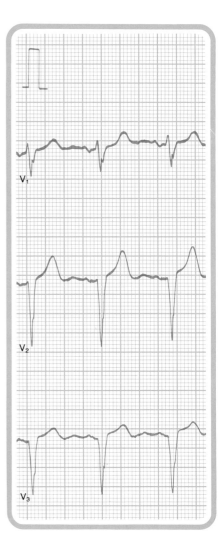

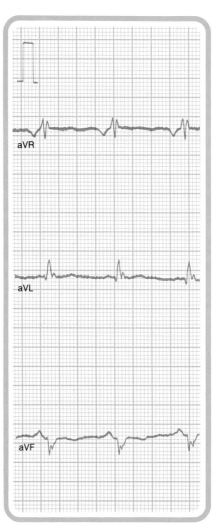

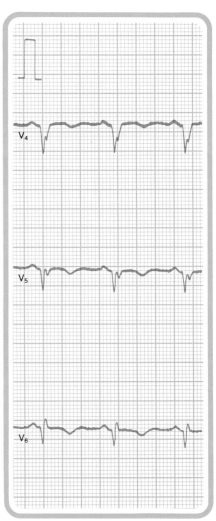

Figure 124

The rhythm is sinus. The r wave in V_1 is normal. The r wave in V_2 is smaller than that in V_1. This may in itself be an abnormality, indicative of infarction, but occasionally in a normal electrocardiogram the r wave in one of the leads V_2, V_3 or V_4 may be smaller than that in the leads immediately to its right in the precordial series in the transition zone area (page 45). V_3, V_4 and V_5 show QS complexes indicative of transmural infarction in the area of myocardium underlying these electrodes. V_6 shows a Qr complex. The r wave is clearly smaller than it should be (even though we cannot "bracket" this r wave with those from leads on either side of it), and the Q wave is abnormally deep (it has a depth exceeding one quarter the height of the ensuing r wave) and is also abnormally wide (in this case it is clearly more than 0.04 sec in duration). On the basis of **either** of these criteria the Q waves are abnormal. Superficial examination suggests that there are abnormal Q waves in Leads II, III and aVF but close examination reveals a small initial r wave in each of these leads (difficult to see in Lead II except in the third QRS complex in that lead). It may well be that these r waves have been reduced in height as a result of infarction, but one cannot be sure of this. In the case of the limb leads such dramatic variations in r wave appearances can simply represent variations in the frontal plane axis. The axis in this case is very abnormal at $-75°$. In the absence of definitive evidence of inferior (see page 180) infarction, this axis most probably indicates left anterior hemiblock (page 197).

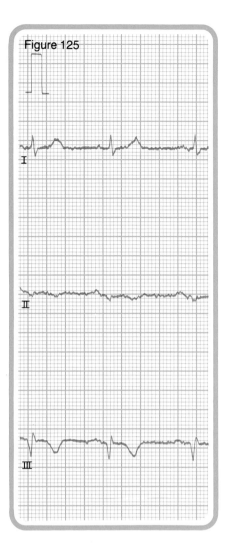

Figure 125

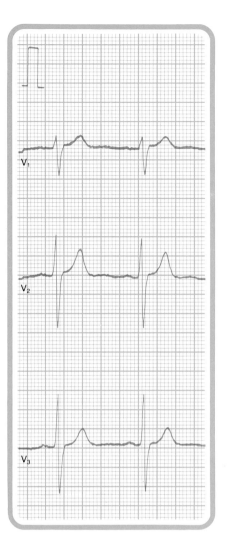

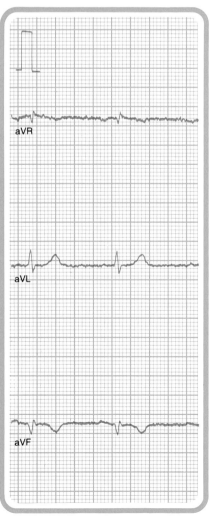

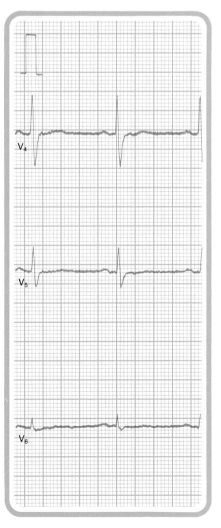

Figure 125

The rhythm is sinus. The R wave in the left precordial leads looks abnormally small but one cannot be **totally** confident of the signficance of this without a previous record for comparison. In the normal ECG the R wave in V_6 is often smaller than that in V_5, and that in V_5 is often smaller than that in V_4 (page 33 and Figure 42). However, it is unusual for the R wave in V_4 to be smaller than that in V_3. In addition the R wave in V_6 is very much smaller than one normally sees. The **probability** therefore is that the R waves in the left precordial leads are abnormally small. This **could** indicate infarction but **one cannot be sure of this.** However, there are definitively abnormal Q waves in Leads II, III and aVF (in each case the Q waves are abnormally deep (more than one quarter of the height of the ensuing R wave) and abnormally wide (clearly exceeding 0.04 sec)). These Q waves therefore indicate infarction.

The S-T Segment Changes of Infarction

It has already been stressed that it is only the QRS changes which provide **definitive** evidence of infarction. However, in the early stages of infarction S-T segment elevation usually occurs and may occasionally be dramatic in degree. Such changes are indicative of **injury** rather than **infarction.** The injury state is an unstable one. Acute S-T segment elevation **always** resolves to some extent (and **usually** resolves completely). The resolution of the acute S-T segment elevation is **usually** accompanied by development of the QRS changes of frank infarction, but **occasionally** the S-T segment elevation may resolve without the development of these diagnostic changes of infarction.

The essential change of myocardial injury is S-T segment elevation above the iso-electric line. The iso-electric line is the horizontal line indicating the position of the recording pen when there is no cardiac activity, i.e. between heart beats (that is between the end of the T wave and beginning of the next P wave). The normal S-T segment does not deviate by more than one millimetre above or below the iso-electric line (page 42). In the early stages of acute myocardial infarction, S-T segment elevation occurs (Figure 126).

The S-T segment shift is produced by injury to the myocardial cell membrane. As a result of that injury the current flow across the membrane is disturbed. The disturbance only occurs in injured myocardium, the pattern in healthy myocardium being unchanged. The normal iso-electric S-T segment in any lead depends upon the balance between normal myocardium in parts of the heart facing (close to) and opposite (remote from) a given lead. When the injury current flows in the cell membrane of part of the myocardium, the balance is disturbed and S-T segment shift occurs.

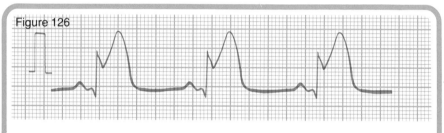

Figure 126

The rhythm is sinus. The rate is relatively slow. Because of the slow rate a clear iso-electric line is visible between the end of each T wave and the beginning of each P wave. The S-T segment is clearly elevated some 5mm above the iso-electric line.

Note 1
As explained earlier (page 42) in the presence of tachycardia, there may be no interval between the end of the T wave and the beginning of the next P wave and no iso-electric line would be visible. In that event, S-T segment elevation may only be regarded as significant if it is striking (Figure 52).

Note 2
Minor degrees of apparent S-T segment elevation may be present in leads in which the S-T segment merges imperceptibly into the T wave. This is often the case in normal records in the right precordial leads. One should be very cautious about regarding minor degrees of S-T segment shift in V_1 and V_2 as being significant (e.g. V_2 Record 11, page 82; V_2 Record 14, page 85; V_2 Record 24, page 95).

Abnormal S-T segment elevation of the type described occurs in leads facing the infarction, both in transmural myocardial infarction and in sub-epicardial infarction. As will be seen later (page 182) **"reciprocal" S-T segment depression** may be seen (at the same time as the above primary changes) in leads precording from positions opposite to the infarct. **Primary S-T segment depression** may be seen in leads facing in the infarct when the infarct is sub-endocardial (page 183).

The T Wave Changes of Infarction

A whole variety of T wave changes may occur in association with myocardial infarction. These include flattening of the T waves, di-phasic T waves, inverted T waves and abnormally tall T waves. None of these changes is specific. There is a tendency to regard non-specific T wave changes as unimportant, i.e. to equate "non-specific" with "not significant". This is quite unjustifiable. "Non-specific" simply means that a specific cause cannot be assigned to a change which is **definitely abnormal.** For example, minor T wave flattening may be the only ECG abnormality in a patient with severe coronary artery disease. Non-specific T wave changes occur in myocardial ischaemia, ventricular hypertrophy, intraventricular conduction defects, myocarditis, cardiomyopathy, pericarditis, electrolyte disturbances (particularly potassium changes) in response to certain drugs (especially digitalis) in hypothyroidism, subarachnoid haemorrhage, occasionally in pregnancy and even in response to drinking cold water. Since changes in body position can affect the physical position of the heart within the thorax, such changes in position can affect the QRS axis and therefore also

the T wave axis. Such slight changes in axis (which are usually of the order of 15-30°) can produce changes in the T waves in the limb leads. By convention, of course, the standard 12-lead electrocardiogram is recorded with the patient in the recumbent position. It can be seen from the list of possible causes of T wave changes given above that though these changes are abnormal (i.e. they are not found in the vast majority of normal persons) they may occasionally (though unusually) have a non-pathological explanation. The most obvious two examples of this are pregnancy and drinking cold water. In these cases the explanation is usually apparent! It would certainly be unwise, for example, to diagnose pregnancy on the basis of such changes! Equally one cannot be **certain** that pregnancy is the cause unless one has a record taken for the pregnancy and one subsequent to the pregnancy, neither of which shows the T wave change in question. This is another example of the importance of primary and secondary interpretation of the electrocardiogram (page 109).

The most typical T wave change of acute myocardial infarction is deep, symmetrical T wave inversion (Figure 127).

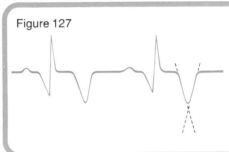

Figure 127

There is an abnormal Q wave. The S-T segment is normal but there is deep, symmetrical T wave inversion. The "symmetry" refers to the equality of the angles downstroke and upstroke of the T wave.

Deep-symmetrical T wave inversion may occur in association with the sequential changes of acute transmural or sub-epicardial myocardial infarction, but may also occur in the absence of

QRS changes (i.e. as a primary change in sub-endocardial infarction). In such a case the T wave changes are usually apparent in many leads.

Abnormal T waves in inferior[*] infarction

The criterion for normality of the T waves in the limb leads was quoted on page 56 as being a T wave axis not differing from the QRS axis by more than ±45°. At that stage (and again on page 58) it was indicated that, **in the special situation of inferior myocardial infarction,** negative (inverted) T waves in II and aVF are regarded as abnormal even if the angle between the mean frontal plane QRS and T axes does not exceed 45°.

Examples are seen in Record 26, page 97 and in Figure 125. Both

examples show abnormal q waves in II, III and aVF indicative of inferior infarction and the T waves are inverted in these leads. This is abnormal even though the frontal plane QRS axis and the frontal plane T axis do not differ by more than 45°. (In Record 26 the QRS axis is −30° and the T wave axis −75°. In Figure 125 the QRS axis is −45° and the T wave axis is −45°.

Note
[*] The location of changes in myocardial infarction is described later (page 180).

The Sequence of Changes in Acute Myocardial Infarction

Although any part or all of the spectrum of changes described above may occur in myocardial infarction, a common, typical sequence of changes is recognised. The more completely the described changes are present and the more closely the usual sequential patterns are followed, the more confident one can be of the diagnosis and of the timing of the infarction. The sequential changes of acute myocardial infarction in a single lead are shown in Figure 128.

Figure 128

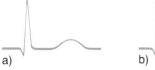 a) 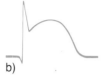 b) 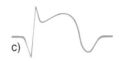 c) 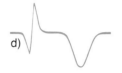 d) 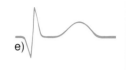 e)

a) Shows the control, normal appearances in a lead, which by the QRS morphology, clearly lies over the left ventricle.

b) Within **hours** of the clinical onset of infarction there is S-T segment elevation. At this stage no QRS changes or T wave changes have occurred. Although such a pattern is frequently spoken of, loosely, as showing "acute infarction", no definitive evidence of infarction is shown. There is evidence of myocardial damage. There is an unstable situation. In the vast majority of cases evolutionary changes of infarction follow. Occasionally the record returns to normal.

c) Within **days** the R wave voltage has fallen and abnormal Q waves (in this case both in duration and in depth relative to the R wave height) have appeared. These changes are sufficient to prove the occurrence of infarction. In addition T wave inversion has appeared. The S-T elevation is less pronounced than in (b).

d) Within **one or more weeks** the S-T segment changes revert completely to normal. The R wave voltage remains reduced and the abnormal Q waves persist. Deep symmetrical T wave inversion may develop at this stage. In some patients this pattern remains permanently, in others it progresses to the appearances shown in (e).

e) **Months** after the clinical infarction the T waves may gradually return to normal. The abnormal Q waves and reduced R wave voltage persist.

Note the following:

1. S-T elevation is an unstable situation and indicates a recent event. It nearly always precedes evolutionary changes of infarction.

2. Reduced R wave voltage and the development of abnormal Q waves indicate infarction. These changes are usually permanent. Occasionally even these changes may regress. When this occurs it does not indicate regeneration of myocardium, but rather shrinkage of the extent of scar tissue underlying the electrode with the pulling closer together of adjacent areas of healthy myocardium. As a result of this shrinkage of scar tissue, leads which after an infarction show either abnormal q wave (or reduced R waves) may subsequently show r waves (or increase in R wave size). This is termed "regeneration of the R waves". As noted above it does not indicate regeneration of myocardium.

3. QRS evidence of infarction with elevated S-T segments indicates recent infarction (i.e. within days). QRS evidence of infarction with normal S-T segments and deep, symmetrical T wave inversion indicates infarction of intermediate age (weeks or a month or two). QRS evidence of infarction with normal S-T segments and T waves indicates old (months to years) infarction.

4. Occasionally, all evidence of infarction may be lost with the passing of time – due to shrinkage of scar tissue.

The Location of Changes in Myocardial Infarction

Primary electrocardiographic changes of the type described will occur in leads overlying the infarct. The leads in which such primary changes occur will, conversely, indicate the location of the infarct. This is shown in Table 4 and illustrated in Figures 129 and 130.

Table 4

Location of Infarction	Leads showing Primary Changes
	Typical Changes
Anterior Infarction Anteroseptal	V_1, V_2, V_3
Anterior	Some of the group V_1-V_3 plus some of the group V_4-V_6
Anterolateral	V_4, V_5, V_6, I, aVL, and possibly II
Extensive anterior	V_1, V_2, V_3, V_4, V_5, V_6, I, aVL
High lateral	aVL (plus high precordial leads)
Inferior Infarction Inferior	II, III, aVF
Inferolateral = (apical)	II, III, aVF, V_5, V_6 and sometimes also I and aVL
Inferoseptal	II, III, aVF, V_1, V_2, V_3
	Other Changes (see text)
Posterior Infarction	V_1, V_2 (Inverse of the usual changes elsewhere)
Subendocardial Infarction	Any lead (usually multiple leads)

High lateral infarcts show in aVL only, but if high precordial leads are used they may show similar changes. These leads are placed in the same horizontal distribution as the standard precordial leads but are placed one (labelled V'1, V'2, V'3 etc) or two (labelled V"1, V"2, V"3 etc) interspaces higher.

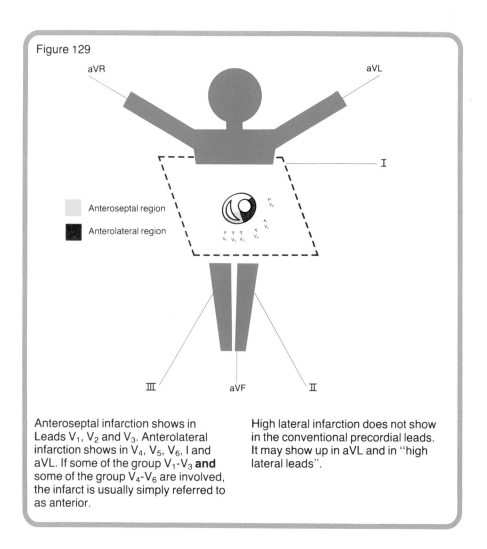

Figure 129

Anteroseptal region

Anterolateral region

Anteroseptal infarction shows in Leads V_1, V_2 and V_3. Anterolateral infarction shows in V_4, V_5, V_6, I and aVL. If some of the group V_1-V_3 **and** some of the group V_4-V_6 are involved, the infarct is usually simply referred to as anterior.

High lateral infarction does not show in the conventional precordial leads. It may show up in aVL and in "high lateral leads".

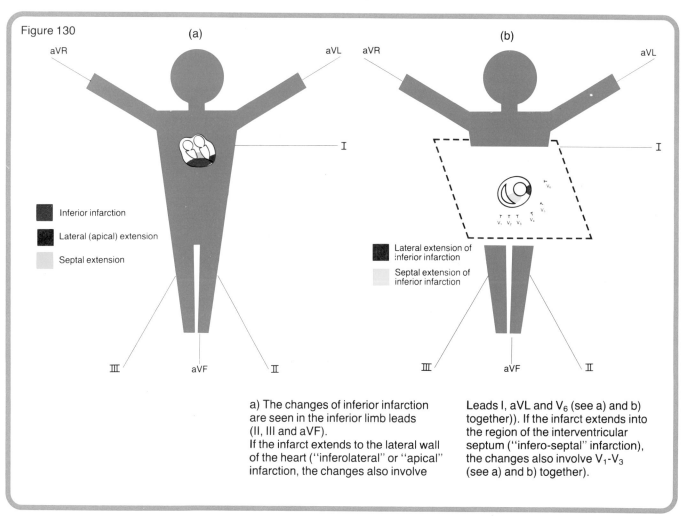

Figure 130

(a)

(b)

Inferior infarction

Lateral (apical) extension

Septal extension

Lateral extension of inferior infarction

Septal extension of inferior infarction

a) The changes of inferior infarction are seen in the inferior limb leads (II, III and aVF).
If the infarct extends to the lateral wall of the heart ("inferolateral" or "apical" infarction, the changes also involve

Leads I, aVL and V_6 (see a) and b) together)). If the infarct extends into the region of the interventricular septum ("infero-septal" infarction), the changes also involve V_1-V_3 (see a) and b) together).

Reciprocal Changes

In addition to the primary changes which occur in leads facing the infarcted area, "reciprocal" changes occur in leads opposite to the infarction. Reciprocal changes are the inverse of primary changes, i.e. S-T segment depression instead of S-T segment elevation and tall-pointed T waves instead of symmetrical T wave inversion. The reciprocal changes can easily be visualised by turning the primary changes upside down (Figure 131).

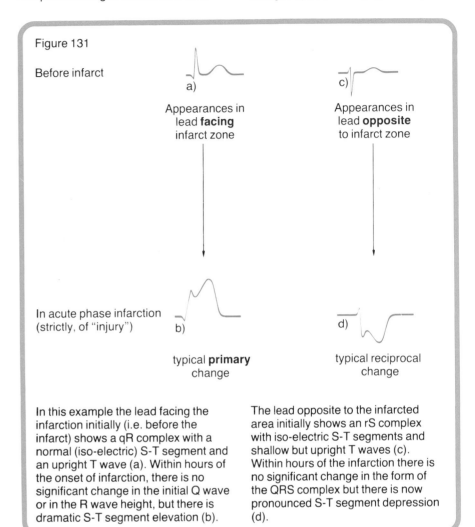

Figure 131

Before infarct

a)

Appearances in lead **facing** infarct zone

c)

Appearances in lead **opposite** to infarct zone

In acute phase infarction (strictly, of "injury")

b)

typical **primary** change

d)

typical reciprocal change

In this example the lead facing the infarction initially (i.e. before the infarct) shows a qR complex with a normal (iso-electric) S-T segment and an upright T wave (a). Within hours of the onset of infarction, there is no significant change in the initial Q wave or in the R wave height, but there is dramatic S-T segment elevation (b).

The lead opposite to the infarcted area initially shows an rS complex with iso-electric S-T segments and shallow but upright T waves (c). Within hours of the infarction there is no significant change in the form of the QRS complex but there is now pronounced S-T segment depression (d).

The inferior limb leads on the one hand and the precordial leads, together with Leads I and Lead aVL, on the other hand are mutually "opposite" in that primary changes in one of these groups will frequently be accompanied by reciprocal changes in the other group. Although, as we shall see later, S-T segment depression may, when present alone, be a primary change, it is safe to assume that **when S-T segment elevation is present in one group of leads and S-T segment depression in another, in the same cardiogram, the elevation is the primary and the depression the secondary change.**

True Posterior Infarction

Infarction showing primary changes in II, III and aVF is properly termed inferior infarction, for these are the "inferior" limb leads. Previous terminology referred to this as "posterior" infarction, but this was anatomically incorrect. **True** "posterior" infarction is relatively rare and is not easily recognised since no leads in the conventional 12-lead recording are posteriorly situated. It can only be recognised by looking in the **anterior** leads for **reciprocal** changes. There are no primary changes since there are no true posterior leads. The evidence of true posterior infarction is therefore the presence of abnormally tall and broad R waves in V_1 (reciprocal to abnormally deep and broad Q in a posterior lead, if one existed). If the infarct is very recent S-T depression may be present in V_1, if it is of intermediate age, tall T waves may be present in V_1, V_2 and V_3 may be similarly affected (Figure 132).

Figure 132

True posterior infarction showing in V_1

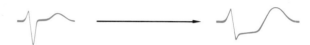

Normal appearance prior to infarction

Appearance in acute stage of true posterior infarction. The r wave has become taller and broader (the reciprocal of abnormally deep and broad q waves in leads showing primary changes). The S-T segment is depressed (the reciprocal of S-T elevation in leads showing primary changes). The T waves are taller than normal (the reciprocal of T wave inversion).

True posterior infarction. This is most easily recognised in V_1. The R wave becomes broader and taller than normal (its breadth exceeds 0.04 sec)

and in the initial stages there is also S-T segment depression and increase in height of the T waves.

True posterior infarction is often accompanied by inferior or by anterolateral infarction. An example is shown in Figure 141.

Subendocardial Infarction

Most infarcts are regional, intramural infarcts (sub-epicardial or transmural). When the term "myocardial infarction" is used without a qualifying adjective, **regional** infarction is implied. **Sub-endocardial** infarcts are relatively rare. When they do occur they not infrequently encircle the interior of the left ventricle and are therefore **zonal** rather than regional infarcts. The electrocardiographic evidence consists of **primary** S-T segment depression (i.e. S-T segment depression in some leads without simultaneous S-T segment elevation in other leads, with the possible exception of cavity leads) or of deep-symmetrical T wave inversion without any change in the QRS complexes. Each of these changes can be produced by myocardial ischaemia without infarction and for this reason the diagnosis of sub-endocardial infarction cannot be made on a single electrocardiogram alone. Either a single such record accompanied by clinical or enzyme evidence of infarction (i.e. necessarily accompanied by secondary interpretation) or serial records which **persistently** show primary S-T segment depression or deep symmetrical T wave inversion is required for the diagnosis to be made. When the primary change is S-T depression it will be visible in all or most leads with the exception of the cavity leads (aVR is always a cavity lead, aVL is a cavity lead when the heart is vertical, and aVF is a cavity lead when the heart is horizontal). The cavity leads alone may show reciprocal S-T segment elevation. This is the only exception to the rule that "when S-T segment elevation and S-T depression are both present in the same recording, it is the elevation which is the primary change" By definition, cavity leads inevitably show QS complexes.

The Changes in Myocardial Ischaemia

Relative hypoxia of the myocardium, from local ischaemia, may occur in the absence of necrosis (infarction). Such changes may occur in relation to **exertion** (physical stress), in response to **emotion** (psychological stress) or **spontaneously** (i.e. in the absence of overt stress). Significant myocardial ischaemia can exist without any recognisable ECG abnormalities. When electrocardiographic changes do occur in relation to myocardial ischaemia they are confined to the S-T segments and T waves. **Myocardial ischaemia, in the absence of infarction, does not give rise to any changes in the QRS complexes.**

The following electrocardiographic changes may occur in myocardial ischaemia:-
1. Flattening of the T waves.
2. Inversion of the T waves.
3. Abnormally tall T waves (i.e. inferred increase in T wave height).
4. "Normalisation" of primarily abnormal T waves.
5. Sloping S-T segment depression.
6. Horizontal S-T segment depression.
7. S-T segment elevation.
8. Combinations of the above.

Flattening of the T Wave

One of the commonest findings in ischaemic heart disease is flattening (i.e. reduction in the voltage of) the T waves. Since there are no **definitive** criteria for the normal T wave height (page 40 and pages 56-58) it can only be stated that the T waves appear to be of low voltage. This is a non-specific change and may be associated with almost any condition affecting the myocardium or pericardium – ischaemia, ventricular hypertrophy, intraventricular conduction problems, electrolyte disturbances, drug effects, myocarditis, cardiomyopathy, hormone disturbances, pericarditis and even obesity. An example of such non-specific T wave flattening is seen in Record 12, page 83 (in Leads V_4, V_5 and V_6 and in all of the limb leads), in Record 22, page 93 (the T waves are of low voltage in all 12 leads of this record, but this is to be expected since the QRS voltages are low. Prominent U waves are seen in V_2 and V_3 – see page 149) and in Record 27, page 98 (in Leads V_4-V_6 and the limb leads). Though such T wave flattening is one of the commonest T wave changes in ischaemic heart disease its presence does not **prove** the existence of ischaemic heart disease, even if the changes occur in relation to stress.

Inversion of the T Wave

The term "T wave inversion" refers to negative T waves in leads in which the T wave is usually upright. The term is most properly applied in the precordial leads where negative T waves are always abnormal if present in any of the Leads V_3-V_6. Negative T waves in either V_1 or V_2 are abnormal if they were formerly upright in those leads (page 40) and negative T waves in V_2 are abnormal if the T waves are upright in V_1.

The term "T wave inversion" is also frequently applied when negative T waves are found in Leads I, II or aVF where the T waves are usually upright. However, it should be remembered that in the limb leads normality or otherwise of the T waves applies to **all** the leads collectively and not to each lead individually (page 58). In this respect the limb leads differ fundamentally from the precordial leads and one should strictly speaking refer not to T wave inversion in any given limb lead but to an abnormal angle between the mean frontal plane and T wave axes (pages 56-58).

T wave inversion is a non-specific change which can occur in myocardial ischaemia, ventricular hypertrophy, intraventricular conduction problems, electrolyte disturbances, drug effects, myocarditis, cardiomyopathy, intracranial haemorrhage, mitral valve prolapse, pulmonary embolism, pericarditis, after episodes of tachycardia and after Stokes-Adams seizures. T waves which are **deeply and symmetrically** inverted are likely to be of ischaemic origin. Abnormal T waves are shown in Record 3 (page 73). The T wave inversion in V_5 and V_6 is abnormal in this record. One may refer loosely to T wave inversion in I and aVL in this record, but more strictly the angle between the mean frontal plane QRS and T wave axes is abnormal (more than 45°) and thus in fact the limb lead T waves are abnormal (i.e. they are all abnormal). There is no QRS abnormality in this record and the T wave changes are therefore, by definition, **primary.** They could still have any of the causes listed above including myocardial ischaemia. They are not **diagnostic** of ischaemia.

In Record 5 (page 75) the T waves in the limb leads are abnormal and there is T wave inversion in V_4-V_6. However, in this case the precordial QRS complexes are abnormal. It is likely that the T wave changes are **secondary** to the QRS abnormality (which in this case is left ventricular hypertrophy).

Abnormally Tall T Waves

Since there are no accepted absolute criteria for normality of T wave height in any lead there can be no definitive criterion for abnormally tall T waves. The term cannot sensibly be applied at all to the limb leads for the T waves in all the limb leads are either (collectively) normal or (collectively) abnormal depending on the relationship of the T wave axis to the QRS axis (pages 56-58).

In the precordial leads the tallest T wave is usually in V_3 or V_4, the smallest in V_1 and V_2 and in general from V_3 to V_6 the T wave is not less than 1/8 and not more than 2/3 of the height of the R wave. Abnormally tall T waves can only be gauged against these approximate criteria. An example of an ECG which shows T waves of definitely abnormal height is shown in Figure 133.

Strikingly tall T waves are not definitely abnormal. They may be found as a normal variation in healthy individuals. In the precordial leads they may be indicative of ischaemia of the posterior wall of the heart (they are the inverse of the T wave inversion which would be shown in posterior leads directly over the ischaemic area if such leads existed). They also occur in the precordial leads in cases of recent true posterior infarction (again as the inverse of the T wave inversion which would be shown in posterior leads over the infarcted area if such leads existed). Tall precordial T waves are also seen in hyperkalaemia, in cases of intracranial haemorrhage, in left ventricular hypertrophy and in left bundle branch block (in both of the latter cases the abnormality of the QRS complex usually clearly indicates the diagnosis).

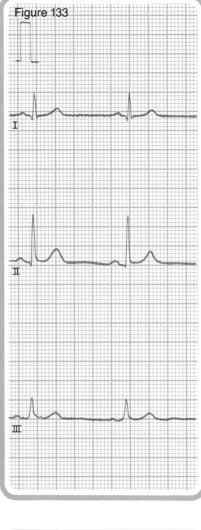

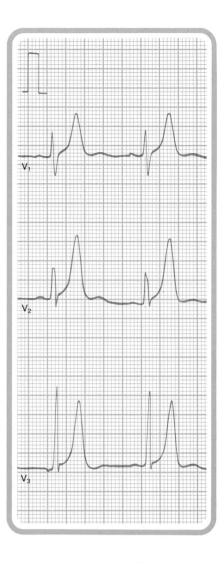

Figure 133

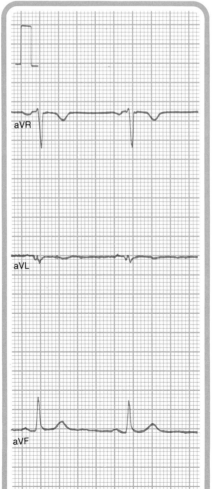

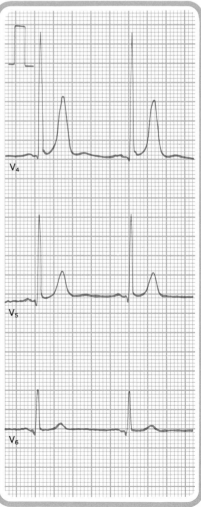

Figure 133

The rhythm is sinus. The T waves are upright in all the precordial leads. This feature is quite normal. The T waves are quite tall from V_1-V_4 and particularly so in V_2 and V_3. The T waves here are abnormally tall. This patient had ischaemia of the posterior wall of the ventricle proved by caesium scanning.

Normalisation of T Waves

If the T waves in certain leads are chronically inverted in a patient with ischaemic heart disease it occasionally happens that the T waves become upright during a further ischaemic episode, whether that ischaemic episode occurs spontaneously or in relation to emotional or physical stress. This process is referred to as "normalisation" of the T wave. It is definitely abnormal and is almost always indicative of myocardial ischaemia.

Primary Sloping S-T Segment Depression

The term "primary" indicates that the S-T segment depression is not secondary to S-T segment elevation in other leads, i.e. there is no simultaneous S-T segment elevation in other leads.

Downward sloping S-T segment depression is a non-specific abnormality which can be produced by ventricular hypertrophy, intraventricular conduction problems, cardiomyopathy, myocarditis, digitalis, hyperkalaemia and pericarditis as well as myocardial ischaemia. Sloping S-T segment depression occurring in association with the QRS changes of ventricular hypertrophy or intraventricular conduction defect should be regarded as part of the diagnosis relevant to the particular QRS abnormality. For example, the sloping S-T segment depression seen in Leads I, II, aVL and V_4–V_6 in Record 5 (page 75) should be seen as part of the appearance of left ventricular hypertrophy for the record shows definite QRS changes of that condition. Likewise the sloping S-T segment depression seen in Leads I, aVL, V_5 and V_6 in Record 7 (page 77) should be seen as part of the appearance of left bundle branch block for the record shows definite QRS changes of that condition. The sloping S-T segment depression seen in V_5 and V_6 in Record 12 (page 83) is seen in the absence of any QRS abnormality and is therefore primary. The cause of the S-T segment depression therefore cannot be determined from the electrocardiogram. Secondary interpretation (page 109) must be used, i.e. the **probable** cause should be assessed from the clinical picture. The **definitive** cause cannot be assessed. For example if the depression occurred in relation to stress and in association with chest pain, if there is no evidence of hyperkalaemia and the patient is not on digitalis, ischaemia is a probable cause.

Primary Horizontal S-T Segment Depression

The term "primary" indicates that the S-T segment depression is not secondary to S-T segment elevation in other leads, (i.e. there is no simultaneous S-T segment elevation in other leads) and is not occurring in association with the kind of QRS changes which often give rise to S-T depression (e.g. those of ventricular hypertrophy or of bundle branch block). (In cases where there are primary QRS abnormalities with appropriate secondary S-T changes, if new S-T segment changes develop without any changes in the QRS complexes these new changes are also deemed primary).

The finding of primary horizontal S-T segment depression is very strongly suggestive of subendocardial ischaemia or infarction. It is not nearly such a non-specific feature as most of the other S-T and T wave changes discussed above. Horizontal S-T segment depression may occur in spontaneous ischaemic episodes or in relation to angina induced by physical or emotional stress. It is not possible from a single record to say whether the S-T segment depression is induced by **ischaemia** of the myocardium or by **infarction** of the subendocardium. When subsequent records show return of the S-T segment to normal, it can be inferred that the horizontal S-T segment depression found in earlier records must have been indicative of ischaemia of the myocardium rather than of infarction of the subendocardium. When the changes are persistent it is likely that there has been infarction of the subendocardium. In addition, secondary interpretation may help. For example, if the levels of cardiac enzymes show an increase, the S-T segment depression is more likely to be indicative of infarction.

Subendocardial infarction is usually zonal rather than regional (page 183) and horizontal S-T segment depression is often seen in many leads – in fact frequently in all leads except those looking into the cavity of the heart.

S-T Segment Elevation

S-T segment elevation is usually part of the pattern of acute myocardial injury and often precedes the development of definitive changes of regional myocardial infarction. Occasionally primary S-T segment elevation may occur in relation to what is known as "Prinzmetal angina" or "variant angina". This is a form of angina which differs from the usual variety in several ways. The pain is not usually aggravated by exertion or by emotion, it tends to be more intense and more prolonged than exertional angina. It often occurs at the same time of day. If an ECG is obtained during an attack there may be transient S-T segment elevation which does not progress through the usual evolutionary changes of infarction (when S-T segment change occurs in relation to the usual form of angina – induced by exertion or emotion – it is usually S-T segment depression). The episodes are often associated with arrhythmias. Coronary angiography in such patients often shows a high grade obstruction in at least one major proximal coronary artery. Where the coronary arteries appear angiographically normal, coronary artery spasm in a similar site is thought to be responsible.

Primary S-T segment elevation in relation to anginal episodes is rare since "Prinzmetal angina" is rare.

Combinations of S-T Segment and T Wave Changes

Various combinations of the above-described S-T segment and T wave changes may occur. Usually such combinations are non-specific and frequently consist of flat or sloping S-T segment depression together with flattening of the T waves or possible inversion of the terminal part of the T wave ("Terminal T wave inversion").

Exercise Stress Testing

The object of stress test electrocardiography (which is almost synonymous with exercise electrocardiography – see below) is to create a haemodynamic situation in which part, at least, of the ventricular myocardium becomes hypoxic if the patient has stenosing atheroma of the coronary arteries. If the extent and severity of the myocardial hypoxia is sufficient to induce diagnostic changes in the electrocardiogram, the stress test will be positive. If not, the stress test will be negative. Depending upon the severity of the stress induced, the false negative rate of the procedure may be in the region of 10-30% (i.e. not infrequently a completely normal electrocardiogram may be obtained at the end of a rigorous stress test procedure despite the presence of significant coronary atheroma. It follows that a negative stress test does **not** exclude significant coronary artery disease).

Although the morbidity and mortality of the test are both extremely low, they are not zero and the physician must realise that there is at least a small risk in stressing a patient, whom he suspects of having ischaemic heart disease, to the point of myocardial ischaemia. If all appropriate precautions (including the provision of **adequate** cardio-pulmonary resuscitative procedures) are available, the mortality rate of the procedure is about 0.01% and the morbidity rate (i.e. the necessity for subsequent hospital admission for non-fatal complications) is about 0.02%. **Adequate** cardio-pulmonary resuscitative procedures include not only the immediate availability of the appropriate equipment and trained personnel, but also adequate in-patient back-up procedures with coronary and respiratory intensive care.

Although some centres do conduct exercise stress tests when the resting electrocardiogram is abnormal, interpretation of records from such tests is even more difficult than when the resting record is normal. Since the **primary** aim of exercise electrocardiography is to look for diagnostic evidence of ischaemic heart disease and since such evidence is often difficult or impossible to evaluate if the resting record is abnormal, in the author's opinion there is no point in exercise stress testing **for diagnostic purposes** if the resting record is abnormal. There is, however, a second reason for exercise stress testing – namely the assessment of a patient's exercise capability. If this is the reason for the test the electrocardiogram is used as a safety monitor rather than as a diagnostic aid. In this event the test can usefully be applied even when the resting record is abnormal (however, see later under "precautions"). These two aims, namely **the diagnosis of ischaemic heart disease** and the **assessment of exercise capability** are often blurred and are obscured by loose thinking. This reduces the precision of the observations and leads to uncertainties about the result.

Types of Stress Test

1. Master Two-step. This test requires only modest equipment. It involves walking up and down a two-step platform (similar to the type used in athletic medal presentation ceremonies). The patient climbs the two steps at one end, descends them at the other end and walks briskly round on the level in a circle to start again. This test is much less frequently used than formerly. The work load remains constant during the test and it is sometimes difficult to obtain a level of exercise sufficient to achieve an adequate heart rate response.

2. Atrial Pacing. In this test cardiac stress is applied by means of controlled tachycardia induced by atrial pacing using a temporary transvenous pacing electrode introduced into the right atrium. It has the advantage of producing rapid and accurate control of the heart rate (and unlike the situation with stress tests, the tachycardia can be stopped abruptly if necessary). However, it has major drawbacks – it is unphysiological (in exercise there is an appreciable peripheral vasodilatation, an increase in cardiac output and in stroke volume whereas in atrial pacing the cardiac output changes little and the stroke volume falls as the heart rate is increased) and it is an invasive procedure requiring full cardiac screening and catheterisation facilities. It is certainly not suitable for general usage.

3. Graded Exercise Test. This is the most commonly used procedure and involves the use of a treadmill or bicycle ergometer. The former is preferable (though more expensive) since all patients are accustomed to walking and few to cycling. The fundamental difference from the Master Two-step is that the work load is graded.

Protocol for a Graded (Treadmill) Exercise Test

There are numerous multistage exercise protocols available. There is no ideal protocol – the needs vary both as far as the patient and as far as the institution are concerned. The initial workload should be well within the patient's normal exercise capability. The final workload should be sufficient to achieve the target heart rate (see below). Intermediate workloads should be sufficient to provide a smooth progression of exercise levels.

The following protocol was devised by the author for use in the Manchester Royal Infirmary.

Manchester Royal Infirmary – Exercise Protocol

Precautions

1. Continuous supervision is necessary during and immediately after the procedure. **The test should only be carried out in the presence of a doctor and a technician or assistant.**

2. A defibrillator in good working order must be available.

3. Emergency drugs must be available, including glyceryl trinitrite, atropine and lignocaine.

4. Full emergency back-up facilities including the possibility of endotracheal intubation and coronary and respiratory intensive care should be available.

5. The patient should have the nature of the test explained to him and his informed consent obtained.

6. The patient should not currently be taking treatment with digitalis or beta-blockers. The former may produce ECG changes which increase during exercise, rendering interpretation of the test difficult. The latter usually precludes the achievement of an adequate heart rate response. Occasionally, diuretics, antidepressants and sedatives may cause false-positive responses.

7. It is important to ensure that the patient has not recently had a heavy meal.

8. It is important to exclude congestive heart failure, severe hypertension, history of myocardial infarction within the preceding 2–3 months and a history of recent (i.e. within weeks) onset of chest pain or recent change in the pattern of pain suggestive of crescendo angina or unstable angina.

9. The heart rate, the precordial ECG (usually a modified V_5 lead) and preferably also the blood pressure should be monitored during the procedure.

If the appropriate (rather more sophisticated) equipment is available the full 12-lead ECG should be monitored during the procedure.

Procedure

1. A standard 12-lead ECG is obtained and inspected by the supervising doctor. If this record shows evidence of S-T segment elevation or depression or serious arrhythmia (including ventricular tachycardia, multiple ventricular ectopics, R-on-T ectopics, atrial tachycardia, atrial flutter and possibly atrial fibrillation) the test must not proceed. As indicated earlier, if the resting record is abnormal the value of proceeding with the test for diagnostic purposes is very limited.

2. After thorough preparation of the skin, the precordial electrode is applied. A modified V_5 electrode is probably best if the equipment only permits a single lead to be monitored during the test. The modified V_5 lead is produced by connecting the positive end of the bipolar system to the usual V_5 location (page 27) and the negative end at some suitable site such as the manubrium sterni. If possible the full 12-lead system should be connected throughout the test. In female patients with large breasts, the breasts may need to be supported by some suitable garment to minimise motion artefact. In male patients with hairy chests local shaving may be necessary. (It is unusual for both of these preparatory steps to be necessary!).

3. A resting record is taken from the monitoring precordial lead. If the standard 12-lead electrocardiogram was satisfactory, the modified V_5 appearances should also be satisfactory. A further rhythm strip is obtained from this modified V_5 lead with the patient standing. (Where monitoring facilities with all 12 leads are available, the full 12-lead record should be taken with the patient standing, at rest, on the treadmill.)

4. If possible, arrangements should be made to monitor the blood pressure during the test. This is best done by the usual sphygmomanometric technique, but it is unreasonable to expect to be able to measure anything other than the **systolic** blood pressure.

5. Exercise then proceeds as indicated in Table 5 below:-

Table 5

Stage	Duration of stage (min)	Total elapsed time (min)	Speed km/h	mph	Gradient (%)	Work load (METS*)	Recreational activities of equivalent level
1	1	1	3	1.9	0	2	Casual walking
2	3	4	3	1.9	10	5	Casual cycling
3	3	7	4	2.5	12	6–7	Jogging
4	3	10	5.5	3.4	14	8–9	Running
5	3	13	7	4.4	16	16	Squash

EXERCISE IS STOPPED
IF AN ABNORMALITY DEVELOPS
or
IF THE TARGET HEART RATE IS ACHIEVED

Otherwise, exercise continues from one stage to another without interruption. The indications for stopping exercise are given on page 190.

6. Following the completion or cessation of exercise the patient is transferred quickly to a bed for the post-exercise observations. If a 3-lead ECG machine is used the 12-lead record is taken in the following order:
first, V_4, V_5, V_6,
then, I, II, III,
then, aVR, aVL, aVF,
finally V_1, V_2, V_3.

Note

* The unit "MET" refers to a metabolic equivalent, i.e. they are multiples of the basal metabolic rate. Healthy, sedentary individuals can usually exercise to 10-11 METS and beyond and healthy, physically active individuals to 16 METS and beyond. Most patients with true angina develop indications for stopping the test at or before the 8 MET level.

If full 12-lead ECG monitoring is available throughout the test a 12-lead record is taken with the patient standing at rest on the treadmill immediately after cessation of exercise and before transfer to the bed.

Where a single channel machine is used the same order is followed i.e. V_4, V_5, V_6, I, ... V_2, V_3.

The reason for this order is that the left precordial leads are the most likely leads to show a positive response, followed by the standard limb leads, then aVL and aVF and finally the right precordial leads. In the immediate post-exercise situation the haemodynamic state is changing rapidly and it is important to use those leads most likely to show changes as soon as possible in case any changes which occur are short-lived.

The full 12-lead recording is repeated 2 minutes, 4 minutes and 6 minutes after the end of exercise. The order of recording the 12 leads is not critical at this juncture.

Indications for stopping the exercise test
1. Development of an abnormality

Clinical Indications
The patient requests it. (He feels he has "had enough").
Excessive fatigue
Excessive dyspnoea
Dizziness
Pallor, clammy skin, exhaustion
Reduction in blood pressure and/or heart rate despite increasing work loads.
Worrying Arrhythmias
Frequent ventricular ectopic beats
Multifocal ventricular ectopic beats
Ventricular tachycardia
Atrial tachycardia
Atrial flutter
Atrial fibrillation

Evidence of Ischaemia
Increasing anginal pain
Significant (more than 1mm) S-T segment shift (depression or elevation)
Equipment Failure
Monitoring system faults
Defibrillator faults
Treadmill faults
2. Achievement of heart rate

The "target" heart rate is related to the age of the patient. The most rigorous tests set a target of 85–90% of the predicted maximal exertional heart rate in normal subjects of the appropriate age. In general, the author prefers to use slightly lower heart rates as given below in Table 6:-
(The 85-90% maximal target rates are also quoted for comparison)

Table 6

Patient age	Target heart rate	("85-90% Maximal" target heart rates)
<40	170	175
40-50	160	170
50-60	155	165
60-70	150	160

Interpretation of the exercise test
1. Features diagnostic of the positive test

The only **definitive** criteria for positive exercise electrocardiograms are:
a) horizontal S-T segment depression of 1mm or more.
b) horizontal S-T segment elevation of 1mm or more.
c) downsloping or upsloping S-T segment elevation or depression of 1mm or more.

In each case the S-T segment shift must persist for 0.08 sec or more in each complex.

When these changes occur they are usually apparent in the early post-exercise record and usually revert to normal within a few minutes.

In 10% of positive cases the changes are seen only **during** exercise and will be missed if, as is often the case, records can only be taken after the end of exercise. (Sophisticated and expensive recording equipment is needed to obtain artefact-free interpretable ECG recordings during exercise). In most positive cases, however, S-T segment shift begins during exertion and continues for the first few minutes at the end of exercise. In a small proportion of positive cases (perhaps 5%) S-T segment shift only appears **after** the completion of the exercise. S-T segment elevation is much less common that S-T segment depression (perhaps 1 or 2% of positive cases). This response is usually indicative of the presence of severe stenoses in major proximal branches of the coronary systems.

S-T segment shift should ideally be measured against the true iso-electric line (the T-P interval (page 42)) but this is not always practicable in the context of exercise electrocardiography for, if the target heart rate is achieved, no T-P interval remains. (The target heart rate is more likely to be achieved when the coronary arteries are normal or when there is only mild coronary atheroma). If the heart rate is very rapid and no T-P interval is visible, the S-T segment can, of necessity, only be assessed against the P-R segment.
In the presence of significant coronary atheroma, left ventricular performance on exercise will often be compromised and the patient will frequently not be able to achieve the target heart rate. In this event it is usually possible to compare the S-T segment with the true iso-electric line – i.e. the T-P interval.

Figure 134 shows a negative exercise test and Figure 135 shows a positive exercise test.

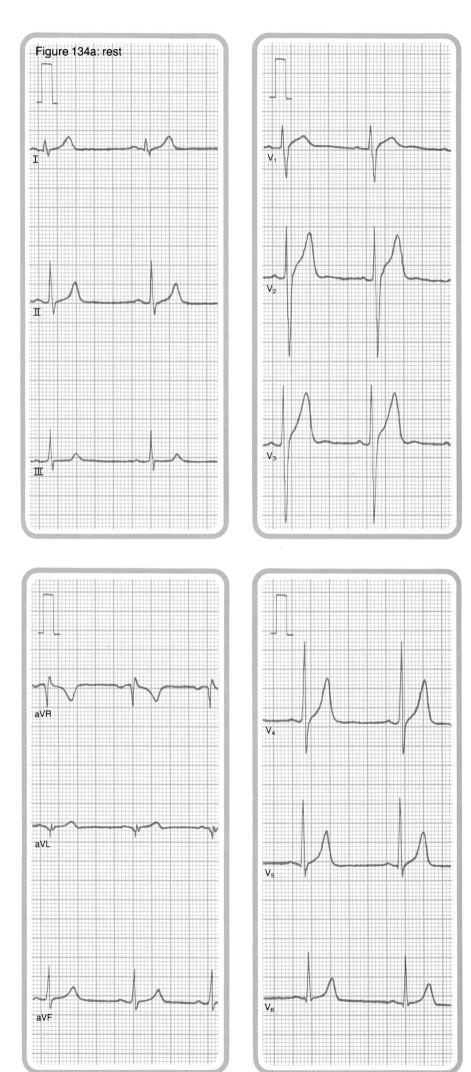

Figure 134a: rest

I

II

III

aVR

aVL

aVF

V₁

V₂

V₃

V₄

V₅

V₆

Figure 134a

The resting record is within normal limits. The q wave in aVL is normal since the heart is vertical (axis +75°) and aVL is therefore a cavity lead (Figure 62, page 55). The resting heart rate is 59/min.

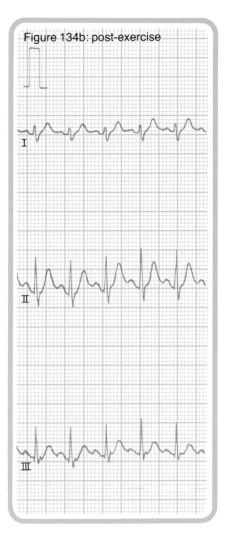

Figure 134b: post-exercise

I

II

III

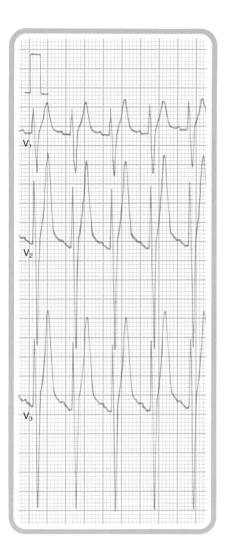

V₁

V₂

V₃

Figure 134b

The immediate post-exercise record is also within normal limits. The patient was a 42-year-old man. The heart rate achieved was 168/min and the patient thus achieved the target heart rate. There were no indications for stopping the exercise prematurely. There is no significant S-T segment shift (see criteria above) and the exercise test is therefore negative. Some changes do occur but these do **not** signify abnormality. Prominent atrial repolarisation (Ta) waves are seen (easily recognised in Leads II, III, aVF and V₆). The T waves in V₁–V₃ are taller following exercise than at rest, but this is not abnormal. (Had the T waves been abnormal, i.e. inverted, before exercise and had become upright following exercise, this would have been abnormal).

Subsequent records taken over the next 10 min after exercise likewise showed no abnormality. The Ta wave gradually diminished and the T waves in the right precordial leads gradually returned to their former size.

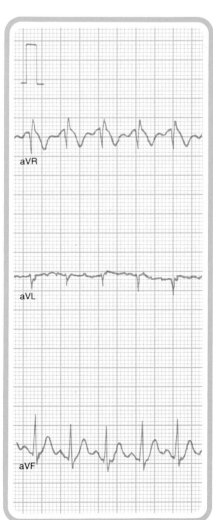

aVR

aVL

aVF

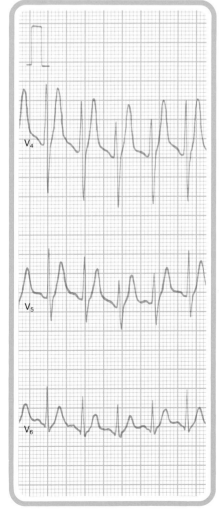

V₄

V₅

V₆

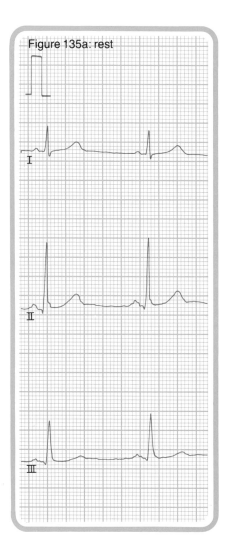

Figure 135a: rest

I

II

III

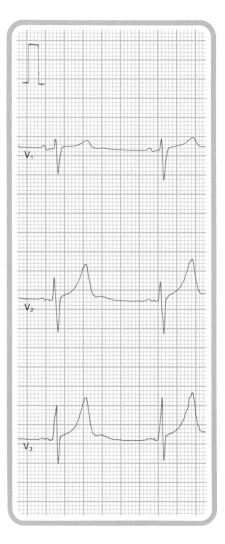

V₁

V₂

V₃

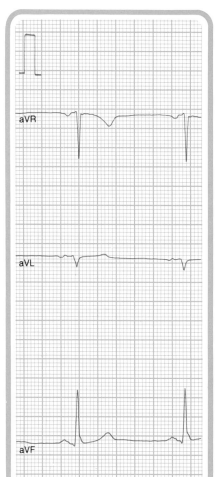

aVR

aVL

aVF

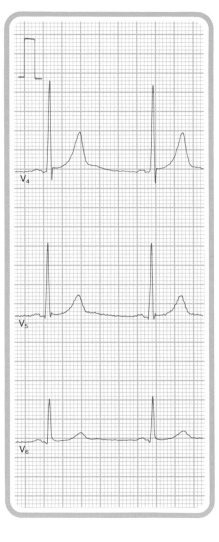

V₄

V₅

V₆

Figure 135a

The resting record is within normal limits (the deep negative wave in the QRS in aVL (it is an S wave since there is a small initial r wave – but it would still be normal even if it were a Q wave) is due to the fact that the heart is vertical – the axis is +75°). The T waves in V_2 and V_3 are rather tall but this is not definitely abnormal. The resting heart rate is 52/min.

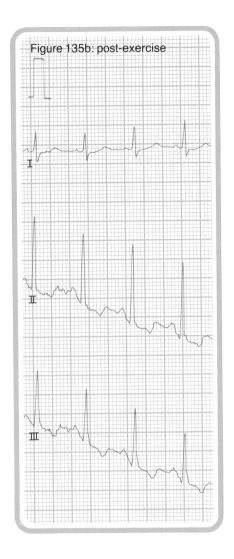

Figure 135b: post-exercise

I

II

III

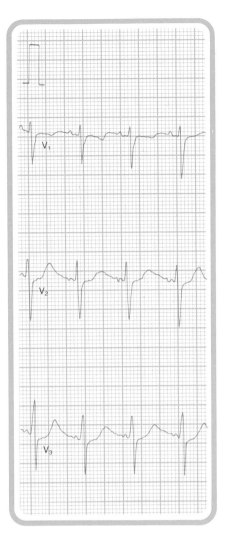

V₁

V₂

V₃

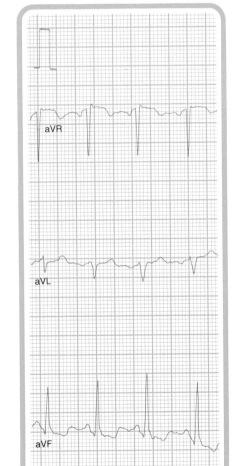

aVR

aVL

aVF

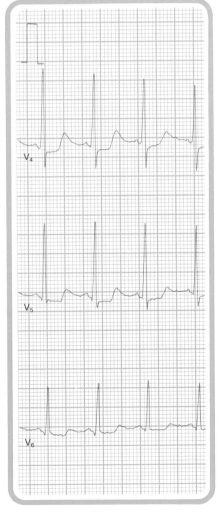

V₄

V₅

V₆

Figure 135b

The immediate post-exercise heart rate is only 115/min. The patient was unable to complete the exercise programme because of the development of anginal pain. There is 2mm S-T depression clearly seen in V_4 and V_5. There is lesser S-T depression in V_6 and aVF. Assessment of S-T changes in II and III is not possible because of the sloping S-T segment.

At coronary angiography the patient had a localised 90% occlusion of the proximal part of the anterior descending branch of the left coronary artery.

2. Factors strongly suggestive of a positive test

a) "Normalisation" of previously inverted T waves.

b) Development of terminal T wave inversion or of U wave inversion (see below).

c) Development of ventricular tachycardia or of multiple ventricular ectopic beats.

d) Development of increased R wave amplitude in the precordial leads.

e) Development of hypotension (a clinical not an electrocardiographic response, of course).

3. Features with no definitive diagnostic value

(i.e. important negative points)

a) Development of atrial or nodal arrhythmia.

b) Development of first degree heart block or Wenckebach phenonomen.

c) Development of intraventricular block – right or left bundle branch block, anterior or posterior hemiblock, bifascicular block etc.

d) T wave flattening or inversion.

e) Increase in U wave height (see below).

f) Sloping S-T segment shift if not both
a) more than 1 mm in height,
and b) 0.08 sec or longer in duration.

g) Changes in P wave morphology.

The U Wave

The U wave is a small, rounded positive deflection occurring immediately after the T wave. It is often seen in normal records but in normal circumstances is almost always inconspicuous. It is part of the repolarisation process (as are the S-T segments and T waves), but its precise mode of genesis is uncertain. The amplitude of the normal U wave is related to that of the preceding T wave. The U wave is normally 5-25% of the height of the preceding T wave. Because of this relationship, it follows that the U wave is usually tallest in V_2, V_3 and V_4. In these leads it may occasionally reach 2 mm in height though the average height of the normal U wave in these leads is less than 0.5 mm. The normal U wave is usually upright in the limb leads except for 'cavity' leads (i.e. in almost all hearts, aVR, in the case of vertical hearts, aVL, and in the case of horizontal hearts, Lead III).

Small (normal) U waves are seen in V_2, V_3, V_4, V_5 and Lead II of Record 2 (page 72). When the U wave is inverted it is abnormal. When the U wave exceeds the height of the preceding T wave it is abnormal – as in Leads V_2 and V_3 of Record 15 (page 86).

Conditions giving rise to increased height of the U wave or to U wave inversion are listed on page 263.

False-positive and false-negative exercise electrocardiograms

There are several factors which may give rise to false-positive or false-negative exercise tests, i.e. which may give rise to tests which wrongly suggest the presence or the absence respectively of ischaemic heart disease. Most of these factors should not present a real problem – for they are usually obvious in advance and when they are so recognised there is little point in going ahead with the investigation for the results are bound to be equivocal.
The factors are as follows:-

1. Factors giving rise to false-positive tests

a) Intraventricular conduction defects.

b) Ventricular pre-excitation (see pages 212 to 220).

c) Overt ventricular hypertrophy.

d) Valve disease (which may be giving rise to "occult" ventricular hypertrophy, i.e. hypertrophy not apparent in the resting record).

e) Hypertension (for reasons given in d) above).

f) Pulmonary hypertension (for reasons given in d) above).

g) Cardiomyopathy (congestive or hypertrophic) and myocarditis.

h) Electrolyte disturbances – especially hypokalaemia.

i) Hypothyroidism.

j) Concurrent drug administration – especially digitalis but also including quinidine, procainamide, diuretics, antidepressants and sedatives.

k) Pericarditis.

l) Mitral valve prolapse.

m) Post-prandial changes.

n) Hyperventilation.

o) Pre-existing and non-specific S-T, T changes.

p) Pectus excavatum.

2. Factors giving rise to false-negative tests

a) Concurrent administration of beta-blocking drugs. The use of these drugs prevents the achievement of the target heart rate which is the commonest cause of false-negative responses.

b) Other anti-anginal drugs may occasionally give rise to false-negative responses.

c) An inadequate exercise level with inappropriately low maximal heart rate.

d) Previous physical training – this may result in a **relative** inadequacy of the maximal heart rate achieved, i.e. a higher heart rate target should be set.

In the absence of the above factors, false-negative exercise electro-cardiograms can still be found despite the presence of significant coronary disease.

Correlation of exercise electrocardiography with the presence of coronary artery disease

Pathological studies reveal that when the test is positive (i.e. there is significant S-T segment shift related to exertion) the patients **usually** have severe and extensive coronary atheroma.

A rigorously conducted negative exercise test does not, however, exclude significant coronary atheroma.

Coronary angiographic studies confirm that the exercise test can be negative despite the presence of significant atheroma in the coronary vessels and it also demonstrates that positive stress tests are more likely to be achieved in multi-vessel rather than in single-vessel disease.

The test does have prognostic value when asymptomatic subjects are screened. Those with positive stress tests have mortality rates 4 or 5 times higher than those with negative tests and the excess of mortality is roughly proportional to the depth of the S-T segment depression produced.

Diagnosis of Myocardial Infarction

At this stage it is appropriate to repeat the diagnostic criteria for myocardial infarction. It will be recalled that myocardial infarction can only be diagnosed on the basis of the appropriate QRS abnormalities (pages 168 *et. seq.*).

Diagnostic criteria[†] for myocardial infarction

A **definitive** diagnosis of myocardial infarction from the electrocardiogram can only be made on the basis of abnormalities of the QRS complex. These diagnostic abnormalities are as follows:-

a) q waves which **either** are 0.04 sec or longer in duration (excluding aVR and III) **or** have a depth which is more than one quarter of the height of the ensuing R wave (excluding aVR and III).

b) qs or QS complexes[*] (excluding aVR and III).

c) local area of inappropriately low R wave voltage (where this can confidently be ascertained).

Additional features frequently associated with myocardial infarction

These changes include S-T segment and T wave changes and also the development of specific changes related to the local effects of infarction (e.g. intraventricular conduction disturbances and cardiac arrhythmias).

a) S-T segment elevation (usually with slight curvature, convex upwards) occurs in leads facing the infarcted zone. This is a transient change often occurring within hours of the onset of symptoms, usually being the first electrocardiographic **manifestation** of acute infarction (though not actually being **diagnostic** of it) and usually lasting for days only. Prolonged (weeks or months) S-T segment elevation of minor degree may occur in extensive infarction and in the presence of a ventricular aneurysm.

b) S-T segment depression (usually with a slight curvature) occurs as a "reciprocal" change in leads "opposite to", i.e. remote from, the infarcted area during the time that primary S-T segment elevation persists.

c) Horizontal S-T segment depression may occur as a primary change (i.e. without concurrent S-T elevation in other leads) in subendocardial infarction.

Note

† These criteria are, strictly speaking, the criteria for loss of viable, electrically active myocardium. The commonest cause is myocardial infarction but any disease directly causing myocardial necrosis or replacement of electrically active by inactive myocardium can give rise to similar appearances. Thus fibrosis induced by cardiomyopathy or replacement of myocardium by amyloid tissue can give rise to similar appearances in the QRS complexes (see pseudo-infarction pattern, page 198). It follows that secondary as well as primary interpretation is important for a definitive diagnosis. The primary interpretation really just defines loss of viable myocardium. However, when the full, evolving, time-sequential pattern of myocardial infarction (page 179) is shown, definitive diagnosis by primary interpretation is possible.

* qs or QS complexes are normal for any lead "looking into" the cavity of the heart ("cavity leads"). aVR is almost always a cavity lead and usually shows a QS complex. Lead aVL is often a cavity lead when the heart is vertical and Lead III is often a cavity lead when the heart is horizontal, and in these respective circumstances aVL or III will usually show a qs complex. V_1 is often and V_2 is occasionally, a cavity lead if there is pronounced clockwise cardiac rotation. In such circumstances V_1 and possibly also V_2 may show QS complexes.

It is by far the most **typical** change of subendocardial infarction but it is not **specific** to it for it occurs also in subendocardial ischaemia and in exertional angina.

d) Downsloping or upsloping S-T segment depression may occur in leads overlying or adjacent to areas of infarction. The change is quite non-specific but in this context probably reflects local myocardial ischaemia.

e) Deep symmetrical T wave inversion frequently occurs overlying and adjacent to areas of acute myocardial infarction. The change does not usually occur in the first 24 hours (being later than the S-T segment change). It may persist for weeks. It is also seen in relation to ischaemia without infarction and may also be the sole manifestation of subendocardial infarction.

f) Shallow or asymmetrical T wave inversion is a non-specific change. It frequently occurs in areas adjacent to infarction but can occur in many other conditions (page 184).

g) Abnormally tall T waves may occur in leads "opposite to" the infarcted area (this change is most frequently seen in the precordial leads in true posterior infarction). This change can occur in true posterior ischaemia without infarction and can also occur in hyperkalaemia and in intraventricular conduction disturbances.

h) Terminal T wave inversion may occur with acute myocardial infarction – usually at about the time when there is recognisable S-T segment elevation. This change may be the same process as U wave inversion.

i) Low voltage T waves or **T wave flattening** is a non-specific change. It frequently occurs in areas adjacent to infarction but can occur in many other conditions.

j) Cardiac arrhythmias frequently occur in relation to infarction. Since any part of the myocardium or conducting tissue may be involved in the infarction, any arrhythmia is possible. There may be **disturbances of function at the sino-atrial node** (sinus tachycardia, sinus bradycardia, sinus arrhythmia, sino-atrial block, sinus arrest, nodal-escape beats, nodal-escape rhythm), **disturbances of conduction** (first, second or third degree atrio-ventricular block, right bundle branch block, left bundle branch block, left anterior hemiblock, left posterior hemiblock), **ectopic arrhythmias** (atrial ectopic beats, atrial tachycardia, atrial flutter, atrial fibrillation, nodal ectopic beats, nodal tachycardia, ventricular ectopic beats, ventricular tachycardia, ventricular fibrillation) and finally there may be any **combination of the above.** (Obviously, in the case of ventricular fibrillation, any concomitant rhythm disturbance would be both occult and irrelevant). The arrhythmias are described in Section 3.

k) Axis shift. Left ventricular depolarisation is the dominant influence in determining the form of the QRS complexes in all normal and in most abnormal electrocardiograms (page 22) and plays by far the most important role in determining the mean frontal plane QRS axis (pages 22-24). Myocardial infarction involves loss of viable myocardium, usually from the left ventricle. In the frontal plane, the mean forces of left ventricular depolarisation are directed downwards and to the left so that a typical normal frontal plane QRS axis is $+60°$ (pages 22-24). The normal range for the frontal plane axis in adults is $-30°$ to $+90°$ (page 53). When there is necrosis of these parts of the left ventricular myocardium which normally give rise to components of the depolarisation wave at extremes of this normal range, the loss of components at **one extreme** tends to give rise to a **mean** QRS axis at or beyond the other **extreme.** Thus since the myocardium of the inferior wall of the left ventricle normally contributes a component of ventricular depolarisation directly inferiorly in the frontal plane (i.e. towards aVF) the loss of this myocardium as in inferior infarction, tends to give rise to a mean frontal plane QRS axis directly more superiorly, but still to the left. Therefore, **the development of inferior infarction is often accompanied by the simultaneous development of abnormal left axis deviation.** This is a direct consequence of loss of the inferiorly directed component of left ventricular depolarisation and does not imply the development of left anterior hemiblock (pages 133 and 175). In like manner, **the development of antero-lateral myocardial infarction is often accompanied by the development of abnormal right axis deviation.** This is a direct consequence of the loss of the superiorly and leftward directed component of left ventricular depolarisation and does not imply the development of left posterior hemiblock (page 137).

(Figure 141 shows an example of inferior infarction giving rise to abnormal left axis deviation and Figure 96 an example of left anterior hemiblock giving rise to abnormal left axis deviation). The essential difference between the two on the frontal plane leads is the presence of an abnormal Q wave (actually QS complex in Figure 141) in aVF in inferior infarction, compared with an rS in aVF in LAH. Figure 137 shows an example of antero-lateral infarction giving rise to an abnormal degree of right axis deviation. (This does not imply the development of left posterior hemiblock).

Pseudo-infarction Patterns

As explained earlier, abnormal q waves or abnormal QS patterns, particularly if associated with S-T segment shift and T wave changes, are the most reliable electrocardiographic indications of myocardial infarction. However, similar changes are occasionally seen in patients without coronary artery disease. It is important to be aware of these "pseudo-infarction patterns".

Conditions associated with absence of, or reduction in the size of, the r waves in the right precordial leads, thus simulating infarction

a) **Chronic lung disease.** As a result of the pronounced clockwise cardiac rotation which occurs in this condition the r waves in the right and mid-precordial leads may be small or absent.

b) **Spontaneous pneumothorax.** This may produce changes similar to those in chronic lung disease.

c) **Left ventricular hypertrophy.** May give rise to reduction in r wave size (and occasionally to absence of r waves) in the right precordial leads. Record 5 (page 75) shows an example of left ventricular hypertrophy in which there are small r waves in V_1-V_3 and a sudden increase in R wave height in V_4. (This type of R wave progression can occasionally be indicative of anteroseptal infarction but in this case is due to left ventricular hypertrophy).

(Left bundle branch block may also give rise to abnormally low r wave voltages in the right precordial leads in just the same way as LVH (e.g. see Record 7, page 77 and compare with Record 5, page 75) but this is not rightfully considered a "pseudo-infarction pattern" since the presence of criteria for the diagnosis of left bundle branch block precludes the diagnosis of myocardial infarction (page 125 and page 250) except in special circumstances (pages 251 and 252)).

It is worthwhile to compare the r wave progression in the precordial leads in Record 4, page 74 (normal), Record 5, page 75 (LVH), Record 7, page 77 (LBBB) and Record 8, page 79 (Anteroseptal infarction).

Conditions in which abnormal q waves may occur, thus simulating infarction

a) **Cardiomyopathy.** In **hypertrophic cardiomyopathy** the interventricular septum may be markedly thickened (substantially increasing the "Phase 1" voltage of ventricular depolarisation). As a result, the septal q waves are increased in size and abnormal q waves may appear – particularly in Leads V_4, V_5, V_6, I and aVL.

In **congestive cardiomyopathy** abnormal q waves may occur in any lead. These q waves are usually the result of patches of fibrosis in localised areas of the myocardium.

Other **myocardial diseases** may give rise to abnormal q waves. These diseases include:-
Amyloidosis
Scleroderma
Primary or secondary tumours
Myocarditis
Friedreich's ataxia
Progressive muscular dystrophy.

b) **Left bundle branch block.** This often gives rise to QS complexes in the inferior limb leads (as in Record 28, page 99) and often in the right precordial leads (Record 28 shows abnormally small r waves in the right precordial leads).

These changes occur because of reversal of the direction of septal depolarisation. For this reason it is unwise to diagnose infarction in the presence of left bundle branch block unless previous records are available showing left bundle branch block **before** the infarction.

c) **Ventricular pre-excitation.** In this condition the direction of septal depolarisation is reversed and abnormal q waves may appear in the limb leads or in the precordial leads (e.g. Figure 150, page 217).

d) **Pulmonary embolism.** In this condition abnormal q waves may develop in III and aVF. This change has been attributed to dilatation of the right ventricle with consequent changes in the orientation of the interventricular septum so that the right side of the septum is directed superiorly. When this happens Phase 1 of ventricular depolarisation is directed away from III and aVF and initial q waves appear in these leads. In contrast to the situation in inferior infarction, such q waves do not usually appear also in II and they tend to be small in aVF. Occasionally, in massive pulmonary embolism, abnormal q waves may appear across the precordial leads.

Conditions in which S-T segment and T wave changes occur, thus simulating infarction

a) **Hyperkalaemia.** This may give rise to very tall T waves in the precordial leads. Sometimes there may be associated S-T elevation and reduction in R wave height. Such changes only occur in severe (pre-terminal) hyperkalaemia.

b) **Intracranial haemorrhage.** The commonest changes associated with intracranial haemorrhage are S-T segment and T wave changes, but abnormal q waves can be seen.

c) **Pericarditis.** The widespread distribution of the S-T, T changes in pericarditis and the absence of QRS changes usually means that confusion with infarction is unlikely (see pages 231 and 232).

d) **Myocardial Contusion.** Non-penetrating injuries of the myocardium may give rise to local injury or necrosis. Accordingly S-T or T wave changes or q wave development may occur. If the conducting tissue is involved A-V conduction problems may develop. The overall picture may closely mimic infarction but the clinical story usually prevents confusion (illustrating again the importance of secondary interpretation).

Most of these conditions will be considered in detail in the section on miscellaneous abnormalities.

Ventricular Aneurysm

It is widely taught that **persistent** S-T segment elevation (i.e. S-T elevation which occurs in relation to acute infarction but which does not settle after the first few days or weeks as is usually the case) is indicative of the presence of a ventricular aneurysm. Since "ventricular aneurysm" is a haemodynamic concept rather than an anatomical one it is not surprising, in the author's view, that electrocardiography provides no reliable basis whatsoever for the diagnosis. All patients who sustain myocardial infarction and survive, develop a fibrous non-contractile scar in the infarcted area. In a normal heart the whole perimeter of the left ventricular wall moves inwards during systole. After myocardial infarction the infarcted zone either moves inwards less than it did formerly (hypokinesia) or not at all (akinesia). An aneurysm exists when the infarcted zone moves **outwards** during systole (dyskinesia). It would, (again in the author's judgement) be a remarkable thing if this difference in mechanical movement of dead tissue (i.e. between akinesia or hypokinesia on the one hand, and dyskinesia on the other hand) were to be conveniently signified by a particular ECG change! There is no denying the fact that persistent S-T segment elevation does show a significant **correlation** with proven ventricular aneurysm (**proof** of the existence of an aneurysm is only possible by ventricular angiography) but the correlation is relatively weak – only two-thirds of patients with definite ventricular aneurysms have persistent S-T segment elevation and probably less than two-thirds of patients with persistent S-T segment elevation have ventricular aneurysms at angiography. The probable reason for the correlation is that the formation of a left ventricular aneurysm is more likely the more extensive the infarct. In the presence of extensive anterior infarction there will be little residual viable myocardium in the anterior cardiac wall. This wall therefore presents an electrical "window" through to the back of the heart. If there is ischaemia of the posterior wall of the heart (which might give S-T segment depression in a posterior lead) it will show S-T elevation in the anterior leads. Persistent S-T elevation in the anterior leads, together with evidence of extensive anterior infarction is thus simply a manifestation of extensive loss of viable myocardium from the anterior wall of the heart and of ischaemia of the posterior wall. Ventricular aneurysm formation is much more likely the more extensive is the loss of myocardium hence there is inevitably some degree of correlation. (This interpretation is by no means widely accepted. It is speculation by the author. The idea was acquired from Dr H B Burchell while the author was spending a year at the Mayo Clinic).

Atrial Infarction

There are no **diagnostic** changes of atrial infarction. Infarction of atrial myocardium is rare without simultaneous evidence of ventricular infarction. The most specific electrocardiographic sign of atrial infarction is elevation or depression of the P-R segment. This is because the atrial repolarisation wave (Ta wave or atrial T wave) which is the atrial equivalent of the ventricular T wave (page 166), tends to occur at the same time as the QRS complex. The P-R interval therefore corresponds in timing to the atrial equivalent of the S-T segment.

Elevation of the P-R interval can therefore indicate acute atrial injury and depression of the P-R interval can indicate ischaemia of the atrium. A less specific but more sensitive indicator of atrial infarction is a bifid P in II or a biphasic P in V_1 with a dominant negative component (i.e. appearances of the type seen in left atrial hypertrophy). The electrocardiogram cannot reliably distinguish among left atrial hypertrophy, left atrial infarction and left atrial ischaemia. The occurrence of atrial arrhythmias also suggests the possibility of atrial infarction.

Examples of the 12-lead ECG in Ischaemic Heart Disease

It is a useful exercise at this stage to work through a range of different electrocardiographic appearances in patients with unequivocal ischaemic heart disease.

Figure 136

Report
"Sinus rhythm, the mean frontal plane QRS axis is +30°. Old anteroseptal myocardial infarction. Left atrial abnormality".

Explanation
The rhythm is sinus, the frontal plane QRS and T axes are normal (i.e. the QRS axis is within the normal range and the T axis (+15°) is within ±45° of the QRS axis). There is a small initial r wave in V_1. The r wave in V_2 should be significantly larger than that in V_1 but it is not. Occasionally this can occur normally in one lead – especially in the transition zone (page 45). However, in this case it is clearly abnormal since the r wave in V_3 is, if anything, smaller still – it is certainly not larger (as it should be). The r wave progression from V_1-V_3 is definitely abnormal. This abnormality cannot be explained by clockwise cardiac rotation since it is apparent in V_1-V_3 and yet there is a tall R wave in V_4 and the transition zone is between V_4 and V_5. It cannot be explained by left bundle branch block (page 124) since the latter is not present (the total QRS duration is normal and there are normal septal q waves in V_6). The only other feature which could account for it is ventricular pre-excitation (page 215). This is not present, for the P-R interval is normal. The appearances are therefore diagnostic of anteroseptal infarction. The age of the infarct cannot be determined with any accuracy. It is certainly "old" but this could indicate that it happened between a few months and many years ago. The area of the negative component of the P wave in V_1 exceeds the area of the positive component. This indicates left atrial abnormality. It could be atrial ischaemia or atrial hypertrophy. Since there is evidence of ventricular infarction and therefore of ischaemic heart disease, it may well be indicative of atrial ischaemia or infarction. The ECG does not distinguish between ischaemia, infarction and hypertrophy of the atria.

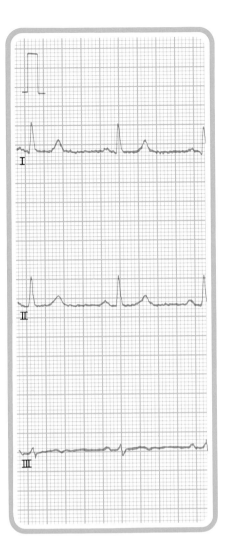

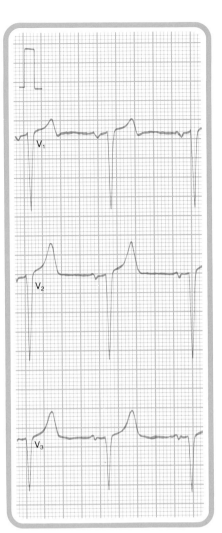

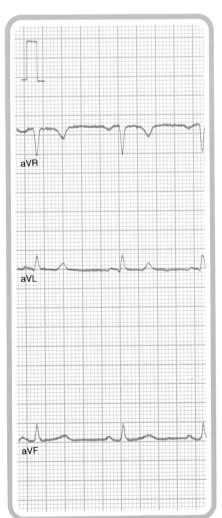

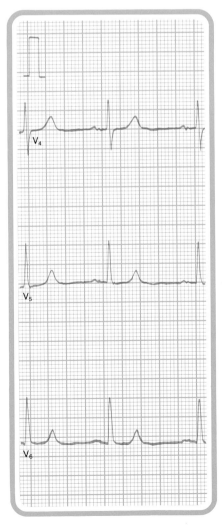

Figure 137

Report

"Sinus rhythm. The mean frontal plane QRS axis is indeterminate. There is evidence of recent extensive anterior myocardial infarction. The appearances are also consistent with true posterior ischaemic damage".

Explanation

There are definitely abnormal Q waves from V_2-V_6 and in I and aVL. (In each clearly indicates necrosis of the myocardium underlying V_2-V_6 and in the antero-lateral area. The pronounced S-T segment elevation in these same leads, with reciprocal S-T segment depression in III and aVF indicates that the necrosis is the result of infarction and that the infarct is recent – probably days old. The S-T segment depression in V_1 cannot be explained on the basis of a reciprocal change since it is very close to a lead showing primary changes (V_2). It could therefore be a primary change in itself and could indicate damage in the posterior wall of the left ventricle. At most the appearances in V_1 indicate ischaemic **damage** to the posterior wall of the left ventricle. There is no definite evidence of true posterior **infarction** since the R wave in V_1 is neither greater in height than the ensuing S wave is in depth, nor is it 0.04 sec or longer in duration.

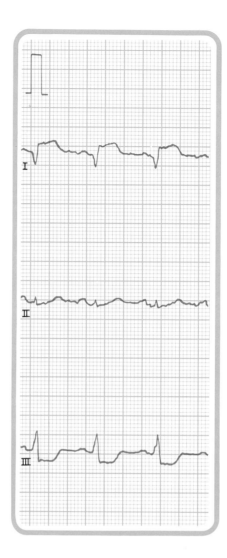

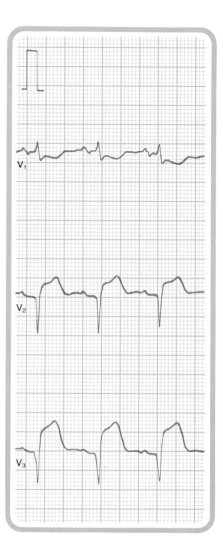

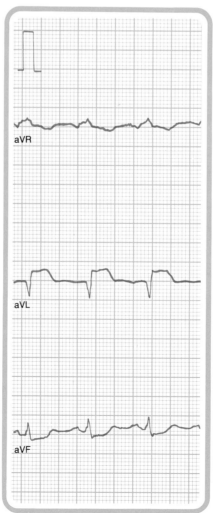

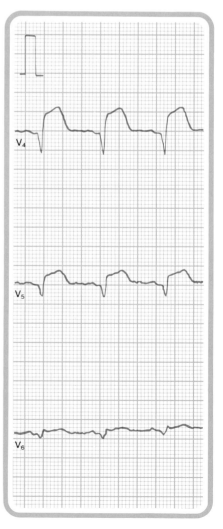

Figure 138

Report
"Sinus rhythm. The mean frontal plane QRS axis is −15°. There is evidence of relatively recent anterior myocardial infarction and of old inferior infarction".

Explanation
There are QS complexes from V_1-V_3 with abnormal q waves in V_4. There is no evidence of left bundle branch block or of ventricular pre-excitation and these appearances are therefore indicative of anterior infarction assuming that none of the causes of pseudo-infarction patterns is present (page 198). The QS complexes indicate transmural infarction underlying V_1-V_3. The abnormal q wave in V_4 indicates less than full thickness infarction underlying the electrodes. The R waves in V_5 and V_6 are probably smaller than they were prior to the infarction but without a record before the infarct, one cannot be confident of this. There is no definite S-T elevation and therefore the infarct is not very recent (i.e. it is more than days old). However, there is T wave inversion from V_1-V_5 and low voltage T waves in V_6, I and aVL. (Note that, as is often the case, the non-specific T wave changes are more widespread than the definitive QRS changes of infarction). The T wave changes indicate that the infarct is of intermediate age (i.e. more than days old but probably less than weeks old). There are QS complexes in aVF without S-T elevation or T inversion in this lead. This indicates the presence of old inferior infarction.

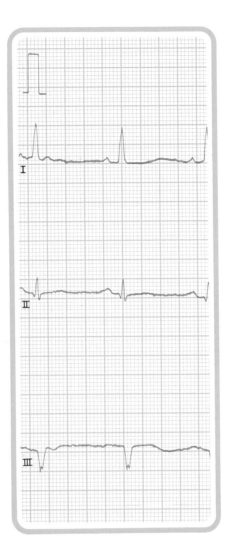

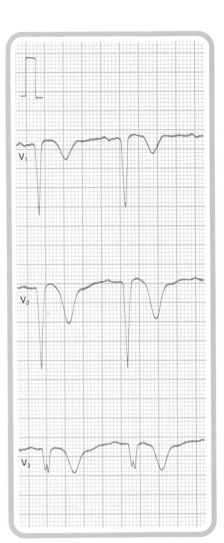

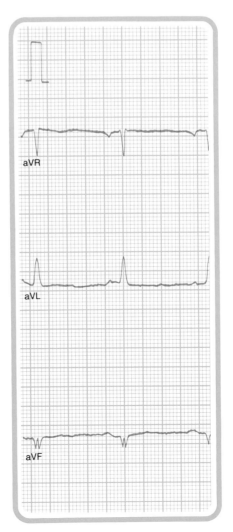

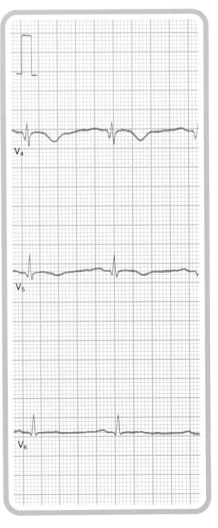

Figure 139

Report

"Sinus rhythm. The mean frontal plane QRS axis is +75°. There is evidence of recent infero-lateral myocardial ischaemic damage."

Explanation

The striking abnormality is the S-T segment elevation. This is most obvious in Leads II, III and aVF (the inferior leads). It is also apparent in V_4-V_6 (the lateral precordial leads). The changes are those of **damage** ("injury") to the myocardium on the inferior wall of the ventricle extending into the lateral wall. (This combination of localisation is sometimes referred to as "apical" (page 180)). There is S-T segment depression in I, aVL and V_1-V_3. This S-T segment depression is "reciprocal". There are no diagnostic QRS changes of infarction, though it is likely that such changes will appear within the next few days (page 179). The R wave voltages in the left precordial leads are smaller than one would expect and it is **possible** there has already been some true infarction in the lateral wall. However, one cannot be **certain** of this since the leads in question are not "bracketed" by undoubtedly normal appearances (for the simple reason that there are no precordial leads further to the left of V_6) and the appearance of the precordial QRS complexes could simply be a manifestation of clockwise cardiac rotation.

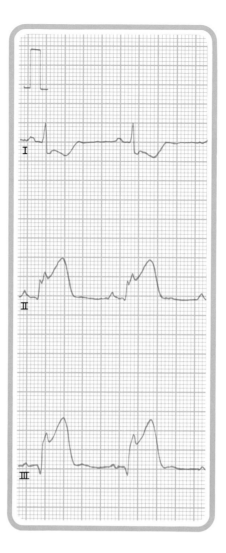
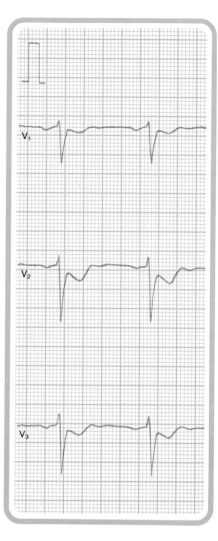
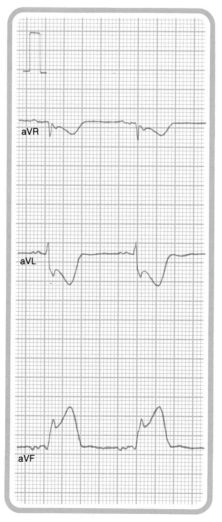
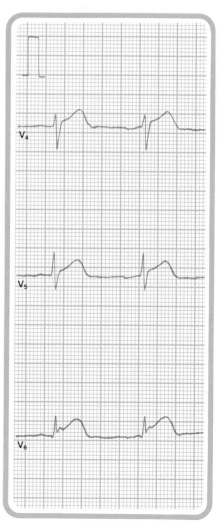

Figure 140

Report

*"Sinus rhythm. The mean frontal plane
QRS axis is −15°. There is evidence of
inferior myocardial infarction of relatively
recent origin. There is minimal S-T
segment elevation in V₅ and V₆ with
terminal T wave inversion in these leads,
suggesting ischaemic damage to the
antero-lateral wall of the ventricle. The
tall T waves in V₂ and V₃ raise the
possibility of true posterior ischaemia".*

Explanation

The Q waves in aVF exceed 0.04 sec in
duration and have a depth which
substantially exceeds one quarter of the
height of the ensuing R wave. In the
absence of ventricular pre-excitation and
left bundle branch block this is diagnostic
of inferior infarction. As is frequently also
the case in inferior infarction, prominent
Q waves are also seen in III. However,
the appearances in Lead III can never be
used to diagnose infarction for the
reasons given on pages 54 and 173 and
174. There is T wave inversion in the
inferior limb Leads II, III and aVF. This is
abnormal in this context (even though the
frontal plane T wave axis, at −15°, is
normal in its relationship to the frontal
plane QRS axis). As explained on page
58, when there is definitive QRS
evidence of inferior myocardial infarction,
T wave inversion in the inferior limb leads
is considered abnormal even if the angle
between the mean QRS and T wave
axes does not lie outside the normal
limits of ±45°. These T wave changes
are secondary to the QRS abnormality
and indicate that the infarction is unlikely
to be more than several weeks old. The
slight S-T segment elevation in V₅ and V₆
is definitely abnormal as is the slight
terminal T wave inversion in these leads.
These changes indicate the presence of
recent antero-lateral myocardial
ischaemic damage. The T waves in V₂
and V₃ are tall. One cannot be sure that
this is an abnormality (unless a prior
record with lower T wave voltages is
available for comparison). They **could**
indicate true posterior ischaemia.

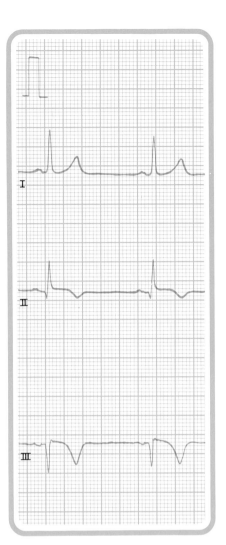

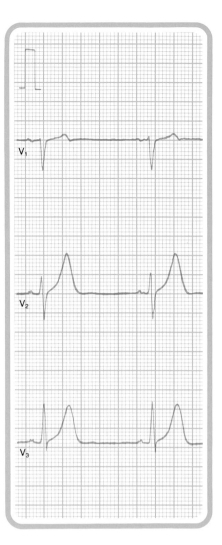

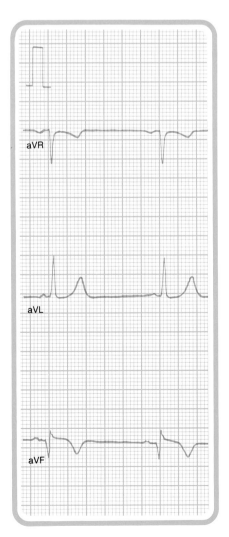

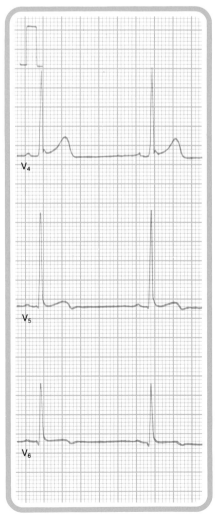

Figure 141

Report

"Sinus tachycardia. The mean frontal plane QRS axis is −45°. This is an abnormal degree of left axis deviation. There is evidence of old infero-lateral myocardial infarction. In addition there are signs of recent true posterior infarction. There is also evidence of left atrial abnormality".

Explanation

The rhythm is sinus but the rate exceeds 100/minute and there is therefore sinus tachycardia. There is an abnormal degree of left axis deviation (−45°). The two commonest causes of this are left anterior hemiblock and inferior myocardial infarction (page 135). There are clearly abnormal Q waves in II and aVF (and also, as is often the case, Lead III) indicating inferior myocardial infarction. This is therefore an adequate explanation for the left axis deviation and there is no need to invoke left anterior hemiblock. The T waves are upright indicating that at least several weeks have elapsed since the infarct occurred. The infarct could be anything from weeks to years in age. V_6 shows a clear infarct pattern, with abnormal Q waves, obvious reduction in R wave height (so striking that it is apparent even without "bracketing" with normal appearances in leads on each side of the one in question). The appearances indicate infarction of the lateral wall of the ventricle. There is still S-T elevation in this lead and the antero-lateral change is therefore recent (days). There is striking S-T depression from V_1-V_4. This cannot be a reciprocal change for it is far more pronounced and extensive than the concurrent S-T elevation (seen only in V_6). It is therefore likely to be a primary change. As such it could indicate subendocardial ischaemia (or infarction) or true posterior ischaemic damage. Since there is an abnormally tall and broad R wave in V_1 there is unequivocal evidence of true posterior infarction. The S-T segment depression is likely to be part of this and to indicate that the true posterior infarct is recent. (Theoretically the dominant R wave in V_1 could suggest right ventricular hypertrophy but there is no supporting evidence for this (right axis deviation, clockwise cardiac rotation, right atrial hypertrophy) and there is impressive evidence of extensive ischaemic heart disease). The form of the P waves in V_1 indicates left atrial abnormality.

Note

(The combination of abnormal left axis deviation and a dominant R wave in V_1 could suggest biventricular hypertrophy (page 157) but there is unequivocal evidence of infero-lateral infarction (abnormal q waves in II, aVF and V_6) and pronounced horizontal S-T changes in V_1-V_4, typical of myocardial ischaemia. There is therefore no need to invoke biventricular hypertrophy).

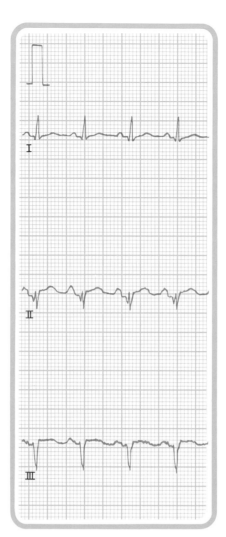

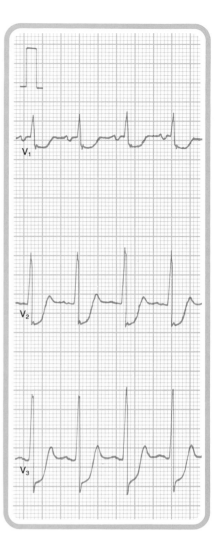

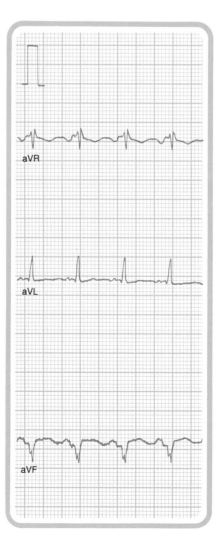

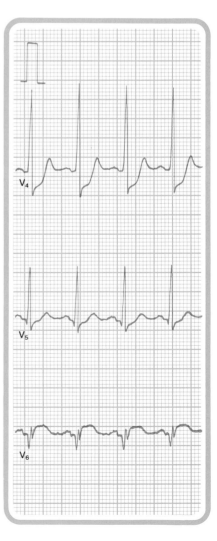

Figure 142

Report
*"Sinus rhythm. The mean frontal plane
QRS axis is +60°. The appearances in
Leads II, III and aVF suggest recent
inferior myocardial infarction. The deep
symmetrical T wave inversion from V_2-V_6
and in I and aVL suggest subendocardial
ischaemia or infarction".*

Explanation
The electrocardiogram is clearly
abnormal and certainly indicates
ischaemic heart disease. There is a
suggestion of S-T elevation in II and aVF,
but the degree of S-T elevation is not
beyond normal limits. There are
pronounced q waves in II and aVF but
they are not definitely abnormal. The
terminal T wave inversion in II and aVF is
definitely abnormal. Collectively these
appearances suggest recent inferior
infarction but the criteria for a definitive
diagnosis have not been fulfilled. The
deep symmmetrical T wave inversion
from V_2-V_6 and in Lead I and aVL
suggest subendocardial ischaemia or
infarction. Only consecutive records or
collateral clinical data (i.e. secondary
interpretation) can distinguish between
these two possibilities. Note that the
upright T wave in aVR is also an
abnormality – the T waves are usually
negative in this lead. (However – the
T waves should be considered
collectively in the limb leads. The mean
frontal plane T wave axis is 180°. The
angle between the frontal plane T wave
axis and the QRS axis is thus abnormal
at +120°). The r wave progression from
V_1-V_3 is very poor and it is therefore
possible that there is partial thickness
regional infarction in this area.

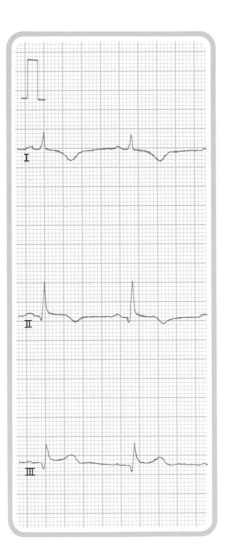

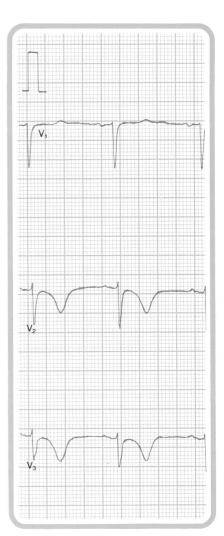

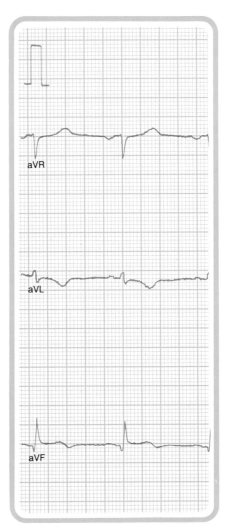

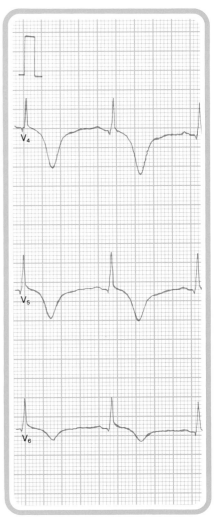

Figure 143

Report
"Sinus rhythm. The mean frontal plane QRS axis is +60°. The T waves in V₁-V₄ are abnormally tall. This is a non-specific change".

Explanation
The T waves are almost certainly abnormally tall in V_2 and V_3. No definitive criteria exist to establish this as a certainty. The possible causes include true posterior myocardial ischaemia, hyperkalaemia and normal variation. The use of relevant clinical data will permit secondary interpretation. This particular patient had been complaining of typical chest pain and it is therefore **likely** that there is true posterior ischaemia. The serum potassium level was normal. Note that the diagnosis cannot be made from the ECG alone. The clinical data do not **prove** that the tall waves indicate ischaemia – though they do suggest that there may well be ischaemia somewhere. The q waves in aVL are more than a quarter of the height of the ensuing r wave, but in this case aVL is almost a cavity lead – aVL is actually just at right angles to the frontal plane axis. The appearances in aVL should therefore be regarded as normal.

The fact that the R/S ratio in V_1 is unity (i.e. the R and S waves are of equal size) is also worthy of comment. Normally in V_1 the r wave is smaller than the S wave (page 32). The causes of an R wave in V_1 **larger** than the S wave include right ventricular hypertrophy and true posterior myocardial infarction (page 262 – of the other two causes, ventricular pre-excitation is ruled out by the ECG appearances (pages 212 to 220) and muscular dystrophy by the clinical picture (secondary interpretation)).

In the absence of an abnormal degree of right axis deviation, right ventricular hypertrophy cannot be diagnosed (page 155). The form of the QRS complexes in V_1 **could** be indicative of true posterior infarction.

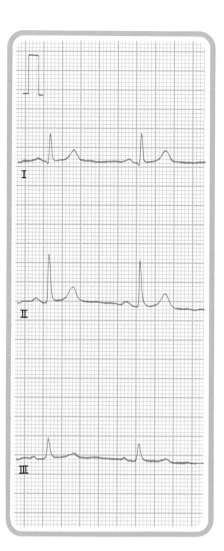

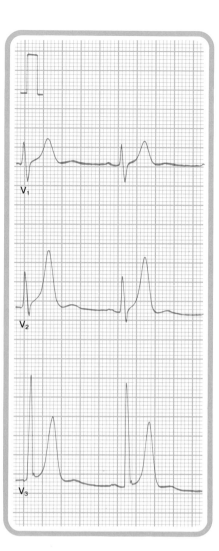

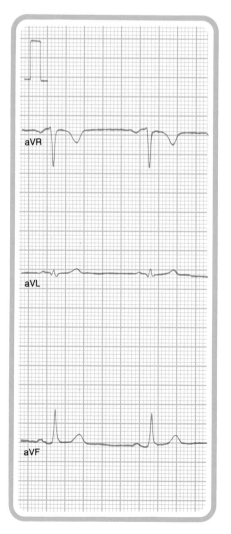

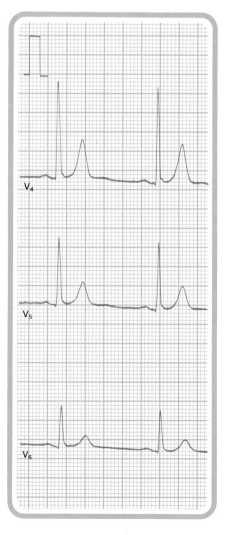

Figure 144

Report

"Sinus rhythm. The mean frontal plane QRS axis is +45°. There is T wave inversion in V_2, V_3 and aVL. The T waves are of low voltage in I, V_4 and V_5 and there is S-T segment depression in Lead I. The record is frankly abnormal but the changes are non-specific".

Explanation

The abnormalities are as listed in the report. The record is definitely abnormal, but a specific cause cannot be assigned. There are non-specific S-T, T changes in the precordial leads and in the limb leads (the mean frontal plane T axis is +105°, therefore the angle between the frontal plane QRS and T axes is abnormal). The patient was complaining of typical chest pain. Secondary interpretation therefore **suggests** but does not **prove** that the changes are ischaemic in origin.

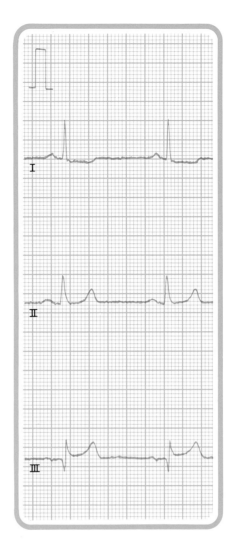

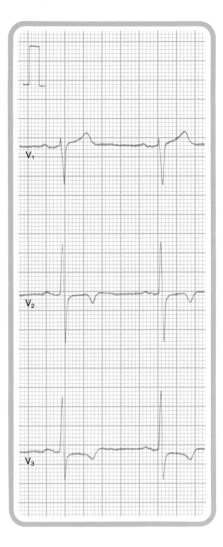

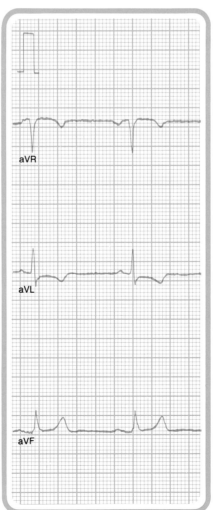

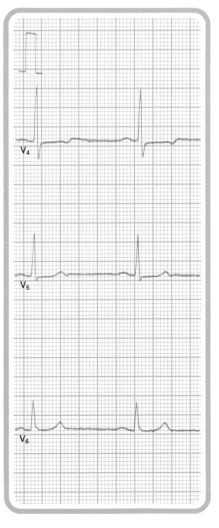

Figure 145

Report
"Sinus rhythm. There is left anterior hemiblock (the mean frontal plane QRS axis is −60°). There are non-specific S-T, T changes in Leads I, II and V_4-V_6. Abnormal U waves are seen in V_3-V_6."

Explanation
The two common causes of abnormal left axis deviation are left anterior hemiblock and inferior infarction. There is no evidence of inferior infarction (there are no q waves in II or aVF) and there is therefore left anterior hemiblock.
The S-T segment depression and T wave inversion in the leads facing the left ventricle are clearly abnormal, but are non-specific changes. The U waves in V_3-V_6 are abnormal since they are taller than the preceded T waves. The patient had a normal serum potassium level and a clinical history of recent ischaemic pain. The **probability** is, therefore, that the S-T, T and U wave changes are ischaemic in origin but one cannot be sure of this from the ECG appearances.

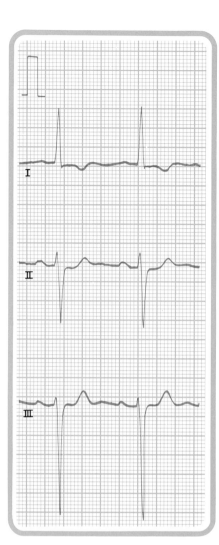

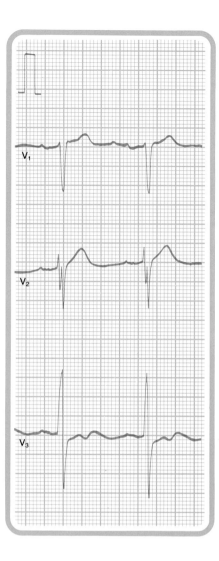

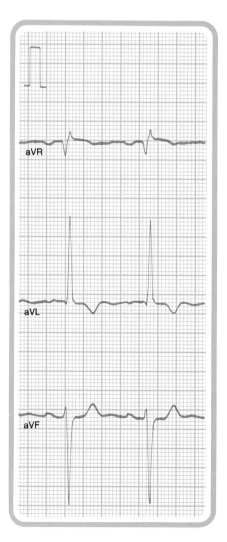

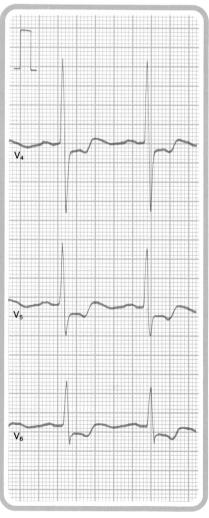

Figure 146

Report

"Sinus rhythm. The mean frontal plane QRS axis is +75°. There is evidence of acute infero-lateral myocardial damage."

Explanation

There is striking S-T segment elevation in II, III and aVF and minimal S-T elevation in V_5 and V_6. These changes indicate infero-lateral (i.e. "apical") myocardial damage. The S-T elevation in the inferior leads is convex upwards. This shape is typical of **ischaemic** damage. The S-T segment depression in I, aVL and V_1-V_3 is reciprocal to the primary S-T elevation. There is no QRS evidence of **infarction.**

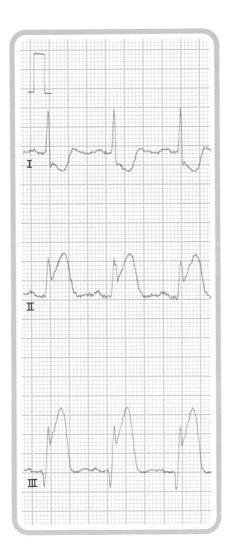

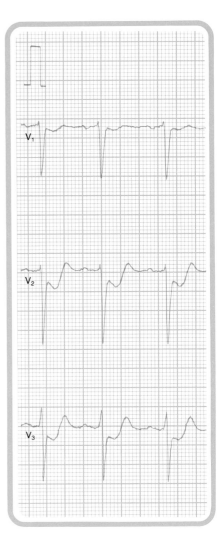

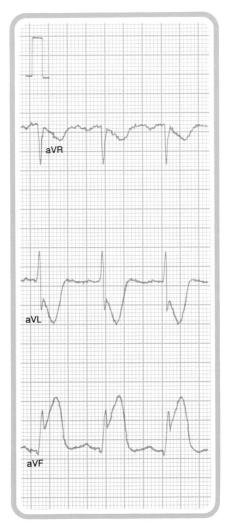

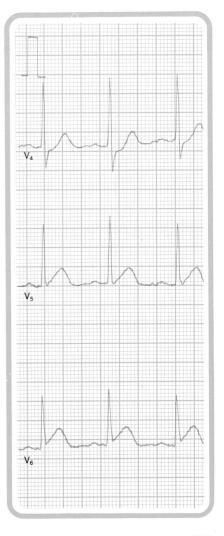

Figure 147

Report
"Sinus rhythm. The mean frontal plane QRS axis is −15°. There is evidence of relatively recent inferior myocardial infarction. There are non-specific S-T, T changes in V₆ and low voltage T waves in V₄ and V₅".

Explanation
There are abnormal Q waves in aVF indicating inferior infarction. There is S-T elevation in the inferior limb leads indicating that the infarct is recent. The T wave inversion in these leads is part of the pattern of recent infarction. There is slight S-T elevation in V_6 indicating involvement of the antero-lateral wall of the left ventricle in the infarction. There are non-specific T wave changes (flattening) in V_4 and V_5. The S-T segment depression in I and aVL is reciprocal.

Record 147 was taken from the same patient as Record 146, one day later. Note the **sequential** changes of inferior infarction. Note that the axis has shifted markedly to the left. Inferior myocardial infarction is one of the two common causes of shift of the axis to the left (in this case it has not actually become an abnormal degree of left axis deviation).

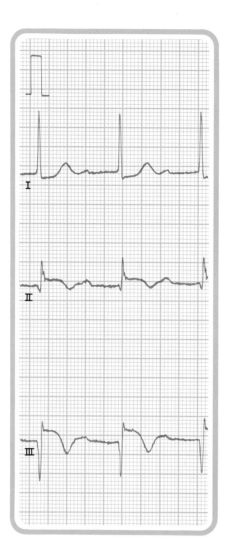

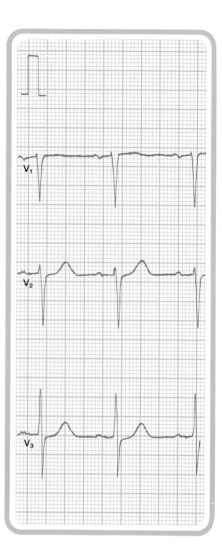

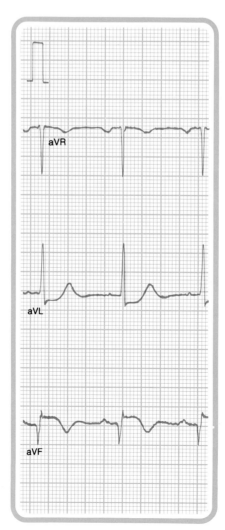

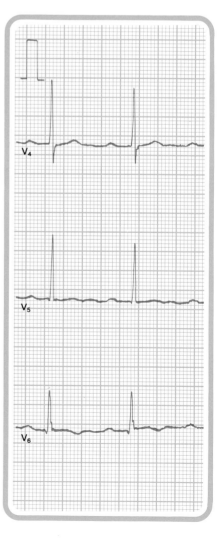

Miscellaneous Abnormalities

Ventricular Pre-excitation

This is a relatively rare condition and because of that fact it is usually dealt with towards the end of textbooks of electrocardiography. However, if the concept is not fully appreciated important diagnostic errors may occur.

The basic abnormality in ventricular pre-excitation is that the depolarisation wave, after passing through the atrial myocardium, activates the ventricles earlier than would be expected if the impulse travelled normally from atria to ventricles via the atrio-ventricular node and His bundle. For this reason ventricular pre-excitation is also known as **accelerated atrio-ventricular conduction.** In its most common form, the condition occurs as a result of the congenital presence of an "accessory" atrio-ventricular conduction pathway which conducts the impulse more rapidly than the A-V node and hence produces a rapid by-pass of the normal slow route. The P-R interval (the time interval between the first recognisable part of the P wave and the first recognisable part of the QRS complex) is shortened by the more rapid transmission of depolarisation, from atrial myocardium (P waves) to ventricular myocardium (QRS complexes).

As a consequence of the more rapid transmission of depolarisation from atrial myocardium to ventricular myocardium the P-R interval is shortened. As a result of the fact that the part of the ventricular myocardium to which the accessory atrio-ventricular pathway passes is the upper part of the right side of the interventricular septum and that this is the first part of the myocardium to be activated (whereas normally the left side of the upper part of the interventricular septum is the first part of the ventricular myocardium to be depolarised) **ventricular activation is interfered with and the QRS complex becomes distorted in shape and prolonged in duration. The combination of a short P-R interval and an abnormally shaped, abnormally long QRS complex comprises the electrocardiographic diagnosis of ventricular pre-excitation.**

The presence of two pathways for atrio-ventricular conduction (the **normal pathway** (through the A-V node, the His bundle and bundle branches) and the **accessory bundle**) leads to the possibility of the depolarisation wave passing from atria to ventricles down one pathway, back to the atria via the other pathway, then back to the ventricles via the first pathway etc. Such a cyclical, repetitive re-entry into the atrial and ventricular myocardium gives rise to paroxysmal tachycardia (e.g. atrial tachycardia or atrial flutter – see Section 3). **Patients with ventricular pre-excitation therefore have a tendency to episodes of paroxysmal tachycardia. This combination of (i) a short P-R interval, (ii) widening of the QRS complex with an abnormal configuration, and (iii) episodes of paroxysmal tachycardia, constitutes the Wolff-Parkinson-White (WPW) syndrome.** Note that the first two criteria are electrocardiographic and the third is clinical. All three are necessary for the diagnosis of the WPW syndrome. The presence of the two electrocardiographic criteria alone is often loosely regarded as diagnostic of the WPW syndrome, but strictly it is only diagnostic of ventricular pre-excitation, the physiological substrate which permits the paroxysmal tachycardia to occur. There are, in fact, several different types of ventricular pre-excitation. The different types have different electrocardiographic appearances and different anatomical substrates. The common type is WPW type pre-excitation.

The Mechanism of Accelerated Atrio-ventricular Conduction

Figure 148 (i) shows the normal pathway of atrio-ventricular conduction and Figure 148 (ii) the pathway in a typical case of ventricular pre-excitation.

(i) In normal conduction the depolarisation wave is initiated at the sino-atrial node and spreads in all directions through the atrial myocardium. That part of the atrial myocardium closest to the sino-atrial node (a) is the first part to be depolarised and this gives rise to the first part of the P wave. That part of the atrial myocardium most distant from the sino-atrial node (b) is the last part of the atrial myocardium to be depolarised and this gives rise to the last part of the P wave. The depolarisation wave reaches the atrio-ventricular node as soon as the myocardium adjacent to the A-V node (c) has been depolarised. This occurs at some time after the depolarisation of (a) and before that of (b), although the actual time at which the impulse reaches the A-V node cannot be recognised from the surface electrocardiogram. The route through the A-V node and His bundle provides the only pathway for depolarisation between atrial and ventricular myocardium. Since Purkinje arborisation begins earlier from the left bundle branch than from the right bundle branch (page 111) the interventricular septum is depolarised from left to right. This upper part of the interventricular septum is the first part of the ventricular myocardium to be depolarised (d) and this gives rise to the first part of the QRS complex (Figure 148 (i)).

(ii) In the presence of an accessory atrio-ventricular pathway (Figure 148 (ii)) there are two possible routes for transmission of depolarisation from atria to ventricles. The accessory pathway is depolarised at about the same time as the A-V node. However, the conduction through the accessory pathway is much faster than that through the A-V node.

Because of this, the first part of the ventricular myocardium to be depolarised is the **right** side of the interventricular septum and the septum is depolarised from right to left (e). The alteration in the initial direction of depolarisation of the ventricular myocardium changes the direction of the initial deflection in the QRS complex (from a negative to a positive wave – Figure 148 – compare e (ii) with d (i)). The initial part of the QRS complex (which begins before the completion of the P wave) is slurred. This premature, slurred initial portion of the QRS complex (e) is called the "delta wave". The total QRS duration is prolonged since the normal pathways of intraventricular conduction are not followed (this is necessarily so since ventricular depolarisation does not start in the normal place). As a result of the simultaneous shortening of the P-R interval and lengthening of the total QRS duration, the total time from the onset of the P wave to the end of the QRS complex is approximately the same as normal (Figure 148 – compare (ii) with (i)). Since ventricular depolarisation is abnormal, ventricular repolarisation is also abnormal and there may be S-T segment depression and/or T wave inversion.

Note

It should be clearly understood that the fact that the QRS complex normally starts well after the completion of the P wave is due to the very slow conduction in the A-V node. The depolarisation wave reaches the A-V node (c) well before the final part of the atrial myocardium is depolarised (b). The conduction velocity in the A-V node is very slow (page 111) and atrial myocardial depolarisation is normally complete before the depolarisation wave leaves the distal end of the A-V node. From this point, conduction through the His bundle and proximal part of the left bundle is very rapid (page 111).

It is illuminating to contrast the situation with that obtaining in complete left bundle branch block (Figure 148 (iii)). In this condition the pathway of atrio-ventricular conduction is normal (and therefore the P-R interval is normal). The septum is depolarised from right to left (and therefore the initial direction of the QRS deflection is opposite to normal). The pathway of ventricular myocardial depolarisation is therefore necessarily abnormal, the time taken for this depolarisation is increased. The total QRS duration is therefore prolonged.

Figure 148 shows the similarities and differences between bundle branch block and ventricular pre-excitation and these features are emphasised in Table 7.

Figure 148

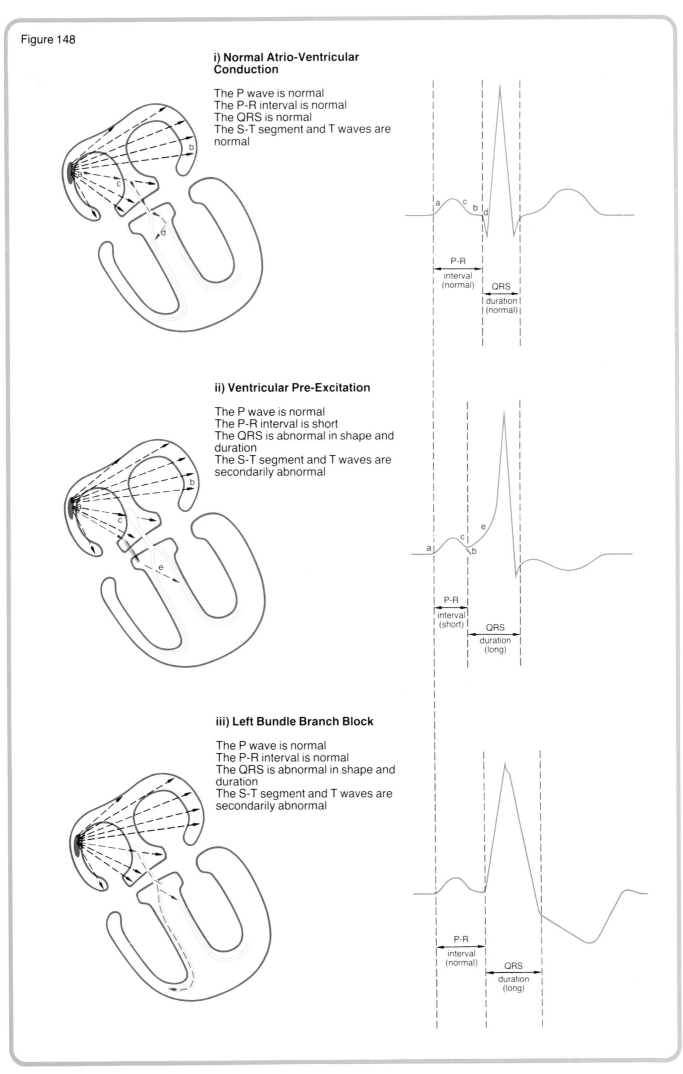

i) Normal Atrio-Ventricular Conduction

The P wave is normal
The P-R interval is normal
The QRS is normal
The S-T segment and T waves are normal

P-R interval (normal)

QRS duration (normal)

ii) Ventricular Pre-Excitation

The P wave is normal
The P-R interval is short
The QRS is abnormal in shape and duration
The S-T segment and T waves are secondarily abnormal

P-R interval (short)

QRS duration (long)

iii) Left Bundle Branch Block

The P wave is normal
The P-R interval is normal
The QRS is abnormal in shape and duration
The S-T segment and T waves are secondarily abnormal

P-R interval (normal)

QRS duration (long)

Table 7

	Normal	Bundle Branch Block	Ventricular Pre-excitation
P wave	Normal	Normal	Normal
P-R interval	Normal	Normal	Abnormally short
Initial direction of QRS	Normal	Reversed	Reversed
Total QRS duration	Normal	Increased	Increased
Slurred delta wave	Absent	Absent	Present
Secondary S-T segment changes	Absent	Present	Present
Secondary T wave changes	Absent	Present	Present

Each of the electrocardiographic features of ventricular pre-excitation has its anatomical substrate as indicated in Table 8.

Table 8

ECG changes in pre-excitation	Anatomical substrate
Short P-R interval	Rapid A-V conduction through accessory pathway
Delta wave	Abnormal site of initiation of ventricular depolarisation
Prolongation of QRS duration	Abnormal site of initiation of ventricular depolarisation

Diagnostic criteria of WPW type pre-excitation

The criteria for the diagnosis of ventricular pre-excitation of the type found in the Wolff-Parkinson-White syndrome are as follows:-

1. A P-R interval of less than 0.12 sec (i.e. 0.11 sec or less*) in the presence of sinus rhythm †.
2. An abnormally wide QRS complex of more than 0.10 sec (i.e. 0.11 sec or more*).
3. The presence of initial (first 0.03 to 0.05 sec) slurring of the QRS complex.

These three criteria must **all** be fulfilled for a diagnosis of pre-excitation of the WPW type.

Additional features frequently present in WPW type pre-excitation
1. S-T segment depression
and/or
2. Low-voltage T wave or T wave inversion.
3. Abnormal q waves or QS complexes may be seen in the absence of myocardial infarction (pages 216 to 220).
4. The r wave progression in the precordial leads may be abnormal (page 217).

Clinical Features Found in Association with the Full Clinical Picture of the Wolff-Parkinson-White Syndrome

1. Paroxysmal supraventricular tachycardia
or
2. Paroxysmal atrial fibrillation.

Note

* The limit of resolution of time measurements on the electrocardiogram recorded at normal speed is one quarter of one small square on the recording paper, i.e. 0.01 sec. (Thus "less than 0.12 sec" is equivalent to "0.11 sec or less" and "more than 0.10 sec" is equivalent to "0.11 sec or more").

†In the presence of atrial ectopic rhythms the P-R interval can be abnormally short simply because of the arrhythmia.

The electrocardiographic findings of WPW type pre-excitation are found in something of the order of 0.5% of routine electrocardiograms.

An example of WPW type ventricular pre-excitation is shown in Figure 149.

Note the superficial resemblance of Figure 149 to the appearances in left bundle branch block – compare Figure 149 with Figure 87 (page 123). The duration and configuration of the QRS complexes and the S-T segment and T wave appearances are virtually identical in the two cases. The fundamental difference lies in the **combination** of the short P-R interval and the delta wave. The delta wave is an early, slurred take-off of the QRS complex before the completion of the P wave (compare also Figure 148). The similarities between the QRS complexes in left bundle branch block and in this type of ventricular pre-excitation occur because in both cases the ventricular depolarisation is initiated abnormally from the upper and **right** side of the interventricular septum.

The delta wave is often directed superiorly (i.e. away from the inferior leads). In such a case the inferior leads will show a broad, slurred q wave (the delta wave in this case) which might lead to a wrongful diagnosis of inferior infarction. An example is shown in Figure 150.

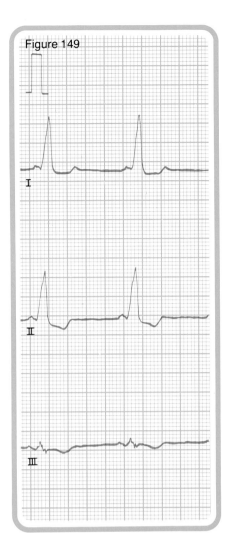

Figure 149

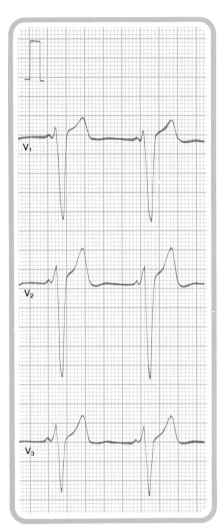

Figure 149

The rhythm is of sinus origin. The P-R interval is abnormally short at 0.06 sec (well seen in the second complex in V_1). The total QRS duration is abnormally long at 0.18 sec (well seen in both QRS complexes in V_2).

The initial slurring of the QRS complex (the delta wave) is well seen in I, V_2, V_3 and V_4. (One might expect that the delta wave would be visible in all leads, but it is always a small wave and is often inconspicuous in leads at right angles to the direction of the depolarisation giving rise to the delta wave). Non-specific S-T segment depression and T wave flattening are seen in I, II, III, aVF, V_5 and V_6.

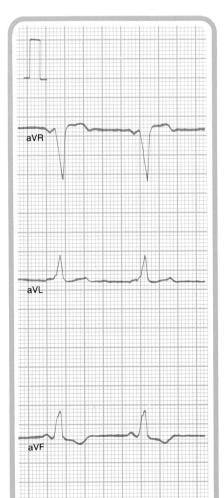

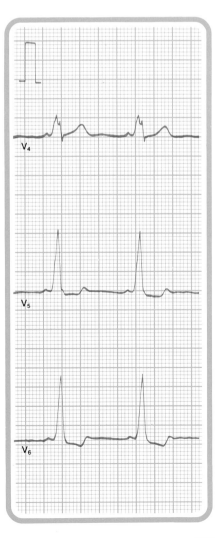

Practical Note

The risks of serious mis-diagnosis of the electrocardiogram are substantially reduced if the following simple rules are followed:-

1. In the presence of left bundle branch block, do not diagnose myocardial infarction.

2. In the presence of pre-excitation, do not diagnose left bundle branch block or myocardial infarction.

In both cases the diagnosis of infarction **can** sometimes be made despite the prior presence of one of the two abnormalities (pre-excitation or bundle branch block), but special conditions may need to be fulfilled (such as the availability of previous records) and for the non-expert, the problem is best avoided. Under-diagnosis of the ECG is a much less serious sin than over-diagnosis.

It has been acknowledged earlier (page 212) that several different types of ventricular pre-excitation exist. Indeed the Wolff-Parkinson-White type pre-excitation has itself been divided into Types A, B and C.

In **Type A** the delta wave vector is directed anteriorly (thus the initial slurred part of the QRS complex will be positive in the anterior leads). In such a case the delta wave is positive in all the precordial leads. The remainder of the QRS is also positive in these leads. The QRS complex in V_1 has a morphology similar to that in right bundle branch block or right ventricular hypertrophy and there is often right axis deviation.

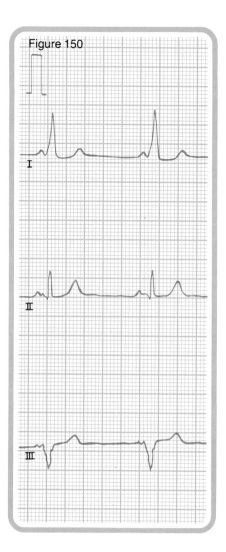

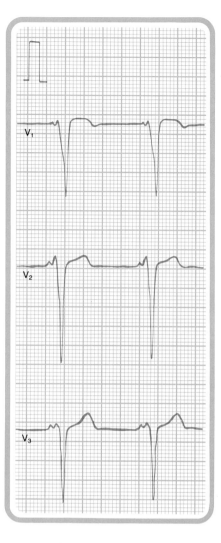

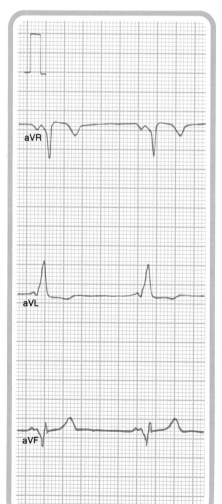

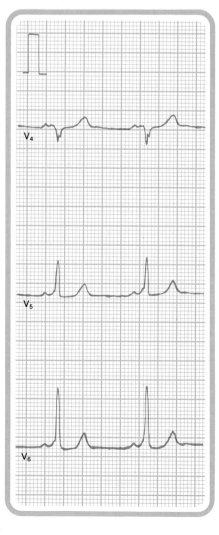

Figure 150

The rhythm is of sinus origin. The P-R interval is short at 0.05 sec (well seen in the second beat in V_2). The QRS duration is prolonged at 0.14 sec (well seen in I). There is a slurred initial part to the QRS complex (the delta wave) well seen in I, aVL and V_6. Abnormal Q waves are seen in aVF. In the absence of ventricular pre-excitation this would indicate inferior infarction. In the presence of pre-excitation it has no such significance. There is nothing in this record to indicate the presence of infarction.

In **Type B** the delta wave vector may be negative or positive in the right precordial leads, but the dominant QRS deflection is negative in the right and positive in the left precordial leads, and the morphology of the QRS complex resembles that of left bundle branch block. Type B is much commoner than Type A and Figures 149 and 150 both show examples of Type B. In each case the delta wave is positive in V_1-V_3. When it is negative in these leads QS complexes will occur. Figure 151 shows an example of Type A. Both the delta wave and the main QRS deflections are upright from V_1-V_5. In both types the r wave progression in the precordial leads will often be abnormal. Unless the presence of ventricular pre-excitation is recognised this too may lead to a false diagnosis of myocardial infarction.

In **either Type A or Type B** the delta wave vector may be directed superiorly – in which case abnormal q waves will appear in any of the Leads II, III and aVF.

Type C is much rarer even than Type A. In this type the delta wave is negative in V_5 and V_6 but positive in V_1 to V_4.

It cannot be emphasised too strongly that abnormal q waves or QS complexes in ANY lead do not indicate myocardial infarction if there is evidence of ventricular pre-excitation.

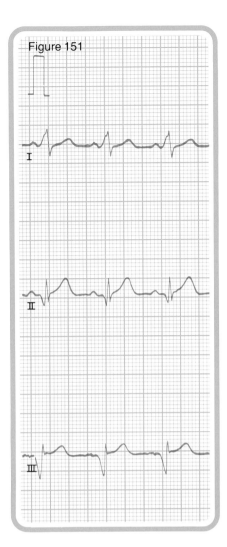

Figure 151

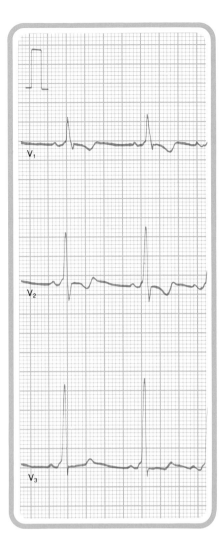

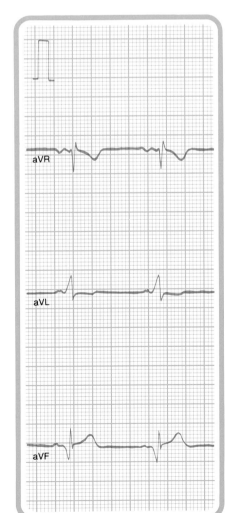

Figure 151

The rhythm is sinus. The P-R interval is abnormally short at 0.08 sec (well seen in V_1 and V_2). The total QRS duration is abnormal at 0.12 sec (well seen in V_2 and V_3) and there is a delta wave (well seen in I, aVL, V_1-V_5). The q waves in II, III and aVF are abnormal but do **not** indicate infarction. The S-T segment abnormalities in V_1-V_3 are a result of the pre-excitation. The dominant R wave in V_1 is not indicative either of right ventricular hypertrophy or of true posterior infarction – it is a result of the ventricular pre-excitation.

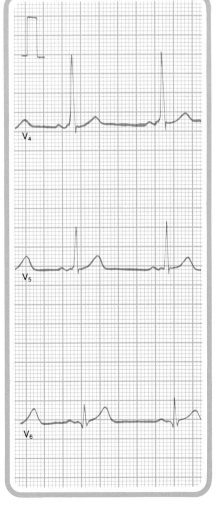

Doubt has recently been expressed about the validity of the classification of ECG patterns in ventricular pre-excitation. Numerous anatomical possibilities, each with its own resulting ECG pattern, are now known to exist.

Other Types of Ventricular Pre-excitation

In addition to the WPW type, other forms of pre-excitation exist. The next most common type is the **Lown-Ganong-Levine (LGL) syndrome.**

> The **electrocardiographic criteria** for the LGL type pre-excitation
> 1. A P-R interval (in the adult) of less than 0.12 sec (i.e. 0.11 sec or less*
> 2. A normal QRS duration with no delta wave.

Patients with pre-excitation of the LGL type have a tendency to episodes of paroxysmal supraventricular tachycardia (in the same way as those with WPW type pre-excitation). Patients who have the electrocardiographic features of LGL type pre-excitation, together with the **clinical criterion** of having had episodes of paroxysmal tachycardia have the LGL syndrome.

Note that since the QRS complexes are normal, the electrocardiographic findings are not confused with bundle branch block or myocardial infarction.

An example of the ECG appearances in LGL syndrome is seen in Figure 152.

In the LGL syndrome the accessory pathway is thought to run from the atrial myocardium to the distal part of the A-V node or to the beginning of the His bundle, thus short-circuiting the normal A-V nodal delay (with consequent reduction in the P-R interval) whilst permitting normal intraventricular conduction (with consequent normality of the QRS complex).

Note
* The limit of resolution of time measurements on the electrocardiogram recorded at normal speed is one quarter of one small square on the recording paper, i.e. 0.01 sec.

Figure 152

The basic rhythm is of sinus origin. The P-R interval is abnormally short at 0.08 sec. The QRS complexes are normal. The P waves are hardly visible in the precordial leads. This indicates that the P wave vector is directed superiorly and inferiorly and therefore has no major component in the horizontal plane.

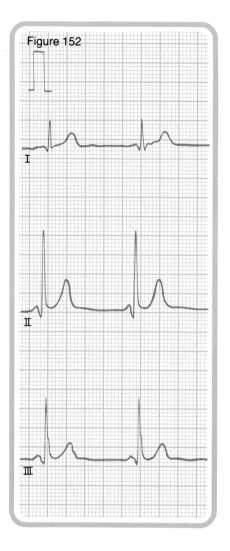

Figure 152

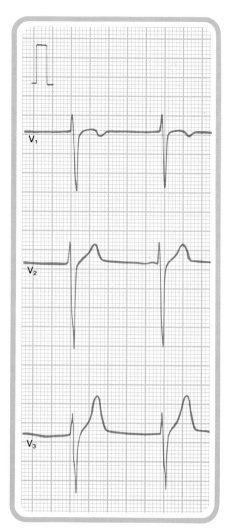

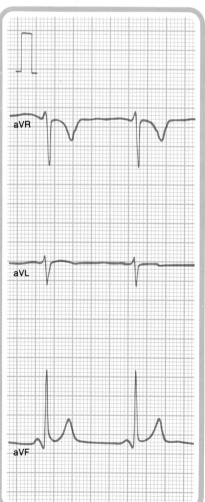

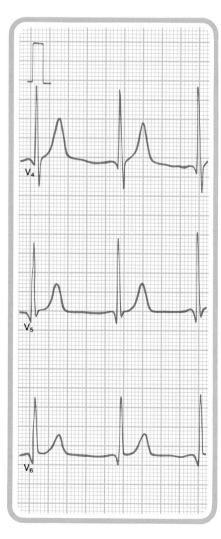

The Significance of Ventricular Pre-excitation

Ventricular pre-excitation is relatively uncommon. In terms of its frequency a totally disproportionate amount of space has been devoted to it in this book. This apparently undue emphasis is, however, justifiable in view of the real risk of mistakenly making a diagnosis of serious heart disease when the ECG shows pre-excitation.

The only real clinical consequence of ventricular pre-excitation is episodic supraventricular tachycardia. These attacks may often be a nuisance and can be temporarily disabling but do not usually constitute a risk to the patient unless the rhythm is atrial fibrillation (this is rare – normally it is atrial tachycardia).

The important diagnoses which can be made in error through misinterpretation of an ECG actually showing pre-excitation include the following:-

1. Inferior myocardial infarction (in Types A, B or C).
2. Anterior myocardial infarction (in Types B or C).
3. Left bundle branch block (in Type B).
4. Right bundle branch block (in Types A and C).
5. Right ventricular hypertrophy (in Types A and C).
6. True posterior infarction (in Types A and C).

Also, during an episode of atrial tachycardia in a patient with ventricular pre-excitation, ventricular tachycardia may be mistakenly diagnosed – see Section 3. About 50% of patients with electrocardiographic evidence of ventricular pre-excitation have episodes of paroxysmal tachycardia.

Digitalis – induced Changes in the ECG

Digitalis has complex effects on the heart. It induces both electrical and mechanical changes **directly** by inhibiting the normal active process of sodium ion transport across the membranes of both myocardial and pacemaker cells. This primary interference with sodium ion transport necessarily results in secondary changes in potassium ion movement across the membranes. Digitalis and potassium ions have mutually antagonistic effects on ion-flux across cell membranes (especially flux involving sodium and calcium ions). Digitalis also has **indirect** effects on the heart by increasing the vagal tone.

When a patient is receiving a digitalis preparation in therapeutic doses the electrocardiogram may show recognisable changes, but need not necessarily do so. When such changes are seen they are referred to as "digitalis effect". Digitalis effect does not indicate overdosage and is in no way synonymous with "digitalis toxicity" (*vide infra*).

The possible changes induced by digitalis on the electrocardiogram are:-

1. Decreased T wave amplitude.
2. S-T segment depression.
3. Increase in U wave amplitude.
4. Shortening of the Q-T interval.

⎱ "digitalis effect"

5. Development of various cardiac arrhythmias – arrhythmias due to digitalis are always a sign of toxicity.
6. Combinations of the above.

Whether or not a patient receiving digitalis develops recognisable changes of digitalis effect depends upon a whole variety of factors including the dose of digitalis, the physical size and age of the patient, the general metabolic state (in particular the thyroid function) the serum potassium level and the presence or absence of ventricular hypertrophy.

T Wave Changes

One of the earliest and commonest changes is reduction in the voltage of the T waves. This is, of course, a non-specific change, which has many other possible causes. When it is present it is certainly not possible by inspecting the electrocardiogram to assert that the changes are due to the action of digitalis though the knowledge that the patient is receiving digitalis makes it a possibility (secondary interpretation). The T wave changes are most often seen in leads facing the left ventricle (left precordial leads and those limb leads orientated in the region of the cardiac axis – i.e. aVL and I when the heart is horizontal and II, aVF and III when the heart is vertical). In the presence of right ventricular hypertrophy the T wave changes induced by digitalis may be most pronounced in the right precordial leads. Occasionally the T wave changes may be so pronounced as to give biphasic or even inverted (negative) T waves.

S-T Segment Change

The most frequently recognised finding of digitalis effect is a downward sloping S-T segment depression. This is often associated with T wave flattening and the combined appearance of the sloping S-T segment and flattened T wave has been said to be similar to a reversed tick (or the tick made by a left-handed person) (Figure 153).

Figure 153

This shows the appearances in a left precordial lead in a normal subject (a) in the presence of mild (b) and more pronounced (c) changes of digitalis effect.

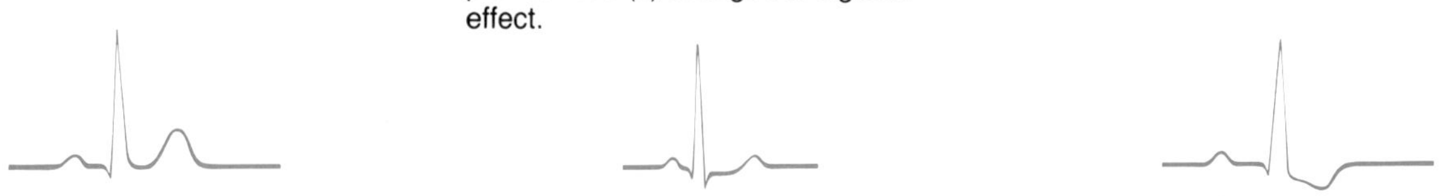

a) Normal QRS complexes, S-T segment and T waves.

b) Non-specific S-T segment depression with reduction in T wave voltage.

c) Downward sloping S-T segment depression with flat T waves – highly typical of, but not diagnostic of, digitalis effect.

Increased U Wave Amplitude

The normal U wave is smaller than the preceding T wave. The U wave becomes more prominent when the patient takes digitalis. The increased U wave height is usually best seen in the mid-precordial leads. The degree of increase in U wave height is usually slight and is less than that found in hypokalaemia or in response to quinidine therapy.

Shortening of the Q-T Interval

The normal Q-T interval bears an inverse relationship to the heart rate. The normality or otherwise of the Q-T interval can only be determined if the Q-T interval measurement is evaluated in relation to the heart rate at the time (see pages 263 and 264). As a rough guide the normal Q-T interval is in the region of 0.36 to 0.44 sec for adults with heart rates in the region of 60-90 per min. As the heart rate increases the Q-T interval falls and vice-versa. The Q-T interval changes in digitalis therapy are slight and rarely recognised unless specifically sought.

The changes in T waves, S-T segments, U waves and Q-T interval described above are the features known as "digitalis effect". An example of "digitalis effect" is shown in Figure 154.

Digitalis Toxicity

The above effects may be found in any patient receiving treatment with digitalis. In the presence of digitalis over-dosage, toxicity occurs. This most frequently presents with gastro-intestinal symptoms such as nausea, anorexia and vomiting and may occasionally present with visual disturbances.

Digitalis-induced arrhythmias are always a manifestation of **toxicity** rather than just digitalis effect. When death occurs as a result of digitalis toxicity, it is always due to ventricular fibrillation.

The common arrhythmias occurring in digitalis toxicity are:-
1. Ventricular premature (ectopic) beats.
2. Coupled ventricular premature beats.
3. Multifocal ventricular premature beats.
4. Nodal (junctional) tachycardia.
5. Sinus bradycardia.
6. Atrial tachycardia with atrio-ventricular block.
7. First-degree heart block (first-degree atrio-ventricular block).
8. Mobitz Type I second-degree atrio-ventricular block (Wenckebach phenomenon).
9. Third-degree atrio-ventricular block.
10. Multifocal atrial premature (ectopic) beats.
11. Ventricular tachycardia.
12. Atrial flutter.
13. Atrial fibrillation.
14. Sino-atrial block.
15. Sinus arrest.
16. Ventricular fibrillation.

The recognition of these arrhythmias will be dealt with in Section 3.

Digitalis toxicity may also occasionally give rise to widening of the QRS complexes even in the absence of arrhythmias.

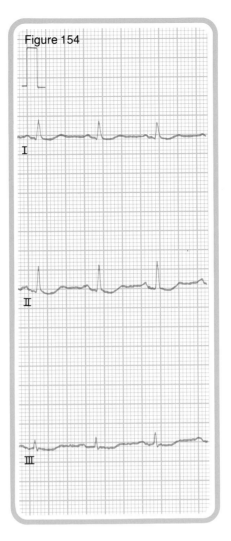

Figure 154

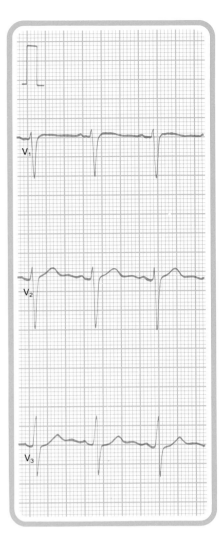

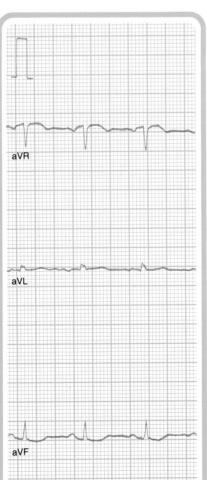

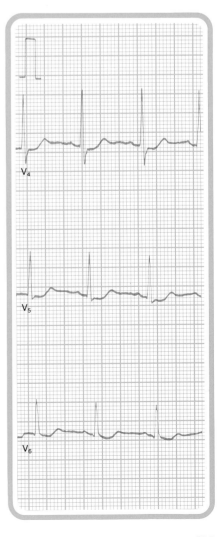

Figure 154

The rhythm is sinus. The record is normal except for the presence of S-T, T changes. There is S-T segment depression in II, III and aVF and in V_4 to V_6. The T waves are of low voltage in the limb leads and in V_5 and V_6. These changes are non-specific. They are **consistent with** but not **diagnostic of** digitalis effect.

Effects of Other Drugs on the ECG

Numerous drugs produce relatively minor changes in the ECG, some of the commoner, more important ones are listed below:-

Quinidine

1. Low voltage T waves (or T wave inversion).
2. S-T segment depression.
3. Prolongation of the Q-T interval.
4. Increased height of U wave.
5. Widening and notching of P waves.

In toxic doses, quinidine gives rise to widening of the QRS complexes and serious arrhythmias, including heart block, ventricular tachycardia and ventricular fibrillation. Sometimes less severe arrhythmias occur such as sinus bradycardia, sinus arrest or sino-atrial block.

Propranolol (and other beta-blocking drugs)

The most obvious effect is the reduction of the sinus rate. No significant changes in the QRS complexes, S-T segments or T waves occur. Rarely the degree of A-V block may be increased in patients with A-V conduction abnormalities. In patients with atrial fibrillation or atrial flutter, the ventricular rate is reduced.

Phenothiazine drugs and Tricyclic antidepressants

These produce changes similar to those of quinidine.

Lignocaine

In therapeutic doses lignocaine has no recognisable effect on the electrocardiogram. In toxic doses sinus tachycardia, sinus arrest or atrio-ventricular block may occur.

Mexiletine

The actions of this drug are similar to those of lignocaine. In therapeutic doses it has no detectable effect on the electrocardiogram. In toxic doses the central nervous system is primarily affected but sinus bradycardia, nodal rhythm or, rarely, A-V conduction disturbances can occur.

Aprindine, tocainide and lidoflazine
are other congeners of lignocaine with similar, minimal effects on the ECG in therapeutic doses. Of the group, lidoflazine has been reported as possibly giving rise to serious ventricular arrhythmias occasionally.

Diphenylhydantoin

In normal doses no noticeable effect on the ECG occurs. Occasionally the P-R interval may be increased and the Q-T interval diminished. In the presence of extensive myocardial disease the intravenous administration of this drug has occasionally been followed by bradycardia, A-V block, asystole or venticular fibrillation.

Procainamide

Therapeutic doses produce only minimal changes. As the dose is increased, prolongation of the P-R interval, QRS duration and Q-T interval occurs. The T wave voltage is reduced and the U wave height increased.

Toxic doses may give rise to gross widening of the QRS complexes, ventricular ectopic beats, ventricular tachycardia, ventricular fibrillation or asystole. These effects are more commonly seen after intravenous administration, than after oral therapy.

Disopyramide

In therapeutic doses the effects are minimal. As the dose is increased, changes similar to those seen with quinidine occur.

Verapamil

This drug acts primarily by inhibiting the slow calcium channel in the myocardial cell membrane. It produces a slowing of the sinus rate and of conduction through the atrio-ventricular node. The latter effect gives rise ultimately to prolongation of the P-R interval. There is no change in the QRS complexes or in the corrected Q-T interval.

The effects of the drug on the sino-atrial and atrio-ventricular nodes are additive with those of beta-blocking drugs and the use of verapamil and beta-blocking drugs simultaneously can give rise to profound and occasionally catastrophic bradycardia.

Nifedipine

This drug is also a slow calcium channel blocker. Its effect on the heart is much less pronounced than that of verapamil, and it has much more effect on the peripheral circulation. No significant changes in the P waves, P-R interval or QRS complexes occur even at doses which produce profound haemodynamic effects.

Perhexilene

This slow calcium channel blocker produces a slowing of the sinus rate, probably by a direct effect on the sino-atrial node. No other significant effects on the electrocardiogram have been noted, but the use of this drug is severely limited by its side effects on liver function and on peripheral nerves.

Amiodarone

Gives rise to prolongation of the Q-T interval and increase in the height of the U waves. This is in keeping with its characteristic electrophysiological effect of prolongation of the action potential.

Electrolyte Disturbances

The normal state of polarisation of cardiac cell membranes is dependent upon the maintenance of normal ionic balance across the membranes. The processes of depolarisation and repolarisation are related to ionic fluxes. It is therefore predictable that disturbance of the normal levels of electrolyte in extracellular or intracellular fluids may give rise to electro-cardiographic changes.

The most important ion in the maintenance of the normal state of polarisation of the membranes is the potassium ion. The resting transmembrane potential is, for all practical purposes, determined by the ratio of intracellular to extracellular potassium ion concentration. The normal extracellular potassium ion concentration lies in the range 3.5 to 5.0mmol/l. The intracellular concentration is of the order of 140mmol/l. Substantial changes in the extracellular levels may occur in disease states. Changes in intracellular levels in diseases are proportionately much smaller. In view of this difference in the degree to which variations in the intracellular and extracellular absolute levels of potassium concentration can occur, together with the fact that it is the **ratio** of intracellular and extracellular levels which determines membrane stability, it follows that the absolute extracellular level of potassium ion concentration is the single most important factor affecting the cell membranes and therefore also the electrocardiogram. The often repeated assertion that the ECG is a guide to **intracellular** potassium ion levels is false and is the result of confused thinking. It is often also stated that the ECG can be used to monitor the potassium state of the patient. Since the correlation of the degree of ECG changes with the degree of abnormality of the extracellular potassium ion concentration is poor, this is not practicable advice. Indeed none of those who give this advice appear to take it themselves. They always measure the serum potassium ion level when they are concerned about the patient's potassium status (and rightly so!).

Note

$$Em = \frac{RT}{F} \ln \frac{[K^+]_o}{[K^+]_i}$$

where
Em = resting membrane potential
T = absolute temperature
F = Faraday's number
R = Universal gas constant

$[K^+]_o$ = extracellular potassium ion concentration
$[K^+]_i$ = intracellular potassium ion concentration

ECG Changes in Hyperkalaemia

Hyperkalaemia produces changes in the electrocardiogram which are increasingly more severe as the potassium ion level rises. There is, in other words, a **direct** correlation between the degree of increase in the serum potassium ion level and the resulting ECG changes. However, this correlation is **neither precise nor totally consistent.**

If hyperkalaemia is suspected the serum potassium ion level should be measured. If hyperkalaemia is to be "monitored", changes in the serum potassium ion level should be followed. Hyperkalaemia is always a serious problem demanding urgent attention in view of the constant risk of ventricular fibrillation.

An enormous range of possible changes occurs in hyperkalaemia. A few of these are listed in Figure 155.

There are no diagnostic changes of hyperkalaemia. All the changes are non-specific and may be seen in myocardial damage arising from other causes, e.g. infarction and drugs. All parts of the ECG – P waves, QRS complexes, S-T segments, T waves and the cardiac rhythm may be affected in hyperkalaemia.

The typical, progressive changes of hyperkalaemia are as follows:-

Development of tall, pointed narrow T waves.

$\downarrow$

Reduction in P wave amplitude, reduction in R wave height, widening of QRS complexes, S-T segment change (elevation in some leads, depression in others), development of hemiblock (especially left anterior hemiblock) development of first degree heart block.

$\downarrow$

More advanced intraventricular block (very wide QRS complexes with right bundle branch block, left bundle branch block, bifascicular or trifascicular block) ventricular ectopic beats.

$\downarrow$

Absent P waves. Very broad and bizarre QRS complexes (often simulating infarction). Atrio-ventricular block, ventricular tachycardia or fibrillation or ventricular asystole.

In modern clinical practice it is unusual for changes more advanced than the earliest change of tall pointed T waves to be seen. Such tall T waves do not necessarily indicate hyperkalaemia for they may be seen in the precordial leads as a normal variant or in true posterior ischaemia. The diagnosis of or exclusion of hyperkalaemia when there is such a finding is by measurement of the serum level of potassium ions.

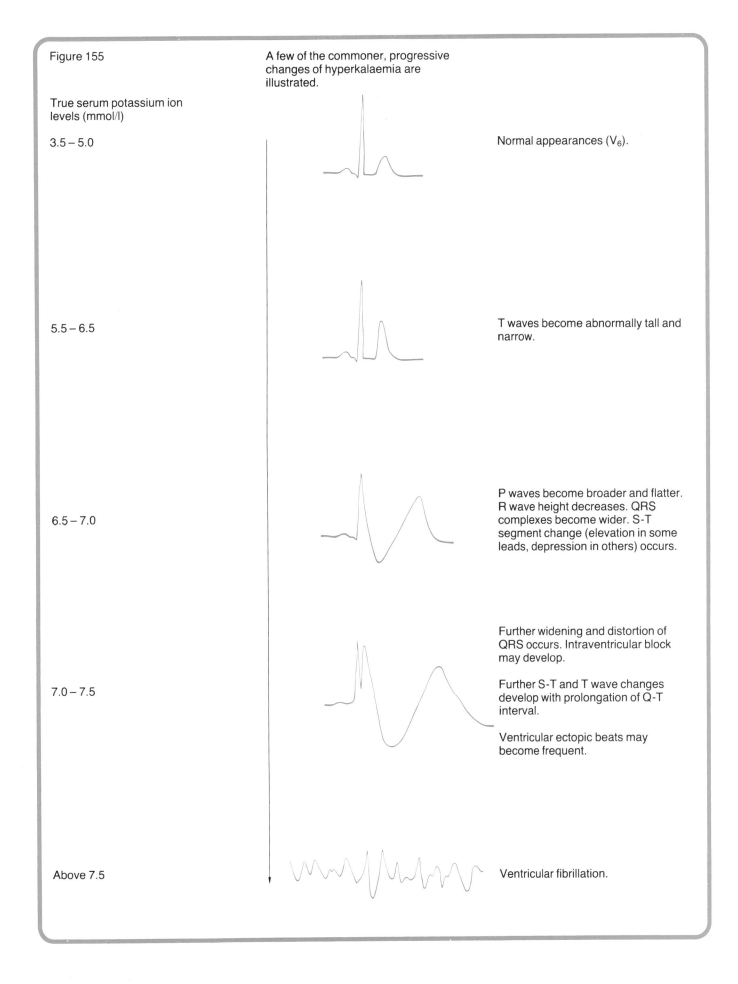

Figure 155

True serum potassium ion levels (mmol/l)

A few of the commoner, progressive changes of hyperkalaemia are illustrated.

3.5 – 5.0

Normal appearances (V₆).

5.5 – 6.5

T waves become abnormally tall and narrow.

6.5 – 7.0

P waves become broader and flatter. R wave height decreases. QRS complexes become wider. S-T segment change (elevation in some leads, depression in others) occurs.

7.0 – 7.5

Further widening and distortion of QRS occurs. Intraventricular block may develop.

Further S-T and T wave changes develop with prolongation of Q-T interval.

Ventricular ectopic beats may become frequent.

Above 7.5

Ventricular fibrillation.

ECG Changes in Hypokalaemia

Significant hypokalaemia can exist without recognisable changes on the electrocardiogram and when such changes are present, the correlation between the extent of the change and the degree of hypokalaemia is very poor. However, hypokalaemia is encountered much more commonly than hyperkalaemia.

The changes found in hypokalaemia (in descending order of frequency) are:

1. S-T segment depression, decreased amplitude of the T waves, increased U wave height.

2. Cardiac arrhythmias.

3. Prolongation of the QRS duration, increase in P wave amplitude and duration.

Figure 156 shows an example of the most commonly seen changes.

The S-T segment, T wave and U wave changes of hypokalaemia illustrated in Figure 156 are by far the commonest changes seen in hypokalaemia.

Less common changes include minimal (and usually unnoticed) prolongation of the QRS complexes and (rarely) increase in amplitude and duration of the P waves.

Many different types of arrhythmia can occur when the serum potassium ion level falls (since the ratio of extracellular to intracellular potassium ion concentration becomes abnormal and the cell membrane becomes less stable). These arrhythmias include atrial ectopic beats, atrial tachycardia, ventricular ectopic beats, ventricular tachycardia, first, second and third degree heart block and ventricular fibrillation. When unexplained arrhythmias develop, it is worth checking the serum potassium ion level.

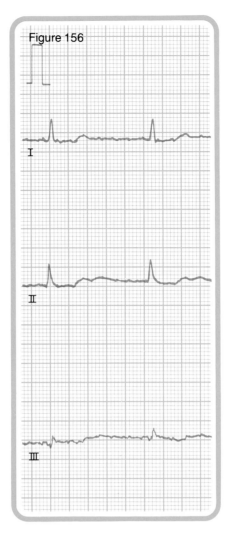

Figure 156

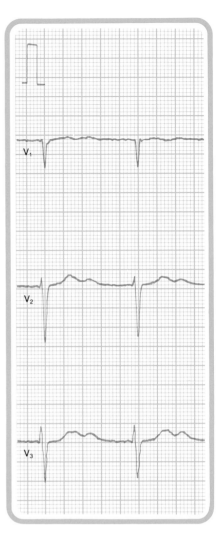

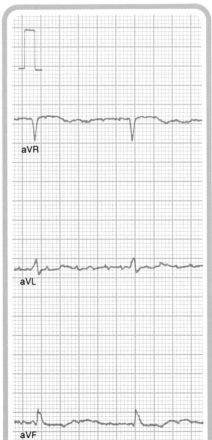

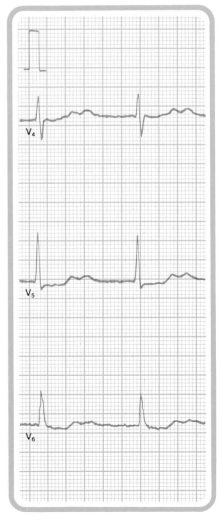

Figure 156

The rhythm is sinus. The T waves are of low voltage in every lead. There is S-T segment depression in I, II, aVF and V_4–V_6. There are abnormally tall U waves seen in II, aVF and V_4–V_6 (in all these leads the U waves are taller than the preceding T waves). The U waves are also prominent in V_1–V_3.

Hypocalcaemia

The main electrocardiographic change in hypocalcaemia is prolongation of the Q-T interval. The duration of the T wave (though it is not usual to measure the T wave duration) is not changed. The S-T segment is prolonged. The degree of prolongation of the Q-T interval is approximately proportional to the degree of lowering of the level of ionic calcium in the serum. It is said that hypocalcaemia is the **only** condition which gives rise to prolongation of the S-T segment without either (i) increased T wave duration or (ii) apparent increased T wave duration due to prominence of the U waves.

Hypothermia may present an exception to this rule.

The ECG changes of hypocalcaemia appear to be of little significance. They are usually unrecognised clinically unless it is known that the serum calcium ion level is low and they are specifically looked for. The P waves, P-R interval and U waves are usually unaltered. The QRS morphology is usually unchanged. The QRS duration may be slightly reduced but it is rare for this to be noticed. Hypocalcaemia does not usually give rise to arrhythmias.

Hypercalcaemia

The main electrocardiographic change in hypercalcaemia is reduction in the Q-T interval. The T wave duration appears unaffected, the reduction being in the duration of the S-T segment. The degree of reduction in the Q-T interval is approximately proportional to the increase in the serum concentration of ionic calcium. At very high levels of serum calcium ions this relationship breaks down because progressive T wave prolongation occurs, offsetting the effect of the reducing S-T duration on the total Q-T interval.

No appreciable change occurs in the P, QRS or T morphology. The dimensions of these deflections are not usually significantly altered except for the above noted tendency for the T wave to become prolonged at very high serum levels of calcium. The U wave amplitude may increase, sometimes contributing to the apparent T wave duration.

Significant cardiac arrhythmias do not often result from hypercalcaemia. However, slight prolongation of the P-R interval and occasionally second or third degree A-V block have been described.

Patients with hypercalcaemia have an increased sensitivity to digitalis. Sinus arrest, sino-atrial block, atrial or ventricular ectopic beats, ventricular tachycardia and ventricular fibrillation have all been described in hypercalcaemic patients taking digitalis. It is said that the intravenous administration of calcium to a fully digitalised patient is potentially dangerous. Fatalities have been recorded in this situation.

Hypo- and Hyper-magnesaemia

Minor electrocardiographic changes are described in both of these electrolyte disturbances. Since there are often simultaneous abnormalities of other electrolytes their specificity is uncertain.

In hypomagnesaemia, changes resembling those of hypokalaemia occur with flattening of the T waves, S-T segment depression, prominence of the U waves and occasionally prolongation of the P-R interval. Like hypokalaemia and hypercalcaemia, hypomagnesaemia aggravates digitalis toxicity. A whole variety of arrhythmias including ventricular fibrillation has been described in association with hypomagnesaemia, but there is frequently associated hypokalaemia and digitalis is often also implicated. Significant arrhythmias induced solely by hypomagnesaemia must be very rare.

The electrocardiographic changes associated with hypermagnesaemia are similar to those in hyperkalaemia. There may be prolongation of the P-R interval and widening of the QRS complexes.

Hypo- and Hyper-natraemia

No significant changes appear in the electrocardiogram in response to changes in the serum level of sodium ions.

Hypothyroidism

Biochemical and clinical hypothyroidism can exist without any recognisable ECG changes. However, when hypothyroidism is severe or prolonged, generalised ECG changes occur. These are the result of interstitial myocardial oedema and often also of the additional presence of a pericardial effusion.

The changes of hypothyroidism are:-
1. **Sinus bradycardia.**
2. **Low voltages of P waves, QRS complexes and T waves.**
3. **Slight S-T segment depression.**
4. **Prolongation of the P-R interval.**
5. **Atrio-ventricular block (occasionally).**
6. **Prominent U waves may occur.**
7. **The Q-Tc interval may be prolonged but measurement of this may be difficult or impossible since the T wave amplitude is diminished and the U wave height may be increased.**

An example is shown in Figure 157.

The changes of hypothyroidism usually resolve within the first few weeks of thyroid replacement therapy. Occasionally improvement may even be apparent within the first few days of treatment.

Arrhythmias are not especially common in hypothyroidism (except for sinus bradycardia) but atrial tachycardia, A-V junctional escape rhythm, A-V block of various degrees and right or left bundle branch block occasionally occur.

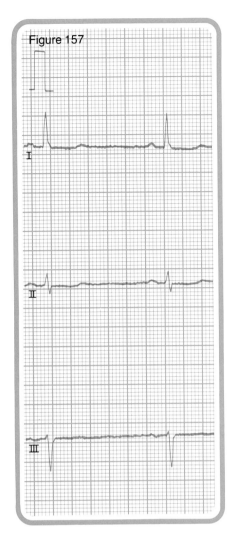

Figure 157

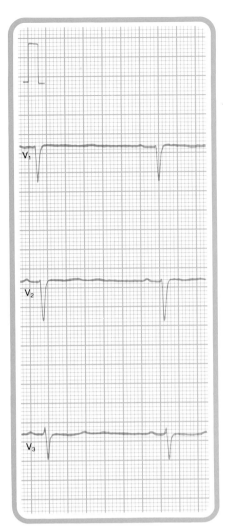

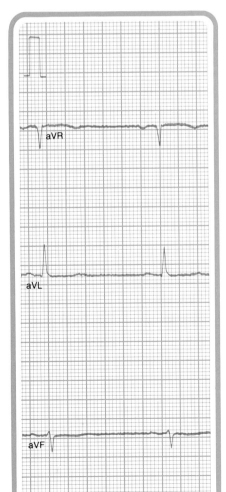

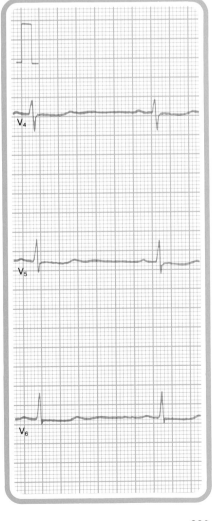

Figure 157

The rhythm is sinus bradycardia. The T waves are of low voltage in every lead. The P waves are of low voltage. The tallest R wave in the precordial leads is 8mm (V_6) – the precordial QRS complexes are therefore of abnormally low voltage (at least one R wave in the precordial series should **exceed** 8mm). There is S-T segment depression in II and V_4–V_6. Prominent U waves (not large but larger than the corresponding T waves) are seen in V_2–V_6.

Hyperthyroidism

This produces no morphological change in the electrocardiogram but arrhythmias may occur. Sinus tachycardia is the rule and atrial tachycardia, atrial fibrillation or atrial flutter may occur.

Pericarditis

Acute pericarditis almost always gives rise to transient ECG changes – of which by far the **most typical and most common is generalised S-T segment elevation.** It is thought that this change is due to inflammation of the myocardium in the sub-epicardial region (adjacent to the inflamed pericardium). The only other common cause of S-T elevation is acute myocardial ischaemic damage. It is widely taught that the main difference between the S-T segment elevation of acute pericarditis and the S-T segment of acute myocardial ischaemic damage lies in the configuration of the S-T segments (which are convex upwards in acute myocardial ischaemic damage, and concave upwards in acute pericarditis). However, a more obvious and reliable discriminator is the fact that the S-T segment change in ischaemic damage is **localised** whereas the S-T segment change in pericarditis is **generalised.** This is simply because acute pericarditis is usually a generalised inflammatory process involving the whole of the pericardium, whereas myocardial ischaemic damage is typically localised to one area. The only form of myocardial ischaemic damage which is generalised is sub-endocardial ischaemia and this usually gives rise to S-T segment depression or to T wave inversion.

In pericarditis, there is S-T segment elevation in all the precordial leads and in all the limb leads except those facing the cavity of the ventricles (i.e. aVR (always), aVL (in vertical hearts), and III (in horizontal hearts)). In limb leads facing the cavity of the heart in this way there will be S-T segment depression. In any limb lead at right angles to the frontal plane axis, there will be no significant S-T segment deviation since there will only be a tiny QRS deviation. An example of the changes in acute pericarditis is shown in Figure 158.

If there is a pericardial effusion associated with the acute pericarditis there may be reduction in the P, QRS and T voltages in all leads, but this is relatively uncommon.

The changes in acute pericarditis are transient. After the acute illness is over the ECG usually returns completely to normal. In a small proportion of cases chronic constrictive pericarditis may develop. The changes associated with chronic pericarditis are non-specific. These include:-

1. Abnormal P waves – notched or abnormally wide.
2. S-T segment depression (in most leads).
3. Low voltage T waves or T wave inversion (in most leads).
4. Atrial arrhythmias (atrial ectopic beats, atrial tachycardia, atrial flutter, atrial fibrillation).
5. Abnormal right axis deviation.
6. Generalised low voltage QRS complexes.

Figure 158

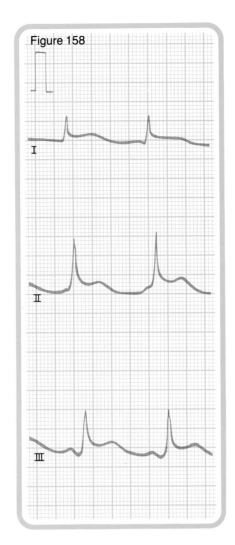
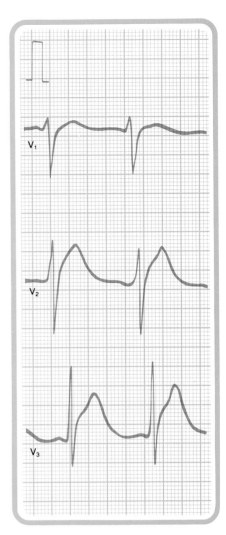
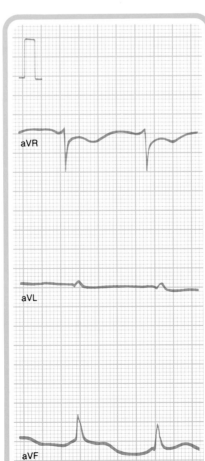
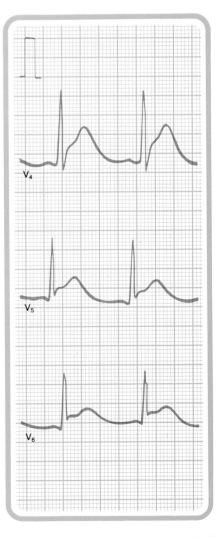

Figure 158

The rhythm is sinus tachycardia. The QRS complexes are normal. There is S-T segment elevation in Leads I, II, III, aVF, and V_1–V_6. The S-T elevation is concave upwards. There is no S-T segment shift in aVL since this lead is at right angles to the frontal plane axis. The only lead in which there is S-T depression is aVR which is a **cavity** lead. The S-T segment deflection in this lead is opposite to that in the surface leads because, and only because, the lead is looking into the cavity of the heart. It is therefore **not** a reciprocal change. Reciprocal changes in myocardial infarction are seen in leads "reciprocal to" the primary changes but the reciprocal leads and the primary leads are both looking at the external surface of the heart (see page 182).

ECG Changes in Acute Disorders of the Central Nervous System

For reasons which are not adequately understood, several types of acute disturbance in the central nervous system give rise to electrocardiographic changes. ECG changes can be seen in relation to infections or tumours in the central nervous system, after head injuries and after neurosurgery, but are most commonly seen in association with subarachnoid haemorrhage and intracranial haemorrhage.

Subarachnoid Haemorrhage

More than 50% of patients with subarachnoid or intracranial haemorrhage develop transient ECG changes.

The most common changes in central nervous system disease are:-
1. **Deep T wave inversion.**
2. **Abnormally tall T waves.**
3. **Prominent U waves.**
4. **S-T segment elevation or depression.**
5. **Prolongation of the Q-T interval.**
6. **Arrhythmias (sinus tachycardia, sinus bradycardia, nodal rhythm, atrial fibrillation, ventricular tachycardia).**

The changes are non-specific but this does not mean that they are necessarily minor or that they are non-significant. The changes can be very impressive indeed. Where there is S-T segment elevation, pericarditis can be wrongly suspected. Where there is extensive, deep, symmetrical T wave inversion, subendocardial infarction can be wrongly suspected. (Occasionally, even abnormal Q waves may develop).

The most generally accepted explanation of the pathogenesis of ECG changes in central nervous system disease is that the changes occur as a result of sympathetic or parasympathetic activity resulting from damage in central areas rich in autonomic connections, but some pathological studies have suggested that subendocardial haemorrhage may occur in acute central nervous system disturbances and that these cardiac effects cause the ECG abnormalities.

Figure 159 shows the appearances in a patient with acute subarachnoid haemorrhage. The patient had no evidence of primary cardiac disease. The record was taken within 24 hours of the onset of symptoms. There was no clinical evidence of pericarditis.

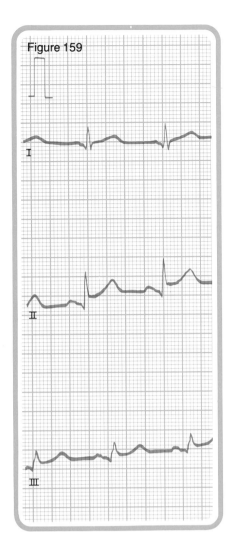

Figure 159

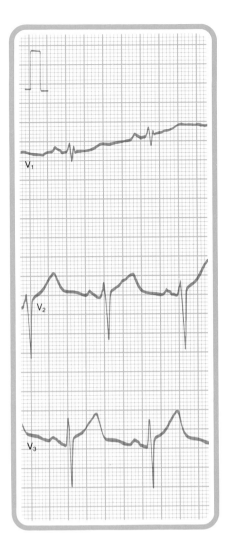

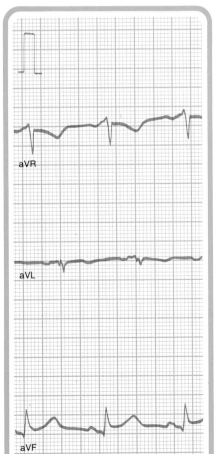

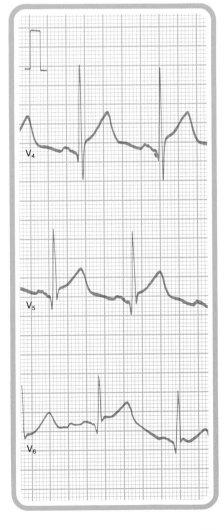

Figure 159

The rhythm is sinus. The mean frontal plane QRS axis is +75°. Since the heart is therefore vertical, the appearance in aVL (with prominent q waves and T wave inversion) is within normal limits. There are prominent but not abnormal q waves in the left precordial leads. There is a small secondary r wave in V_1 (incomplete right bundle branch block – see page 119). The striking abnormality is S-T elevation in I, II, III, aVF and V_2-V_6. The changes resemble those of acute pericarditis (compare Figure 158). Figure 160 shows the appearances in the electrocardiogram taken from the same patient, one week later.

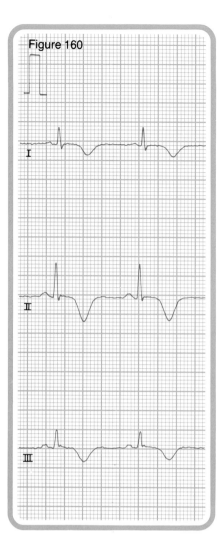

Figure 160

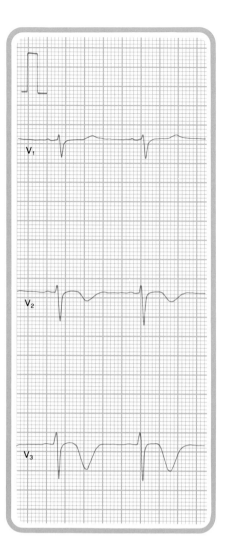

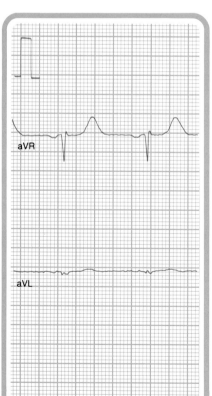

Figure 160

The rhythm is sinus. The mean frontal plane QRS axis is +60°. The QRS complexes are within normal limits (the differences in QRS complexes between this record and the previous one may not be significant – the earlier record was taken on a machine with an inferior frequency response, under adverse conditions when the patient was acutely distressed.) The S-T segments are normal.

The striking abnormality is the deep symmetrical T wave inversion in I, II, III, aVF and V₂–V₆. (The tall T waves in aVR are part of the same pattern – the T waves are upright in this lead because it is a cavity lead).

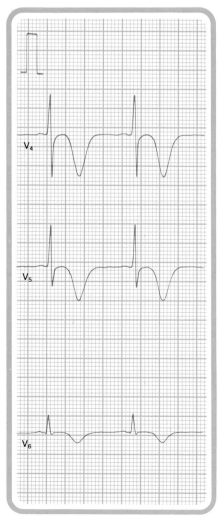

235

Note that these records could easily be misinterpreted as indicating ischaemic heart disease. **Primary interpretation** of the record of Figure 159 might be as follows:-

"Sinus rhythm. The mean frontal plane QRS axis is +75°. There are prominent but not definitely abnormal q waves in the left precordial leads. There is a small secondary r wave in V_1 suggesting incomplete right bundle branch block. There is significant S-T segment elevation in I, II, III, aVF and V_2-V_6. This is frankly abnormal. The changes are non-specific but raise the possibility of pericarditis".

In the light of the clinical information that the patient had acute subarachnoid haemorrhage the **secondary interpretation** would acknowledge that the findings are **consistent with** subarachnoid haemorrhage and do not prove the presence of pericarditis (equally, of course, they do not prove the presence of subarachnoid haemorrhage!).

Likewise, the **primary interpretation** of the record of Figure 160 might be as follows:-

"Sinus rhythm. The mean frontal plane QRS axis is +60°. The QRS complexes are within normal limits. There is deep, symmetrical T wave inversion in I, II, III, aVF and V_2-V_6. The record is frankly abnormal. Changes of this type may be seen in subendocardial ischaemia or infarction and in pericarditis, but other causes cannot be excluded."

In the light of the clinical diagnosis of subarachnoid haemorrhage, the **secondary interpretation** would acknowledge that the findings are **consistent** with subarachnoid haemorrhage.

At no time was there any clinical evidence that the patient (a 25-year-old woman) had any cardiac abnormality. The changes occurring with subarachnoid haemorrhage may persist for weeks after the acute event.

Hypothermia

A drop in the body temperature is associated with a reduction in the sinus rate and with prolongation of the P-R and Q-T intervals. When the temperature falls below 25°C an additional and highly characteristic change occurs. This is the development of an extra deflection occurring at the end of the QRS complex and just overlapping the beginning of the S-T segment. This deflection is called the "J wave". It is usually upright in the leads facing the left ventricle and it increases in size as the temperature falls. It is often mistakenly interpreted as a prolongation of the QRS duration. The broad, second part of the QRS complex (which, in V_1, may superficially resemble right bundle branch block) is also known as the "camel hump sign" and it is accompanied by S-T segment depression and low voltage T waves or T wave inversion. Atrial fibrillation may develop. The Q-T interval may be prolonged. The signs usually reverse as the patient is warmed up. An example of a case of profound hypothermia (from an elderly patient exposed to the cold) is shown in Figure 161.

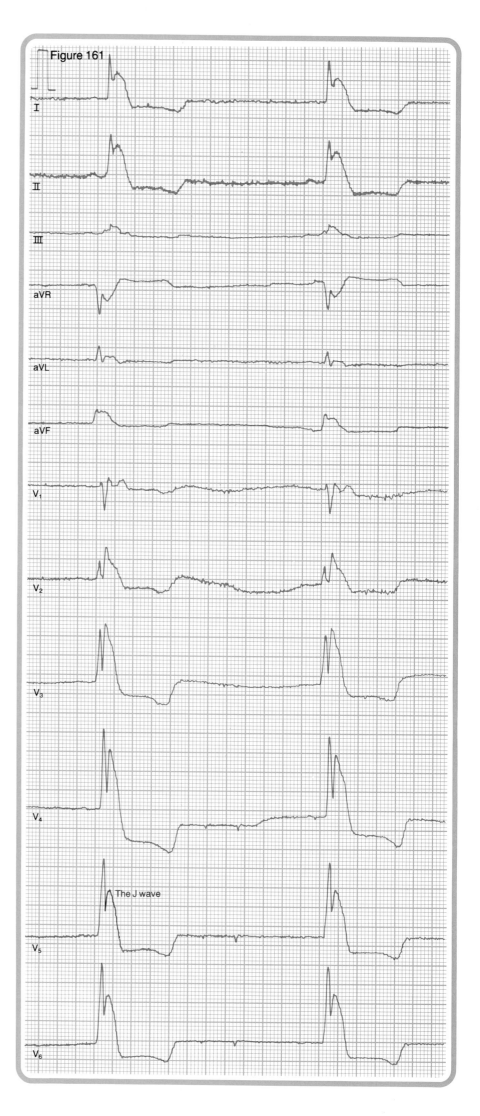

Figure 161

The rhythm is sinus bradycardia. The rate is 28 per min. The P-R interval is 0.20 sec (best seen in Lead II). Broad, slurred J waves are seen adjacent to the initial QRS deflection in all leads, but most obviously in Leads I, II and V_2–V_6. There is pronounced S-T segment depression and T wave inversion.

The Electrocardiogram Associated with Artificial Pacing of the Heart

The commonest indications for cardiac pacing currently are (a) Stokes-Adams syndrome associated with chronic atrio-ventricular block and (b) the sick sinus syndrome (the "brady-tachy syndrome"). There are now many different systems available for temporary or for permanent artificial pacing of the heart. The heart may be paced regularly irrespective of whether or not there is any spontaneous excitation ("fixed rate pacing") or the heart may receive pacing stimuli only when spontaneous activity does not occur ("demand pacing"). Usually, pacing is achieved by stimulation of the ventricle (**ventricular fixed rate** or **ventricular demand pacing).** Occasionally (if atrio-ventricular conduction is known to be normal) **atrial fixed rate** or **atrial demand pacing** may be used. Occasionally, **atrio-ventricular sequential pacing** may be used – the atrium being paced initially, and the ventricles some 0.2 sec later – the delay approximating to the normal atrio-ventricular conduction delay. A more sophisticated system still uses the spontaneous atrial depolarisation (the P wave) to initiate (after a suitable delay) ventricular depolarisation. This is called **atrial synchronous pacing.** These various types of pacing systems and the ECG appearances associated with their normal and with their faulty functioning will be discussed in Section 3, but it will be helpful at this stage to review the appearances of the 12-lead electrocardiogram during sustained ventricular pacing.

During ventricular pacing, depolarisation of the ventricular myocardium is initiated by an artificial stimulus applied directly to the ventricular myocardium from the pacemaker box via the pacing electrode.

Although the electrode may occasionally be stitched onto the surface of the heart, it is much more usual for it to be passed via a proximal vein through the superior vena cava and right atrium into the right ventricle.

During artificial ventricular pacing, a "pacemaker spike" is seen initially, followed immediately by an abnormally wide and abnormally shaped QRS complex. When (as is usual) the pacemaker electrode is situated at the apex of the right ventricle, depolarisation of the interventricular septum necessarily passes from right to left as in left bundle branch block. The induced precordial QRS complexes therefore resemble those in left bundle branch block. In addition, since the ventricular depolarisation begins low down in the right side of the interventricular septum, the predominant pathway of left ventricular depolarisation is upwards and to the left, and this gives rise to an abnormal degree of left axis deviation. Since the QRS complexes are abnormal, the S-T segments and T waves are abnormal, as in left bundle branch block.

An example is shown in Figure 162.

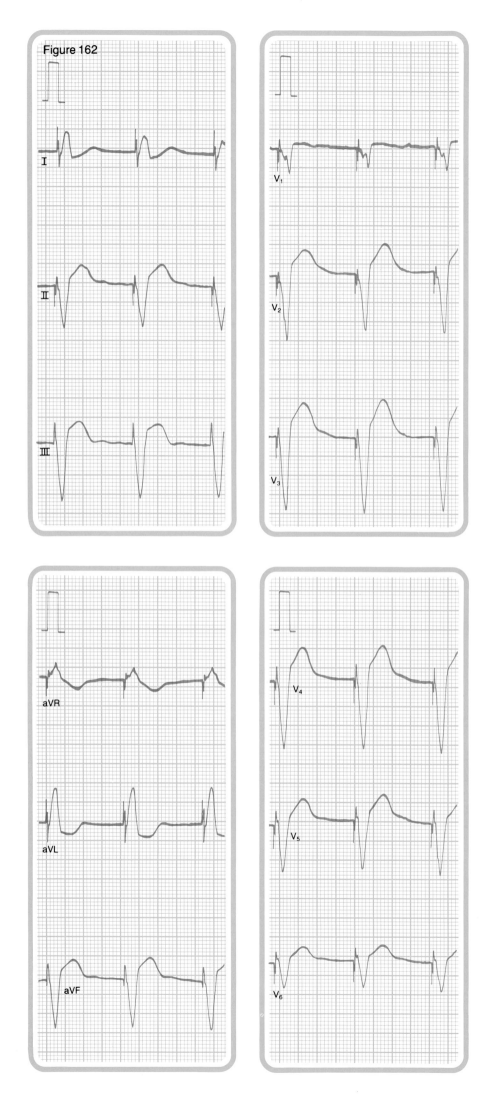

Figure 162

Figure 162

Regular ventricular pacing. The sharp pacemaker spike is seen in all leads preceding the abnormal QRS complexes. The precordial QRS complexes have the left bundle branch block configuration (there is no initial negative (q) wave in V_6 – the initial negative deflection in this lead is part of the pacemaker spike). The mean frontal plane QRS axis is −75°, i.e. there is an abnormal degree of left axis deviation.

Pericardial Effusion

The most common electrocardiographic finding in the presence of pericardial effusion is a general reduction in the voltages of all deflections in all leads. Low voltage QRS complexes are also seen in emphysema and in a variety of diffuse myocardial disorders such as haemochromatosis and amyloidosis. The two most common causes of generalised low voltages are hypothyroidism and pericardial effusion. The most obvious electrocardiographic difference between the two is that there is usually a bradycardia with hypothyroidism and a tachycardia with pericardial effusion. However, there are usually very striking clinical differences between the two which render their distinction by electrocardiography superfluous. Occasionally the amplitude of the P, QRS and T waves may be alternately high and low in consecutive beats in patients with large pericardial effusion.

Cor Pulmonale

There are no diagnostic features of cor pulmonale on the electrocardiogram, but the common findings are a combination of abnormal right axis deviation and clockwise cardiac rotation in the absence of definitive evidence of right ventricular hypertrophy.

There may, in addition, be evidence of right atrial hypertrophy. Non-specific S-T, T changes may appear, most commonly in the inferior limb leads and there may occasionally be complete right bundle branch block.

Pulmonary Embolism

The electrocardiogram is widely regarded as being a very helpful investigation in the diagnosis of pulmonary embolism, but this is far from the truth. The findings which are most commonly quoted as being very strongly suggestive of pulmonary embolism are the development of the so-called S_1, Q_3, T_3 pattern (i.e. the presence of large S waves in Lead I, large Q waves in V_3 and T wave inversion in Lead III), abnormal right axis deviation, transient right bundle branch block and T wave inversion in the right precordial leads. However, only in a small minority of cases (something of the order of 5%) do these appearances develop in pulmonary embolism. Most cases of pulmonary embolism are unsuspected clinically. Most cases which are suspected clinically either have no electrocardiographic changes at all or only minimal changes. The more massive the pulmonary embolism, the more likely are ECG changes to occur. However, even in massive pulmonary embolism, large-scale studies have shown that the development of the S_1, Q_3, T_3 syndrome, right bundle branch block, right axis deviation and tall pointed P waves in Lead II is seen only in approximately one quarter of the patients. By far the most common electrocardiographic abnormalities are non-specific T wave changes (which may be found in any of the precordial leads) and non-specific elevation or depression of the S-T segment. Right axis deviation only occurs in 5-10% of patients with pulmonary embolism, and the development of left axis deviation is actually equally as common. Likewise only a minority of patients with pulmonary embolism develop atrial fibrillation or atrial tachycardia. Occasionally the Q-T interval is prolonged.

The electrocardiogram thus contributes very little to the diagnosis of pulmonary embolism, and normal electrocardiographic findings should never be held to refute the possibility of pulmonary embolism.

Mitral Valve Prolapse

This is an extremely common congenital abnormality, being present in something of the order of 10% of the female population. The patients often have a late systolic click, followed by short systolic murmur and there are characteristic findings on the echocardiogram. The electrocardiogram often shows non-specific abnormalities. The most common abnormalities are flattening or inversion of the T waves in Leads II, III and aVF. These changes are sometimes accompanied by slight S-T segment depression and they may be wrongly interpreted as evidence of inferior myocardial ischaemia. Sometimes the T waves may be of low voltage in the left precordial leads or there may be shallow T wave inversion in some of the precordial leads. The changes in the precordial leads may be seen either together with, or independently of, changes in the inferior leads. Occasionally prominent U waves may be visible. The Q-T interval may be prolonged. Ventricular pre-excitation is found more commonly in subjects with mitral valve prolapse than in those without. The condition may also be associated with frequent ventricular or atrial premature beats. Supraventricular tachycardia may also occur and occasionally atrial flutter or fibrillation may develop. In the majority of patients the syndrome is innocent and has no effect on a patient's functional state or his life expectation. A minority of patients may have significant mitral incompetence and occasionally sudden death (thought to be due to paroxysmal ventricular tachycardia or ventricular fibrillation) may occur. The most important aspect of the electrocardiogram in patients with valve prolapse is that non-specific S-T, T changes in the inferior limb leads may be mistakenly thought to be evidence of inferior myocardial ischaemia if the existence of the mitral valve prolapse syndrome is not recognised. Of course the presence of mitral valve prolapse does not prove that any S-T, T changes are due to the mitral prolapse but at least it admits the possibility.

Heredofamilial Neuromyopathic Disorders

Three major hereditary and familial neuromyopathic disorders are usually associated with cardiac involvement and may give rise to electrocardiographic changes. These conditions are the progressive muscular dystrophies, dystrophia myotonica and Friedreich's ataxia.

Progressive Muscular Dystrophy

There are various different forms of progressive muscular dystrophy and all may show electrocardiographic changes. **Many of them show sinus tachycardia, sometimes with an unusual degree of lability of the heart rate. They may also be associated with the sick sinus syndrome, with atrial ectopic beats, ventricular ectopic beats, atrial flutter, atrial tachycardia, atrial fibrillation, paroxysmal ventricular tachycardia, right or left bundle branch block and various degrees of heart block. In addition the Duchenne type of progressive muscular dystrophy frequently has an abnormal R/S ratio in V_1 (i.e. the R wave is dominant in V_1). There may also be prominent q waves in the limb leads or the left precordial leads and these may simulate infarction.**

Dystrophia Myotonica

In dystrophia myotonica there may be a variety of cardiac arrhythmias including sinus bradycardia, atrial fibrillation, atrial flutter, atrial ectopic beats, ventricular ectopic beats and ventricular tachycardia. There may also be disturbances of conduction with prolongation of the P-R interval, left or right bundle branch block, left anterior hemiblock or complete heart block. The abnormal R/S ratio in the Duchenne type of muscular dystrophy does not appear to occur in dystrophia myotonica.

Friedreich's Ataxia

In Friedreich's ataxia, inappropriate sinus tachycardia, supraventricular or ventricular ectopic beats, atrial tachycardia, atrial fibrillation, atrial flutter and ventricular ectopic beats are the commonest arrhythmias and the commonest abnormalities in morphology are non-specific S-T, T changes (flattening and possible inversion of the T waves and slight S-T segment depression) occasionally the electrocardiogram may satisfy the voltage criteria for left ventricular hypertrophy and rarely bi-ventricular hypretrophy can be found.

Obesity

The most common electro-cardiographic manifestations of obesity are a **generalised reduction in voltages of the P waves, QRS complexes and T waves. Sometimes there is persistent sinus tachycardia.**

Pregnancy

Minor electrocardiographic changes may occur in relation to pregnancy. **Sinus tachycardia is common. As pregnancy advances there is usually a leftward shift of the mean frontal plane QRS axis** (as a result of the shift in the physical position of the heart with the abdominal distension). Prominent q waves may be seen in Lead III in pregnancy (but this should never be taken as an indication of an abnormality in any event, see Section I, pages 53 and 54). In patients subject to paroxysmal supraventricular tachycardia the episodes may be more frequent during pregnancy than in the non-pregnant state. The author does not reccommed the diagnosis of pregnancy from the appearance of the electrocardiogram!

Post-myocardial Infarction Syndrome (Dressler's Syndrome)

This is a syndrome in which pleuro-pericarditis occurs within the first 12 weeks following an episode of acute myocardial infarction. The pericarditis is secondary to the myocardial infarction and is induced by an abnormal auto-immune mechanism.

Anti-myocardial antibodies may be present in the serum of the affected patients. **The electrocardiogram shows the typical diffuse S-T segment elevation as in pericarditis of other causes. Later there may be T wave flattening and minor S-T changes.**

Post-cardiotomy Syndrome

This syndrome is very similar to the post-myocardial infarction syndrome. It occurs usually within the first 12 weeks following cardiac surgery and in some degree may be present in 20-30% of patients following cardiac surgery. As in the post-myocardial infarction syndrome the mechanism is thought to be an auto-immune response and there is pleurisy and pericarditis. In addition there may be a fever and a raised erythrocyte sedimentation rate. **The electro-cardiogram shows widespread S-T segment elevation as in acute pericarditis of any origin. Later, low voltage T waves may occur and there may be minor S-T segment changes.**

Connective Tissue Disease

The heart may be involved in any of the connective tissue diseases, the commonest ones to involve the heart are scleroderma and systemic lupus erythematosus. The electrocardiogram is abnormal in about half of patients with scleroderma.

Scleroderma

The commonest abnormalities are non-specific S-T, T changes but evidence of right or of left ventricular hypertrophy may occur. Occasionally bi-ventricular hypertrophy is seen. Sometimes there is generalised reduction in the QRS voltage or the development of abnormal q waves simulating myocardial infarction. Right or left bundle branch block may occur, and there may be abnormalities of the P wave configuration.
Various arrhythmias including atrial and ventricular ectopic beats and conduction disturbances may be present.

Systemic Lupus Erythematosus

Similar changes may be apparent in systemic lupus erythematosus, but more often the electrocardiographic changes in this condition are confined to non-specific S-T, T changes with reduction in the T wave voltage and occasionally with S-T segment elevation, indicative of pericarditis. Supraventricular and ventricular ectopic beats and tachycardias may occur.

Haemochromatosis

In this condition the electrocardiogram may show generalised low voltage of the QRS complexes, with low voltage T waves or T wave inversion. Ventricular and supraventricular ectopic beats and tachycardia may occur and there may be right bundle branch block, left bundle branch block or first, second or third degree heart block.

Amyloidosis

This condition is by no means always associated with cardiac involvement, but when there is cardiac involvement the electrocardiogram may well be abnormal. There may be left axis deviation, right or left bundle branch block, complete heart block or absence of initial r waves in V_1-V_3 (simulating antero-septal myocardial infarction). In addition, there may be generalised low voltage of the QRS complexes and T waves.

Myocarditis

Transient acute myocarditis is very common in systemic viral infections. It occurs in association with influenza, poliomyelitis, mumps, viral hepatitis and infectious mononucleosis.

Viral Myocarditis

In the majority of cases the electrocardiographic changes involve non-specific flattening of the T waves, minimal S-T segment depression and the occurrence of frequent atrial or ventricular premature beats. Occasionally abnormal q waves, simulating myocardial infarction, may occur.

Acute Rheumatic Myocarditis

In the myocarditis of acute rheumatic fever the commonest abnormality is prolongation of the P-R interval, but second degree heart block of the Wenckebach type may occur and minor non-specific S-T changes are also common.

Cardiomyopathy

In congestive cardiomyopathy (which is usually of unknown aetiology) there may be abnormalities of the P waves, QRS complexes, the S-T segments, the T waves and the cardiac rhythm. In other words, almost any form of electrocardiographic abnormality may occur. The appearances may simulate left or right ventricular hypertrophy or myocardial infarction. Left anterior and left posterior hemiblock may occur and there may also be heart block. The single most characteristic feature of the ECG in cardiomyopathy is evidence of involvement of all four chambers, e.g. left ventricular hypertrophy plus right atrial abnormality plus right bundle branch block plus ectopic beats arising in the left atrium. Figure 163 shows an electrocardiogram from a patient with congestive cardiomyopathy.
The widespread nature of the changes, involving P waves, QRS complexes, S-T segments, T waves and the cardiac rhythm is typical of the findings in cardiomyopathy.

Similar changes may occur in **hypertrophic obstructive cardiomyopathy.** The earliest changes in this condition are those of **left ventricular hypertrophy and left atrial hypertrophy, but subsequently arrhythmias (atrial or ventricular) left or right bundle branch block and either left anterior or left posterior hemiblock may occur. Not uncommonly in this condition** abnormal q waves which, in other circumstances, would suggest myocardial infarction, may be seen.

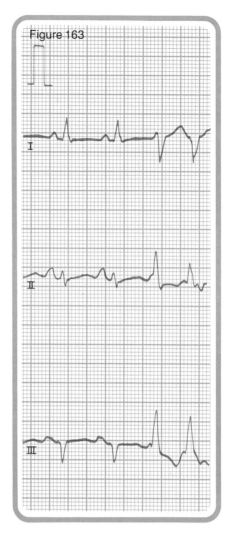

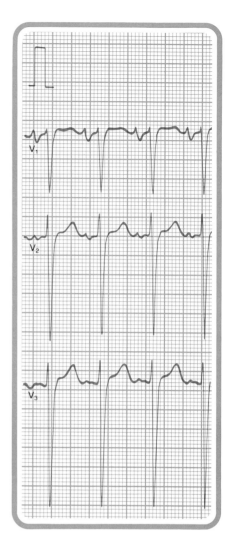

Figure 163

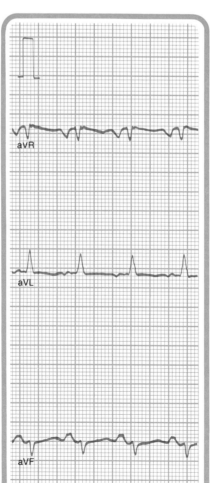

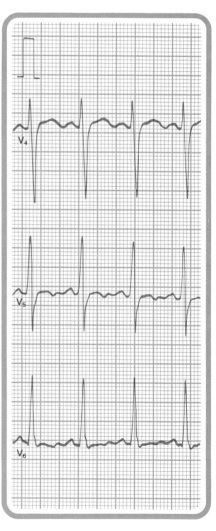

The basic rhythm is sinus tachycardia (the heart rate is often raised in congestive cardiomyopathy owing to the reflex sympathetic drive which occurs consequent upon decreased ventricular output). Two ventricular ectopic beats are seen (the third and fourth beats seen in Leads I, II and III). The P waves show evidence of right atrial abnormality (abnormally tall P waves in II) and of left atrial abnormality (dominant negative component to the P wave in V_1). The precordial QRS complexes satisfy the voltage criteria for left ventricular hypertrophy. There are non-specific S-T, T changes in the limb leads and in the left precordial leads. The mean frontal plane QRS axis is at the extreme left hand side of the normal range at $-30°$.

Dissecting Aneurysm

This may be associated with **non-specific S-T segment depression, low voltage of the T waves and occasionally T wave inversion. It may** actually give rise to myocardial infarction, in which case the usual changes of this condition would be seen.

Chest Deformities

Abnormalities of the anatomy of the thorax may induce secondary changes in the electrocardiogram, usually because of the change in the physical position of the heart. If there is appreciable depression of the sternum the heart may be displaced to the right or to the left.

Pectus Excavatum

Pectus excavatum may be associated with **counter-clockwise or clockwise cardiac rotation.**

Pulmonary Atalectasis

With collapse of the left lung or with the presence of a large right pleural effusion, the mean frontal plane QRS axis may be shifted to the left.

Pleural Effusion

Conversely, in the presence of a large left pleural effusion, the frontal plane axis can be shifted to the right.

Congenital Heart Disease (In the adult)

Atrial Septal Defect

This condition is usually associated with **borderline abnormal right axis deviation and complete or incomplete right bundle branch block**. There may also be **clockwise cardiac rotation** (this applies to the common, ostium secundum type of atrial septal defect. In the case of the less common ostium primum type of atrial septal defect, complete or incomplete right bundle branch block is seen in association with **left** axis deviation).

Ventricular Septal Defect

The electrocardiogram is normal in cases of ventricular septal defect associated with a small shunt. If there is a very large defect with a resulting large left-to-right shunt, the electrocardiogram may shows signs of **left ventricular hypertrophy**. In cases associated with pulmonary hypertension, there may be right ventricular hypertrophy or bi-ventricular hypertrophy.

Patent Ductus Arteriosus

In the majority of cases the electrocardiogram is normal. If the shunt is large there may be evidence of left ventricular hypertrophy and possibly of left atrial hypertrophy. In the presence of pulmonary hypertension, abnormal right axis deviation and ultimately right ventricular hypertrophy may be seen.

Coarctation of the Aorta

The common findings are those of **left ventricular and left atrial hypertrophy**. Occasionally there may be an abnormal degree of left axis deviation. For reasons which are not understood a complete or incomplete right bundle branch block pattern may also be found.

Pulmonary Stenosis

The electrocardiographic changes here are simply those of **right ventricular hypertrophy and right atrial hypertrophy.**

Fallot's Tetralogy

The vast majority of patients with this condition have an abnormal electrocardiogram. There is nearly always evidence of **right ventricular hypertrophy and right atrial hypertrophy**. In addition, a **right bundle branch block pattern is sometimes seen.**

Ebstein's Anomaly

This is a relatively rare congenital abnormality in which the tricuspid valve is displaced downwards from its normal position towards the apex of the right ventricle. The electrocardiogram frequently shows **atrial ectopic beats, atrial tachycardia, atrial flutter, atrial fibrillation or nodal tachycardia.** When the patient is in sinus rhythm, **the P waves are often abnormally tall and abnormally wide and the P-R interval may be prolonged.** Sometimes **second or third degree heart block may be present.** The QRS complexes may show a **right bundle branch block configuration and sometimes ventricular pre-excitation of the Wolff-Parkinson-White variety** (most commonly Type B) **can be found.**

244

Dextrocardia

"Situs inversus" describes a congenital developmental "abnormality" in which every organ in the body develops as a left-to-right mirror image of the usual pattern. The heart lies in the right side of the chest with the "left", i.e. systemic, ventricle to the right and the "right", i.e. pulmonary, ventricle to the left. When all the organs in the body are transposed in this way the heart is usually normal, apart from its position. The "dextrocardia" is then part of the "situs inversus". Isolated dextrocardia (in which the heart is the **only** organ to be transposed) may also occur. This too can occur with a heart which is, in respects other than its position, normal but complex congenital cardiac abnormalities of great functional significance are much more likely to occur in association with isolated dextrocardia than with dextrocardia which is part of the pattern of "situs inversus".

In the presence of dextrocardia (whether isolated or part of "situs inversus") striking changes are seen in the ECG and if the electrocardiogram is recorded in the normal way (i.e. using the standard recording positions as recommended by the British Cardiac Society and the American Heart Association (Section I, page 27)), then profound "abnormalities" of the electrocardiogram will be seen. These "abnormalities" are in no way indicative of disease. They merely reflect the abnormal anatomical relationship of the heart to the usual recording positions. Figure 164 shows an example of the kind of appearances which may be found.

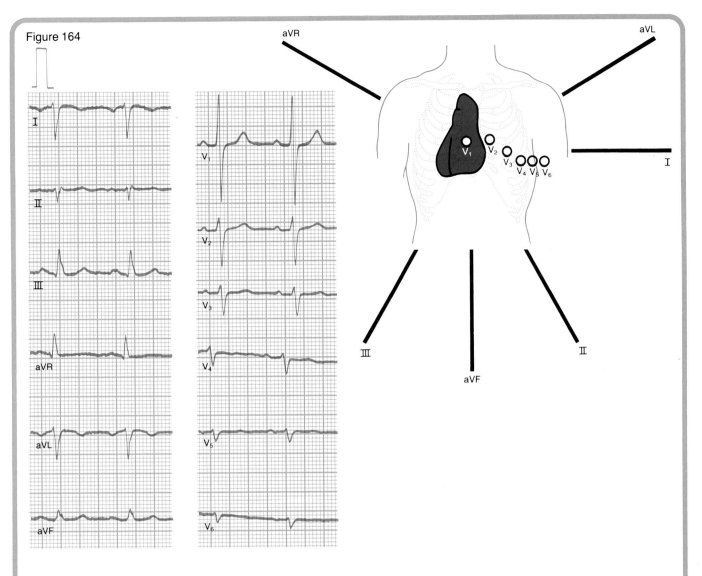

Figure 164

The ECG recording on the left is from a patient with mirror-image dextrocardia. There was no evidence of organic heart disease. The patient was simply born with left/right inversion of the body organs. When the conventional electrocardiographic recording is made (i.e. the precordial electrodes positioned in their conventional sites and the limbs connected according to the normal convention) appearances similar to those in the left-hand side of the figure are seen.

As usual (page 15)
    I = +L−R
    II = +F−R
    III = +F−L

Lead 1 shows an inverted P wave, QRS complex and T wave which is a very unusual finding. The only alternative explanation for this finding is "technical dextrocardia" – see later. The appearances in V_1 are consistent with normality, but from V_2-V_6 the r waves become progressively

smaller rather than larger and there is T wave inversion. These are very abnormal findings. These abnormal findings do not indicate structural abnormality within the heart for the conventional electrode positions are not suitable for obtaining an electrocardiogram when the heart is mirror-image inverted. The diagram on the right shows the position of the heart (in dextrocardia) in relation to the position of the recording electrodes.

The conventional positions for the recording electrodes are therefore inappropriate for patients with dextrocardia. For this reason the recording system used in Figure 165 is chosen. In this system the right and left arm connections are deliberately reversed and the precordial connections are also right/left inverted.

Thus:
(inverted commas are used to indicate the lead achieved by the deliberately "false" connections. The corresponding conventional connections are expressed without quotation marks).

$$\text{"L"} = R$$
$$\text{"R"} = L$$
$$\text{"F"} = F$$

Since therefore
$$\text{"I"} = +\text{"L"} - \text{"R"}$$
$$\text{"I"} = +R - L$$
$$= \text{I turned upside down}$$

Similarly
$$\text{"II"} = +\text{"F"} - \text{"R"}$$
$$= +F - L$$
$$= III$$

and
$$\text{"III"} = +\text{"F"} - \text{"L"}$$
$$= +F - R$$
$$= II$$

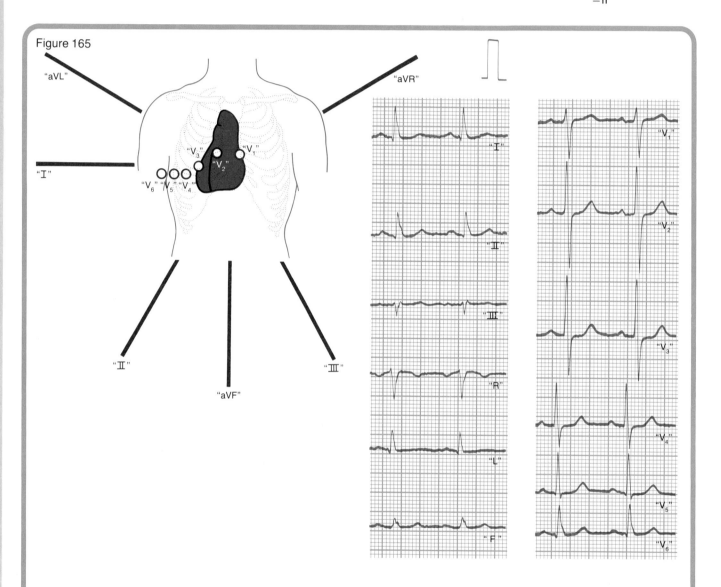

Figure 165

This figure shows the position of the heart in the patient with mirror-image dextrocardia as in Figure 164, however, a "mirror-image" recording system is used in which the precordial leads are left/right inverted (they are sited exactly as quoted in Figure 34, page 27, except that all right-sided positions become left, and all left-sided positions become right). The limb lead connections are mirror-image inverted simply by reversing the right and left arm connections. The foot lead connection is a central connection and does not need to be inverted. Leads recorded in this way are shown between inverted commas to distinguish them from the conventional recording system.

Note that the appearances in "V₁" (Figure 165) are identical to those in V_2 (Figure 164) and the appearances in "V₂" (Figure 165) are identical to those in V_1 (Figure 164).

The remainder of the precordial leads in Figure 165 have no counterpart in Figure 164 for the leads in Figure 164 are inappropriately placed, distant from the heart.

In the limb leads "I" (Figure 165) is the same as I (Figure 164) upside down, "II" (Figure 165) is identical with III (Figure 164) and "III" (Figure 165) is the same as II (Figure 164). Likewise "L" (Figure 165) equals R (Figure 164) and "R" (Figure 165) equals L (Figure 164). "F" (Figure 165) equals F (Figure 164).

It should be noted that the electrocardiogram in dextrocardia looks very abnormal if recorded in the conventional way. **The great clue to its presence is the fact that the P waves, the QRS complexes and T waves are all negative in Lead 1 and that the precordial leads show a completely abnormal R wave progression with the R wave voltages getting** **progressively smaller from V_1-V_6 for** these electrodes are progressively further and further away from the heart. **The greatest clue lies in the negative P wave in I**. This is very rarely seen in the presence of sinus rhythm except in dextrocardia. The only condition with which it is likely to be confused is technical dextrocardia.

Technical Dextrocardia

Technical dextrocardia refers to the electrocardiographic appearances which are obtained as a result of an **error** in the ECG recording technique. The error involves the accidental connection of the right arm to the left arm lead, and the left arm to the right arm lead. Thus the appearances in aVR and in aVL are interchanged, and those in aVF are unchanged. The appearances in Leads II and III are also interchanged and the appearances in Lead I are inverted. The result is that in the **limb leads** the appearances are identical to those in true dextrocardia. However, the appearances in the **precordial leads** are entirely normal. An example is shown in Figure 166.

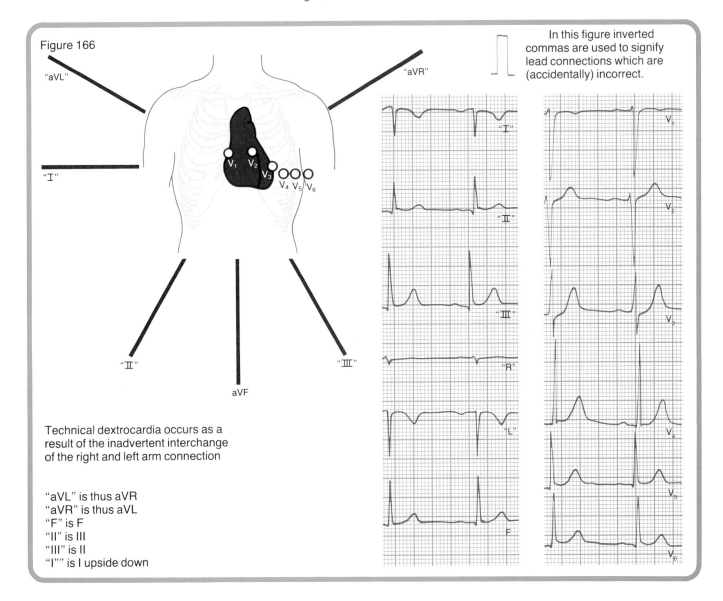

Figure 166

In this figure inverted commas are used to signify lead connections which are (accidentally) incorrect.

"aVL"
"aVR"
"I"
"II"
"III"
aVF

Technical dextrocardia occurs as a result of the inadvertent interchange of the right and left arm connection

"aVL" is thus aVR
"aVR" is thus aVL
"F" is F
"II" is III
"III" is II
"I"" is I upside down

"I"
"II"
"III"
"R"
"L"
F

V_1
V_2
V_3
V_4
V_5
V_6

The Recognition of Dextrocardia

When the P wave is inverted in Lead I in the presence of sinus rhythm the only likely explanations are dextrocardia or technical dextrocardia. The latter is considerably more common than the former. When the precordial R wave progression is normal the explanation is technical dextrocardia. The true appearances of the record are then already shown in the precordial leads. The true appearances in the limb leads can be ascertained by interchanging aVL and aVR, interchanging II and III, turning I upside down and leaving aVF as it is. When the R wave voltage progressively decreases from V_1 to V_6 there is true dextrocardia. The true appearances can be assessed in the limb leads by interchanging aVR and aVL, interchanging II and III, turning I upside down and leaving F alone. The true appearances in V_1 and V_2 can be determined by interchanging them but the true appearances in V_3-V_6 can only be determined by recording again using right-sided V_3-V_6 placements. By far the simplest approach in true dextrocardia is to obtain a record using **appropriate** electrode placings, i.e. deliberately to interchange the R and L connections and to use right-sided precordial leads as indicated in Figure 165.

Multiple and Complex Abnormalities

In this book, as in most other text books of electrocardiography, abnormalities have been explained and demonstrated individually – and this is necessary in the interests of clarity. However, in real life, abnormalities of the electrocardiogram are not necessarily conveniently "packaged" into individual types. Combinations of abnormalities may occur by coincidence (for example, if a patient with right ventricular hypertrophy due to congenital pulmonary stenosis develops acute viral pericarditis) but much more commonly combinations of abnormalities may occur because of common aetiology (e.g. when there is left ventricular hypertrophy on the basis of hypertension and the patient develops either acute myocardial infarction or atrial fibrillation). Some combinations of abnormalities are virtually inevitable, for the development of one abnormality gives rise to the development of a second abnormality. The most obvious example in this category is that in the presence of ventricular hypertrophy, hypertrophy of the corresponding atrium is inevitable. Thus **left ventricular hypertrophy** is **usually** accompanied by **left atrial hypertrophy** (left atrial hypertrophy can only be recognised if the rhythm is sinus) – an example is shown in Figure 104 – and **right ventricular hypertrophy** is **usually** accompanied by **right atrial hypertrophy** (which latter can likewise only be recognised if the rhythm is sinus). An example is shown in Figure 108.

Other combinations of abnormalities, whilst by no means inevitable, are nevertheless common – for the disease process may involve more than one area. Examples include:-

1. Right bundle branch block with left anterior hemiblock – for degenerative disease commonly affects these two fascicles of the conductive system. An example is shown in Figure 100.

2. Left atrial hypertrophy with right ventricular hypertrophy. This combination (in the absence of left ventricular hypertrophy) usually implies obstruction at the mitral valve orifice (most commonly due to mitral stenosis, and rarely due to atrial myxoma).

3. Anterior myocardial infarction and right bundle branch block. When the infarct involves the myocardium of the interventricular septum carrying the bundle branches, block of either bundle branch may occur. Anterior myocardial infarction and right bundle branch block can both be diagnosed from the same electrocardiogram since neither interferes with the diagnostic processes involved in the other (Figure 169).

4. Anterior myocardial infarction with left bundle branch block. If left bundle branch block and myocardial infarction co-exist, usually only the left bundle branch block is apparent for this so distorts the electrocardiogram that the normal criteria for infarction cannot be applied (see page 125). It is **sometimes** possible to diagnose myocardial infarction in the presence of left bundle branch block but this is **always** difficult and is **never** completely reliable.

Diagnosis of Myocardial Infarction in the Presence of Left Bundle Branch Block

It must be repeated that (a) it may prove impossible to diagnose myocardial infarction in the presence of left bundle branch block, and (b) when the diagnosis is attempted, subsequent autopsy examination indicates that the diagnosis may be in error in a significant number of cases (i.e. the specificity of the criteria for myocardial infarction in the presence of left bundle branch block is very low).

The criteria which have been applied by various authors are:-

1. Abnormal Q waves in I, aVL, V_4–V_6 (i.e. a q wave of 0.04 sec or more in duration or more than ¼ of the height of the ensuing R wave). This is probably the most reliable indicator of infarction in the presence of left bundle branch block, but it will immediately be seen that this defies one of the two "essential" criteria for the diagnosis of left bundle branch block in the first place! The diagnosis of left bundle branch block is then dependent upon (a) a prolonged QRS duration of 0.12 sec or more (b) dominant positive waves in V_6, and (c) displacement of the S-T segment and T waves in a direction opposite to the dominant deflection of the QRS complex in any lead, and (d) absence of a secondary R wave in the right precordial leads (thus demonstrating that there is no right bundle branch block).

The form of the QRS complex in V_6 in the presence of left bundle branch block, complicated by anteroseptal infarction, is shown in Figure 167.

2. QS or W-shaped deflection in II, III and aVF
This is usually an indication of inferior infarction, but it is not a totally reliable criterion. The criteria for LBBB listed (a) to (d) in 1 above must still obtain.

3. Primary S-T or T wave changes
In uncomplicated left bundle branch block the S-T segments and T waves are usually opposite in sign to the dominant QRS deflection. These are the expected "secondary" changes (i.e. they are secondary to the QRS abnormality, page 124). When, in leads with upright QRS complexes, there is S-T segment elevation and the T waves are tall and upright, infarction is possible. These are "primary" S-T or T changes, i.e. they are changes not induced inevitably by the QRS abnormality. S-T depression or T inversion in leads in which the dominant QRS deflection is negative have the same significance.

Several examples of combined abnormalities are now shown.

Figure 167

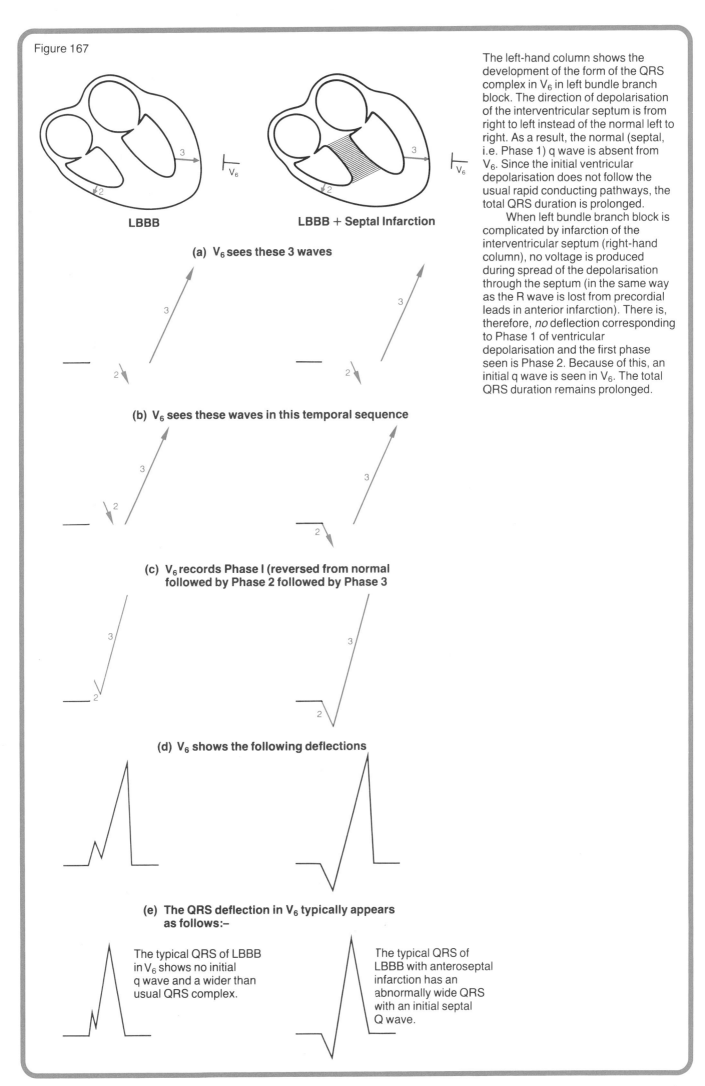

LBBB

LBBB + Septal Infarction

(a) V₆ sees these 3 waves

(b) V₆ sees these waves in this temporal sequence

(c) V₆ records Phase I (reversed from normal followed by Phase 2 followed by Phase 3

(d) V₆ shows the following deflections

(e) The QRS deflection in V₆ typically appears as follows:–

The typical QRS of LBBB in V₆ shows no initial q wave and a wider than usual QRS complex.

The typical QRS of LBBB with anteroseptal infarction has an abnormally wide QRS with an initial septal Q wave.

The left-hand column shows the development of the form of the QRS complex in V₆ in left bundle branch block. The direction of depolarisation of the interventricular septum is from right to left instead of the normal left to right. As a result, the normal (septal, i.e. Phase 1) q wave is absent from V₆. Since the initial ventricular depolarisation does not follow the usual rapid conducting pathways, the total QRS duration is prolonged.

When left bundle branch block is complicated by infarction of the interventricular septum (right-hand column), no voltage is produced during spread of the depolarisation through the septum (in the same way as the R wave is lost from precordial leads in anterior infarction). There is, therefore, *no* deflection corresponding to Phase 1 of ventricular depolarisation and the first phase seen is Phase 2. Because of this, an initial q wave is seen in V₆. The total QRS duration remains prolonged.

1. Left Bundle Branch Block, with Left Atrial Hypertrophy and Left Anterior Hemiblock (Figure 168)

Figure 168

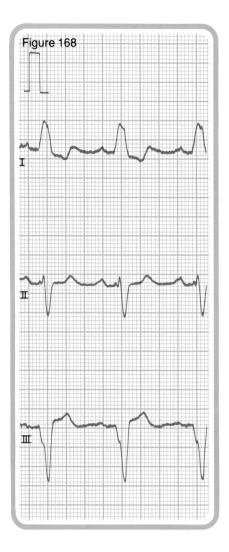

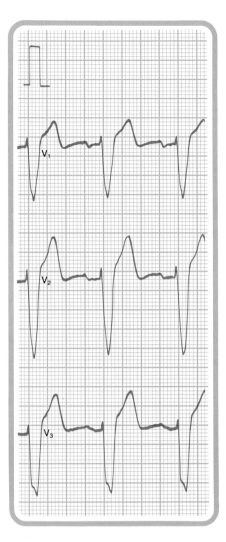

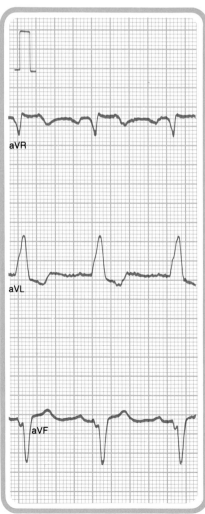

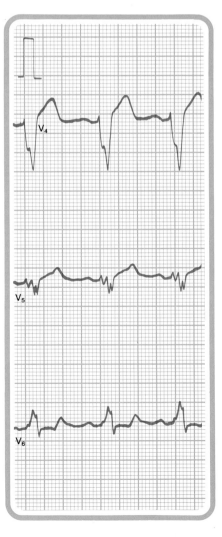

Figure 168

The rhythm is sinus. The total QRS duration is abnormal at 0.16 sec. There is no secondary R wave in V_1 to indicate right bundle branch block. There is no initial q wave in V_6, I or aVL and there is therefore **left bundle branch block**. The mean frontal plane QRS axis is abnormal at $-75°$. The two common causes of such an axis are inferior infarction and left anterior hemiblock. The former cannot be confidently diagnosed in the presence of left bundle branch block. There may well be distal disease in the anterior division of the left bundle branch as well as a proximal lesion in the main left bundle branch and the **probability** is that there is **left anterior hemiblock** as well as left bundle branch block (left bundle branch block alone **does not** cause left axis deviation). The form of the P waves in V_1 suggests left atrial hypertrophy.

A suitable report on this record would be:-

"Sinus rhythm. There is complete left bundle branch block. There is an abnormal degree of left axis deviation ($-75°$) suggesting additional left anterior hemiblock. The form of the P waves in V_1 suggests left atrial hypertrophy."

This patient had hypertrophic obstructive cardiomyopathy.

2. Anterior Myocardial Infarction, Inferior Myocardial Infarction and Right Bundle Branch Block (Figure 169)

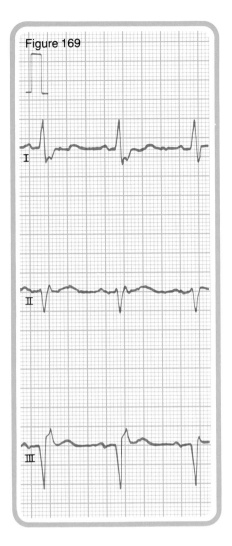

Figure 169

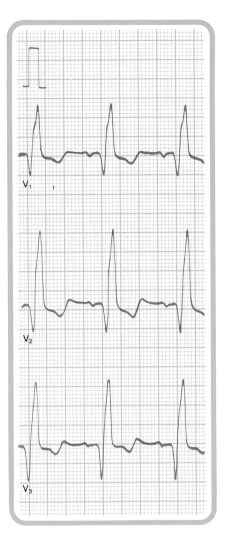

Figure 169

The rhythm is sinus. There are abnormal Q waves in aVF, indicative of inferior infarction. There are abnormal Q waves from V_1–V_4 indicating anteroseptal infarction. The frontal plane QRS axis is abnormal at $-60°$ (due to the inferior infarction). The total QRS duration is prolonged indicating bundle branch block. There is a large, "secondary" R wave in V_1 to indicate the presence of right bundle branch block. (Even though there is no initial q wave in V_6, this does not indicate *left* bundle branch block (page 124)). The "secondary" r wave is visible but the "primary" r wave is lost because of the anteroseptal infarction (remember, the initial part of the QRS complex is normal in all leads in right bundle branch block and the criteria for infarction can be applied – page 118, Figure 82).

A suitable report on this record would be:-

"Sinus rhythm. Inferior myocardial infarction (resulting in abnormal degree of left axis deviation). There is anteroseptal infarction and complete right bundle branch block.".

This patient had unequivocal clinical evidence of ischaemic heart disease.

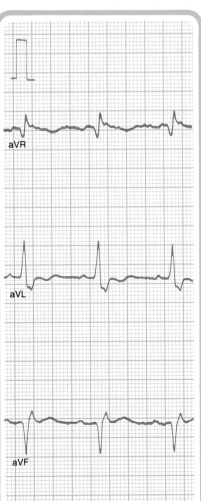

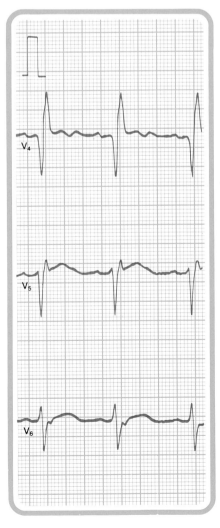

254

3. Left Ventricular Hypertrophy, Left Atrial Hypertrophy, Right Atrial Hypertrophy (Figure 170)

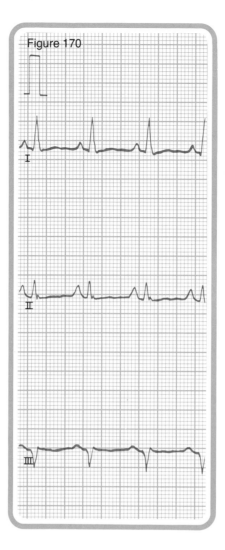

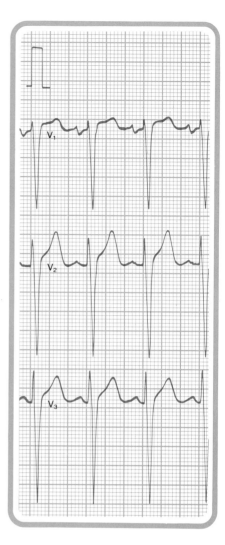

Figure 170

The rhythm is sinus (at about 100/min). The precordial QRS complexes satisfy the voltage criteria for left ventricular hypertrophy. There is T wave inversion in V_5 and S-T segment depression in V_6. These are non-specific changes which could well be secondary to the QRS abnormalities. The P waves in V_1 have a dominant negative component indicative of left atrial hypertrophy (strictly "abnormality"). The P waves in II are abnormally tall and pointed and indicate right atrial hypertrophy (strictly "abnormality"). The mean frontal plane QRS axis is $-15°$. The frontal plane T wave axis is indeterminate. Since the QRS axis is determinate and the T wave axis indeterminate, the frontal plane T waves are abnormal (page 58). A suitable report for this record would be as follows:-

"Sinus tachycardia. The mean frontal plane QRS axis is $-15°$, but the frontal plane T wave axis is indeterminate indicating that the frontal plane T waves are abnormal. This is a non-specific abnormality. There is evidence of left and right atrial abnormality and of left ventricular hypertrophy. There are non-specific S-T, T changes in the left precordial leads".

This patient had a congestive cardiomyopathy, thought to be due excessive alcohol consumption.

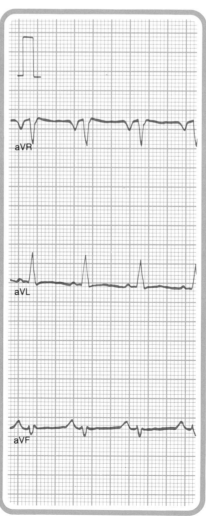

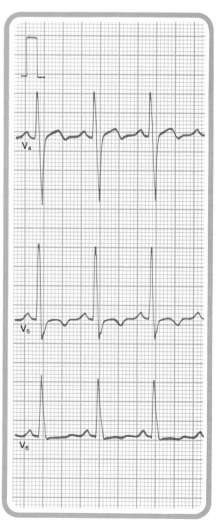

4. Anteroseptal Infarction with Left Anterior Hemiblock (Figure 171)

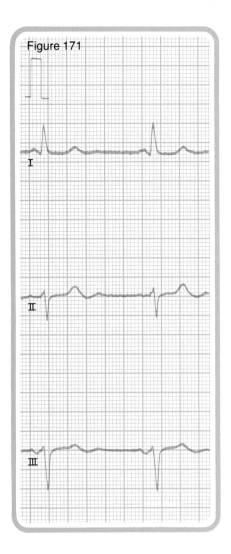

Figure 171

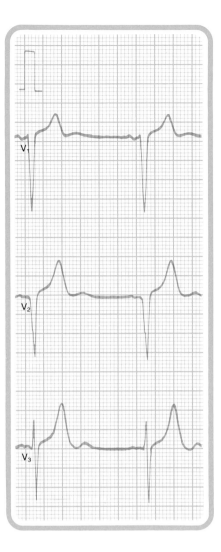

Figure 171

The rhythm is sinus. The r wave in V_1 is small. There is no r wave at all in V_2 (there are deep QS complexes) and the appearances are those of an old anteroseptal infarction. The mean frontal plane QRS axis is $-45°$. This is an abnormal degree of left axis deviation. Abnormal left axis deviation is not a feature of anteroseptal infarction. There is no evidence of inferior infarction (initial r waves are seen aVF) and the likely cause is therefore left anterior hemiblock, which may indicate that the infarct involves the anterior division of the left bundle branch in the interventricular septum. There are prominent, but not abnormal (see page 195) U waves in II, III, aVF and V_1-V_6.

A suitable report for this record would be as follows:-

"Sinus bradycardia. The form of the QRS complexes in V_1 and V_2 is very strongly suggestive of an old anteroseptal infarction. There is an abnormal degree of left axis deviation ($-45°$) indicative of left anterior hemiblock. The U waves are prominent, but not definitely abnormal, in most leads. The possibility of hypokalaemia should be considered".

The patient had clear clinical evidence of ischaemic heart disease. The serum potassium ion level was 3.2 mmol/l.

Note

This serum potassium ion level is abnormally low but it does not follow that the prominent U waves were necessarily related to this.

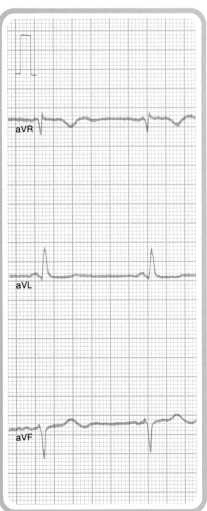

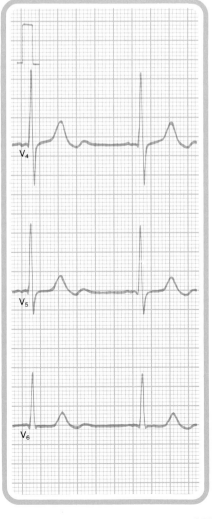

5. Right Bundle Branch Block with Lateral Infarction (Figure 172)

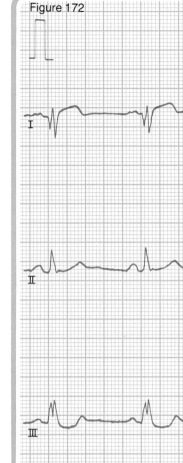

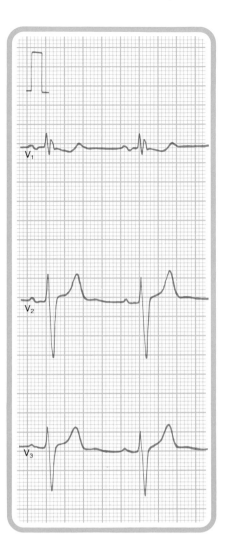

Figure 172

Figure 172

There is an Rsr' complex in V_1 with a total QRS duration of 0.13 sec (well seen in V_2 and V_3). There is therefore complete right bundle branch block. There are abnormal Q waves in I and aVL (more than one quarter of the height of the ensuing R wave and also more than 0.04 sec in duration).

Since the mean frontal plane QRS axis is $+105°$, the abnormal Q waves in aVL could simply be related to the heart position (i.e. aVL is a cavity lead). However, this cannot explain the abnormal Q waves in I, which indicates a lateral infarction. No evidence of infarction is seen in the precordial leads but some evidence might be found if high lateral leads were used (Table 4, page 180). There is S-T segment elevation and terminal T wave inversion in I and aVL suggesting **recent** infarction. The S-T segments and T waves in V_6 are minimally abnormal. The abnormal degree of right axis deviation could be due to right inferior hemiblock, but abnormal right axis deviation has many causes including anterolateral infarction without involvement of the inferior division of the left bundle. In this case there is actually probably a different reason altogether – see below[*].

A suitable report for this record would be as follows:-

"Sinus rhythm. The mean frontal plane QRS axis is abnormal at $+105°$. There is complete right bundle branch block. There are abnormal q waves in I and aVL, indicating lateral myocardial infarction. The form of the S-T segments and T waves in these leads and in V_6 suggest that the infarct is recent".

Note

[*] This patient had just suffered acute myocardial infarction. The physical signs suggested the presence of an atrial septal defect. The latter – a congenital lesion unrelated to the infarction and previously unsuspected – was subsequently confirmed by cardiac catheterisation. Coronary angiography revealed occlusive disease in the diagonal branch of the left coronary artery.

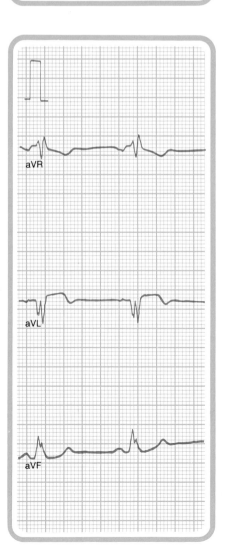

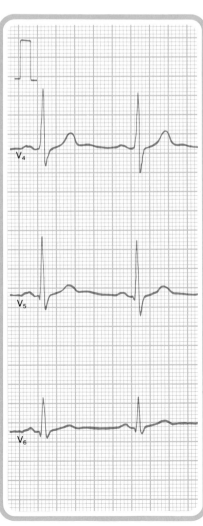

6. Right Ventricular Hypertrophy with Acute Pericarditis (Figure 173)

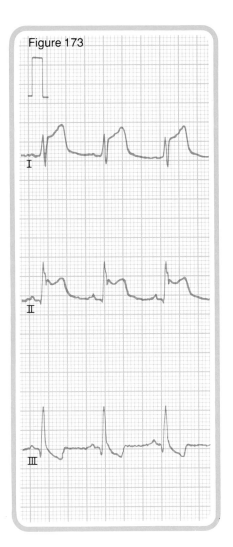

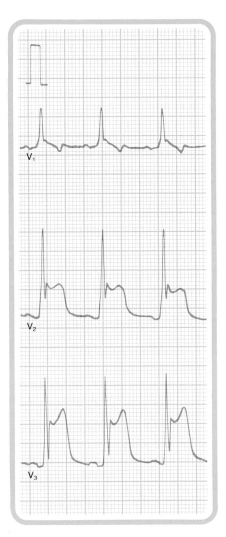

Figure 173

Figure 173

The rhythm is sinus. There is striking S-T segment elevation in virtually all leads (aVR, being a cavity lead, naturally shows S-T segment depression. This is **not** a reciprocal change). Such widespread S-T elevation is usually indicative of acute pericarditis. The S-T elevation is concave upwards which is also typical. The R wave in V_1 is dominant and the total QRS duration is normal. This is powerfully suggestive of right ventricular hypertrophy. One would expect right ventricular hypertrophy to be associated with S-T segment depression in V_1 and the apparently neutral S-T segment in this lead may be the result of the cancelling out of opposite effects – S-T segment depression, anticipated due to the right ventricular hypertrophy and S-T segment elevation anticipated due to the pericarditis.

A suitable report for this record would be as follows:-

"Sinus rhythm. There is widespread S-T segment elevation indicative of acute pericarditis. The form of the QRS complexes in V_1 is indicative of right ventricular hypertrophy."

The patient had an atrial septal defect. The record was taken in the immediate post-operative period. The pericarditis was a reaction to the operation.

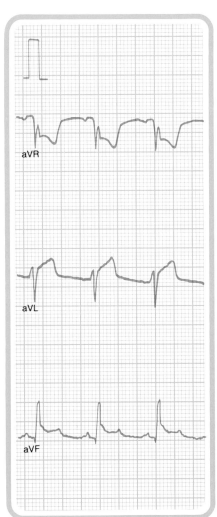

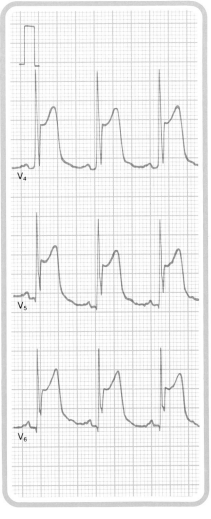

7. Non-specific T Wave Changes with Left Anterior Hemiblock and Technical Dextrocardia (Figure 174a)

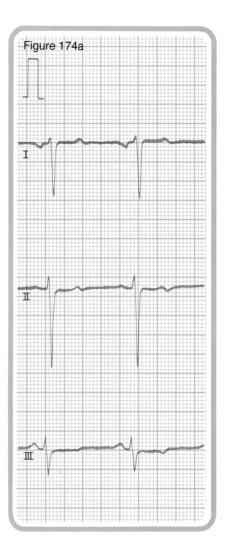
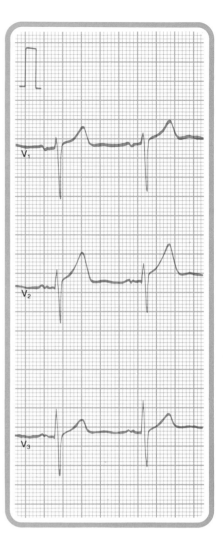

Figure 174a

The P wave is negative in I and the QRS deflection is dominantly negative in this lead. This raises the suspicion that the right and left arm leads have been inadvertently interposed. When this happens the T wave in I is usually also inverted so the present appearances are not typical. However, the reason for this will emerge later. This record is actually an example of accidental right/left arm lead interposition, i.e. of technical dextrocardia. Figure 174b shows a further record, taken within minutes of the first one with the right and left arm leads correctly arranged. Comparison between 174a and 174b shows the effects of technical dextrocardia and how the two appearances can be judged without retaking the record:-

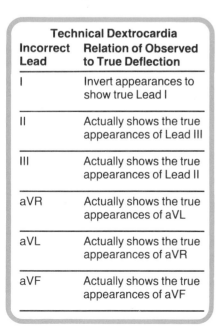

Technical Dextrocardia	
Incorrect Lead	Relation of Observed to True Deflection
I	Invert appearances to show true Lead I
II	Actually shows the true appearances of Lead III
III	Actually shows the true appearances of Lead II
aVR	Actually shows the true appearances of aVL
aVL	Actually shows the true appearances of aVR
aVF	Actually shows the true appearances of aVF

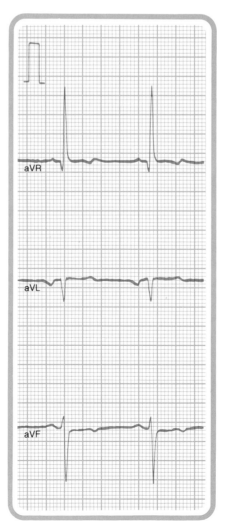
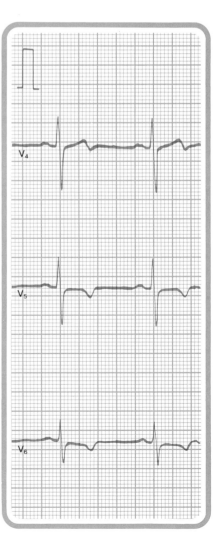

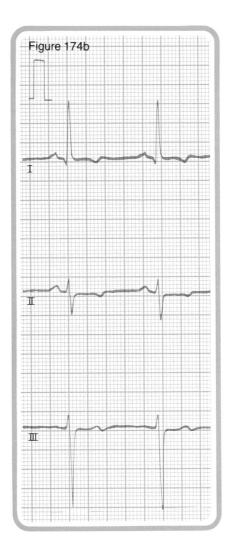

Figure 174b

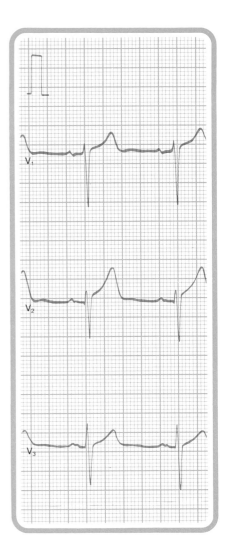

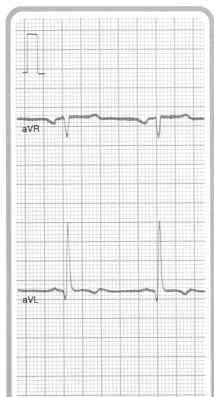

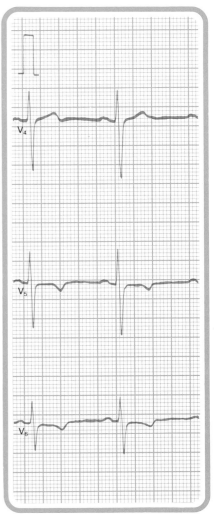

Figure 174b

Figure 174b shows why the T waves were not negative in I when there was technical dextrocardia – because the T wave is actually abnormal (inverted) in I. Record 174b might be reported as follows:-

"Sinus rhythm. The mean frontal plane QRS axis is −45° indicating left anterior hemiblock. The frontal plane T axis is −150°. The angle between the frontal plane QRS and T wave axes is therefore abnormal, indicating that the frontal plane T waves are abnormal. There is T wave inversion in V_5 and V_6 which is frankly abnormal. The T wave changes are non-specific. There is pronounced clockwise cardiac rotation."

8. Arrhythmias together with Morphological Abnormalities

Such combinations are extremely common. They will be dealt with in Section 3.

Practical Aids in ECG Interpretation

This section does not present a systematic approach to a single topic – rather it points to several useful topics which are helpful to bear in mind during ECG interpretation. In most aspects of medicine, there are diagnostic possibilities which are easily forgotten – perhaps because the signs are subtle or because the condition is relatively uncommon. Examples of such syndromes in clinical medicine in the author's experience include, for example, amyloidosis and haemochromatosis. To consider these possibilities when presented with a clinically obscure problem takes little time and may occasionally be very rewarding. These examples are not necessarily optimal for everyone. Each has blind spots or weak spots in his own diagnostic approach and it is useful to recognise when this has happened and to add this diagnosis to one's list of such possibilities so that subsequently, at each diagnostic level, the contents of the list may be considered in the diagnostic process. The same principle applies in electrocardiography and it is in this spirit that this section is presented.

Causes of QS Complexes in the Right Precordial Leads

1. Clockwise cardiac rotation (V_1 only).
2. Anteroseptal myocardial infarction.
3. Left bundle branch block.
4. Ventricular pre-excitation.

Causes of Dominant R Waves in V_1

1. Right ventricular hypertrophy.
2. True posterior myocardial infarction.
3. Ventricular pre-excitation.
4. Duchenne-type muscular dystrophy.
5. Pronounced counter-clockwise cardiac rotation (very occasionally). (Dominant R waves may also be seen as part of the RBBB pattern but this should not cause confusion since the presence of the secondary R wave and of prolongation of the total QRS duration is easily recognised).

Conditions which may give rise to an Incorrect Diagnosis of Myocardial Infarction

1. Ventricular pre-excitation.
2. Left bundle branch block.
3. Left anterior hemiblock.
4. Hypertrophic obstructive cardiomyopathy (abnormal q waves may occur in this condition without infarction).
5. Congestive cardiomyopathy (abnormal q waves may occur in this condition without infarction).
6. Extreme clockwise cardiac rotation.
7. Left ventricular hypertrophy (occasionally the r wave in the right precordial lead may be so small as to suggest infarction).
8. Pulmonary embolism.
9. Hyperkalaemia.
10. Intracranial haemorrhage.

Useful Advice

Remember
It is **always difficult, often impossible,** and **sometimes dangerous** to diagnose myocardial infarction in the presence of left bundle branch block.

Remember
Ventricular pre-excitation is easily missed and can give rise to a false diagnosis of left bundle branch block or of myocardial infarction.

Causes of a Mean Frontal Plane QRS Axis more positive than $+90°$

1. Right ventricular hypertrophy
2. Anterolateral infarction
3. Left posterior hemiblock
4. Normal finding in infants and children (90° to 120°)
5. Normal finding occasionally in tall slim adults (90° to 105°)
6. Chronic lung disease
7. Pulmonary embolism
8. Atrial septal defect (ostium secundum type)
9. During coronary angiography (injection of contrast into right coronary artery)

Causes of a Mean Frontal Plane QRS Axis more negative than $-30°$

Common Causes

1. Left anterior hemiblock
2. Inferior myocardial infarction

Rare Causes

3. Ventricular pre-excitation
4. Hyperkalaemia
5. Tricuspid atresia

6. Atrial septal defect (ostium primum type)
7. Artificial cardiac pacing from apex of right or left ventricles

Easily Recognisable Cause

8. During coronary angiography (injection of contrast into left coronary artery)

Conditions giving rise to Prominent U Waves	1. Hypokalaemia. 2. Hypomagnesaemia. 3. Hypercalcaemia. 4. Bradycardia. 5. Following exercise. 6. Left ventricular hypertrophy. 7. Mitral valve prolapse. 8. Central nervous system disorders. 9. Hyperthyroidism. 10. During treatment with digitalis, quinidine, procainamide or phenothiazines.	
Conditions giving rise to U Wave Inversion	1. Left ventricular hypertrophy. 2. Myocardial ischaemia.	
Conditions giving rise to Prolongation of the Q-Tc Interval	Ischaemic heart disease. Myocarditis. Cardiomyopathy. Hypocalcaemia. Hypothermia. Mitral valve prolapse. Intracranial haemorrhage. Drugs (quinidine, disopyramide, procainamide, amiodarone, tricyclic antidepressants, phenothiazines). Hypothyroidism (but see page 229).	Acute cor pulmonale. Post Stokes-Adams seizures. Long Q-T syndrome. (This is a syndrome consisting of a long Q-Tc interval, episodes of syncope and sudden death. It is often referred to as the Romano-Ward syndrome. When there is also congenital deafness it is referred to as the Jarvell and Lange-Nielsen syndrome).
Conditions giving rise to Shortening of the Q-Tc Interval	Hypercalcaemia. Digitalis therapy.	

Evaluation of the Q-T Interval

The Q-T interval is the time interval from the first recognisable part of the QRS complex to the final recognisable part of the T wave in the same lead. Since the QRS deflections are usually sharp the onset of the Q-T interval is usually easy to measure. However, the terminal part of the T wave is often a rather gentle slope and the precise position of the final part of the T wave may be difficult or even impossible to determine with total confidence. In the presence of a prominent U wave the difficulty is increased. The Q-T interval is therefore a relatively difficult measurement to make.

In addition to the difficulties in making the **measurement** of the Q-T interval there are considerable difficulties in **interpreting** the significance of measurement. This is because the Q-T interval varies inversely with the heart rate. There are two ways of overcoming this problem. The first is to consult a table of known values for the upper and lower limits of the Q-T duration at various heart rates. Several such tables are available in the literature. A second approach is to "correct" the measured Q-T interval at the observed heart rate to that which would be predicted for the same electrocardiogram if the heart rate were the "standard" rate of 60/minute. This corrected heart rate, or Q-Tc, can be obtained from nomograms which show Q-Tc in terms of observed heart rate and observed Q-T interval or can be obtained by the application of Bazett's formula (described in 1920):-

$$Q\text{-}Tc = \frac{\text{Measured Q-T interval}}{\sqrt{\text{R-R interval}}}$$

[The units of the variable "Q-Tc" are usually expressed as "seconds", whereas strictly speaking they should be "seconds$^{1/2}$" i.e. "$\sqrt{\text{seconds}}$"].

There is some disagreement among various authorities on the range of normality of Q-Tc. The values are less for men than for women and are less for children than for adults.

Table 9 shows the predicted upper limits of normal for the Q-T intervals in men and women at various heart rates. The heart rate values are chosen on the basis of there being an integral number of 0.04 sec intervals (and therefore a precise number of small squares of the ECG graticule) in each chosen R-R interval. The maximum Q-T interval is that predicted by the Bazett formula using a maximum Q-Tc for men of 0.42 sec and for women of 0.43 sec. In practice it is more convenient to count the number of small squares (on the ECG graticule) between consecutive R waves (the "cycle time") and to use this to obtain the upper limit of normal for the Q-T duration rather than to work out the heart rate itself.

Table 9

Heart rate (per min)	Cycle time (number of 0.04 sec units)	Maximum Q-T (sec) (Males)	(Females)
300	5	.19	.19
250	6	.21	.21
214	7	.22	.23
187	8	.24	.24
166	9	.25	.26
150	10	.27	.27
136	11	.28	.29
125	12	.29	.3
115	13	.3	.31
107	14	.31	.32
100	15	.33	.33
93	16	.34	.34
88	17	.35	.35
83	18	.36	.36
78	19	.37	.37
75	20	.38	.38
71	21	.38	.39
68	22	.39	.4
65	23	.4	.41
62	24	.41	.42
60	25	.42	.43
57	26	.43	.44
55	27	.44	.45
52	28	.44	.46
51	29	.45	.46
50	30	.46	.47
48	31	.47	.48
46	32	.48	.49
45	33	.48	.49
43	34	.49	.5
42	35	.5	.51
41	36	.5	.52
40	37	.51	.52
39	38	.52	.53
38	39	.52	.54
37	40	.53	.54
36	41	.54	.55
35	42	.54	.56
35	43	.55	.56
34	44	.56	.57
33	45	.56	.58
32	46	.57	.58
32	47	.58	.59
31	48	.58	.6
30	49	.59	.6
30	50	.59	.61

The majority of conditions which alter the Q-T interval do so by causing Q-T prolongation. For that reason the upper limits of normality are more often required in detail than the lower limits. Significant shortening of the Q-T interval is less common and such a detailed table for the lower limits of normality is unnecessary. The following simple Table (10) gives the lower limits of normal for the Q-T interval at various ranges of heart rate.

Table 10

Heart Rates (per min)	Minimum 'Q-T interval' (sec)
45–55	.39
55–65	.36
65–75	.34
75–85	.32
85–105	.30

A Systematic Approach to the Interpretation of the ECG ("Updated")

We are now in a position to re-formulate the systematic approach to ECG interpretation which was first presented in Section I (pages 62–69). The basic approach is unchanged, but we can now graft on to it some additions and refinements as a result of our understanding of some electrocardiographic abnormalities.

Documentation and Recording Quality

It remains obligatory to ensure that the record **documentation** is satisfactory, i.e. that the **patient's name**, the **date** (and preferably also **time**) of the recording and the **lead labelling** and **gain calibration** are correctly entered on the record.

It remains obligatory also to ensure that the recording **quality** is adequate. In particular, baseline drift, skeletal muscle interference and mains frequency interference should be absent or minimal and the frequency response of the machine should be adequate (and preferably up to American Heart Association standards).

Provided the above preliminary requirements have been satisfactorily fulfilled, interpretation may proceed.

It is useful at this stage to review the systematic approach to ECG interpretation and to repeat the more important guidelines to the commoner and more significant abnormalities. The contents of the next four pages are repeated on the pull-out card in the flap at the back of this book.

Preliminary Assessment of Record Quality

Check
Name, date, lead labelling, normal gain calibration, paper recording speed.
Ensure
Minimal baseline drift, skeletal muscle interference, and muscle frequency interference and adequate machine frequency response.

Systematic Interpretation of ECG and Normal Criteria for Adults

1A. Determine Cardiac Rhythm

Criteria for normality of P waves only apply if rhythm is of sinus origin. Criteria for normality of QRS complexes, S-T segments and T waves only apply if rhythm is of supraventricular origin.

1B. Check P-R Interval

If 0.11 sec or less, consider pre-excitation. If pre-excitation is present (defined by (a) P-R interval is 0.11 sec or less, plus (b) total QRS duration is 0.11 sec or more, plus (c) slurring of initial 0.03 to 0.05 sec of QRS complex) **normal criteria for QRS complexes, S-T segments and T waves do not apply.**

2. Assess QRS Morphology in Precordial Leads

a) V_1 should have rS;

rS

V_6 should have qR but may have R, Rs or qRs.

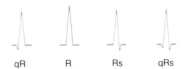

qR   R   Rs   qRs

(In the presence of clockwise rotation there may be no initial q in V_6 but a normal initial q may be seen in leads farther to left, i.e. I and aVL).

b) r wave should progressively increase in size from V_1 to V_6. However, it is quite normal for the R wave in V_6 to be smaller than that in V_5 and it is also normal for the R wave in V_5 to be less than that in V_4 provided the R wave in V_6 is also less than that in V_5 (compare Figure 42).
c) Transition (from right ventricular to left ventricular complexes) zone in precordial leads marked either by change from initial r to initial q (e.g. V_3-V_4 below) or by development of dominant R wave (V_3 below).

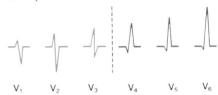

V_1 V_2 V_3 V_4 V_5 V_6

3. Check QRS Dimensions in Precordial Leads

a) Total QRS duration should not exceed 0.10 sec (2½ small squares).

> If QRS duration is 0.12 sec or more and there is no initial q wave in V_6, I and aVL and there is no secondary R wave in V_1 (and assuming the rhythm is supraventricular), there is left bundle branch block. In this situation the normal criteria for the QRS complexes, S-T segments and T waves do not apply.

b) At least one R wave should exceed 8 mm.

c) The tallest R wave should not exceed 27 mm.
d) The deepest S wave should not exceed 30 mm.
e) The sum of the tallest R and deepest S should not exceed 40 mm.
f) The ventricular activation time should not exceed 0.04 sec.
g) Any q wave seen should not have a depth exceeding ¼ of the height of the ensuing R wave.
h) Any q waves seen should not equal or exceed 0.04 sec in duration.

4A. Assess Precordial T Waves

a) The T wave in V_1 may be upright, flat or inverted. If upright in earlier records, it must be still upright.
b) The T wave in V_2 may be upright, flat or inverted. If upright in earlier records or if upright in V_1, it must be upright.
c) The T wave in V_3–V_5 must be upright. **In general** the T wave should be more than ⅛ but less than ⅔ of the R wave height.

4B. Assess the U Waves

The normal U wave is upright in all leads in which the T wave is upright. It should also be upright in the right precordial leads, even if the T waves are inverted here. Its average amplitude is less than 0.5mm. It tends to be largest in V_2 and V_3 where it may occasionally reach 2mm in height. In general it is less than 25% of the height of the preceding T wave. It is definitely abnormal when it is taller than the preceding T wave. Some authorities regard U waves taller than 1.5mm as abnormal. U wave inversion is abnormal.

---

5. Assess Precordial S-T Segments

The S-T segments must not deviate from the iso-electric line by more than ±1mm. Note that this should not be rigidly applied in V_1 and V_2. Caution should also be exercised in the presence of a tachycardia which may render assessment of the iso-electric position difficult or impossible.

---

6. Assess QRS Complexes in Limb Leads

a) A q wave in aVL*,I, II or aVF should not equal or exceed 0.04 sec in duration.
b) A q wave in aVL*,I, II or aVF should not have a depth greater than ¼ of the height of the ensuing R wave.
Note
   *q waves exceeding this criterion are acceptable in aVL if the frontal plane axis is more positive than +60° (i.e. +75° or more).

c) The R wave in aVL should not exceed 13 mm and that in aVF should not exceed 20 mm.
d) The frontal plane axis should not lie outside the range −30° to +90°.

7A. Assess T Waves in Limb Leads

a) The mean frontal plane T wave axis should not differ from the frontal plane QRS axis by more than ±45°.

b) In the presence of abnormal q waves in II, III, and aVF, T wave inversion in these leads is abnormal even if the above criterion is not fulfilled.

7B. Assess the U Waves

The U waves should be upright where the T waves are upright. The criterion for U wave size is as given in 4B above.

---

8. Assess S-T Segment in Limb Leads

These should not deviate by more than 1 mm above or below iso-electric line (see precautions under **5** above).

---

9. Assess P Waves

a) The P waves should not exceed 0.12 sec in duration in II.
b) The P waves should not exceed 2.5mm in height in II.

c) Any negative component to the P wave in V_1 should not have a greater area than the positive component.

---

10. Measure Q-T Interval

Make sure not to include a U wave. The number of 0.04 sec intervals (i.e. small squares on the ECG graticule) between consecutive R waves should be counted and the normality or otherwise of the measured Q-T interval in relation to the observed R-R interval determined by reference to Tables 9 and 10 on page 264.

Note
   *Q-T interval measurement is a difficult measurement to make and is often unrewarding. In the author's experience most abnormalities of Q-T duration are discovered in retrospect when the primary abnormality (e.g. hypocalcaemia) is already apparent.

Criteria for some of the Commoner or More Important Abnormalities

Ventricular Pre-excitation (WPW type)

a) P-R interval of 0.11 sec or less
plus
b) QRS duration of 0.11 sec or more
plus
c) Slurring of initial 0.03–0.05 sec of QRS complex.

> In the presence of ventricular pre-excitation the normal criteria for QRS complexes, S-T segments and T waves do not apply.
> TAKE CARE NOT TO MAKE AN INCORRECT DIAGNOSIS OF LEFT BUNDLE BRANCH BLOCK OR MYOCARDIAL INFARCTION.

Left Bundle Branch Block (LBBB)

a) Total QRS duration of 0.12 sec or more
plus
b) Absence of initial q wave in V_5, V_6 I and aVL
plus
c) Absence of secondary R wave in V_1 to indicate RBBB.

> In the presence of LBBB the normal criteria for QRS complexes, S-T segments and T waves do not apply. The normal criterion for the frontal plane axis does apply.
> TAKE CARE NOT TO MAKE AN INCORRECT DIAGNOSIS OF MYOCARDIAL INFARCTION OR LEFT VENTRICULAR HYPERTROPHY

Right Bundle Branch Block (RBBB)

a) Total QRS duration of 0.12 sec or more
plus
b) Secondary R wave in V_1.

> In the presence of RBBB the normal criteria for the QRS complexes and for the frontal plane axis apply.

Left Anterior Hemiblock (LAH)

a) Mean frontal plane QRS axis more negative than $-30°$
plus
b) Absence of q wave evidence of inferior infarction (i.e. initial r waves are visible in II and aVF).

> Left anterior hemiblock and inferior infarction are the two commonest causes of left axis deviation. The criteria for LAH are based on this. Other less common causes of left axis deviation include ventricular pre-excitation, hyperkalaemia, tricuspid atresia, ostium primum atrial septal defect and artificial cardiac pacing.

Left Ventricular Hypertrophy (LVH)
One or more of:-

a) R in V_4, V_5 or V_6 exceeds 27mm
b) S in V_1, V_2 or V_3 exceeds 30mm
c) R in V_4, V_5 or V_6 plus S in V_1, V_2 or V_3 exceeds 40mm
d) R in aVL exceeds 13mm
e) R in aVF exceeds 20mm
f) Ventricular activation time exceeds 0.04 sec
g) S-T segment depression, T wave flattening, T wave inversion in leads facing left ventricle.

> The reliability of the electrocardiographic diagnosis of left ventricular hypertrophy is directly related to the number of criteria fulfilled. Abnormal left axis deviation is not an expected finding in LVH.

Right Ventricular Hypertrophy (RVH)

a) Dominant R in V_1 (i.e. R, Rs, RR′, qR or qRs)
plus
b) Frontal plane axis more positive than $+90°$

> Dominant R in V_1 can occur in true posterior infarction, ventricular pre-excitation and Duchenne-type muscular dystrophy.

Left Atrial "Hypertrophy"

(Strictly "abnormality")

a) P duration longer than 0.12 sec or P wave bifid in I, II, aVF and aVL
or
b) P wave in V_1 has negative component with area greater than that of positive component.

Right Atrial "Hypertrophy"

(Strictly "abnormality")

a) P wave height 3.0mm or more in II, III or aVF.

Myocardial Infarction

a) q waves 0.04 sec or more in duration (excluding always Leads aVR and III, and, when the frontal plane QRS axis +75° or more positive, excluding also aVL).
or
b) q waves more than ¼ the height of the ensuing R wave (excluding always Leads aVR and III and, when the frontal plane QRS axis is +75° or more positive, excluding also aVL).
or
c) qs or QS complexes (excluding always Leads aVR and III and, when the frontal plane QRS axis is +75° or more positive excluding also aVL).
or
d) Inappropriately low R wave voltage in local area (when the facts can confidently be ascertained).

The concomitant presence of significant S-T elevation suggests that the infarct is not more than days old. If the S-T segments are normal but there is still T inversion, it suggests that the infarct is not more than several weeks old.
IT IS ALWAYS DIFFICULT, OFTEN IMPOSSIBLE, AND SOMETIMES DANGEROUS TO DIAGNOSE INFARCTION IN THE PRESENCE OF LBBB OR VENTRICULAR PRE-EXCITATION.

Note

The above "diagnostic criteria" for myocardial infarction can occasionally be fulfilled in certain particular conditions which gives rise to "pseudo-infarction" patterns (pages 198 and 242). The most likely such condition is cardiomyopathy. The diagnosis of myocardial infarction is extremely unlikely to be incorrect if the full **sequence** of changes (S-T elevation, QRS changes, T wave changes and restoration of normality to the S-T segments) is seen.

Conditions in which "Normal" Criteria do not apply

In the presence of supraventricular arrhythmias the normal criteria for P waves do no apply.

In supraventricular arrhythmias atrial depolarisation begins from an abnormal site. The normal pathway for atrial myocardial depolarisation cannot therefore be followed and the P waves are, in consequence, abnormal. Assuming there is normal intraventricular conduction the normal criteria for QRS complexes, S-T segments and T waves continue to apply.

In the presence of ventricular arrhythmias or of ventricular pre-excitation the normal criteria for the QRS complexes do not apply.

In ventricular arrhythmias ventricular depolarisation begins from an abnormal site and the normal pathway for ventricular myocardial depolarisation cannot be followed. In consequence the QRS complexes are abnormal. The S-T segments and T waves are usually also abnormal in this situation for primary depolarisation (QRS) abnormalities often result in secondary repolarisation (S-T segments and T wave) abnormalities.

The 12-Lead ECG : Annotated Records

This final chapter will review a series of 40 12-lead electrocardiograms. These are referred to as "Records" rather than figures for they may be used either for instruction or for audit. A similar approach was used at the end of Section 1, where 30 "records" were presented. To prevent confusion the first record described here in Section 2 will be labelled "Record 31". For each of the first 10 records, each detailed step of the systematic interpretation originally described on pages 66–69 and subsequently modified on pages 266 to 268 will be followed and described using the same numbering for the paragraphs. Abnormalities will be shown in **heavy type**. Records 41 to 70 then appear without any supporting text. On page 321 each of these last 30 records will be defined as being normal or abnormal. For those records which are abnormal, a list of the abnormal features will appear on pages 322 to 326. This list will use the paragraph headings corresponding to the systematic approach described on pages 266 to 268 (as modified from the list which originally appeared in Section I on pages 67 to 69). The student may use this section either for further systematic tuition or for self-evaluation. Finally, an interpretation of Records 1-30 from Section I will be given on pages 327 to 329. Abnormalities will be expressed in **heavy type**.

Record 31

Normal Record

1. Sinus rhythm. The P-R interval is normal at 0.12 sec (well seen in II).

2. a) V_1 has an rS complex. V_6 has a qR complex.

b) V_1–V_6 shows normal r wave progression from V_1–V_4, with the slight fall-off between V_4 and V_5, and again between V_5 and V_6 which is entirely normal.

c) The transition zone is between V_2 and V_3 (using criterion of dominant R wave, or between V_4 and V_5 using criterion of development of q wave).

3. a) Total QRS duration equals 0.07 sec.

b) The r waves in V_3, V_4, V_5 and V_6 all exceed 8mm.

c) The tallest r wave in the left precordial lead (V_4) measures 17mm.

d) The deepest S wave in the right precordial leads (V_2) measures 13mm.

e) $S_{V_2} + R_{V_4} = 30$mm.

f) Ventricular activation time (well seen in V_5) = 0.03 sec.

g) q waves are seen in V_5 and V_6. They are obviously less than one quarter of the height of the ensuing r waves in the same lead.

h) q waves in V_5 and V_6 are clearly less than 0.04 sec in duration.

4A. The T waves are upright and of normal voltage throughout the precordial leads. The tallest T waves in this case are seen in V_2 and V_3 which is usually the case in normal records and the T wave height in the left precordial leads is not less than ⅛th and not more than ⅔rds of the height of the preceding R wave.
4B. Normal (low voltage but upright) U waves are seen in V_1–V_5.

5. The precordial S-T segments are iso-electric. Note that it is easier to see discrete S-T segments in V_4, V_5 and V_6 than it is in V_1 and V_2. This is usually the case.

6. a) Small q waves are seen in Leads I, II and aVF. They are less than 0.04 sec in duration.

b) The q waves seen in I and II are not greater than one quarter of the height of the ensuing R wave. The q wave in aVF is at the extreme upper end of the normal range in depth, but is not definitively abnormal. (q waves in Lead III which are broader or deeper than the normally accepted criteria are not significant unless abnormal q waves are also present in Lead II or aVF).

c) The R wave in aVL does not exceed 13mm and the R wave in aVF does not exceed 20mm.

d) The mean frontal plane QRS axis is $+60°$. This is within normal limits.

7A. The mean frontal plane T wave axis is $+45°$. The difference from the QRS axis is $15°$, which is within the normal range.
7B. No U waves are visible in the limb leads. This is quite normal.

8. The S-T segments in the limb leads are iso-electric.

9. a) The P wave duration in II is 0.10 " sec.

b) The P wave height in II is 1.5mm.

c) There is no dominant negative component to the P wave in V_1.

10. The Q-T interval is 0.42 sec. The heart rate is 57 per min but it is unnecessary to work this out. The "cycle time" (see page 263) is 26 (i.e. there are 26 small squares (on the ECG graticule) between consecutive R waves. Table 9 (page 264) shows that the upper limit of normal of the Q-T interval appropriate to this heart rate (or cycle time) is 0.43 sec for men or 0.44 sec for women. The Q-T interval is therefore normal.

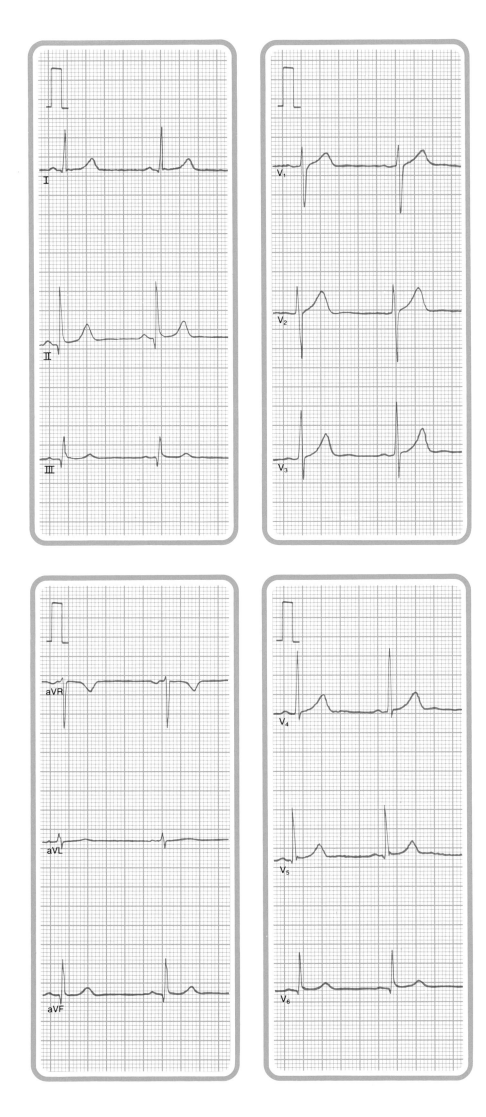

Record 32

Abnormal Record

1. Sinus rhythm. The P-R interval is normal at 0.18 sec.

2. a) **V_1 has a qR complex.** This is frankly abnormal. V_6 has a qRS complex. The S wave is much larger than one would normally expect, but this does not constitute a definite abnormality in its own right. (It is the result of the pronounced clockwise cardiac rotation which obtains in this record).

b) The r wave progression from V_1–V_6 is completely abnormal, but this is due entirely to the fact that the R waves are abnormally tall in the right precordial leads, i.e. it does not constitute an additional abnormality over and above that indicated by the abnormal R wave height in V_1.

c) **The transition zone is beyond (i.e. further to the left than) V_6. This indicates extreme clockwise cardiac rotation.**

3. a) The total QRS duration is within the normal range at 0.09 sec (well seen in V_6).

b) All the R waves in the precordial leads exceed 8mm.

c) The tallest R wave in the left precordial lead (V_4) is within the normal range at 18mm.

d) The S waves in the right precordial leads are much smaller than are usually seen and they certainly are not abnormally deep.

e) The sum of the deepest S waves (V_3) and the tallest R waves (V_4) is 37mm. This is within the normal range.

f) No true estimate of the ventricular activation time can be obtained since no true left ventricular complexes are possible in the precordial series (again due to the pronounced clockwise cardiac rotation).

g) The q waves in V_6 are manifestly not deeper than ¼ of the height of the following r wave.

h) The q waves in V_6 are certainly less than 0.04 sec in duration.

4A. The T waves are inverted from V_1-V_5. This is definitely abnormal. **The T waves are iso-electric in V_6.** This is also abnormal.

4B. No definite U waves are visible in the precordial leads. This is not an abnormality.

5. The S-T segments are depressed from V_1-V_5. This is frankly abnormal.

6. a) Small q waves are visible in aVF. They are less than one quarter of the height of the following r wave.

b) The q waves in aVF are less than one small square in duration (i.e. less than 0.04 sec).

c) The R wave in aVL does not exceed 13mm nor does that in aVF exceed 20mm.

d) **The mean frontal plane QRS axis is +120°.** This is frankly abnormal.

7A. The mean frontal plane T wave axis is +90°. The difference between the frontal plane QRS and T wave axes is within the normal range at 30°. The limb lead T waves are therefore within normal limits.

7B. No definite U waves are visible. This is not abnormal.

8. There is minimal S-T segment depression in Lead III and the foot-lead, but this is not beyond the normal permitted limits of ± 1mm from the iso-electric line.

9. a) The P wave duration in Lead II is 0.11 sec.

b) The P wave height in Lead II is 2mm.

c) **The negative component of the P waves in V_1 is larger than the positive component, indicating left atrial abnormality.**

10. The Q-T interval is 0.38 sec. The cycle time (page 263) is 20 (i.e. heart rate 75) and the Q-T interval is therefore normal.

The combination of a dominant R wave in V_1 with abnormal right axis deviation indicates **right ventricular hypertrophy**. *The S-T segment depression and T wave inversion in the precordial leads and the pronounced clockwise cardiac rotation are frequent accompaniments of right ventricular hypertrophy. In addition there is* **left atrial abnormality**.

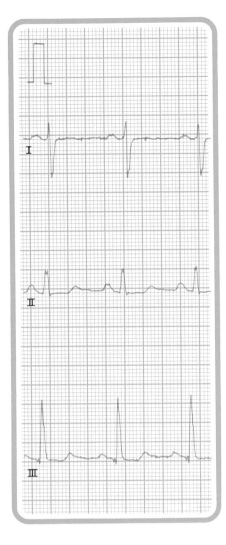

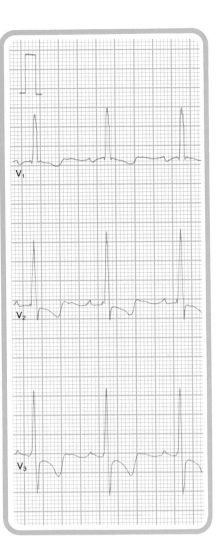

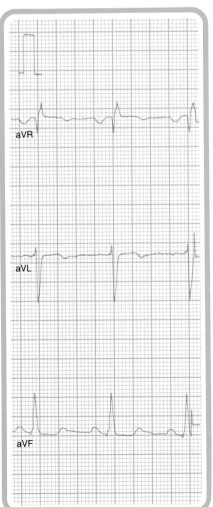

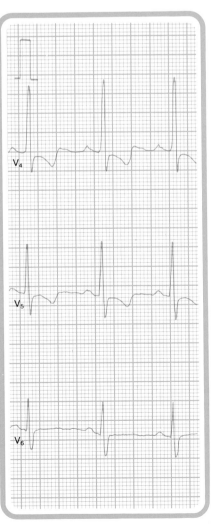

274

Record 33

Abnormal Record

1. Sinus rhythm. The P-R interval is 0.16 sec.

2. a) V_1 has a rS complex. V_6 has a qR complex.

b) V_1–V_6 has a **relatively** normal R wave progression, but the R waves in the left precordial leads are not as tall as one would expect, i.e. the R wave progression does not appear to have developed as well as usual.

c) The transition zone is between V_4 and V_5.

3. a) The total QRS duration is 0.07 sec.

b) The r wave in V_3 is 9mm, i.e. it just exceeds the minimum requirement of 8mm.

c) The tallest R wave is well within the normal range at 9mm (in V_3).

d) The deepest S wave is seen in V_2 and this is within the normal range of 7mm.

e) The sum of the S in V_2 and the R in V_3 is well within the normal range at 15mm.

f) The ventricular activation time is of the order of 0.02 sec.

g) q waves are seen in V_6, and these are clearly less than one quarter of the height of the ensuing r wave in the same lead.

h) q waves in V_6 are clearly less than 0.04 sec in duration.

4A. T waves in V_1, V_2 and V_3 are normal. **The T waves in V_4, V_5 and V_6 are of abnormally low voltage (they are almost iso-electric).**
4B. Prominent U waves are seen in these leads and in **V_5 the U wave is bigger than the P wave which precedes it, which is definitely abnormal.**

5. The S-T segments from V_1 to V_4 are iso-electric. The S-T segments in V_5 and V_6 are minimally depressed but not beyond the normal permitted range of $\pm$ 1mm.

6. a) q waves are seen in Leads I, II and aVL. In all cases they are less than 0.04 sec in duration.

b) **The q wave in Lead II has a depth which is greater than one quarter of the height of the R wave following it, which is abnormal.**

c). The R wave in aVL does not exceed 13mm and the r wave in aVF does not exceed 20mm.

d) The mean frontal plane QRS axis is $-15°$, which is within the normal range.

7A. The mean frontal plane T wave axis is $-45°$. **Although the angle between the mean frontal plane QRS axis and T wave axes is within the normal range, the negative T waves in Leads II, III and the foot-lead should be regarded as being abnormal since there is an abnormal q wave in Lead II, indicative of inferior myocardial infarction** (pages 60 and 178).
7B. Small upright (normal) U waves are seen in I and aVL.

8. The S-T segments in the limb leads are iso-electric.

9. a) The P wave duration is within the normal range at 0.10 sec.

b) The P wave height is within the normal range in Lead II at 1.5mm.

c) The negative component of the P wave in V_1 is about equal to that of the positive component. This is not abnormal.

10. The Q-T interval is 0.44 sec. For a cycle time of 27 (heart rate 55) this is within normal limits.

There is unequivocal evidence of inferior myocardial infarction of intermediate age. It has not occurred within the last few days since there is no residual S-T segment elevation. It is not more than a few weeks old since there is still T wave inversion. The low voltage T waves in the left precordial leads and the prominent U waves there, are non-specific abnormalities. The probability is that they are related to ischaemia in the lateral wall of the ventricle, but one cannot be dogmatic on this point.
Note that aVF shows rS complexes. Even though the r waves are very small, they preclude the diagnosis of inferior infarction from the QRS configuration in this lead. It is possible that these small r waves have "regenerated" (page 179), i.e. that QS complexes were formerly apparent in this lead.

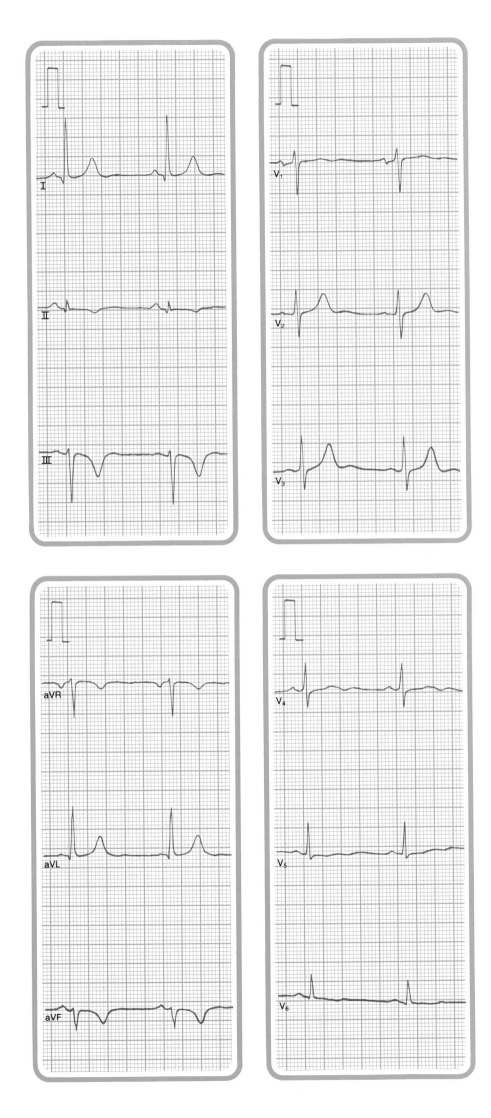

Record 34

Abnormal Record

1. The rhythm is sinus. The P-R interval is within the normal range at 0.12 sec (well seen in V_2).

2. a) V_1 has a rS complex. The r wave is very small indeed and it might be thought that there is a QS complex in this lead, however, there is a definite r wave in V_2 and even if there were no initial r wave in V_1, it would not actually constitute an abnormality .
V_6 shows a qR complex. The q wave is again very small and is perhaps best seen in the second QRS complex of V_6.
   b) The r wave progression from V_1–V_6 is normal.
   c) The transition zone is between V_3 and V_4.

3. a) The total QRS duration is normal at 0.09 sec (well seen in the third QRS complex in V_2).
   b) The R waves in the left precordial leads all exceed 8mm.
   c) The tallest R wave (V_5) is within the normal range at 18mm.
   d) The deepest S wave (V_2) is abnormal at 34mm.
   e) The sum of S in V_2 and R in V_5 is abnormal at 52mm.
   f) The ventricular activation time is 0.04 sec (well seen in V_5).
   g) The q waves in V_6 are not deeper than one quarter of the height of the ensuing r waves.
   h) The q waves in V_6 are less than 0.04 sec in duration.

4A. The T waves are inverted from V_4–V_6. This is frankly abnormal.
4B. Small, upright (normal) U waves are seen in V_2 and V_3.

5. The S-T segments are depressed in V_4, V_5 and V_6. This is frankly abnormal. The S-T depression is sloping rather than flat. It is therefore non-specific.

6. a) Small q waves are seen in aVF. They are less than 0.04 sec in duration.
   b) The q waves in aVF are not deeper than a quarter of the height of the ensuing r wave.
   c) The R wave in aVL does not exceed 13mm and the R wave in aVF does not exceed 20mm.
   d) The mean frontal plane QRS is +45°.

7A. The mean frontal plane T wave axis is indeterminate. Since the mean frontal plane QRS axis is highly determinate, the T waves in the limb leads are abnormal.
7B. No significant U waves are seen in the limb leads.

8. There is S-T segment depression in Lead II and the foot-lead. This is beyond the acceptable limit of one millimetre (well seen in both of these leads) compared with the T-P interval.

9. a) The P wave duration in Lead II is within normal limits at 0.10 sec.
   b) The P wave height is normal at 1.5mm.
   c) The negative component of the P wave in V_1 does not exceed the positive component.

10. The Q-T interval is 0.32 sec. The cycle time is 16 (heart rate 93) for which the upper limit of normal for the Q-T interval is 0.34 sec.

The changes are those of left ventricular hypertrophy. The voltage criteria for left ventricular hypertrophy are fulfilled in the precordial leads. The S-T, T changes in the left precordial leads are probably secondary to the primary QRS abnormality. The S-T, T changes in the limb leads are non-specific, but the probability is that these too are secondary to the abnormal QRS complexes. Note the superficial similarities of the morphology of the QRS complexes to that in left bundle branch block. However, there is no left bundle branch block since:-
a) the total QRS duration is well within the normal range, and
b) the small initial q waves are seen in V_6.

Note
Occasionally the normal ECG has no recognisable r waves in V_1 (page 45).

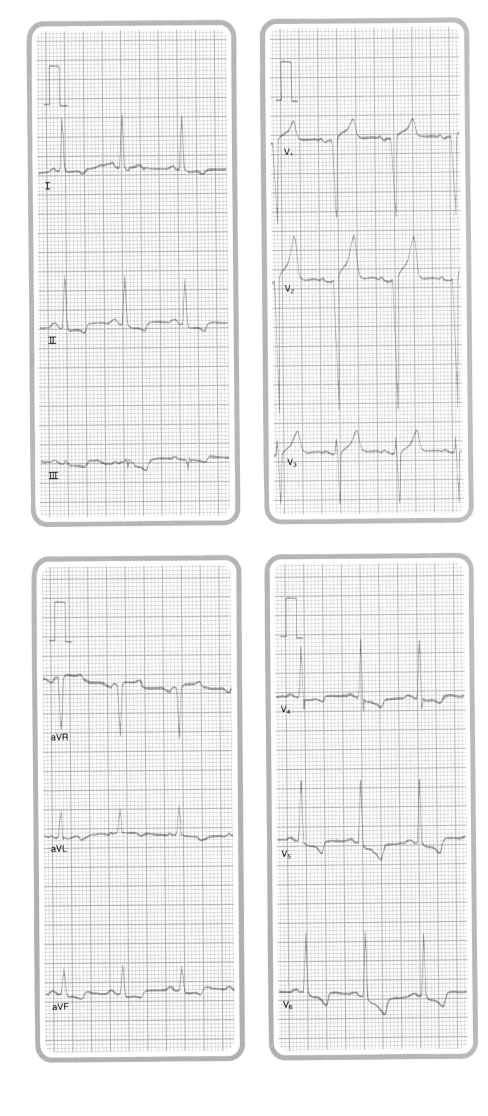

278

Record 35

Abnormal Record

1. The rhythm is sinus. The P-R interval is within the normal range at 0.12 sec (well seen in Lead II). The P-R interval in the left precordial lead looks to be abnormally short on casual inspection (especially in V_5). However, note that the P waves are bifid and that the true origin of the P waves is earlier than initially suspected. The P waves in Lead II are also bifid and the normal length of the P-R interval is readily visible in this lead.

2. a) V_1 has an rS complex. V_6 has a qR complex.

b) **The r wave progression from V_1–V_6 is not normal.**
There is a normal r wave in V_1, **but V_2 shows a QS complex (i.e. complete absence of the r wave) and V_3 shows a qrS complex. The r wave progression in V_2 and V_3 is therefore frankly abnormal.**

c) The transition zone is in the region of V_4.

3. a) The total QRS duration is within the normal range at 0.10 sec (well seen in V_3).

b) The R waves in the left precordial leads clearly exceed 8mm.

c) The tallest R wave in the left precordial leads (V_5) is within the normal range at 19mm.

d) The deepest precordial S wave (V_1) is 22mm.

e) $S_{V_1} + R_{V_5}$ is 41mm, which is strictly speaking just beyond the normal range.

f) The ventricular activation time is 0.04 sec.

g) **There are QS complexes in V_2. This is frankly abnormal.** (By definition, the q waves in a QS complex exceed ¼ of the ensuing R wave since there is no r wave).
The q wave in V_3 is clearly much larger than one quarter of the height of the ensuing r wave, and these q waves are therefore abnormal.

h) **The q waves in V_2 and V_3 are also abnormal in terms of their duration, which exceeds 0.04 sec.**

4A. The T waves are normal from V_1 to V_5. T waves in V_6 are upright, but are of rather lower voltage than one would expect. It is possible (but not certain) that this is an abnormality.
4B. Small, but upright (i.e. normal) U waves are seen in V_2–V_5.

5. The precordial S-T segments are within normal limits. The slight degree of S-T segment elevation seen in the right precordial leads, whilst possibly consistent with the presence of anteroseptal infarction, is also quite possibly within the normal range. Minimal degrees of S-T segment elevation are frequently seen in these leads.

6. a) Initial q waves are seen in Lead I and aVL. In neither case are the q waves 0.04 sec or more in duration.

b) The q waves seen in I and aVL do not have a depth exceeding one quarter of the height of the ensuing r wave.

c) The R wave in aVL does not exceed 13mm and the r wave in aVF does not exceed 20mm.

d) The mean frontal plane QRS axis is −30°. This is at the extreme left hand end of the normal range. There is therefore borderline abnormal left axis deviation.

7A. **The mean frontal plane T wave axis is of the order of +90°. It is not highly determinate, but is certainly in this region. The T waves in the limb leads are therefore abnormal either because the angle between the frontal plane T and QRS axes is beyond the normal range, or because the frontal plane T wave axis is not highly determinate whilst the frontal plane QRS axis is highly determinate.**
7B. Small (normal U waves are seen in II, III and aVF.

8. **The S-T segments are depressed in Leads I and aVL.** The degree of **depression is minimal but probably abnormal.** It may well be that this S-T segment depression has developed as a result of the presence of ischaemic heart disease but one cannot, from the electrocardiogram, with total confidence say that the S-T segment depression is abnormal since it is not beyond the normally accepted range.

9. a) The P wave duration in II is 0.12 sec which is at the extreme upper end of the normal range.

b) The P wave height in II is normal at 1 mm.

c) The P wave in V_1 does not have a dominant negative component.

10. The Q-T interval is 0.46 sec. The cycle time is 31 (heart rate 48) for which the normal upper limit for the Q-T interval is 0.47 sec.

The electrocardiogram shows a definite abnormality of the QRS complexes in V_1 - V_3. This abnormality is indicative of loss of viable myocardium in this area. The most likely cause is an old anteroseptal infarction but other causes (pseudo-infarction patterns) can occur in various cardiomyopathies or infiltrative lesions. In addition there are non-specific S-T, T changes in the limb leads and in V_6. These could well be related to the same basic cause as the abnormal QRS complexes in the precordial leads, but one cannot be totally confident of this. The precordial QRS complexes just satisfy the voltage criteria for left ventricular hypertrophy but it is unwise to make this diagnosis when these criteria are only just fulfilled and there are no additional criteria for the condition fulfilled.

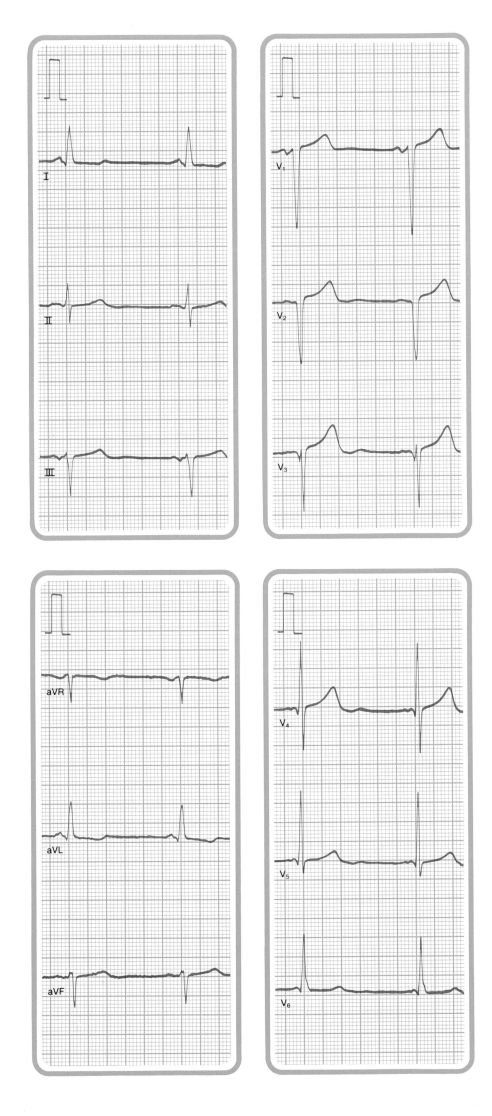

280

Abnormal Record

1. The rhythm is sinus. The P-R interval is 0.19 sec (well seen in Lead II).

2. a) V_1 has an rS complex. V_6 does not have a qR complex. No initial q wave is seen in V_6. **It is obvious also at this stage that the total QRS duration is prolonged. The total QRS duration is 0.18 sec (well seen in V_6). Since there is no initial septal q wave in V_6 the total QRS duration is prolonged and there is no secondary r wave in the right precordial leads, there is therefore left bundle branch block. In view of this, there is no point in making any further assessment of the precordial QRS complexes, S-T segments or T waves. The deep S waves in V_1 and the deep QS complexes in V_2 and V_3 are all part of the left bundle branch block pattern. The depressed S-T segments in V_6 and T wave inversion in this lead and the elevated S-T segments in the right precordial leads are also part of the left bundle branch block pattern.**

Once left bundle branch block has been diagnosed, no further diagnostic processes should be applied to the QRS complexes, the S-T segments or the T waves in the precordial leads. In the limb leads the only diagnostic process which should be applied is the determination of the mean frontal plane QRS axis.

6. d) This is seen to be abnormal at $-45°$. There is therefore an abnormal degree of left axis deviation and this might imply peripheral disease in the anterior division of the left bundle branch system in addition to the proximal lesion causing complete left bundle branch block.

9. The normal criteria can be applied to the P waves and it can be seen that the **P wave in V_1 has a dominant negative component. This indicates left atrial abnormality.**

The only other feature for comment is the presence of a small initial q wave in aVL. This is unusual in left bundle branch block and indeed is normally part of the criteria that initial q waves should be absent not only in V_5 and V_6, but also in Leads I and aVL. This raises the possibility of myocardial infarction as well as left bundle branch block, but as stressed in the text this diagnosis can only rarely be made with confidence and should always be applied with very great caution.

This record is best considered as showing complete left bundle branch block, an abnormal degree of left axis deviation and abnormal P waves indicating left atrial abnormality. (The patient was actually suffering from congestive cardiomyopathy).

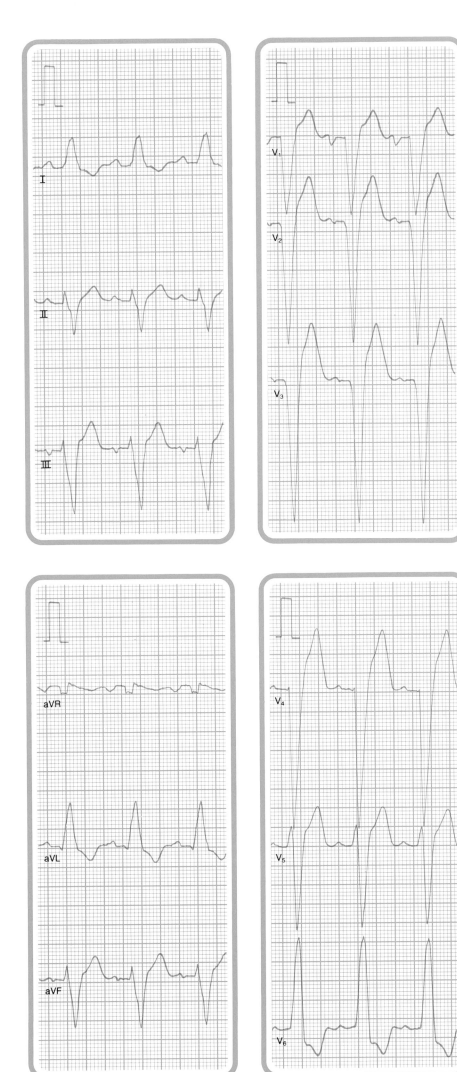

282

Record 37

Abnormal Record

1. The rhythm is sinus. The P-R interval is 0.14 sec.

2. a) There is no initial r wave in V_1 which shows a QS complex. There is no initial q wave in V_6. This leads one to consider the possibility that the interventricular septum might be depolarising in the wrong direction (complete or incomplete left bundle branch block). There is clearly no complete left bundle branch block since the total QRS duration can be seen to be normal. When no initial q wave is seen in V_6, one should inspect other leads looking at the left ventricle. When the heart is horizontal, as is usually the case, this will be Leads I and aVL. In this case the heart is almost vertical (with, as we shall see later, a frontal plane QRS axis of $+75°$) and the left ventricular facing limb leads are therefore Leads II and aVF. These both show small initial q waves and we may therefore conclude that the interventricular septum is depolarising in the normal direction. The absence of a q wave in V_6 is therefore not abnormal.

b) **The r wave progression in the precordial leads is clearly abnormal. No r wave is visible from V_1–V_4. Normal R waves "suddenly" appear in V_5 and V_6.**

c) The transition zone is between V_4 and V_5. Since the R wave progression is abnormal the transition zone has little meaning.

3. a) The total QRS duration is within the normal range at 0.08 sec.

b) The R waves in V_5 and V_6 both satisfy the minimal voltage criterion of 8mm.

c) The tallest precordial R wave (V_5) is well below the maximum permitted normal at 11mm.

d) The deepest S wave is actually seen in V_5. (The negative waves from V_1 to V_4 are not S waves, they are QS complexes and the S wave criteria do not apply to these). The S wave in V_5 is not abnormally deep.

e) $S_{V_5} + R_{V_5} = 14$, which is well within the permitted range.

f) The ventricular activation time cannot be determined since no qR complex is visible in the left precordial leads.

g) **The q waves from V_1 to V_4 are clearly abnormal. In each case they are QS complexes and they are clearly therefore more than a quarter of the height of the ensuing r wave.**

h) **The q waves from V_1 to V_4 are also abnormally long. They are well in excess of the permitted maximum of 0.03 sec . This criterion would itself be sufficient to indicate the presence of infarction.**

4A. There is terminal T wave inversion in V_2, V_3 and V_4, and low voltage T waves in V_5.
4B. Small, upright (normal) U waves are seen in V_5.

5. There is clear-cut, definitive S-T segment elevation from V_1–V_4 and minimal S-T segment elevation in V_5.

6. a) Small q waves are seen in Leads II and aVF. In no case is their depth more than one quarter of the height of the ensuing R wave.

b) Likewise the q waves in II and aVF do not equal or exceed 0.04 sec in duration.

c) The r wave in aVL does not exceed 13mm and the R wave in aVF does not exceed 20mm.

d) The mean frontal plane QRS axis is $+75°$ (it could be interpreted as being $+60°$. It depends whether or not one thinks that the algebraic sum of QRS deflections in aVL is actually zero or slightly negative).

7A. The mean frontal plane T wave axis is $+75°$. The frontal plane T waves are therefore normal.

The T waves in Lead I are flat and those who interpret the electrocardiogram via pattern recognition approach would probably regard them as abnormal. However, they do not actually fulfil the criteria for abnormality. The T waves are flat in Lead I simply because the repolarisation vector is almost at right angles to this lead.
7B. No significant U waves are seen in the limb leads.

8. The S-T segments in the limb leads are iso-electric.

9. a) The P wave duration is normal at 0.10 sec.

b) The P wave height is normal at 1mm.

c) The P waves in V_1 do not have a dominant negative component.

10. The Q-T interval is 0.34 sec (well seen in aVF). The cycle time is 16 (heart rate 93) and the maximum Q-T interval at this heart rate is 0.34 sec.

The record shows unequivocal evidence of recent anteroseptal myocardial infarction.

The record shows relatively recent anterior myocardial infarction. The QS complexes from V_1 - V_4 indicate "through and through" (transmural) infarction. The presence of S-T elevation from V_1 - V_4 (with, in addition, minimal S-T elevation in V_5) indicates that the infarct is relatively recent – probably less than one week old. The terminal T wave inversion in V_2, V_3 and V_4 and the low voltage waves in V_5 are also consistent with the diagnosis of recent anterior infarction.

Note

To say that a "q wave is in excess of 0.03 sec" is the same as saying that its "duration is 0.04 sec or more" since the best temporal resolution in the ECG is 0.01 sec.

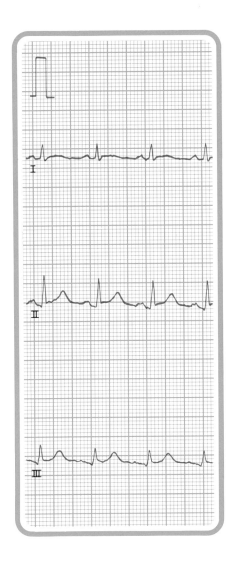
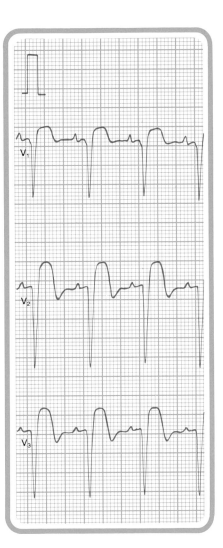
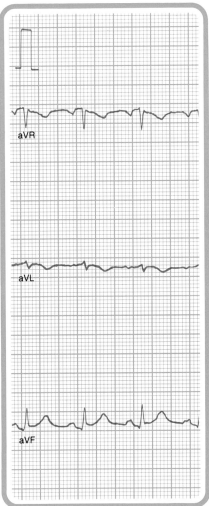
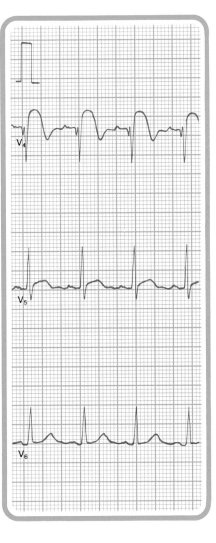

Record 38

Abnormal Record

1. The rhythm is sinus. The P-R interval is 0.14 sec.

2. a) **V_1 has an rsR′ complex. This is abnormal.** V_6 has a qRs complex.

b) The progression from V_1–V_6 of the initial r waves in each lead is normal.

c) The transition zone is between V_4 and V_5 (assessed by development of initial q waves).

3. a) **The total QRS duration is abnormal at 0.18 sec (well seen in V_1). The combination of the rsR′ pattern in V_1 with an increase in the total QRS duration indicates right bundle branch block.**

b) The R waves in V_4, V_5 and V_6 all satisfy the minimal voltage criterion of 8mm.

c) The maximum R waves in the left precordial leads (V_4) are within the normal range at 17mm (V_4).

d) The deepest S wave is seen in V_4 and in this lead it is 7mm.

e) $S_{V_4} + R_{V_4} = 24$mm, which is well within the normal maximum of 40mm.

f) The ventricular activation time is seen in V_6 to be 0.03 sec.

g) The q waves in V_5 and V_6 are not deeper than one quarter of the height of the r waves in the same lead.

h) The q waves in V_5 and V_6 are less than 0.04 sec in duration.

4A. The T waves in the precordial leads are within normal limits.
4B. No significant U waves are seen in the precordial leads.

5. There is S-T segment depression in V_1, but in the other precordial leads the S-T segments are within the normal range. The S-T segment depression in V_1 is almost certainly secondary to the QRS abnormality (right bundle branch block).

6. a) Small q waves are seen in aVL. Their depth does not exceed a quarter of the height of the ensuing r wave.

b) The q waves in aVL are less than 0.04 sec in duration.

c) The R wave in aVL does not exceed 13mm and that in aVF does not exceed 20mm.

d) The mean frontal plane QRS axis is indeterminate. (This is not abnormal).

7A. The mean frontal plane T wave axis is +30°. **Since the frontal plane QRS axis is indeterminate and the frontal plane T wave axis is determinate, the T waves are abnormal in the frontal plane leads. This abnormality is almost certainly also secondary to the right bundle branch block.**
7B. No significant U waves are visible in the limb leads.

8. The S-T segments in the limb leads are iso-electric.

9. a) The P wave duration in Lead II is 0.12 sec.

b) The P wave height is 0.5mm.

c) The negative component of the P wave in V_1 does not exceed the positive component in area.

10. The Q-T interval is 0.41 sec. The cycle time is 24 (heart rate 62) and the maximum Q-T interval corresponding to this rate is 0.41 sec.

The appearances are those of straightforward, uncomplicated, complete right bundle branch block.

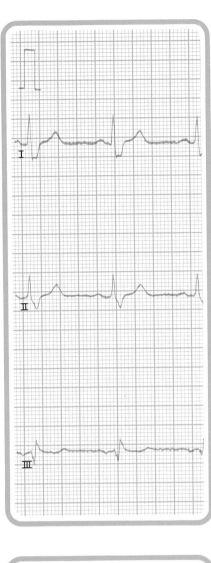

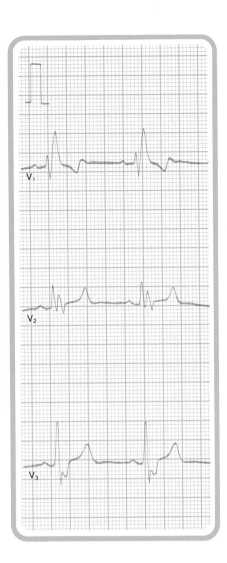

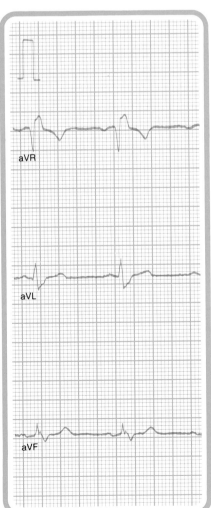

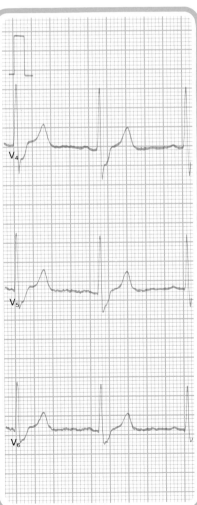

Record 39

Abnormal Record

1. The rhythm is sinus tachycardia. The P-R interval is 0.14 sec.

2. a) The QRS morphology in V_1 is normal (rS). The morphology in V_6 is also normal (qR).

b) The r wave progression appears normal from V_1–V_3, but the R waves in V_4, V_5 and V_6 are smaller than would be expected. (The minimal voltage criterion for the precordial r waves is not in fact satisfied, see 3b below).

c) The transition zone is between V_4 and V_5.

3. a) The total QRS duration is normal at 0.10 sec.

b) **The tallest R wave in the precordial leads is in V_3, where it is 8 mm. The criterion for normality is that at least one r wave should exceed 8 mm. This is therefore an abnormality.**

c) The tallest precordial r wave certainly does not exceed the maximal permitted level for normality (27 mm).

d) The deepest precordial S wave is seen in V_2 and is 26 mm. This is well below the maximum normal of 30 mm.

e) The sum of the tallest R and deepest S waves is well below the maximum of 40 mm.

f) The ventricular activation time is seen in V_6 to be 0.04 sec.

g) q waves are seen in V_5 and V_6. In neither case do they have depth exceeding one quarter of the height of the ensuing r wave.

h) The q waves in V_5 and V_6 do not equal or exceed 0.04 sec in duration.

4A. The T waves in V_1, V_2 and V_3 are normal. **The T waves in V_4, V_5 and V_6 are of low voltage. This is a non-specific abnormality.**
4B. Normal, (low voltage and positive) U waves are seen in V_1–V_4.

5. The S-T segments are normal from V_1–V_4. **There is minimal, but significant S-T segment depression in V_5 and V_6. This is just beyond the normal accepted limit of 1 mm below the iso-electric line.**

6. a) Initial q waves are seen in Leads II and aVF. Their duration is less than 0.04 sec.

b) The depth of the q waves in II and aVF is less than one quarter of the height of the ensuing r wave.

c) The r wave in aVL does not exceed 13 mm and the R wave in aVF is at the extreme upper end of the normal range at 20 mm.

d) The mean frontal plane QRS axis is +90°. This is at the extreme right hand end of the normal range.

7A. The T wave axis in the frontal plane leads is indeterminate. Since the frontal plane QRS axis is highly determinate, the frontal plane T waves are abnormal.
7B. No significant U waves are seen in the limb leads.

8. The S-T segments in the limb leads appear to be depressed in Leads II, III and aVF. However, closer inspection indicates that the apparent S-T segment depression begins before the QRS complex (i.e. immediately after the P wave). These appearances in Leads II, III and aVF are actually due to a prominent atrial repolarisation wave. This is a normal accompaniment of sinus tachycardia.

9. a) The P wave duration is 0.13 sec.

b) **The P wave height in Lead II is 3 mm. This is abnormal and suggests right atrial hypertrophy.**

c) No significant negative component to the P wave in V_1, is visible.

10. The Q-T interval is 0.33 sec. (The Q-T interval is only really measurable in the right precordial leads). The cycle time is 15 (heart rate 100). The maximum Q-T interval corresponding to this rate is 0.33 sec.

The record shows sinus tachycardia, right atrial hypertrophy with a prominent atrial repolarisation wave and borderline abnormal right axis deviation. These features are non-specific but suggest the possibility of chronic lung disease. There are non-specific S-T, T changes in the left precordial leads. The QRS complexes are low voltage in the left precordial leads. This could be due to obesity, emphysema or pronounced clockwise cardiac rotation.

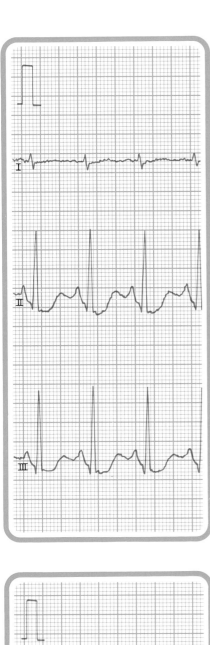

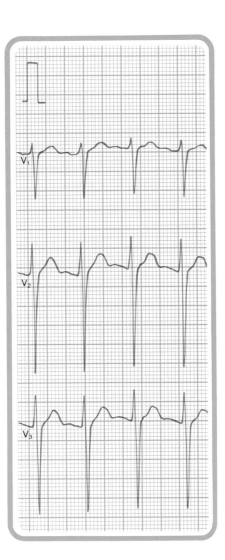

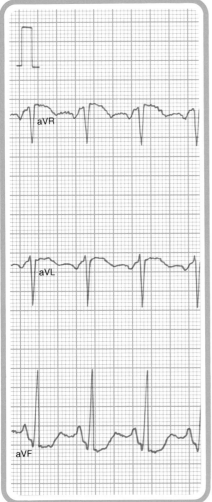

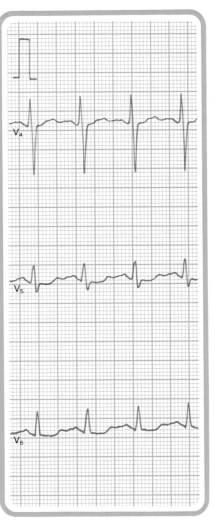

Record 40

Abnormal Record

1. Sinus rhythm. The P-R interval is 0.12 sec.

2. a) **The QRS waveform is abnormal in V_1. Instead of having rS there is an Rs complex. The QRS waveform is also abnormal in V_6 in that instead of having qR, there is Qr.**

b) **The r wave progression from V_1–V_6 is abnormal. After V_2 the R wave disappears completely and this is frankly abnormal.**

c) Since the R wave progression is so abnormal, the term "transition zone" has no meaning.

3. a) The total QRS duration is within the normal range at 0.10 sec (well seen in V_6).

b) **No precordial r wave exceeds the minimum voltage of 8 mm. This is abnormal.**

c) The tallest r wave obviously does not therefore exceed 27 mm.

d) The deepest S wave (V_2) is 15 mm (the negative wave in V_3 is not an S wave, it is a QS complex).

e) The sum of the tallest r and deepest S waves certainly does not exceed 40 mm.

f) The ventricular activation time cannot be measured since this is dependent upon the presence of a normal configuration qR complex in the left precordial leads.

g) **q waves are seen V_3–V_6. In V_3 and V_4 these are actually QS complexes. From V_2–V_6 the q waves in all cases grossly exceed in depth one quarter of the height of the ensuing r wave. This is abnormal and indicates infarction in the myocardium underlying the electrodes.**

h) **From V_4–V_6 the q waves are more than 0.03 sec in duration. This is frankly abnormal and indicates infarction of the subjacent myocardium.**

4A. The T waves are normal from V_1–V_3, **but from V_4–V_6 the T waves are abnormally flat. This is a non-specific abnormality.** It is probably secondary to the extensive QRS abnormalities in the precordial leads which indicate extensive anterior myocardial infarction extending from V_1–V_6.

4B. Small, upright (normal) U waves are seen in V_2 and V_3.

5. The precordial S-T segments are within normal limits, indicating that the infarct is not less than a week old.

6. q waves are seen in Leads I, II and aVF.

a) **The q waves in Leads I and II are greater than one quarter of the height of the ensuing r wave and this is probably also true of the q waves in the foot-lead.**

b) **The q waves in I are certainly in excess of 0.03 sec. The abnormal q waves in Lead I are part of the anterolateral infarction which is also shown in the precordial leads. The q waves in Lead II and also the q waves in aVF (if the latter are actually abnormal), almost certainly indicate additional inferior myocardial infarction.**

c) The r waves in aVL and aVF certainly do not exceed the maximum permissible voltage of 13 and 20 mm respectively.

d) **The mean frontal plane QRS axis is very abnormal at +150°. This is due to the extensive anterolateral infarction which removes electrical forces directed upwards and to the left leaving the predominant direction of ventricular depolarisation as downwards and to the right. It is therefore not necessarily indicative of left posterior hemiblock.**

7A. The mean frontal plane T wave axis is indeterminate. Since the frontal plane QRS axis is hightly determinate, the T waves in the frontal plane leads are abnormal.

7B. No significant U waves are seen in the limb leads.

8. The S-T segments in the frontal plane leads are normal.

9. a) The P waves in Lead II have a normal duration of 0.10 sec.

b) The P wave height in Lead II is within the normal range at 1.5 mm.

c) **The P waves in V_1, have a dominant negative component indicative of left atrial hypertrophy.**

10. The Q-T interval is 0.35 sec. The cycle time is 19 (heart rate 78) which is associated with a maximum Q-T interval of 0.37 sec.

The abnormal q waves from V_3–V_6 and also in Lead I indicate extensive anterolateral myocardial infarction. The abnormal q waves in Leads II and the foot-lead indicate inferior infarction. In this context the dominant r wave in V_1 probably indicates true posterior infarction. The abnormal P waves in V_1 indicate left atrial abnormality. This could be the result of left atrial hypertrophy or of left atrial ischaemia.

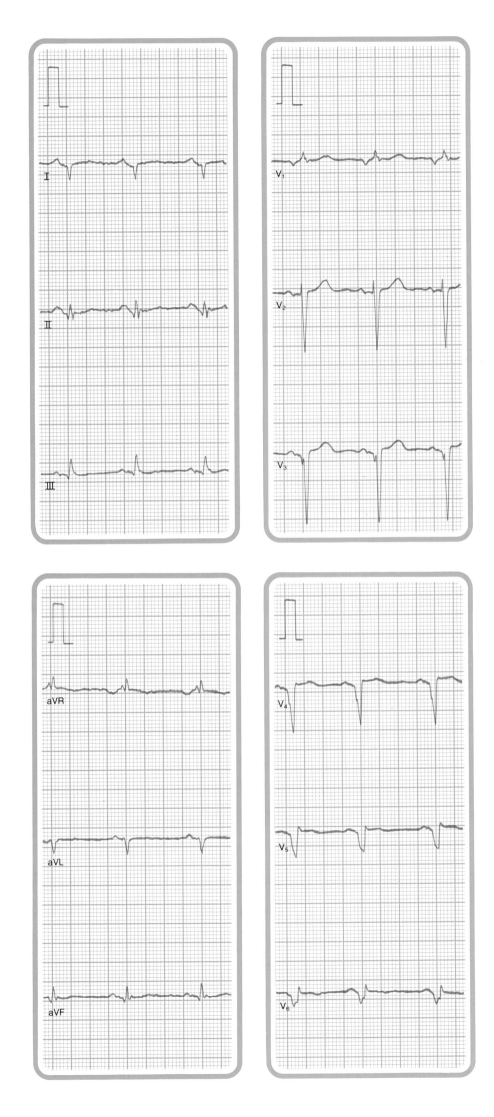

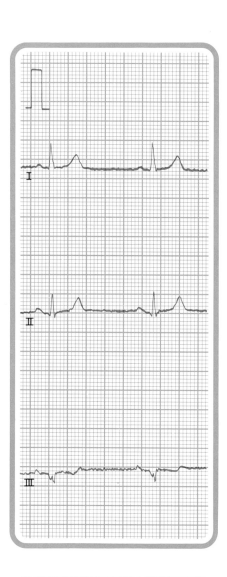

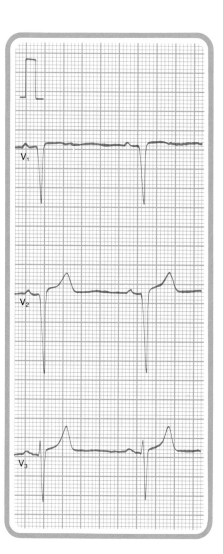

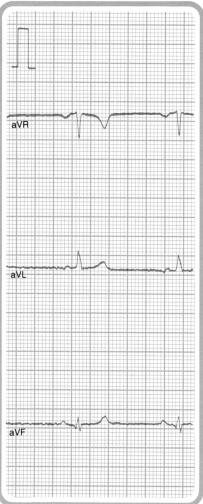

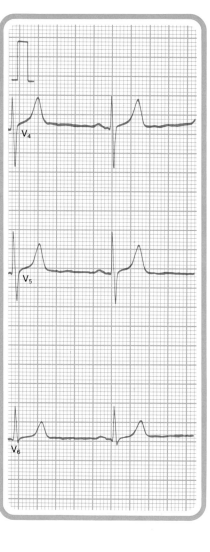

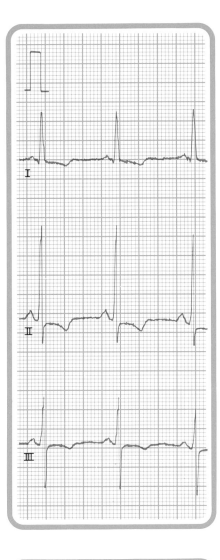

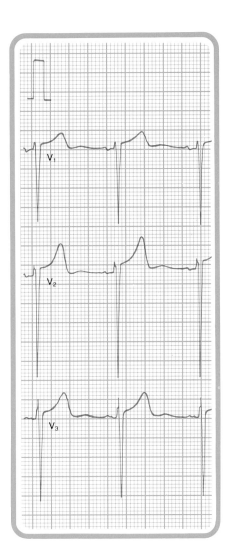

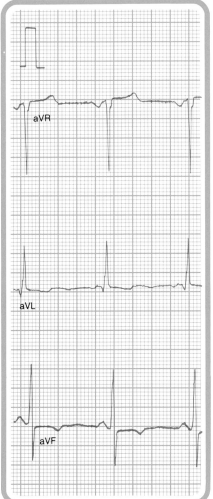

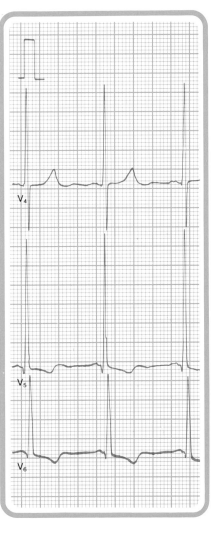

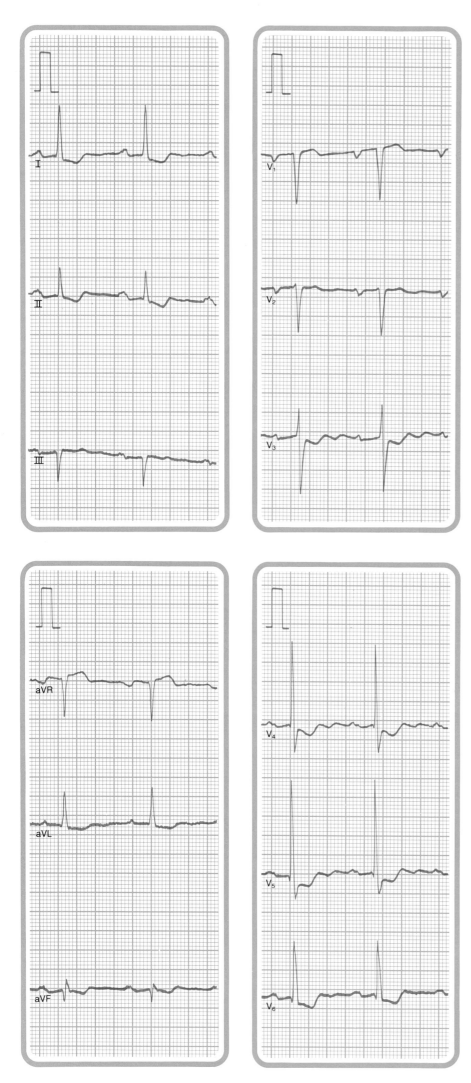

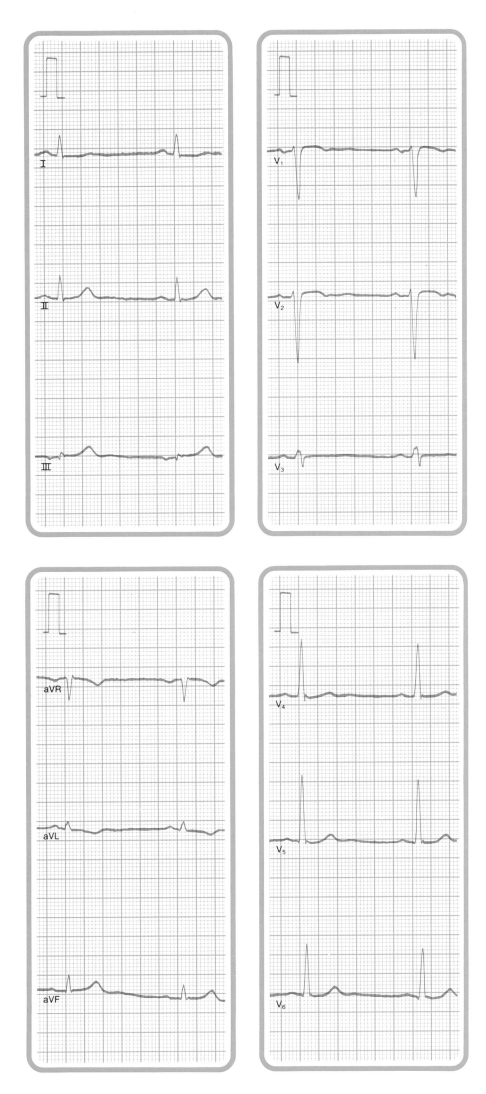

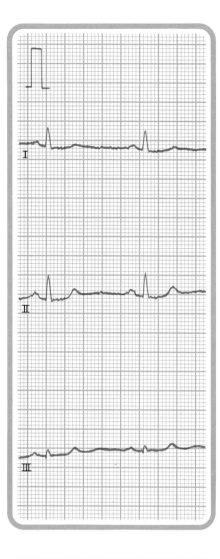

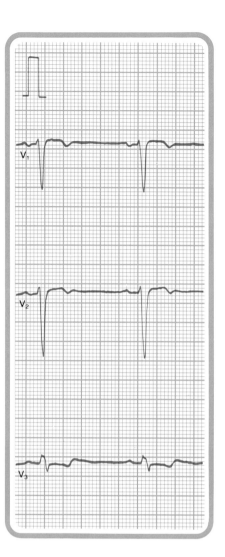

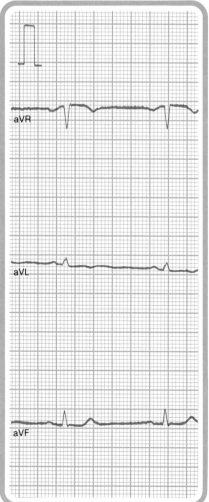

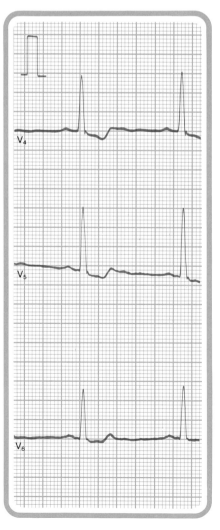

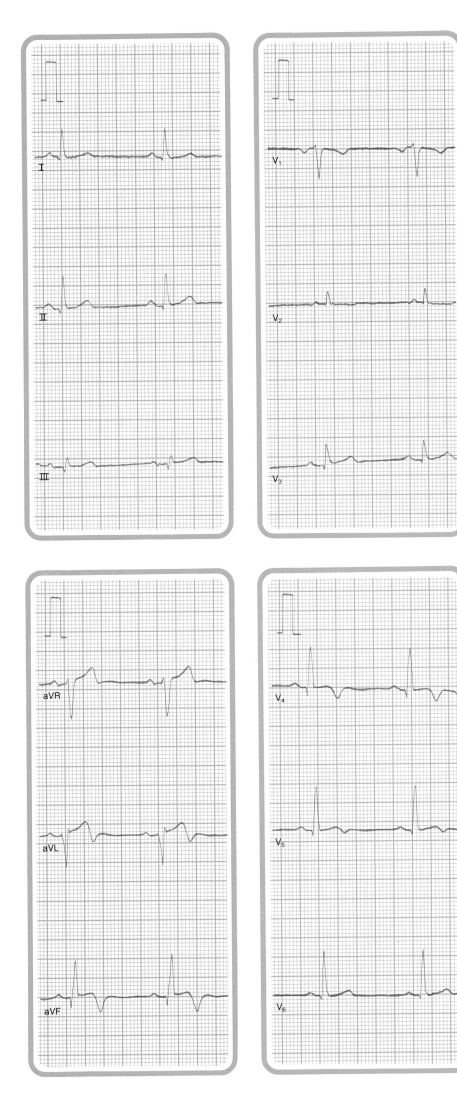

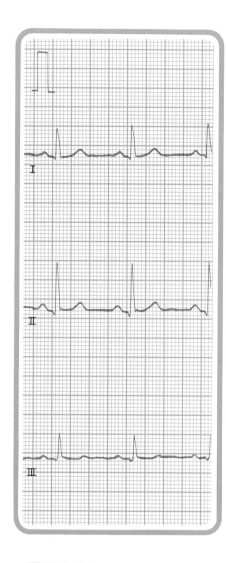

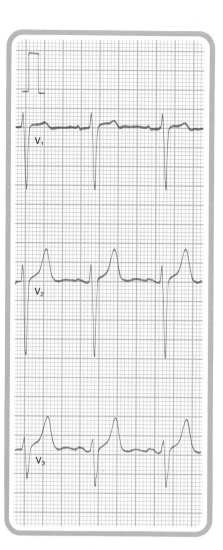

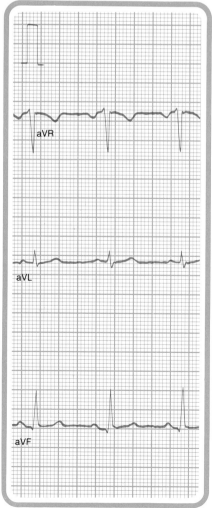

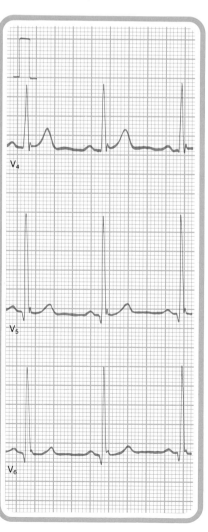

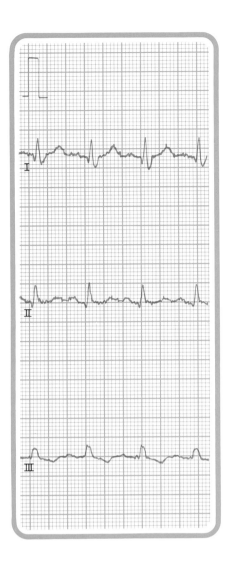

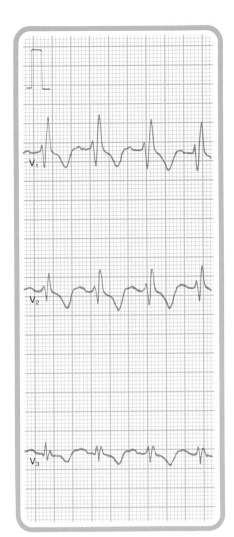

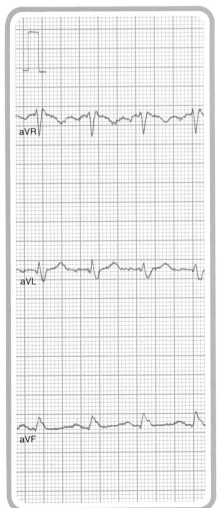

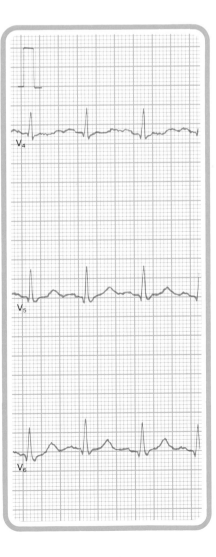

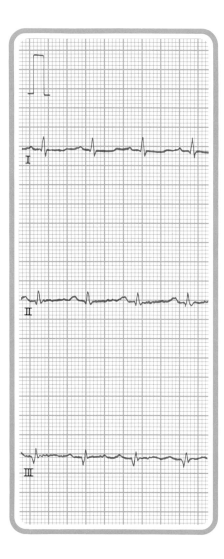

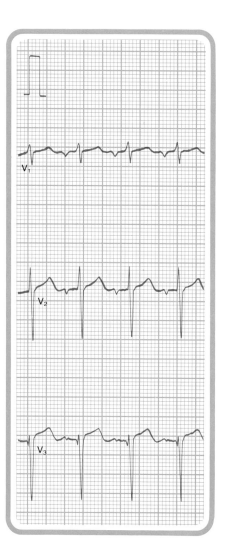

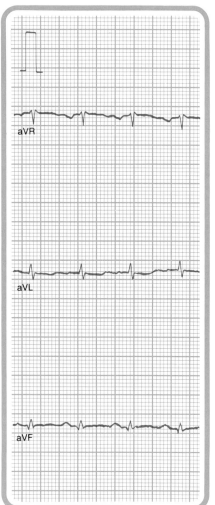

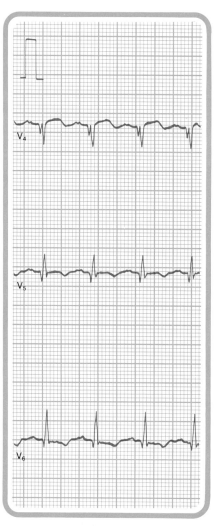

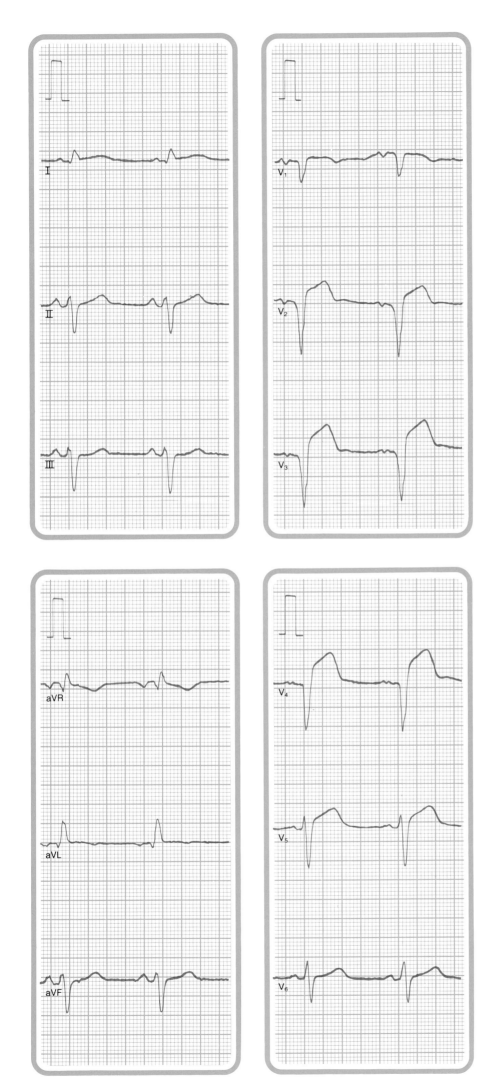

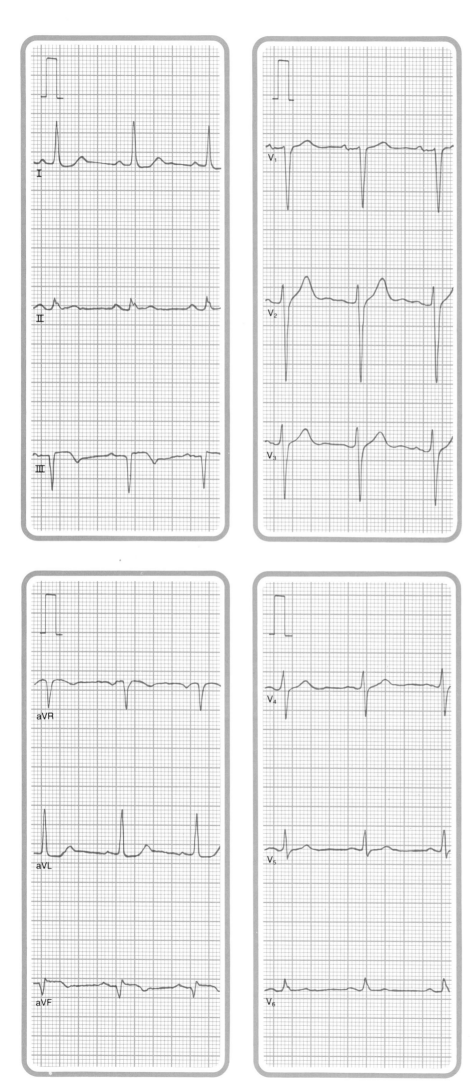

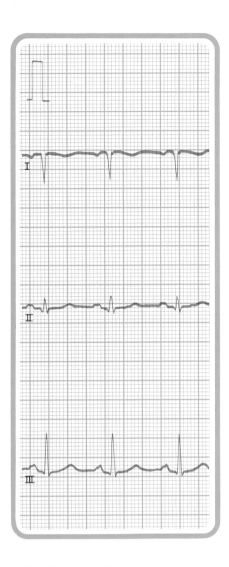

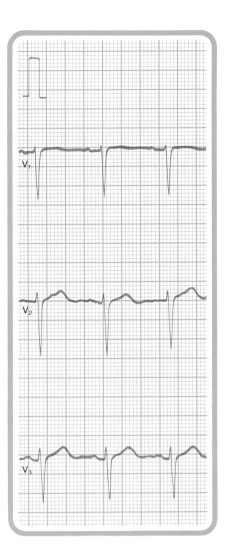

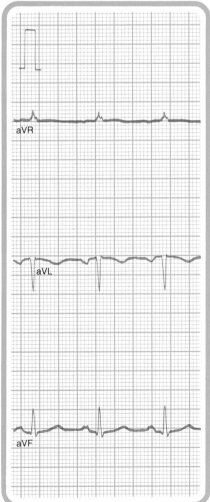

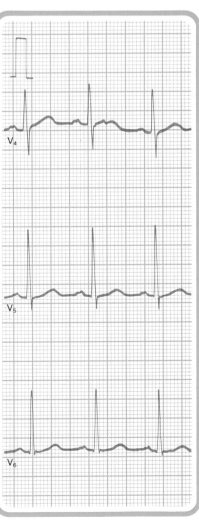

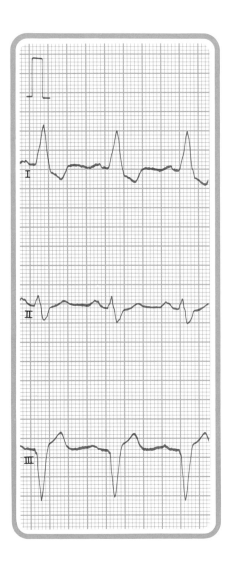

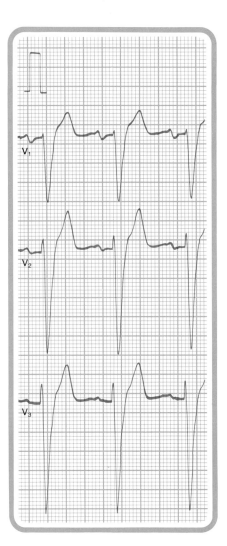

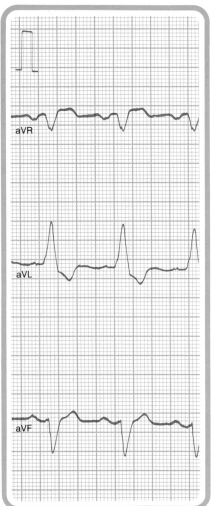

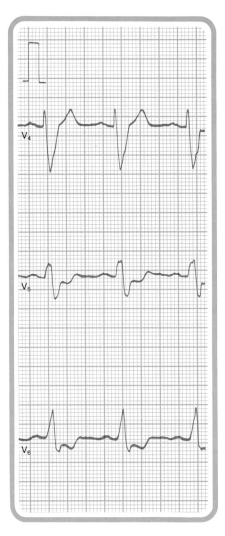

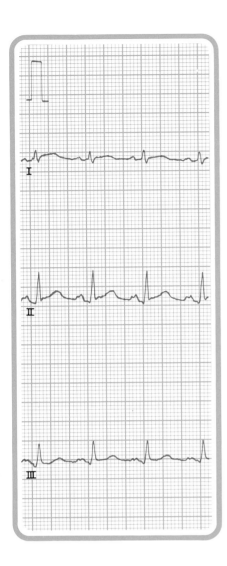

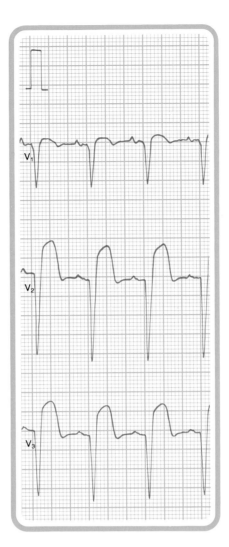

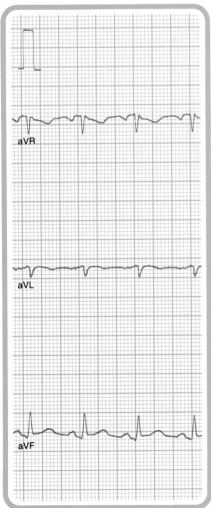

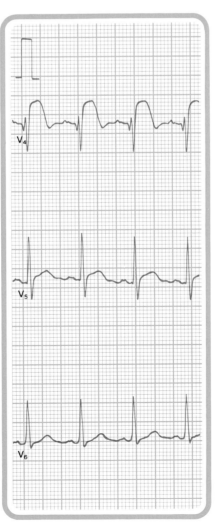

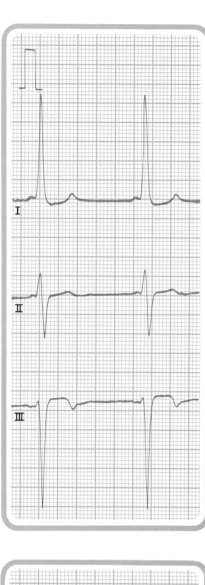

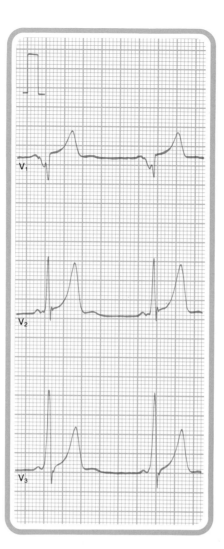

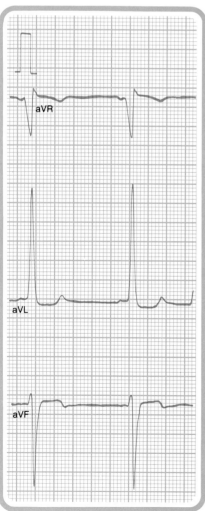

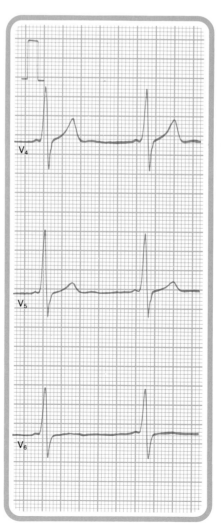

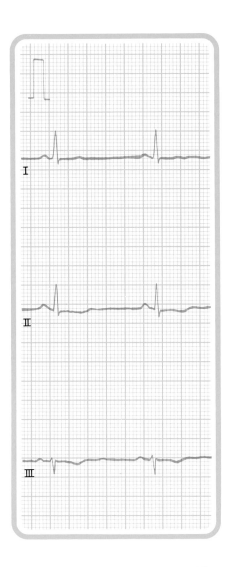

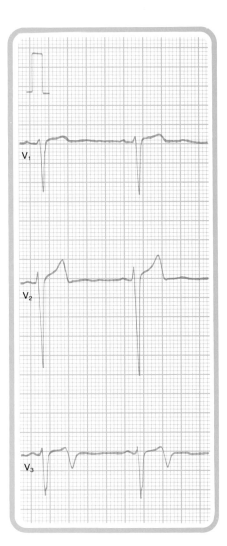

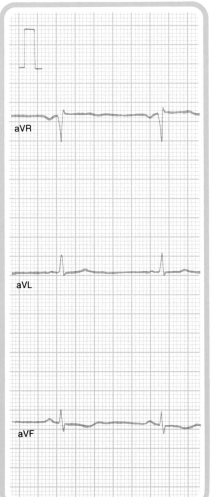

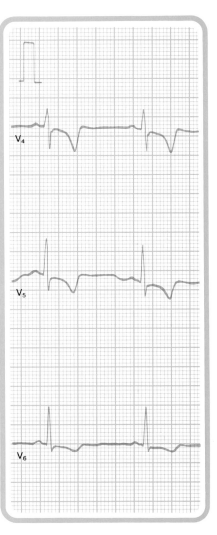

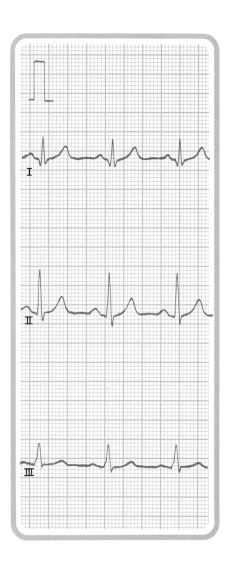

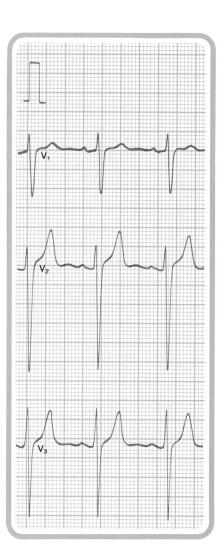

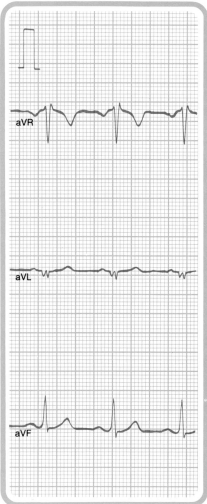

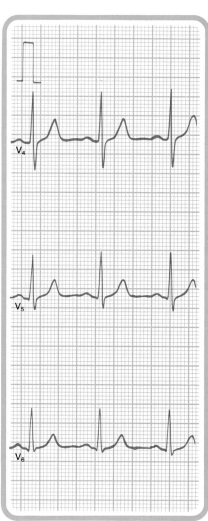

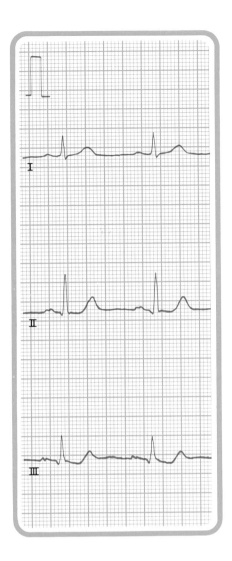

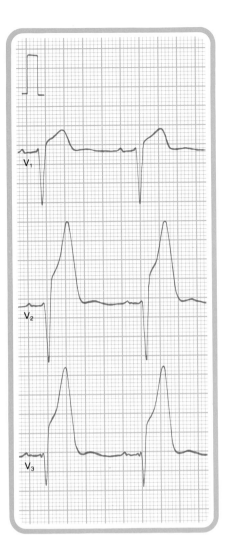

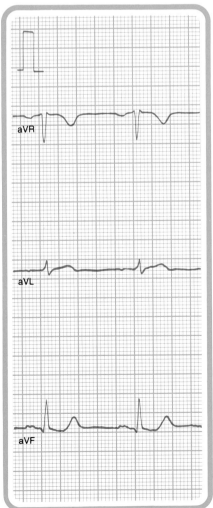

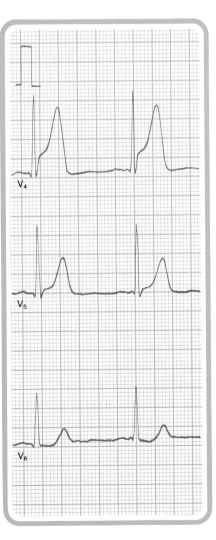

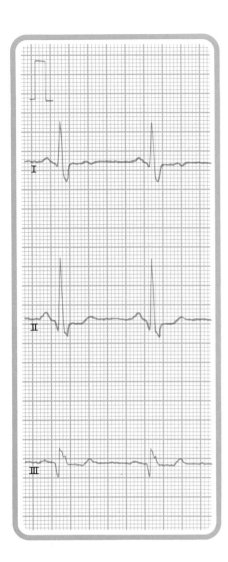

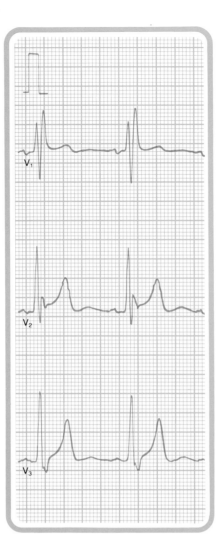

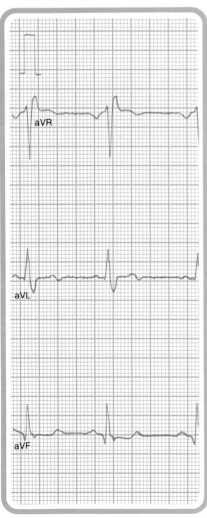

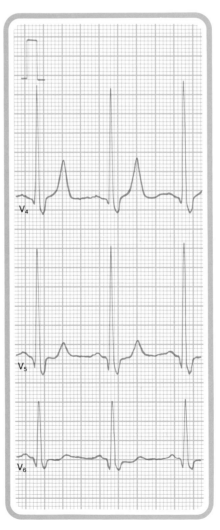

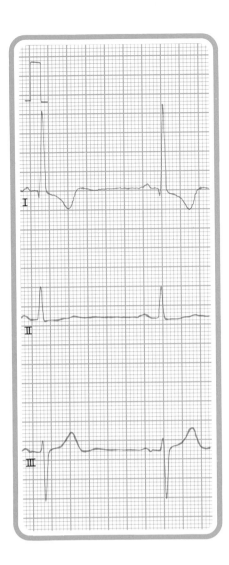

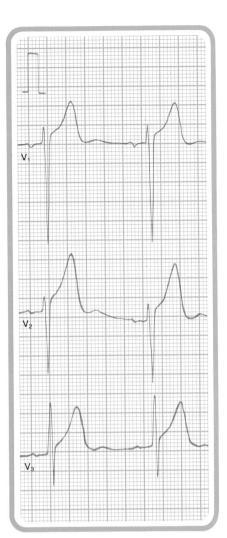

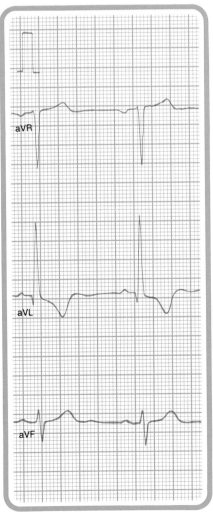

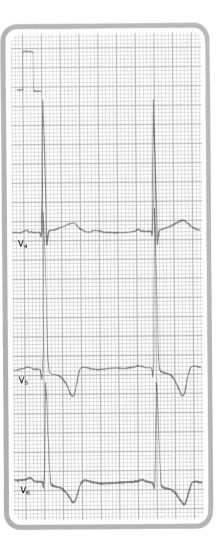

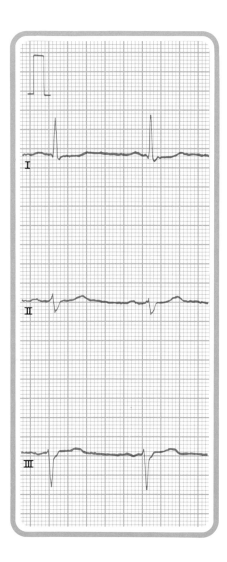
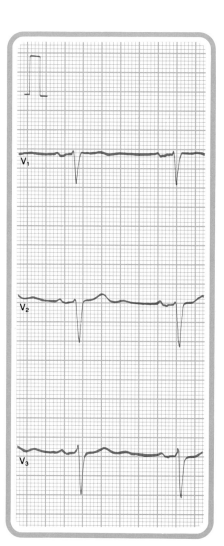
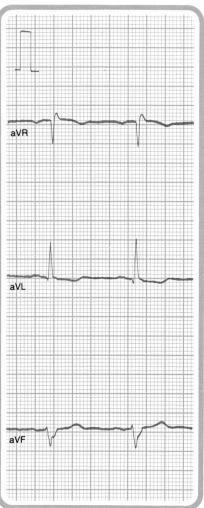
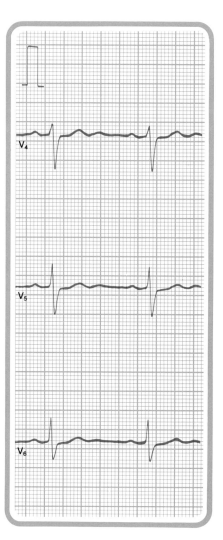

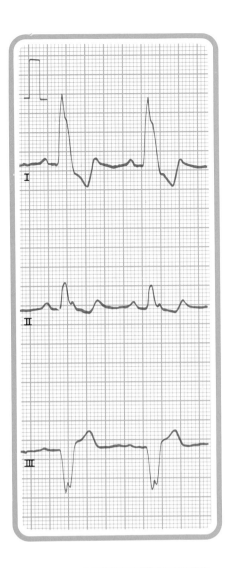

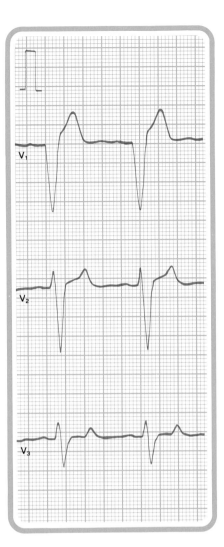

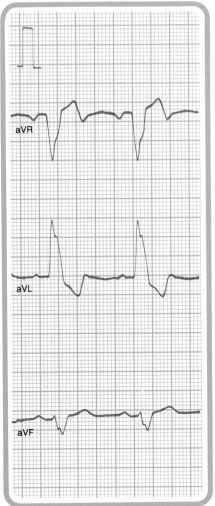

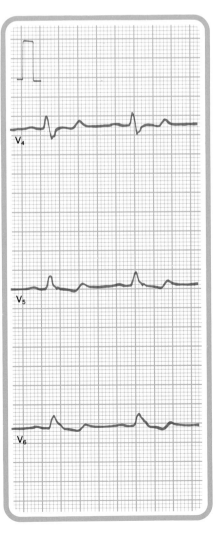

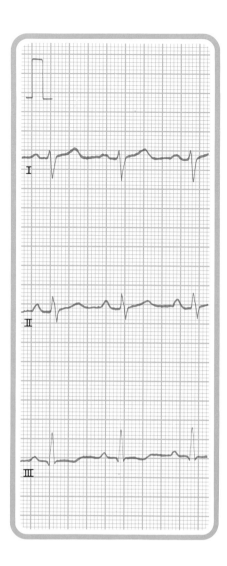

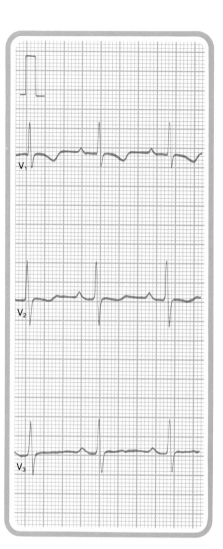

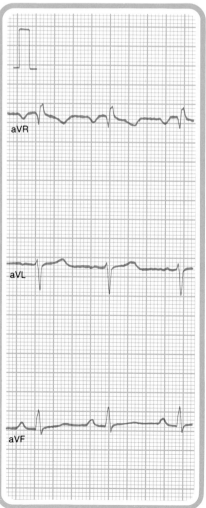

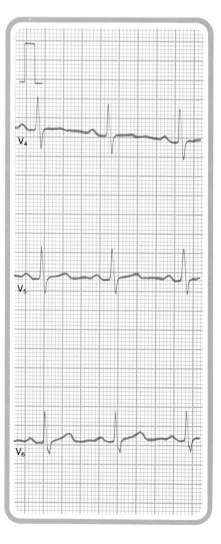

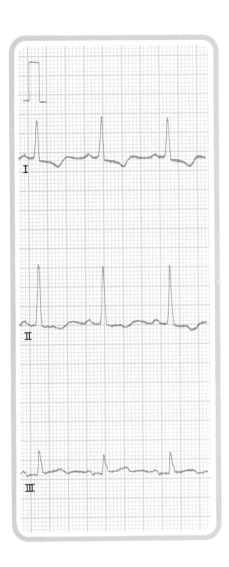

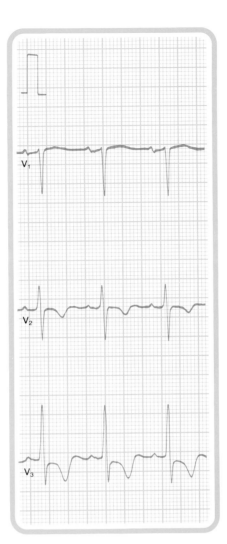

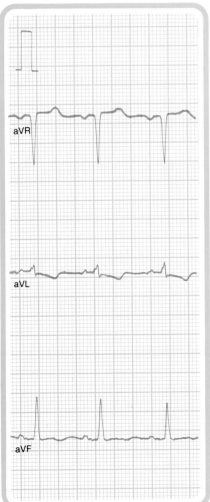

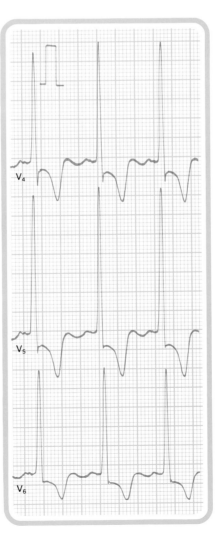

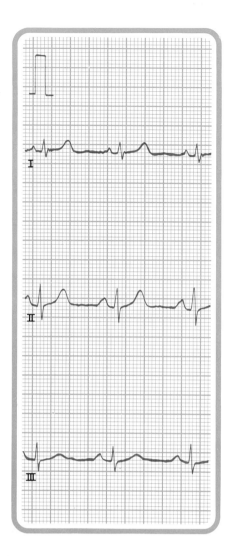

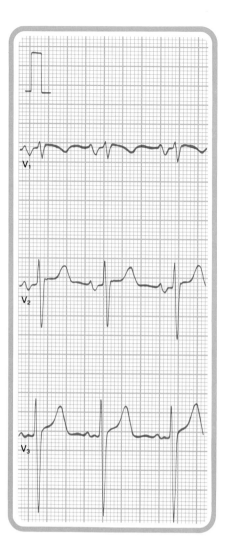

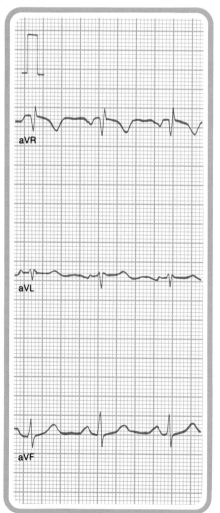

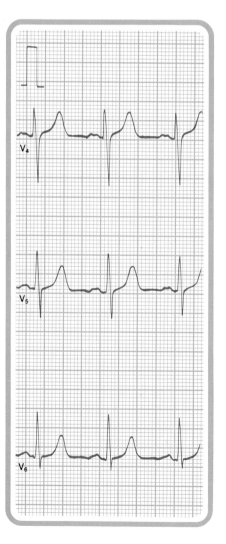

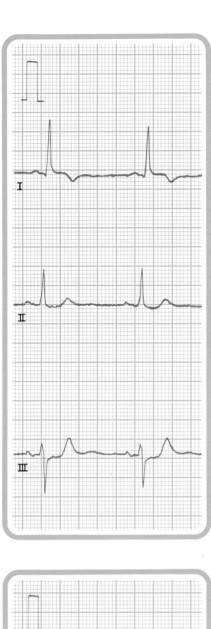

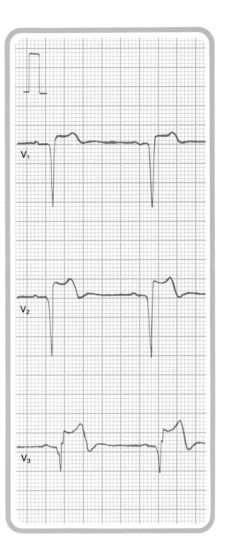

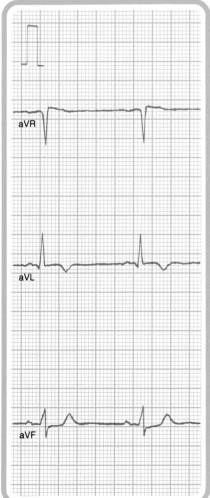

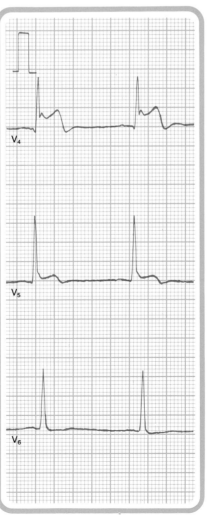

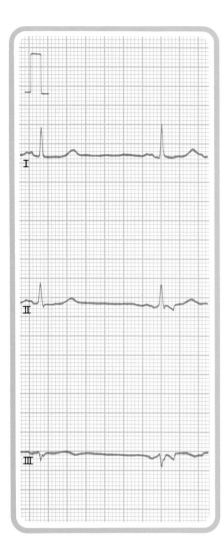

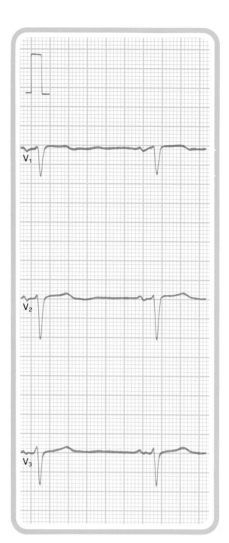

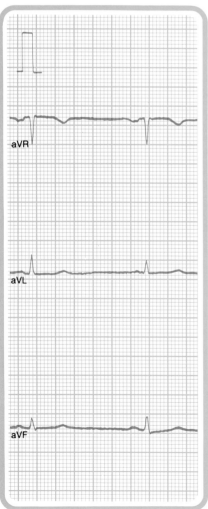

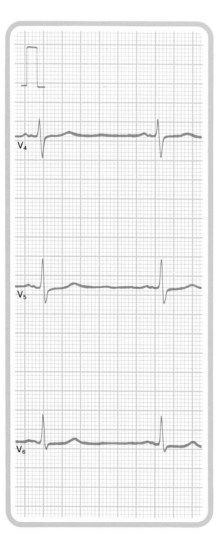

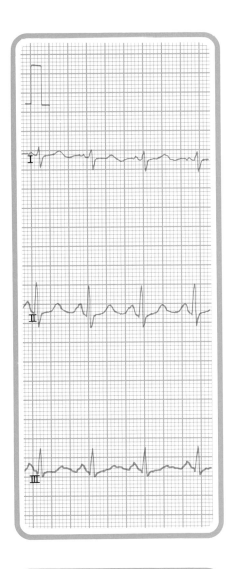

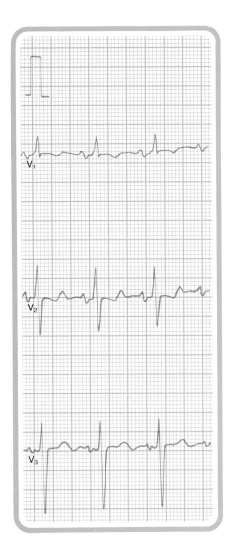

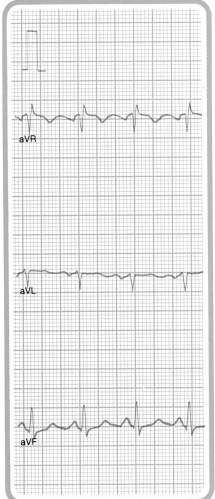

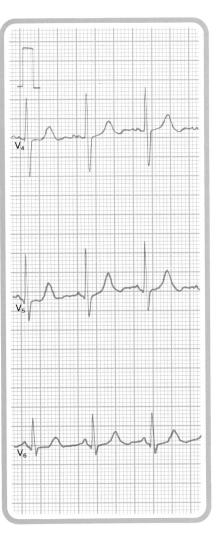

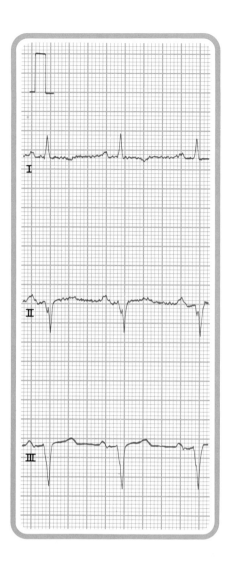

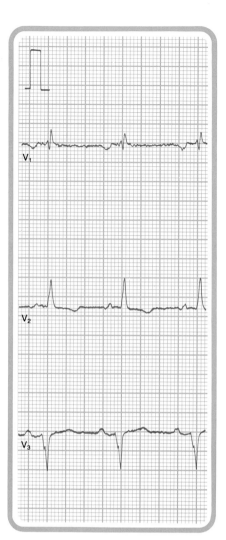

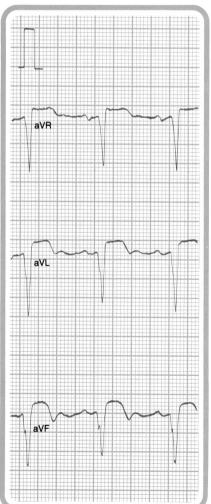

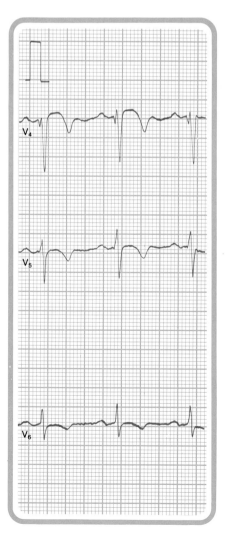

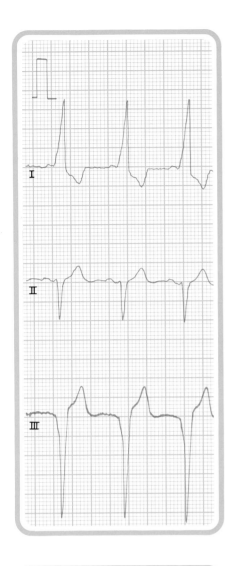

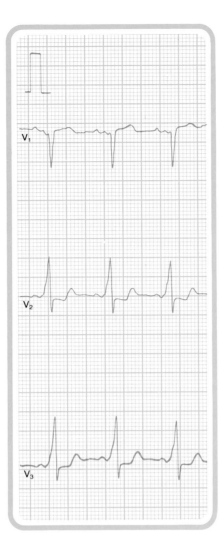

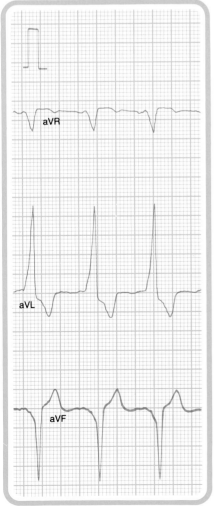

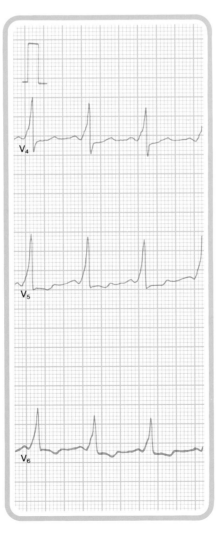

Records 41 to 70

Record 41
Old anteroseptal infarction.
Old inferior infarction.

Record 42
Left ventricular hypertrophy.
Possible left atrial hypertrophy.

Record 43
**Left atrial hypertrophy. Non-specific
S-T, T and U changes – digitalis effect,
hypokalaemia.
First degree heart block.
Old inferior infarction.**

Record 44
Non-specific S-T, T changes.

Record 45
**Non-specific S-T, T changes.
Acute ischaemic S-T segment
depression.**

Record 46
**Recent anterior infarction. Possible
recent inferior ischaemic damage.**

Record 47
Left ventricular hypertrophy.

Record 48
Right bundle branch block.
Sinus tachycardia.

Record 49
Anterior myocardial infarction
(intermediate age).
**Old inferior infarction.
Left atrial abnormality.**

Record 50
**Recent anterior myocardial infarction.
Left anterior hemiblock.**

Record 51
**Relatively recent inferior myocardial
infarction.
Possible anterolateral infarction.**

Record 52
Normal (apart from possible left atrial
abnormality). **Technical dextrocardia.**

Record 53
**Left bundle branch block.
Abnormal left axis deviation.
Left atrial abnormality.**

Record 54
Recent anteroseptal infarction.

Record 55
Ventricular pre-excitation
(WPW type B).

Record 56
Ischaemic S-T, T changes.

Record 57
Normal (Normal Q in aVL).

Record 58
Recent anterior infarction.

Record 59
Right bundle branch block.

Record 60
Left ventricular hypertrophy.
Left atrial hypertrophy.

Record 61
**Left anterior hemiblock.
Non-specific S-T, T and U wave
changes.**
Clockwise cardiac rotation.

Record 62
Left bundle branch block.

Record 63
Right ventricular hypertrophy.
Right atrial hypertrophy.

Record 64
Left ventricular hypertrophy.

Record 65
Left atrial abnormality.

Record 66
**Recent anteroseptal myocardial
infarction.**

Record 67
Myoedema.

Record 68
Right ventricular hypertrophy.
Right atrial hypertrophy.

Record 69
Anterior myocardial infarction
(probable old inferior infarction)
Left axis deviation.

Record 70
Old inferior myocardial infarction
Non-specific S-T, T changes
(digitalis effect).

Listing of abnormalities in record examples 41–70

Record 41

2. a) V_1 has QS (should have rS).

b) No r wave has developed in V_2 – still QS. These two features indicate anteroseptal infarction.

6. b) The Q wave in aVF is more than one quarter of the height of the ensuing R wave. This indicates an inferior infarction.

ECG diagnosis
Old anteroseptal infarction.
Old inferior infarction.

Record 42

3. c) The R wave in V_5 measures 35 mm (well in excess of the permitted 27 mm).

e) $R_{V_5} + S_{V_5} = 62$ mm (well in excess of the permitted 40 mm).

f) The intrinsic deflection time (well seen in V_6) is 0.05 sec.

4. c) There is T wave inversion in V_5 and V_6.

5. There is S-T segment depression in V_5 and V_6.

7. The frontal plane T wave axis is $-135°$ (the QRS axis is $+15°$ and the angle between the two is therefore abnormal).

8. There is S-T segment depression in Leads I, II and aVL.

These changes indicate left ventricular hypertrophy.

9. The P waves in V_1 have a dominant negative component suggesting a possible left atrial abnormality (probably hypertrophy).

ECG diagnosis
Left ventricular hypertrophy.
Possible left atrial hypertrophy.

Record 43

1. The rhythm is sinus. The P-R interval is abnormally long at 0.26 sec. This indicates the presence of first degree heart block (see Section 3).

4A. The T waves are of low voltage throughout the precordial series.

4B. Prominent (and abnormal) U waves are seen from V_3 to V_6. They are definitely abnormal but are non-specific. They suggest hypokalaemia.

5. There is S-T segment depression from V_3–V_6. These are abnormal but non-specific changes. This patient was actually receiving digitalis and this is probably relevant.

6. The q waves in aVF exceed one quarter of the height of the ensuing R waves. This indicates the presence of inferior infarction.

7A. The frontal plane T axis is indeterminate. Since the frontal plane QRS axis is highly determinate at $0°$, the frontal plane T waves are abnormal.

8. There is S-T segment depression in I, II, aVL and aVF.

9. The P waves are abnormally wide and bifid in II and have a dominant negative component in V_1. These changes indicate the presence of left atrial hypertrophy.

10. It is impossible to assess the Q-T interval since the T waves are of abnormally low voltage and the U waves are prominent.

ECG diagnosis
First degree heart block, left atrial hypertrophy, non-specific S-T, T changes, probable hypokalaemia, possible digitalis effect.

Record 44

4A. c) The T waves are flat in V_3 and of low voltage in V_4. This is a non-specific abnormality.

4B. Prominent U waves are seen in the precordial leads but they are not definitely abnormal.

7. The frontal plane T axis is $+90°$. Since the frontal plane QRS axis is $+30°$, the angle between the two axes is abnormal and the frontal plane T waves are therefore minimally abnormal.

The record shows non-specific (but significant) T wave changes.

ECG diagnosis
Non-specific T wave changes.

Record 45

4A. The T waves are of low voltage from V_3–V_6.

5. There is S-T depression from V_3–V_6. This is of borderline significance in V_3 and V_6, but is definitely abnormal in V_4 and V_5.

The record is frankly abnormal but the changes are non-specific.

(This record was taken from the same patient as Record 44 and within 5 minutes of it. During the taking of Record 44 the patient was asymptomatic. During the recording of Record 45 the patient was complaining of spontaneous anginal pain. The S-T segment depression in the left precordial leads is an example of ischaemic change occurring during spontaneous angina).

ECG diagnosis
Non-specific S-T, T changes occurring in association with chest pain.

Record 46

2. b) The r wave in V_2 is smaller than that in V_1.

3. g) The q wave in V_3 has a depth more than one quarter of the height of the ensuing R wave. This is probably true also in V_4.

These two features indicate the presence of anterior myocardial infarction.

4A. b) There is terminal T wave inversion in V_2.

c) There is T wave inversion from V_2–V_5.

5. There is significant S-T elevation in V_2.

8. There is minimal S-T elevation in III and aVF.

The QRS changes are those of anterior infarction. The S-T and T changes in the precordial leads indicate that the infarct is relatively recent – probably one to four weeks. The S-T segment elevation in III and aVF suggests the possibility of recent inferior ischaemic damage.

ECG diagnosis
Recent anterior infarction. Possible inferior ischaemic damage.

Record 47

2. b) The r wave progression in the precordial leads is not "smooth". There is little or no progression from V_1–V_3 and then a sudden increase. Such appearances can be seen in the presence of an old anteroseptal infarction, but the appearances can also be normal and it is always better to under-interpret (and report) rather than to over-interpret (and report) the electrocardiogram.

3. e) $S_{V_2} + R_{V_5} = 44$ mm.

f) The ventricular activation time is 0.05 sec.

These changes indicate the presence of left ventricular hypertrophy.

9. The P waves are bifid in V_2 or V_3. This suggests possible left atrial hypertrophy, but the criteria for this condition have not actually been fulfilled.

ECG diagnosis
Changes suggestive of left ventricular hypertrophy.

Record 48

1A. The rhythm is sinus. The rate is 107 per min and there is therefore sinus tachycardia.

2. a) V_1 has an rSR' complex.

3. a) The total QRS duration is 0.14 sec. These changes indicate the presence of right bundle branch block.

4. There is T wave inversion from V_1–V_3 and the T waves are of low voltage in V_4. These are non-specific changes and are likely to be secondary to the QRS abnormality of right bundle branch block.

ECG diagnosis
Right bundle branch block.

Record 49

2. b) The r wave progression is abnormal. The r wave in V_2 is taller than that in V_1 (normal), but the r wave in V_3 is smaller and there is **no** r wave in V_4 (the smaller r wave in V_3 would be acceptable if the r waves in V_4 were normal (page 45)).

3. g) The q waves in V_3, V_4 and V_5 have a depth exceeding one quarter of the height of the ensuing R wave.
These changes indicate the presence of anterior infarction.

2. h) The q waves in V_4 exceed, and those in V_5 equal 0.04 sec in duration. This, too, indicates infarction.

4A. There is T wave inversion in V_5 and V_6. This is a non-specific abnormality. It is likely to be related to ischaemia in the area adjacent to the infarct.

5. There is minimal S-T elevation in V_3 and V_4, suggesting that the anterior infarct is recent.

6. b) The q wave in aVF has a depth exceeding one quarter of the height of the ensuing r wave. This indicates the presence of inferior infarction.

7. No comment of any significance can be made on the T waves in the frontal plane leads since both the frontal plane QRS axis and the frontal plane T axis are indeterminate.

9. There is a dominant negative component to the P wave in V_1 indicating left atrial abnormality. One cannot be sure whether this is related to ischaemia or to hypertrophy.

ECG diagnosis
Old inferior infarction. Left atrial abnormality.

Record 50

2. a) V_1 has no initial r wave. It has a QS complex. V_6 has an RS instead of qR. This is related to the abnormal R wave progression (see below).

b) The r wave progression is grossly abnormal. No r wave appears from V_1–V_4 and the r waves in V_5 and V_6 are smaller than one would expect.

3. a) The total QRS duration is abnormal at 0.14 sec. There is no rSR' pattern in V_1 to suggest right bundle branch block. There is no initial (septal) q wave in V_6 suggesting the presence of left bundle branch block. However, there is an initial q wave in I and aVL indicating that the septal depolarisation is occurring in the normal direction. This could indicate "through and through" infarction of the interventricular septum with complete left bundle branch block, but this is never a diagnosis one can make with total confidence (page 000). Alternatively the abnormal QRS duration could be indicative of intraventricular block (of the type for which the terms "parietal block" and "peri-infarction block" have been used – see page 000).

b)No r wave exceeds 8 mm. This is due to the presence of anterior infarction – see below.

g) The q waves from V_1–V_4 all have a depth exceeding one quarter of the height of the ensuing R wave. This indicates anterior infarction.

h) The q waves from V_1–V_4 all have a duration exceeding 0.03 sec. This also indicates anterior infarction.

5. There is S-T elevation from V_2–V_5 indicating that the infarction is recent.

6. The frontal plane QRS axis is $-60°$. This indicates an abnormal degree of left axis deviation. There is no evidence of inferior infarction so that the abnormal axis cannot be due to loss of viable myocardium on the inferior wall of the heart. The most likely explanation therefore is block in the anterior division of the left bundle branch system (probably induced by the anterior infarction, though this is speculative).

ECG diagnosis
Recent anterior myocardial infarction.
Left anterior hemiblock.
Additional intraventricular block (possibly parietal block, possibly LBBB).

Record 51

3. b) No r wave in the precordial leads exceeds 8 mm. This can be due to extracardiac causes reducing the voltage (e.g. obesity, emphysema, pleural effusion), or cardiac causes (e.g. pericardial effusion or anterior myocardial infarction).

6. a) The q wave in aVF exceeds 0.03 sec in duration. This indicates the presence of inferior myocardial infarction.

b) The q waves in aVF have a depth exceeding one quarter of the height of the ensuing r wave. This too indicates inferior infarction.

7. Although the angle between the mean frontal plane QRS and T wave axes is not outside the permitted normal range of $\pm45°$ (QRS axis = $-15°$, T axis = $-15°$) the T waves in aVF are considered to be abnormal since they are inverted in this lead in association with QRS evidence of infarction in the same lead. These changes suggest that the infarct is relatively recent (i.e. within weeks).

8. There is slight, but significant S-T elevation in aVF and III, suggesting that the inferior infarct is less than a week old.

ECG diagnosis
Relatively recent inferior infarction.
Possible anterolateral infarction (on the basis of the low voltage R waves in the left precordial leads).

Record 52

6. a) There are QS complexes in I. It is important to recognise that the P waves are also negative in I. The combination of negative P waves and negative QRS complexes in V_1 is usually due either to technical dextrocardia or to true dextrocardia. Since the form of the QRS complexes in the precordial leads are entirely normal, true dextrocardia can be ruled out.

9. The P waves are bifid in the limb leads. They do not fulfil the criteria for abnormality but raise the possibility of left atrial abnormality.
Apart from the possible left atrial abnormality this is a normal record with technical dextrocardia. (The technician had inadvertently mixed up the right and left arm connections).

The true appearances can be deduced as follows:–

true Lead I = recorded Lead I turned upside down

true Lead II = recorded Lead III

true Lead III = recorded Lead II

true Lead aVR = recorded Lead aVL

true Lead aVL = recorded Lead aVR

true Lead aVF = recorded Lead aVF

true precordial leads = recorded precordial leads

ECG diagnosis
Allowing for the recording error (technical dextrocardia) the record is within normal limits.

Record 53

2. a) V_6 has no initial q wave. No initial q wave is seen in I or aVL either. This suggests that the interventricular septum is depolarised in an abnormal direction.

b) The r wave progression is less pronounced than usual but not definitely abnormal.

3. a) The total QRS duration is abnormal at 0.16 sec.

The combination of an abnormal QRS duration and absence of the normal septal q wave (in the absence of (i) an rSR′ complex in V_1 to indicate right bundle branch block, and (ii) any evidence of ventricular pre-excitation) indicates the presence of left bundle branch block. Further evaluation of the QRS complexes, S-T segments, and T waves (apart from the frontal plane axis) should not therefore be undertaken (unless previous records are available for comparison).

6. d) The frontal plane QRS axis is $-45°$. This is an abnormal degree of left axis deviation. It may indicate defective conduction in the peripheral branches of the anterior division of the left bundle branch system.

9. a) The P wave duration in II is abnormal at 0.14 sec and the P waves are bifid in this lead. This indicates the presence of an abnormality of the left atrium.

c) The P waves are biphasic and have a dominant negative area in V_1. This also indicates an abnormality of the left atrium.

ECG diagnosis
Left atrial abnormality.
Complete left bundle branch block.
Abnormal left axis deviation.

Record 54

2. a) There is no r wave in V_1. It shows a QS complex.

b) The r wave progression from V_1–V_4 is abnormal. No r wave is seen in V_1, V_2 or V_3 and only a small r wave in V_4.

3. g) The depth of the q waves in V_1–V_4 exceeds one quarter of the height of the ensuing r waves indicating anteroseptal infarction.

h) The q waves (actually QS complexes) in V_1, V_2 and V_3 exceed 0.03 sec in duration and are therefore abnormal. The abnormal q waves are indicative of anteroseptal infarction in this case (there is no evidence of left bundle branch block or ventricular pre-excitation).

4A. The precordial T wave cannot really be assessed except in V_6 for in all the other leads the T waves are incorporated in the elevated S-T segment.

5. There is significant S-T elevation in V_1–V_5, indicating that the anterior infarct is recent.

8. There is minimal S-T elevation in I, II and aVF.

9. The P waves are bifid in II. They are not abnormally wide and are therefore not definitely abnormal but they suggest the possibility of left atrial abnormality (e.g. ischaemia or hypertrophy).

ECG diagnosis
Recent anterior infarction.

Record 55

1. The P-R interval is abnormally short at 0.10 sec. This feature, combined with the fact that the total QRS duration is abnormally long (at 0.14 sec), indicates the presence of ventricular pre-excitation.

Because of this finding, the normal criteria cannot be applied to the analysis of the QRS complexes, S-T segments and T waves, and the electrocardiographic interpretation is best ended at this point, **unless either** a previous record is available for comparison **or** the interpreter is skilled and experienced in electrocardiography.

ECG diagnosis
Ventricular pre-excitation.

Record 56

4A. There is T wave inversion in V_3, V_4 and V_5.

5. There is S-T depression in V_5 and V_6. These are non-specific but definite and highly significant changes. The deep, symmetrical T wave inversion in V_3 is very suggestive of an ischaemic origin.

7. The mean frontal plane T wave axis is indeterminate. The mean frontal plane QRS axis is highly determinate ($+15°$). The T waves in the limb leads are therefore abnormal.

ECG diagnosis
Non-specific S-T, T changes in the limb leads and from V_3–V_6. The appearances in V_3 are suggestive of an ischaemic origin for these changes.

Record 57

6. a) The q waves in aVL exceed 0.03 sec in duration.

b) The q waves in aVL have a depth exceeding one quarter of the height of the ensuing R wave (inevitable – since there are no R waves!).

These changes **can** indicate the presence of anterolateral infarction. However, the mean frontal plane QRS axis in this case is $+75°$ and because of this aVL is a cavity lead and the q waves in aVL are therefore normal.

ECG diagnosis
Within normal limits.

Record 58

2. b) The r wave progression from V_1 to V_3 is abnormal. The r wave in V_2 is smaller than that in V_1, and the r wave in V_3 is smaller still and is actually preceded by a small q wave.

3. g) The q wave in V_3 has a depth exceeding one quarter of the height of the ensuing r wave. Although such a feature can occasionally occur in a normal record in one single precordial lead in the transition zone, it will be most unwise to accept it as normal in this case because of the obvious S-T segment elevation in the precordial series (see below).

The q wave in V_3 is probably indicative of anterior infarction.

5. There is obvious S-T elevation from V_1–V_4, indicative of acute anterior myocardial ischaemic damage.

There is minimal S-T segment depression in V_6 (not actually beyond the limits of normal).

8. There is slight S-T segment depression in II, III and aVF and slight S-T elevation in I and aVL.

The S-T elevation from V_1 to V_4 and in I and aVL is the primary change and the S-T depression in II, III, aVF and V_6 is a reciprocal change.

9. The P waves in II, III and aVF are bifid. This is not a definite abnormality but raises the possibility of left atrial abnormality.

ECG diagnosis
Acute anteroseptal myocardial ischaemic damage.

Record 59

2. a) V_1 has an RSR′ complex.

3. a) The total QRS duration is 0.14 sec. The combination of these two findings indicates the presence of right bundle branch block. The right bundle branch block accounts for the presence of the broad, slurred R′ wave in V_1 and the broad, slurred S wave from V_3–V_6 and in I and aVL.

ECG diagnosis
Complete right bundle block.

Record 60

3. c) The tallest precordial R wave (V_5) = 41 mm (well in excess of the normal maximum of 27 mm).

e) $R_{V_5} + S_{V_1}$ = 67 mm (well in excess of the normal maximum of 40 mm).

f) The ventricular activation time is abnormal at 0.05 sec.

4A. The T waves are inverted in V_5 and V_6. This is frankly abnormal.

5. There is S-T segment depression in V_5 and V_6. This is frankly abnormal. The S-T depression is asymmetrical and therefore is non-specific. It is not the typical S-T depression of myocardial ischaemia and is likely to be secondary to the QRS abnormalities which are indicative of left ventricular hypertrophy.

6. c) The R wave in aVL measures 20 mm (in excess of the normal maximum).

7. The mean frontal plane T wave axis is +150°. The frontal plane QRS axis is −15°. The angle between the two is therefore abnormal and the frontal plane T waves are abnormal.

8. There is significant, non-specific S-T depression in I and aVL.

9. The P waves in V_1 have a dominant negative component indicating left atrial abnormality.

ECG diagnosis
Left ventricular hypertrophy with left atrial abnormality (probably hypertrophy).

Record 61

2. a) No initial q wave is seen in V_6. However, there is a q wave in I and aVL and therefore the interventricular septum is being depolarised in the normal direction.

c) The transition zone is further to the left than V_6 (using the definition that the transition zone is reached when a septal q wave develops) or is between V_5 and V_6 (using the definition of the development of a dominant R wave). There is therefore pronounced clockwise cardiac rotation.

3. The tallest R wave in the precordial series (V_6) is only 6 mm. This is abnormally small but this is probably due to the pronounced clockwise rotation.

4A. The precordial T waves in V_5 and V_6 are of low voltage but the voltage is entirely appropriate to the size of the R wave and the T waves are therefore normal.

4B. The U waves are prominent (but not abnormal) in the precordial leads.

6. d) The mean frontal plane QRS axis is abnormal at −45°. Since the presence of initial r waves in aVF does not permit an ECG diagnosis of inferior infarction, the abnormal left axis deviation indicates the presence of left anterior hemiblock.

7. The mean frontal plane T axis is +75°. The angle between the T and QRS axes is therefore abnormal and the frontal plane T waves are therefore abnormal.

8. There is S-T segment depression in I and aVL.

ECG diagnosis
Left anterior hemiblock, clockwise cardiac rotation, non-specific S-T, T changes in the limb leads.

Record 62

2. a) No initial r wave is seen in V_1. No initial q wave is seen in V_6, I or aVL.

3. The total QRS duration is prolonged at 0.18 sec.

In view of the prolongation of the total QRS duration and absence of septal q waves (with no rSR′ complex in V_1 to indicate right bundle branch block) and since there is no evidence of ventricular pre-excitation, there is complete left bundle branch block. This precludes any further assessment of the QRS complexes, S-T segments or T waves (except for the assessment of the mean frontal plane QRS axis). If a previous record is available for comparison, or if the interpreter is highly experienced, further interpretation may be possible.

ECG diagnosis
Left bundle branch block.

Record 63

2. a) V_1 has an Rs complex. This is abnormal. It should be an rS complex. Because of this abnormality the r wave progression across the precordial series cannot be normal. There is pronounced clockwise cardiac rotation.

4A. The T waves are iso-electric or minimally inverted in V_3 and V_4 and are of low voltage in V_5.

5. There is S-T depression in V_1 and V_2.

6. The frontal plane QRS axis is +120°. This is abnormal.

The combination of a dominant R wave in V_1 with an abnormal degree of right axis deviation indicates right ventricular hypertrophy.

7. The frontal plane T wave axis is 0°. This is separated from the frontal plane QRS axis by an abnormal angle and therefore the frontal plane T waves are abnormal.

8. There is minimal S-T segment depression in Lead III.

9. b) The P wave height in II is 3 mm. This indicates right atrial hypertrophy.

ECG diagnosis
Right ventricular hypertrophy. Right atrial hypertrophy.

Record 64

2. a) No initial q wave is seen in the left precordial leads or in Lead I or aVL. This can indicate that the interventricular septum is being depolarised in the wrong direction. However, since the total QRS duration is entirely within normal limits, this variation is acceptable. If the QRS duration had been 0.10 or 0.11 sec the ECG diagnosis would have been incomplete left bundle branch block.

3. a) The total QRS duration is within normal limits.

c) The R waves in V_4 and V_5 are abnormally tall (measuring 42 mm in V_5).

f) The ventricular activation time cannot be measured since there is no qR complex in the left precordial leads.

4A. There is T wave inversion from V_2 to V_6.

5. There is S-T segment depression from V_2 to V_6.

7A. The frontal plane T wave axis is +180°. Since the frontal plane QRS axis is +60°, the angle between the two is abnormal and the frontal plane T waves are abnormal.

8. There is S-T depression in I, II and aVL.

The combination of abnormally tall R waves in the left precordial leads, with S-T segment and T wave changes in the precordial leads and S-T, T changes in the limb leads is indicative of left ventricular hypertrophy. It is surprising that there is no evidence of left atrial hypertrophy.

ECG diagnosis
Left ventricular hypertrophy.

Record 65

6. d) The frontal plane QRS axis is indeterminate, but this is not an abnormality, even though the frontal plane T wave axis is determinate (+45°).

9. a) The P wave duration in Lead II is abnormal at 0.13 sec.

c) There is a dominant negative component to the P wave in V_1. These changes indicate left atrial abnormality.

ECG diagnosis
Left atrial abnormality.

Record 66

2. a) No initial r wave is seen in V_1 (or in V_2 or V_3).

3. g) q waves are seen in V_1–V_3 with a duration in excess of 0.03 sec.

h) The q waves in V_1–V_3 have a depth exceeding one quarter of the height of the ensuing R wave.

4A. There is terminal T wave inversion from V_3–V_5 and the T waves are of low voltage in V_6.

5. There is S-T elevation from V_1–V_5. These changes indicate recent anteroseptal infarction.

7. The frontal plane T wave axis is $+120°$. This is at an abnormal angle to the mean frontal plane QRS axis (which is $+15°$). It follows that the T waves are abnormal in the frontal plane leads.

8. There is slight S-T segment elevation in Lead I.

ECG diagnosis
Recent anteroseptal infarction.

Record 67

1. The rhythm is sinus bradycardia.

2. b) No r wave in the precordial series exceeds 8 mm. The precordial R waves are therefore of abnormally low voltage.

4A. The T waves are of low voltage throughout the precordial leads.

9. The P waves are bifid in Lead II and in the precordial leads. This is not a **definite** abnormality, but is sometimes found in left atrial abnormalities.
The overall appearances are abnormal. The combination of sinus bradycardia with low voltage QRS and T waves suggests hypothyroidism.

ECG diagnosis
Sinus bradycardia. Generalised low voltages, suggesting possible hypothyroidism.

Record 68

2. a) V_1 has an Rs complex. This is abnormal. Because of this the R wave progression in the precordial series cannot be normal.

6. d) The mean frontal plane QRS axis is $+105°$.
The combination of a dominant R wave in V_1 with an abnormal degree of right axis deviation indicates the presence of right ventricular hypertrophy.

9. b) The P wave height in II is 3 mm. This is indicative of right atrial hypertrophy.

ECG diagnosis
Right ventricular hypertrophy. Right atrial hypertrophy.

Record 69

2. a) It is not clear whether or not there is a small r wave in V_1 – however –

b) There is no progression of the R wave from V_1–V_4 and this is frankly abnormal.

3. b) No precordial R wave exceeds 8 mm in height.

h) The q wave in V_4 has a height exceeding one quarter of the height of the subsequent R wave.

4A. There is T wave inversion from V_4–V_6.

5. There is S-T segment elevation from V_1–V_4.
These changes indicate the presence of recent anterior infarction. (The main criterion for the diagnosis of infarction in this case is the loss of R wave height from V_1–V_4).

6. a) It is difficult to be sure whether or not there is an initial r wave in Lead II – if not, the QRS complex would be of the QS type and this would be indicative of inferior infarction. However, there is clearly a small r in aVF. In this situation one cannot be confident that there is inferior infarction. It is possible that there has been an inferior infarct and that small r waves have subsequently been generated in place of the initial QS complexes associated with this condition.

d) The frontal plane QRS axis is abnormal at $-60°$.

7A. The frontal plane T wave axis is $+120°$. This is at an abnormal angle to the mean frontal plane QRS axis and the frontal plane T waves are therefore abnormal.

ECG diagnosis
Recent anterior infarction. There is an abnormal degree of left axis deviation. This could be due to old inferior infarction or to left anterior hemiblock. It is not possible with confidence to distinguish between these two possibilities.

Record 70

1. The P-R interval is abnormally short at 0.09 sec. The presence of this feature should lead one to look for the presence of a prolonged QRS duration.

3. (a) The total QRS duration is prolonged at 0.13 sec.
There is slurring of the initial part of the QRS complex. The combination of an abnormally short P-R interval and an abnormally long QRS complex with slurring of the initial part of the QRS complex indicates the presence of ventricular pre-excitation.
Unless a previous record is available for comparison, no further evaluation of the QRS complexes, S-T segments or T waves should be made. (Note, therefore, that the presence of ventricular pre-excitation produces even more severe limitations on ECG interpretation than does the presence of LBBB – for in the presence of the latter condition at least it is justifiable to proceed to the assessment of the frontal plane QRS axis (page 125), whereas this is not so in the case of ventricular pre-excitation). One cannot, therefore, assign any significance to the frontal plane axis (which would otherwise indicate left anterior hemiblock) or to the presence of QS complexes in aVF or V_1 (which would otherwise indicate inferior or anteroseptal infarction).

ECG diagnosis
Ventricular pre-excitation.

Annotated Records from Section 1: Reports

Appropriate reports for the 30 annotated records from Section I (pages 71–101) are given below:-

Record 1

Sinus rhythm. The P-R interval is normal at 0.18 sec. The mean frontal plane QRS axis is +60°. The record is within normal limits.

Record 2

Sinus rhythm. The P-R interval is normal at 0.12 sec. The mean frontal plane QRS axis is +75°. The record is within normal limits. (Note that the q waves which are apparent in aVL, are normal since aVL is, in this case, a cavity lead).

Record 3

Sinus rhythm. The P-R interval is normal at 0.18 sec. The mean frontal plane QRS axis is −15°. **There is a shallow T wave inversion in V_5 and V_6. The angle between the mean frontal plane QRS and T wave axes is abnormal at +135° (the mean frontal plane T wave axis being +120°). There are therefore frankly abnormal T wave changes in the limb leads and in the left precordial leads. These are non-specific abnormalities.**
The U waves are prominent but not abnormal in the left precordial leads. (No specific cause can be assigned to the electrocardiographic abnormalities here. Possibilities include myocardial ischaemia and hypokalaemia. It would be unwise to diagnose left ventricular hypertrophy simply on the basis that the R wave height in aVL is minimally above the accepted voltage criteria.)

Record 4

Sinus rhythm. The P-R interval is normal at 0.16 sec. The mean frontal plane QRS axis is +30°. **The precordial QRS complexes just satisfy the voltage criteria for left ventricular hypertrophy. The ventricular activation time is increased at 0.05 sec. These changes are indicative of left ventricular hypertrophy. There is a dominant negative component to the P wave in V_1, indicating left atrial abnormality (quite possibly hypertrophy). There is significant S-T segment elevation in Leads II, III and the foot-lead, and S-T segment depression in Leads I, the left arm-lead and in V_2 and V_3. These changes are indicative of acute inferior myocardial (ischaemic) damage. (The changes in Leads II, III and the foot-lead are primary, those in I, aVL, V_2 and V_3 are secondary.)**

Record 5

Sinus rhythm. The P-R interval is normal at 0.16 sec. The mean frontal plane QRS axis is +45°. **There are unequivocal changes of left ventricular hypertrophy. The precordial voltage criteria for this condition are fulfilled and there are secondary S-T, T changes in leads facing the left ventricle (in this case V_4 to V_6, Leads I, II and aVL). The form of the P waves in V_1 is indicative of left atrial abnormality (probably hypertrophy).**

Record 6

Sinus rhythm. The P-R interval is normal at 0.14 sec. **The mean frontal plane QRS axis is +165° and there is a dominant R wave in V_1. These changes are indicative of right ventricular hypertrophy. The P waves are abnormally tall in the foot-lead (3 mm) indicating right atrial hypertrophy.** (This criterion is normally used in Lead II but can be applied in whichever frontal plane lead is most closely related to the axis of the P wave. This is usually Lead II, but in this case the P wave axis is +75° which is halfway between Leads II and the foot-lead and either of these leads may be chosen). (The other point for comment in this electrocardiogram is the presence of very deep S waves in V_2 and V_3. Deep S waves in the **left** precordial leads are very much part of the pattern of right ventricular hypertrophy, but deep S waves in the **right** precordial leads are not routinely found in this condition. They raise the possibility of additional left ventricular hypertrophy but they are not totally diagnostic).

Record 7

Sinus rhythm. The P-R interval is normal at 0.16 sec. The mean frontal plane QRS axis is −15°. **There is complete left bundle branch block** (the left bundle branch block accounts for the absence of appropriate r wave progression across the precordial leads and for the S-T, T changes in Leads I, aVL and the left precordial leads).

Record 8

Sinus rhythm. The P-R interval is normal at 0.16 sec. **The mean frontal plane QRS axis is −45° indicating an abnormal degree of left axis deviation. There is evidence of an old anteroseptal myocardial infarction** (there is loss of the r waves from V_1–V_3 and inappropriately small r waves from V_4–V_6. It is likely, but not certain, that the abnormal left axis deviation is due to ischaemic damage to the anterior division of the left bundle branch system giving rise to left anterior hemiblock).

Record 9

Sinus rhythm. The P-R interval is normal at 0.20 sec. The mean frontal plane QRS axis is +75°. There is no significant abnormality in the form of the QRS complexes, the S-T segments or the T waves. **There is clear evidence of left atrial hypertrophy in that the P waves in Lead II are broad and bifid and the P waves in V_1 have a dominant negative component.** The combination of left atrial hypertrophy and a mean frontal plane QRS axis towards the right hand end of the normal range in the absence of any other electrocardiographic abnormality suggests the possibility of obstruction at the mitral valve. (This is very commonly due to mitral stenosis and extremely rarely due to the presence of an atrial myxoma).

Record 10

Sinus rhythm. The P-R interval is normal at 0.13 sec. The mean frontal plane QRS axis is +75°. **The form of the QRS complexes in V_1 is borderline abnormal in that the R/S ratio is unity. The form of the P waves in V_1 indicates the presence of left atrial hypertrophy.** A prominent atrial repolarisation wave is seen in the left precordial leads. (The diagnostic criteria for right ventricular hypertrophy are not fulfilled but the presence of an R/S ratio of unity in V_1, together with a mean frontal plane QRS axis, towards the right hand end of the normal range suggests the possibility of minimal right ventricular enlargement). **The P waves in Lead II are also slightly pointed and the possibility of right atrial hypertrophy should be considered although the appearances are not definitive.** The apparent S-T segment depression in the left precordial leads is part of a prominent atrial repolarisation wave which can be seen to begin before the QRS complex. As in Record 9, the most likely clinical accompaniment of such an electrocardiogram is mitral valve obstruction.

Record 11

Sinus rhythm. The P-R interval is normal at 0.12 sec. The mean frontal plane QRS axis is +30°. The record is within normal limits.

Record 12

Sinus rhythm. The P-R interval is normal at 0.20 sec. The mean frontal plane QRS axis is +15°. **There are non-specific S-T, T changes in the limb leads and the left precordial leads.** (The record is frankly abnormal but no specific cause for the abnormality can be assigned. There is no primary abnormality in the QRS complexes and the S-T, T changes are therefore primary). Abnormalities of this type can be found in association with myocardial ischaemia, myocarditis, cardiomyopathy, pericarditis, hypokalaemia and hypothyroidism. The latter is rendered less likely but by absence of a bradycardia.

Record 13

Sinus rhythm. The P-R interval is within normal limits at 0.12 sec. The mean frontal plane QRS axis is +75°. **There is evidence of recent anterior myocardial infarction. (Definitive evidence of infarction appears from V_1–V_4 and there is also S-T segment elevation in V_5 and Lead I. The q waves in aVL are not necessarily abnormal themselves because the frontal plane QRS axis is +75° and aVL is therefore a cavity lead).

Record 14

Sinus rhythm. The P-R interval is normal at 0.12 sec. The mean frontal plane QRS axis is +45°.
The record is within normal limits. (Note that the T wave inversion in Lead III is not abnormal. The mean frontal plane T wave axis is +15°. The angle between the frontal plane QRS and T wave axes is thus well within the normal range at 30° and it follows that the frontal plane T waves are all within normal limits).

Record 15

Sinus rhythm. The P-R interval is normal at 0.14 sec. The mean frontal plane QRS axis is −15°. **The precordial QRS complexes satisfy the voltage criteria for left ventricular hypertrophy** (note that the precordial leads are half-standardised). **There are non-specific S-T, T changes in the left precordial leads, Leads I, II and aVL. These S-T, T changes are definitely abnormal.** No specific cause for them can be assigned. They may well be secondary to the primary QRS abnormality and thus be part of the picture of left ventricular hypertrophy. However, alternative additional abnormalities may need to be considered as in Record 12.

Record 16

Sinus rhythm. The P-R interval is normal at 0.12 sec. The mean frontal plane QRS axis is 0°. **There is evidence of left ventricular hypertrophy and of inferior myocardial infarction of intermediate age. The precordial QRS complexes satisfy the voltage criteria for left ventricular hypertrophy and the intrinsic deflection time is abnormal. The S-T, T changes in V_4, V_5 and V_6 are probably secondary to the primary QRS abnormality of left ventricular hypertrophy.** The form of the QRS complexes in V_4 could be indicative of a localised anterior infarction (since there is appreciable reduction in the r wave compared with that seen in V_3 and that seen in V_5), but it would be unwise to make a confident diagnosis of this since the r wave can occasionally be inappropriately small in a single lead in the precordial series in the transition zone (page 45). **There is definitive q wave evidence of infarction in aVF where the q waves are abnormally deep and abnormally broad. The T wave inversion in Leads II, III and aVF is probably part of the pattern of inferior infarction. If so it indicates that the infarct is of intermediate age.** It is not a very recent infarction since there is no residual S-T segment elevation. However, one cannot be sure that the T wave changes in the inferior limb leads are related to the infarction. They could also be related to the left ventricular hypertrophy.

Record 17

Sinus rhythm. The P-R interval is normal at 0.16 sec. **The mean frontal plane QRS axis is −45°. This is an abnormal degree of left axis deviation.** The deviation is probably due to left anterior hemiblock. **There is evidence of old anteroseptal myocardial infarction. Small initial r waves are seen in V_1 but the r wave is smaller or absent in V_2, and V_3 shows q waves. The QRS configuration in V_1, V_2 and V_3 therefore unequivocally represents an anteroseptal infarction** (the total QRS duration being within the normal range). The abnormal degree of left axis deviation occurring in the absence of QRS evidence of inferior myocardial infarction indicates the presence of left anterior hemiblock. There is minimal S-T segment depression in V_6 but one cannot be sure of the significance of this since the baseline is not truly horizontal.

Record 18

Sinus rhythm. The P-R interval is normal at 0.15 sec. The mean frontal plane QRS axis is +15°. **There is evidence of left ventricular hypertrophy with counterclockwise cardiac rotation (the precordial QRS complexes satisfy the voltage criteria for left ventricular hypertrophy and the ventricular activation time is prolonged. There are non-specific S-T, T changes from V_3–V_6.** These are almost certainly secondary to the primary QRS abnormality. The transition zone is between V_2 and V_3, indicating pronounced counterclockwise cardiac rotation. **There are non-specific S-T, T changes also in the limb leads.** These too are almost certainly secondary to the primary QRS abnormality).

Record 19

Sinus rhythm. The P-R interval is normal at 0.16 sec. The mean frontal plane QRS axis is +45°. The record is within normal limits.

Record 20

Sinus rhythm. The P-R interval is normal at 0.15 sec. The mean frontal plane QRS axis is +15°. The record is within normal limits.

Record 21

Sinus rhythm. The P-R interval is normal at 0.19 sec. The mean frontal plane QRS axis is +30°. **There is evidence of left ventricular hypertrophy and left atrial hypertrophy. (The S-T, T changes in the left precordial leads and in the limb leads are almost certainly secondary to the primary QRS abnormality).**

Record 22

Sinus rhythm. The P-R interval is normal at 0.16 sec. The mean frontal plane QRS axis is indeterminate. The complexes in all these leads are of low voltage and **no precordial R wave satisfies the minimum voltage criterion of 8 mm. This is a non-specific feature, but raises the possibility of anterior infarction. The q wave in aVF is abnormal and indicates the presence of an old inferior infarction.** (The abnormally low r wave voltage across the precordial leads could be due to obesity or emphysema. Hypothyroidism should also be considered, but this is relatively unlikely in view of the lack of sinus bradycardia).

The generalised low voltage of the T waves is not of any separate significance for the T waves are bound to be of low voltage since the QRS complexes are of low voltage. The significance of the low voltage in the precordial leads can only be assessed by secondary interpretation. It is conceivable that there has been extensive loss of R wave voltage as a result of previous infarction, but in the presence of obesity or emphysema it would be most unwise to make such a deduction. The q waves in aVF, which are easily missed, are indicative of inferior infarction. This is perhaps best seen in the third QRS complex in aVF.

Record 23

Sinus rhythm. The P-R interval is normal at 0.16 sec. The mean frontal plane QRS axis is +75°. **There is complete right bundle branch block** (the "splintering" of the QRS complexes in V_2, V_3 and V_4 is simply part of the right bundle branch block).

Record 24

Sinus rhythm. The P-R interval is normal at 0.14 sec. The mean frontal plane QRS axis is +15°. The record is within normal limits. (The q wave in aVL is at the upper end of the normal range, but is not definitely abnormal).

Record 25

Sinus rhythm. The P-R interval is normal at 0.12 sec. The mean frontal plane QRS axis is +15°.
There is evidence of an old anterior myocardial infarction. (There are QS complexes in V_1 and V_2, abnormally deep and wide q waves with very small r waves in V_3, and abnormally deep and wide q waves in V_4. There are non-specific S-T, T changes throughout the precordial leads. These are almost certainly secondary to the primary QRS abnormality. Non-specific S-T, T changes are also seen in these limb leads).

Record 26

Sinus rhythm. The P-R interval is normal at 0.13 sec. The mean frontal plane QRS axis is −30°.
There is evidence of inferior myocardial infarction of intermediate age. Non-specific S-T, T changes are seen in the left precordial leads suggesting apical extension of the ischaemic or infarcted zone (inferior myocardial infarction is not infrequently associated with ischaemic changes in the left precordial leads, the area of infarction or ischaemia being referred to either as "apical" or "inferolateral". There is no definitive evidence of lateral myocardial infarction in this case although the R waves are rather lower in voltage in the left precordial leads than one would expect).

Record 27

Sinus rhythm. The P-R interval is normal at 0.19 sec. The mean frontal plane QRS axis is +45°.
There are non-specific S-T, T changes in the left precordial leads and in the limb leads. (There is no abnormality in the form of the QRS complexes. The non-specific S-T, T changes are therefore primary). As usual therefore, it is not possible to assign a specific cause for the abnormality.

Record 28

Sinus rhythm. The P-R interval is normal at 0.14 sec. The mean frontal plane QRS axis is −15°.
There is complete left bundle branch block. (Note that the QS complexes in the inferior limb leads do not signify inferior myocardial infarction since there is left bundle branch block. In the same way, the absence of r wave progression in V_1–V_3 does not signify myocardial infarction. Both these features are part of the left bundle branch block pattern).

Record 29

Sinus rhythm. The P-R interval is normal at 0.20 sec. **The mean frontal plane QRS axis is +120°. There is evidence of right ventricular hypertrophy** (the dominant r wave in V_1 together with the abnormal degree of right axis deviation indicates right ventricular hypertrophy. **The pronounced clockwise cardiac rotation is simply part of the pattern of right ventricular hypertrophy as are the S-T, T changes which are present in this record from V_1–V_4.** Prominent U waves are seen in V_3 and V_4 but these are not definitely abnormal).

Record 30

Sinus rhythm. The P-R interval is normal at 0.17 sec. The mean frontal plane QRS axis is +45°.
The record is within the normal limits although the QRS complexes in V_1 and V_2 could be consistent with an old anteroseptal infarction (the r wave progression from V_1–V_3 is not typically normal and there is no doubt that it is possible that there is an old anteroseptal infarction. However, appearances of this type are sometimes seen in normal records and as a general rule it is best to under-report rather than to over-report the electrocardiogram. It must be remembered that not only may **this** pattern be associated with an anteroseptal infarction, so may a completely normal electrocardiogram!).

Epilogue

Every effort has been made, in the writing of this text, to encourage the development of confidence in electrocardiographic interpretation on the part of the reader. It is, nevertheless, essential also to remember that the electrocardiogram has severe limitations as a diagnostic tool. It provides information about depolarisation and about repolarisation of myocardium. Information about disease in the coronary arteries is not directly provided by the electrocardiogram, though it may often be inferred if the electrocardiogram is abnormal. A normal electrocardiogram in no way excludes significant stenosing atheroma of the coronary arteries.
The following two cases illustrate this.

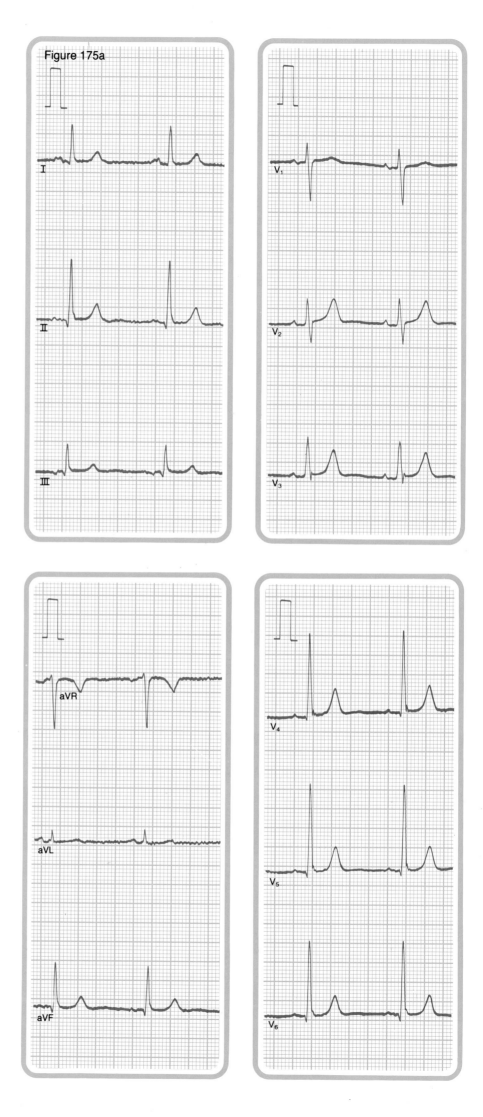

Figure 175a

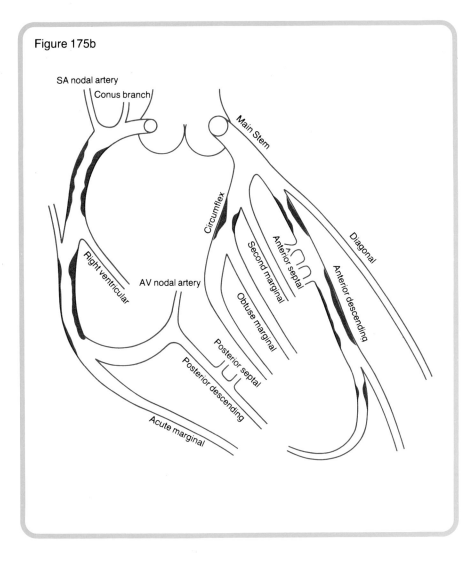

Figure 175b

Case 1

J.R. A 54-year-old lady with an unequivocal story of angina pectoris. The electrocardiogram is shown in Figure 175a. This ECG would be reported as follows:-
"Sinus rhythm. The mean frontal plane QRS axis is +45°. The record is within normal limits".

Figure 175b shows the coronary angiographic appearances in this patient. There is evidence of severe, stenosing atheroma in the anterior descending and circumflex branches of the left coronary artery, and in the main right coronary artery.
This patient thus has involvement of all three major coronary arteries without any electrocardiographic abnormality whatsoever.

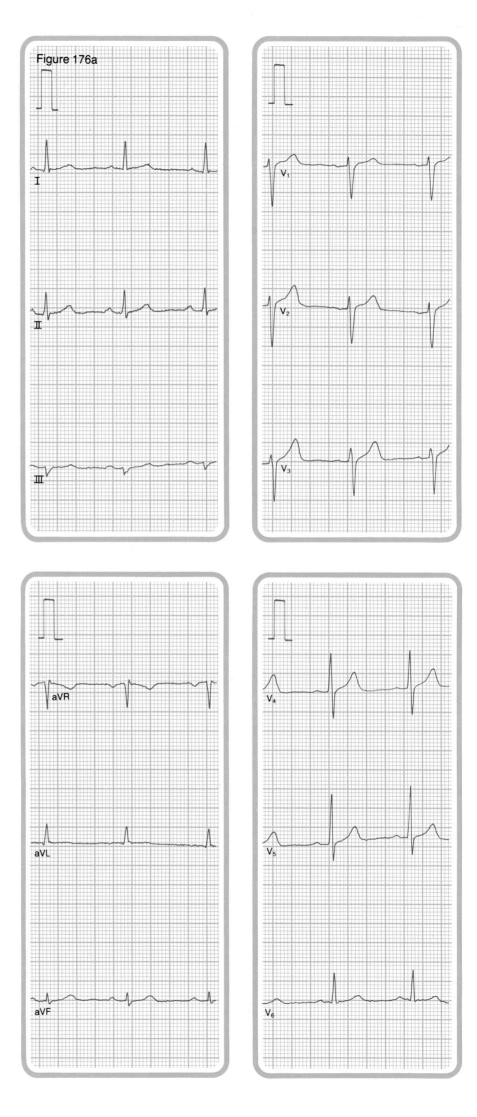

Figure 176a

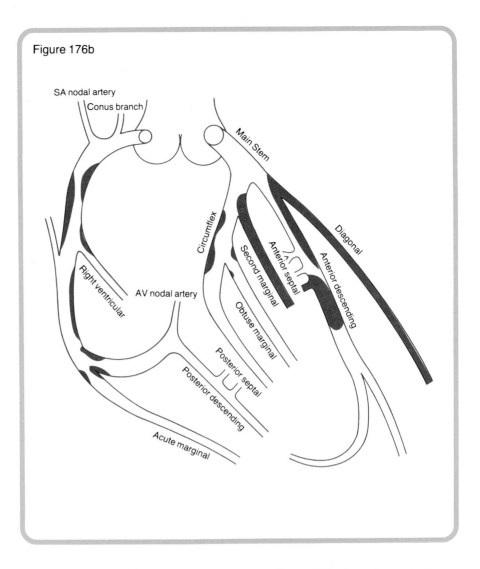

Figure 176b

Case 2

A.A. A 50-year-old man with severe, disabling angina pectoris and repeated hospital admissions with episodes of chest pain. The electrocardiogram is shown in Figures 176a. This electrocardiogram would be interpreted as follows:-
"Sinus rhythm. The mean frontal plane QRS axis is +15°. The record is within normal limits".

Figure 176b shows the coronary angiographic appearances in this patient. There is very extensive disease in the right coronary artery, there is complete occlusion of the diagonal branch of the left coronary artery and of the distal part of the anterior descending branch of the left coronary artery. There is complete occlusion of the second marginal branch of the circumflex coronary artery and significant narrowing in the main circumflex artery itself. In addition, this patient had actually already received four coronary saphenous by-pass grafts, two of which were completely blocked, one of which was severely narrowed and one of which was working normally.

It is hoped that these two cases will provide a cautionary tale sufficient to discourage anyone from believing that a normal electro-cardiogram in any way excludes significant disease in the coronary arteries.

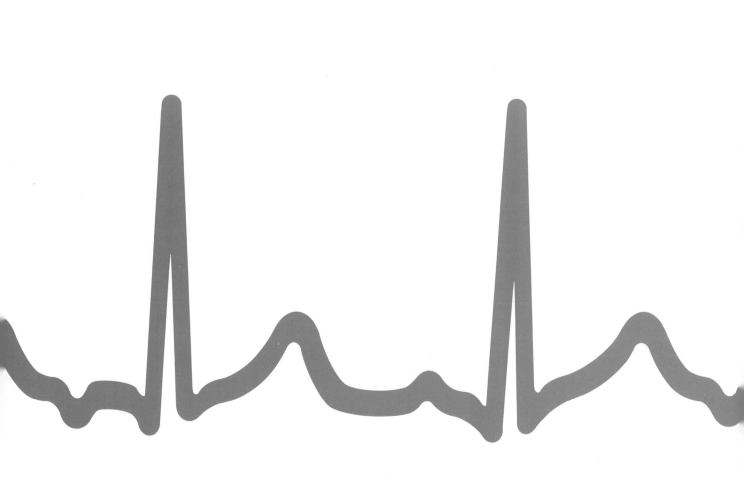

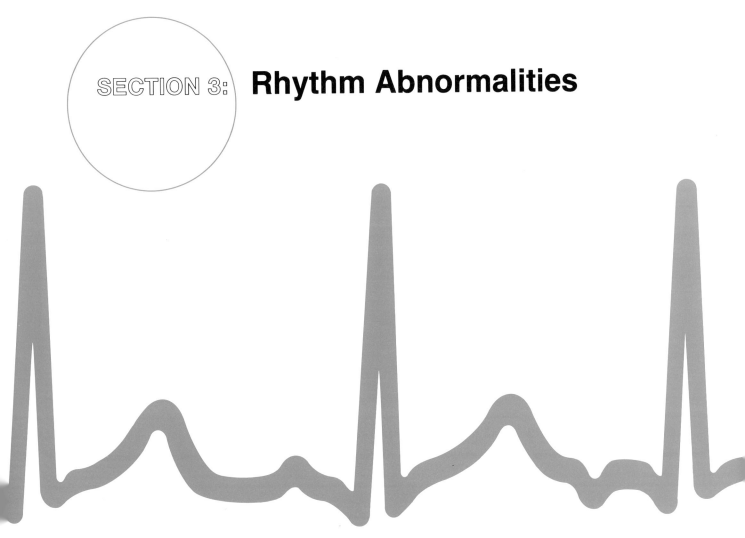

SECTION 3: **Rhythm Abnormalities**

Introduction

The Cardiac Rhythm

The term "rhythm of the heart" describes the ordered sequence of depolarisation of the myocardium with respect to time. "The cardiac rhythm" therefore describes the location of the first depolarisation which initiates the cardiac cycle, the sequence of spread of that depolarisation to other parts of the heart within that cycle and the relationship in time of all the depolarisations within that cycle to those in adjacent cardiac cycles. The term "cardiac rhythm" appears in all textbooks of electrocardiography, but almost always without a formal definition of its meaning. The implication is that the meaning is clear, but without definition ambiguities necessarily develop. It is often also implied that the term refers merely to the **initiation** of depolarisation. This does not seem to be sufficient. The **unqualified** phrase "the heart is in sinus rhythm" is best taken to imply that depolarisation is initiated, at the sino-atrial node, regularly and with rates between 60 and 100 beats per minute that the depolarisation spreads through the atrial myocardium, through the atrio-ventricular node (with normal delay) and then through the specialised conducting tissue to the ventricular myocardium. Since the cardiac rhythm can change (and in pathological states frequently does change) between one cycle and the next, any question about the nature of the cardiac rhythm in a given subject must be asked (and answered) in respect of a particular time period. Furthermore, conclusions about the nature of the cardiac rhythm in a given subject are valid only for the duration of the period of observation.

As indicated in the Introduction to Section 2 of this trilogy (see page 107), the electrocardiogram provides both morphological and rhythm information and these two areas of information are almost discrete. Figure 177 shows a Venn diagram representation of the relationship between morphological and rhythm information in the electrocardiogram.

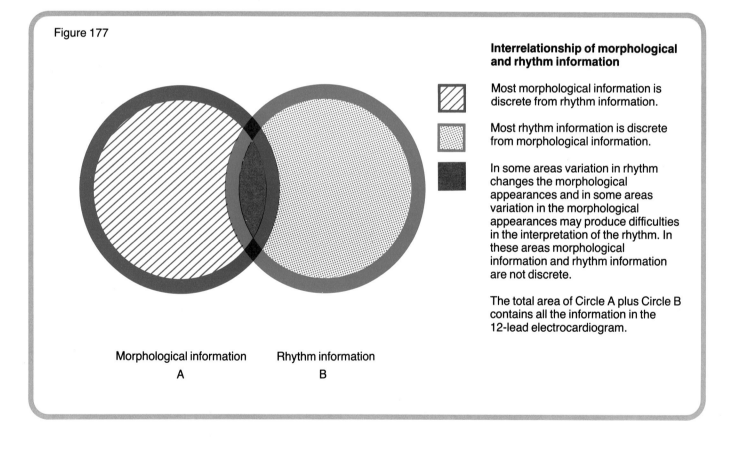

Figure 177

Interrelationship of morphological and rhythm information

Most morphological information is discrete from rhythm information.

Most rhythm information is discrete from morphological information.

In some areas variation in rhythm changes the morphological appearances and in some areas variation in the morphological appearances may produce difficulties in the interpretation of the rhythm. In these areas morphological information and rhythm information are not discrete.

The total area of Circle A plus Circle B contains all the information in the 12-lead electrocardiogram.

Morphological information
A

Rhythm information
B

The Normal Cardiac Rhythm (Sinus Rhythm)

The normal rhythm of the heart is sinus rhythm with a regular rate of 60 to 100 beats per minute. This definition is accepted by the Criteria Committee of the New York Heart Association. The term "regular" is taken to mean that the cycle length (P to P interval) does not vary by more than 10 per cent (longest, with respect to the shortest). Figure 178 shows an example of sinus rhythm.

Note that a **very large number of criteria must be fulfilled before the simple statement "the heart is in sinus rhythm" is a justifiable and sufficient description of the rhythm, as follows: There must be P waves. The P waves must be morphologically usual for that person** (see Note 1). **All P waves must have the same morphology. The P wave rate must be constant** (see Note 2). **The P wave rate must not lie outside the limits 60 to 100 beats per min. There must be QRS complexes. The QRS complexes must have the morphology usual for that person** (see Note 1). **There must be one P wave to each QRS complex. The P waves must be in front of each QRS complex. The P-R interval must be normal (within the limits 0.12 to 0.22 sec). The P-R interval must be constant.**

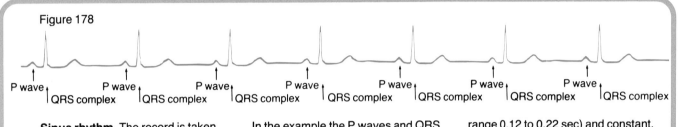

Figure 178

P wave | QRS complex | P wave | QRS complex | P wave | QRS complex | P wave | QRS complex | P wave | QRS complex | P wave | QRS complex | P wave | QRS complex

Sinus rhythm. The record is taken from a lead which shows well the P waves and QRS complexes (for rhythm analysis it is not necessary to recognise the S-T segments or T waves).

In the example the P waves and QRS complexes are morphologically normal (though these are not **requirements** for sinus rhythm). The P waves are regular at 60 per minute, the P-R interval is both normal (in the range 0.12 to 0.22 sec) and constant. Since the P-R interval is constant and the P wave rate is constant, the QRS rate is also constant.

Note 1

The P waves will normally be smooth and rounded and will be upright in II (and usually also in I and aVL). They will often be biphasic in V_1 (and possibly also in V_2) and will usually be upright (though often small) in the other precordial leads. If a patient has a morphological abnormality of the atria (hypertrophy, ischaemia, infarction, etc) the P waves will have an abnormal shape despite the fact that the rhythm is sinus. An abnormal rhythm of atrial origin (e.g. an atrial ectopic beat) will have a P wave shape differing from the usual form for that person. Similar considerations apply to the QRS morphology. Thus in the presence of sinus rhythm the QRS complexes will be abnormal in morphology if there is, for example, ventricular hypertrophy, bundle branch block, myocardial infarction etc. In these circumstances, as also when there is sinus rhythm and the QRS complexes are morphologically normal, abnormal beats of ventricular origin (e.g. a ventricular ectopic beat) will have QRS shape different from the usual form for that person.

Note 2

"Constancy" of the P wave rate has been defined in two ways:

a. (The maximum P-P interval minus the minimum P-P interval) divided by the minimum P-P interval multiplied by 100% is less than 10%

i.e. $\dfrac{(P\text{-}P)_{max} - (P\text{-}P)_{min}}{(P\text{-}P)_{min}} \times 100\% \not> 10\%$

b. The maximum P-P interval does not exceed the minimum P-P interval by more than 0.12 sec

i.e. $(P\text{-}P)_{max} - (P\text{-}P)_{min} \not> 0.12$ sec.

Since it is a requirement of "normal sinus rhythm" that the P-R interval be constant, "constancy" of the P wave rate implies similar constancy of the R wave rate.

This repetitive cycle is dependent upon repetitive spontaneous depolarisation of the SA node (Figure 181).

When the heart is in sinus rhythm, the depolarisation sequence (Figure179a) is initiated at the sino-atrial (SA) node, spreads to and subsequently through the atrial myocardium to the atrio-ventricular (AV) node, down the common bundle, into both bundle branches and into the Purkinje network and then to the ventricular myocardium over which it spreads (sequence 1, 2, 3, 4, 6, 7, 8, 9, 10 in Figure 179b). The sequence is repeated when the SA node depolarises again. When the depolarisation passes over the atrial myocardium the P wave is generated, and when it passes over the ventricular myocardium the QRS complex is generated. **Since the rhythm of the heart is the ordered sequence of DEPOLARISATION of the myocardium the S-T segment and the T wave (which are part of the repolarisation process) play no part in the analysis of the cardiac rhythm. In the same way, the atrial T wave (the Ta wave) plays no part in rhythm analysis.**

The repetitive sequence of atrial depolarisation – ventricular depolarisation – atrial depolarisation – ventricular depolarisation – etc is represented in a typical rhythm strip by the alternating P waves and QRS complexes (the S-T, T sections being, for the purposes of rhythm analysis, ignored (Figure 180)).

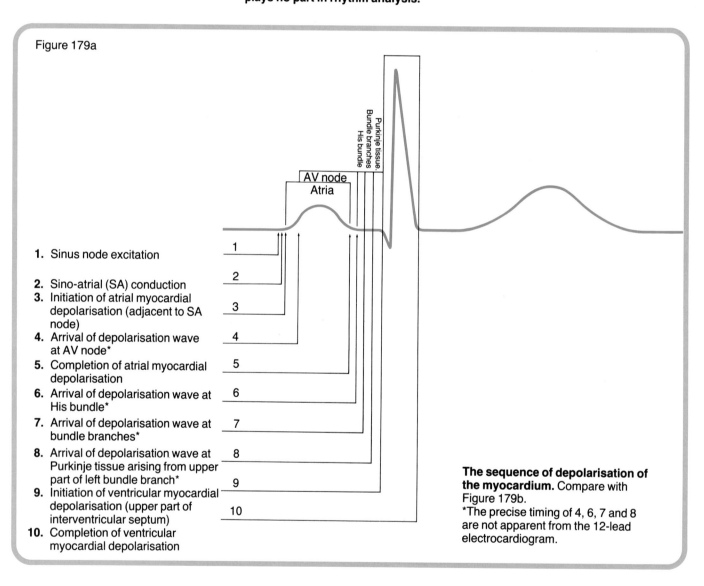

Figure 179a

Purkinje tissue
Bundle branches
His bundle

AV node
Atria

1. Sinus node excitation
2. Sino-atrial (SA) conduction
3. Initiation of atrial myocardial depolarisation (adjacent to SA node)
4. Arrival of depolarisation wave at AV node*
5. Completion of atrial myocardial depolarisation
6. Arrival of depolarisation wave at His bundle*
7. Arrival of depolarisation wave at bundle branches*
8. Arrival of depolarisation wave at Purkinje tissue arising from upper part of left bundle branch*
9. Initiation of ventricular myocardial depolarisation (upper part of interventricular septum)
10. Completion of ventricular myocardial depolarisation

The sequence of depolarisation of the myocardium. Compare with Figure 179b.
*The precise timing of 4, 6, 7 and 8 are not apparent from the 12-lead electrocardiogram.

Figure 179b

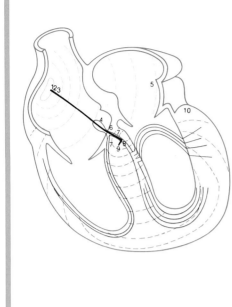

The depolarisation sequence begins with spontaneous depolarisation of the sino-atrial node (1), followed by conduction to the atrial myocardium (sino-atrial conduction, (2)) then atrial myocardial depolarisation (3). The depolarisation process then spreads over the myocardium of both atria (green interrupted lines). During the spread of activation over the atria the P wave occurs. 3 and 5 indicate those parts of the atria, depolarisation of which gives rise to the initial (3) and to the terminal (5) parts of the P wave. At some point during the inscription of the P wave the depolarisation process reaches the AV node (4). After a substantial delay (during which period atrial myocardial depolarisation is completed (5)) the depolarisation reaches the common bundle (bundle of His) (6), spreads down both bundle branches (7) and into the proximal part to the Purkinje network (8). In the upper, left part of the interventricular septum the depolarisation spreads into the ventricular myocardium (9). The depolarisation process then spreads over the myocardium of both ventricles (blue interrupted lines). During the spread of activation over the ventricles the QRS complex occurs. 9 and 10 indicate those parts of the ventricles, depolarisation of which gives rise to the initial (9) and the terminal (10) parts of the QRS complexes. Note that all parts of the atrial myocardium are in electrical continuity with all other parts of the atrial myocardium, that all parts of the ventricular myocardium are in electrical continuity with all other parts of the ventricular myocardium but that the atria and ventricles are electrically isolated from each other except for the bridge provided by the common bundle (bundle of His).

Figure 180

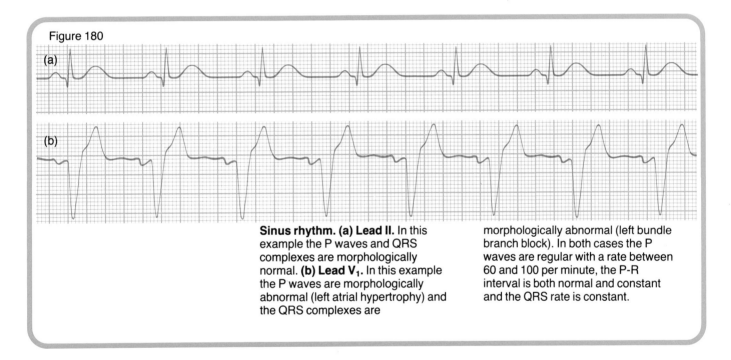

Sinus rhythm. (a) Lead II. In this example the P waves and QRS complexes are morphologically normal. **(b) Lead V$_1$.** In this example the P waves are morphologically abnormal (left atrial hypertrophy) and the QRS complexes are morphologically abnormal (left bundle branch block). In both cases the P waves are regular with a rate between 60 and 100 per minute, the P-R interval is both normal and constant and the QRS rate is constant.

Sinus node depolarisation takes place spontaneously and repetitively as a result of the cells within the node repeatedly undergoing a "ramp" function of charge and discharge (Figure 181).

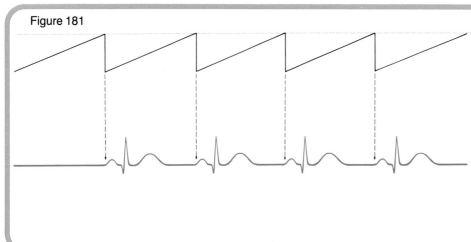

Figure 181

Threshold potential of SA node.

SA node potential climbs ramp to threshold, when threshold is reached the SA node depolarises.

Depolarisation of the SA node initiates atrial myocardial depolarisation. This gives rise to the P wave. Subsequent spread of the depolarisation to the ventricles results in production of the QRS complexes.

If the term "the heart is in sinus rhythm" is used without qualification it implies not only that the depolarisation is initiated at the SA node with a frequency between 60 and 100 beats per min, but also that each depolarisation spreads through the atrial myocardium and thence to the ventricles via the conducting system with a normal delay at the AV node and that this pattern remains constant during the period for which the description is applied. Thus if, even for part of the period in question, the impulse is initiated irregularly, too frequently or too slowly from the SA node, is initiated from a site other than the SA node or fails to conduct normally to the bundle of His and to at least one of the bundle branches and thence to the Purkinje network and ventricular myocardium, the rhythm is, for the period of deviation from these constraints, abnormal. In the terms of this definition intraventricular blocks (e.g. left and right bundle branch block) are not considered to be rhythm abnormalities but atrio-ventricular blocks are so considered.

Arrhythmias : Dysrhythmias

The chosen title for this section of the trilogy ("Rhythm Abnormalities") avoids the problem encountered by choosing between "Dysrhythmias" and "Arrhythmias". The former is preferred by purists as a more appropriate term since the prefix "dys" (Greek δυσ, a prefix meaning "bad" or "ill") implies abnormality of the rhythm whereas the prefix "a" (Greek α, a prefix meaning "no" or "not") implies absence of rhythm! Despite this etymological objection, the latter term is in widespread use. Arguments concerning this terminology are sterile. Accuracy is, of course, an essential quality but pedantry satisfies a few and irritates many. Both terms are, in practice, synonymous with "rhythm abnormalities".

Determinants of Cardiac Rhythm: Assessing the Cardiac Rhythm

The cells which **determine** the rhythm of the heart are the cells of the **pacemaking and conducting tissue** (SA node, AV node, bundle of His (common bundle), bundle branches, Purkinje network) as seen in Figure 182. However, none of these cell groups generates sufficient voltage to give a recognisable deflection on the surface electrocardiogram. The cardiac rhythm can only be assessed from information concerning **myocardial** depolarisation contained in the surface electrocardiogram (the P waves or QRS complexes). From this information the function of the pacemaker and conducting tissue is inferred.

Anatomy of the Normal Cardiac Rhythm

The cardiac rhythm is determined by the behaviour of the pacemaker and conducting tissue of the heart.
An understanding of the normal function of this tissue requires a knowledge of its anatomical arrangement.

Overall Anatomy of the Specialised Pacemaking and Conducting Tissue

The overall layout of the specialised tissue of the pacemaking and conducting tissue was described in Section 2, page 111 and shown in Figure 74, which is repeated as Figure 182.

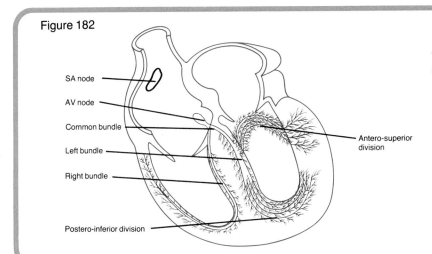

Figure 182

SA node
AV node
Common bundle
Left bundle
Right bundle
Antero-superior division
Postero-inferior division

The anatomy of the pacemaking and conduction tissue. The SA node and the AV node (AV junction) lie in the right atrium. The common bundle (bundle of His) perforates the central fibrous body to reach the interventricular septum, where it divides into the right and left bundle branches. From these the Purkinje network arises.

Sino-atrial Node (SA Node)

The sinus node is a cigar-shaped structure consisting of pacemaker cells in a fibrous matrix. It is 1 to 2cm long and 2 to 3mm in diameter. It lies 1mm deep to the epicardial surface in the right atrial sulcus terminalis at the junction of the superior vena cava and the right atrium.

Atrio-ventricular Node (AV Node)

This is situated at the base of the atrial septum, just beneath the endocardium of the right atrium, anterior to the ostium of the coronary sinus and directly above the insertion of the septal leaflet of the tricuspid valve. The "**atrio-ventricular junctional area**" has three recognisable regions:

1. The "**transitional cell zone**" or "**nodal approaches**" consists of atrial myocardial fibres interdigitating into the proximal part of the AV node.

2. The "**compact region**" or **AV node itself** is superficial and located as described above.

3. The "**penetrating part of the AV bundle**" (**bundle of His**) runs through the central fibrous body (which provides electrical isolation between the myocardium of the atria and that of the ventricles) to reach the upper part of the trabecular interventricular septum where it divides into the right and left bundle branches.

The term "junctional" is often nowadays generally preferred to the term "nodal" since tachycardias arising in the AV junctional area may be initiated in the AV node alone or may be initiated in a zone involving both the AV node and also nodal bypass tracts.

342

Internodal Conduction

Some authorities maintain that "specialised tracts" run from the SA node to the AV node. Others find no anatomical evidence of any such specialised tracts. Electrophysiological studies unequivocally demonstrate preferential pathways of internodal conduction and the only real argument is whether the anatomical substrate of such preferential conduction is served by cells which are histologically specialised or are merely distinct only by their alignment or by the closeness with which they are packed. The weight of evidence is against the presence of histologically specialised tracts but in favour of preferential routes of internodal conduction.

Interatrial Conduction

A large muscle bundle (Bachmann's bundle) runs from the right atrium, round the back of the aorta, to the left atrium and appears to facilitate preferential conduction of depolarisation from the right to the left atrium. Again the weight of evidence suggests that this is functionally but not histologically discrete from the rest of the atrial myocardium.

This bundle is the true anatomical substrate for the known initiation of left atrial depolarisation relatively soon after the onset of right atrial depolaristion. This feature was described (for simplicity at that stage) in Figures 54 and 65 (see Section 1, pages 43 and 59 respectively) as being on the "shortest route" between the SA node and the left atrial myocardium.

Bundle of His

This has already been described as the penetrating part of the atrio-ventricular junctional area.

Bundle Branches

When the common bundle reaches the junction between the membranous and the trabecular (muscular) parts of the interventricular septum it divides into the right and left bundle branches. The **left bundle branch** fibres form a broad cascade or fan giving rise to an interweaving subendocardial sheet. The **right bundle branch** is the continuation of the main bundle after the extensive left bundle branch fibres have left it and it continues initially as an unbranched fasciculus in the subendocardial layer of the myocardium on the right side of the interventricular septum. Its earliest branches arise lower in its course than those from the left bundle.

The left bundle branch, whilst spreading into a very broad, fan-like structure, does have recognisable divisions. Controversy exists concerning the question of whether two or three such divisions are recognisable anatomically but from the point of view of recognising distinctions of electrocardiographic significance it is adequate to consider the existence of two such divisions (see Section 2, pages 129 to 138).

Purkinje Network

This arises from the ends of the bundle branches and forms an interweaving network on the subendocardial surface of the ventricles. The fibres pass into the inner third of the myocardium and transmit the impulse from the bundle branches to the myocardial cells. The very rapid conduction of the bundle branches and Purkinje network results in almost simultaneous depolarisation of the endocardial part of the myocardium throughout the right and left ventricles.

Innervation of the Specialised Pacemaking and Conducting Tissue

SA Node

This receives a rich innervation from the sympathetic (adrenergic, transmitter substance noradrenaline) and the parasympathetic (cholinergic) nervous systems. The discharge rate at the SA node responds briskly to sympathetic stimulation (which induces tachycardia) and to parasympathetic stimulation (which induces bradycardia).

AV Node

This also receives a generous sympathetic and parasympathetic innervation. The rate responses are of the same type as, though less pronounced than, those of the AV node. Sympathetic stimulation, however, not only increases the discharge rate of the AV node, it also shortens the AV nodal conduction time and the duration of the AV nodal refractory period. Conversely, parasympathetic stimulation not only decreases the discharge rate from the AV node, it also prolongs the AV nodal conduction time and refractory period. (Sympathetic stimulation also shortens and parasympathetic stimulation also prolongs the refractory period of atrial myocardium).

In general the innervation of the nodes displays a side preference. Stimulation of the sympathetic or parasympathetic on the right predominantly affects the SA node whereas stimulation on the left predominantly affects the AV node.

His-Purkinje Network

In contrast to their effects on the SA and AV nodes, sympathetic and parasympathetic stimulation have relatively minor effects on the His-Purkinje discharge rate, system conduction time or refractory period. Nevertheless sympathetic stimulation does increase the discharge rate and shorten the conduction time and refractory period, and parasympathetic stimulation has the opposite effects, though in all cases the changes are of modest degree. Stimulation of the right-sided sympathetic or parasympathetic fibres predominantly affects the Purkinje network on the anterior and stimulation of the left-sided sympathetic or parasympathetic fibres predominantly the posterior parts of the right and left ventricles. For many years it was felt that there was no parasympathetic innervation of the ventricular part of the conducting tissue, but it is now known that such innervation does exist.

The Blood Supply of the Specialised Pacemaker and Conducting Tissue

SA Node

This receives its blood supply from the right coronary artery or from the circumflex branch of the left coronary artery (with roughly equal frequency) and occasionally from both of these arteries.

AV Node

This node, like the SA node, has a specific and rich blood supply. The AV nodal artery arises from the right coronary artery in about 95 per cent of persons and from the circumflex branch of the left coronary artery in five per cent. Again there is sometimes a dual supply.

His Bundle and Bundle Branches

Unlike the SA and AV nodes, each of which has its own individual artery which is disproportionately large for the mere metabolic needs of the tissue, the His bundle and bundle branches do not have dedicated arteries. The most important supply comes from the anterior septal perforating branches of the anterior descending division of the left coronary artery with a lesser supply from the posterior septal perforating branches of the posterior descending branch of the right coronary artery.

Purkinje Network

Like the His bundles and bundle branches the Purkinje network has no specific arterial supply. Supply is from the artery serving adjacent myocardium. Some limited flow may occur from the ventricular cavities into the subendocardial area of myocardium (which contains the Purkinje network) but the subendocardial zone is known to be strikingly vulnerable to myocardial ischaemia.

Physiology of the Normal Cardiac Rhythm

The Basis of the Resting Membrane Potential

The voltage difference across the myocardial cell membrane is dependent upon the cell membrane structure which determines the permeabilities of the membrane to the ions and the ionic gradients across the membrane.

The Myocardial Cell Membrane (The Sarcolemma)

This consists of a double layer of phospholipid molecules. The outer layer has the polar (and hydrophilic) component of the phospholipid molecules on the outside, in contact with the extracellular fluid and the inner layer has these components on the inside, in contact with the intracellular fluid. Both layers thus have the non-polar (and hydrophobic) components of the molecules towards the centre of the membrane (Figure 183).
The phospholipid, hydrophobic core of the sarcolemma provides a high resistance insulating cover around the cell. This wrapping exhibits differential ionic permeability.

The phospholipoprotein elements in the sarcolemma act as gates or channels, through which ionic movement can occur. These gates are influenced by adjacent electric fields and change with time. These two variations result in "opening" and "closing" of selective ion gates.

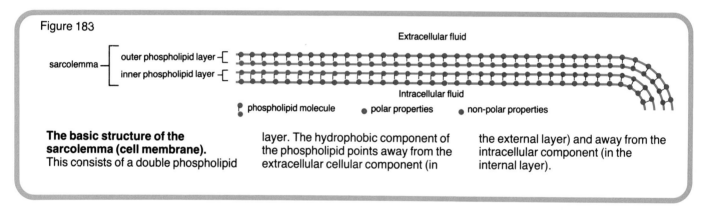

Figure 183

sarcolemma — outer phospholipid layer
inner phospholipid layer

Extracellular fluid

Intracellular fluid

● phospholipid molecule   ● polar properties   ● non-polar properties

The basic structure of the sarcolemma (cell membrane).
This consists of a double phospholipid layer. The hydrophobic component of the phospholipid points away from the extracellular cellular component (in the external layer) and away from the intracellular component (in the internal layer).

Transmembrane Ionic Gradients and Permeabilities

All cardiac cells at rest are polarised, that is the inside of the cell is negatively charged with respect to the outside (see Section 1, page 8). The transmembrane voltage which results from this state of polarisation of the membrane can be measured in experimental situations by introducing a microelectrode tip through the membrane into the cavity of the cell. The transmembrane voltage of the resting myocardial cell (the "resting membrane potential") measured in this way is found to be of the order of −90mV (inside negative with respect to outside). This potential is some hundred times larger than that recorded on the surface of the body as the electrocardiogram. This resting membrane potential arises as a result of the unequal distribution of ions across the cell membrane combined with unequal permeabilities of the membrane to the given ions. The **permeabilities** and the **concentrations** of the ions are independently relevant to the developed membrane potential.

The respective concentrations of the important ionic constituents of intracellular and of extracellular fluid are given in Table 11.

Table 11			
	Concentration		
Ion	Extracellular (E)	Intracellular (I)	Ratio (E/I)
Na^+	145	15	9.7
K^+	4	150	0.027
Cl^-	120	5	24
Ca^{++}	2	10^{-4}	2×10^4

Ions differ from one another in their physical size and in the charge which they carry. Ions which have a large positive charge and a small surface area have a high surface charge density. This feature enables them to attract further electrons (negative charges) and to hold them within their sphere of influence. Water presents a readily available source of electrons since the oxygen atom in the water molecule is electron-rich. An ion with a high surface charge density may surround itself by an organised arrangement of water molecules. These are held in position by electrical attraction and the ion is said to be "hydrated". The state of hydration increases the effective size of the ion. This is particularly important in respect of sodium and potassium ions. Sodium ions have a smaller ionic radius than potassium ions. Both ions have the same charge and therefore sodium ions have a greater surface charge density. The size of the hydrated sodium ion is therefore larger than that of the hydrated potassium ion and its mobility is therefore less.

The uneven distribution of ions across the cell membrane results in chemical gradients (i.e. gradients of ionic concentration) across the membrane. The fact that the membrane is polarised and that the ions carry a charge results in the presence of electrical gradients across the membrane. The presence of non-diffusible (protein) anions within the cell plays an important part in establishing the dynamic equilibrium which exists. The relation which in practice obtains between the various important variables is expressed in the Goldman equation:

$$E = -\frac{RT}{nF} \ln \frac{P_K[K^+]_o + P_{Na}[Na^+]_o + P_{Cl}[Cl^-]_i}{P_K[K^+]_i + P_{Na}[Na^+]_i + P_{Cl}[Cl^-]_o}$$

Where

E is the transmembrane potential

R is the universal gas constant

F is Faraday's number

n is the ionic charge and sign

P_K is the membrane permeability to potassium

P_{Na} is the membrane permeability to sodium

P_{Cl} is the membrane permeability to chloride

$[K^+]_o$ and $[K^+]_i$ are the extracellular and intracellular potassium ion concentrations, respectively.

$[Na^+]_o$ and $[Na^+]_i$ are the extracellular and intracellular sodium ion concentrations, respectively.

$[Cl^-]_o$ and $[Cl^-]_i$ are the extracellular and intracellular chloride ion concentrations, respectively.

When the known values for the constants and appropriate normal values for the ionic permeabilities and concentrations are inserted into the equation the voltage obtained is of the order of −90mV which is very close to that obtained in practice by direct measurements using microelectrodes.

Under normal physiological conditions with the membrane at rest P_K >>P_{Na}. Therefore, for a first order approximation P_{Na} may be equated to zero and the equation simplifies to:

$$E \simeq -\frac{RT}{nF} \ln \frac{P_K[K^+]_o + P_{Cl}[Cl^-]_i}{P_K[K^+]_i + P_{Cl}[Cl^-]_o}$$

Since $P_K \simeq P_{Cl}$

$$[K^+]_o \simeq [Cl^-]_i$$

and $[K^+]_i \simeq [Cl^-]_o$

This may be further simplified to:

$$E \simeq -\frac{RT}{nF} \ln \frac{2 P_K[K^+]_o}{2 P_K[K^+]_i}$$

and therefore to

$$E \simeq -\frac{RT}{nF} \ln \frac{[K^+]_o}{[K^+]_i}$$

This is known as the Nernst equation. If known values for the constants and the physiological variables of the resting membrane are inserted into this equation, a value for E of −98mV is obtained, again close to the observed value. **Thus the voltage across the membrane at rest is predominantly determined by the internal and external potassium concentrations.**

Action Potential

When the membrane is at rest the voltage is effectively determined by the ratio of intra- to extracellular potassium concentrations and remains at a steady level of approximately −90mV. This "resting membrane potential" (Phase 4, Figure 184) is disturbed when the cell is stimulated sufficiently to induce "depolarisation". During depolarisation the inside of the cell becomes transiently positive with respect to the outside (Phase 0, Figure 184). Although this process is called depolarisation it is actually a transient partial reverse polarisation. This **induced** depolaristion is inevitably followed by the **spontaneous** process of repolarisation (Phases 1, 2 and 3, Figure 184) which is a slow and complicated process by which the status quo of the resting potential is restored. The whole polarisation – repolarisation process (Phase 0, 1, 2 and 3) is called the **action potential.**

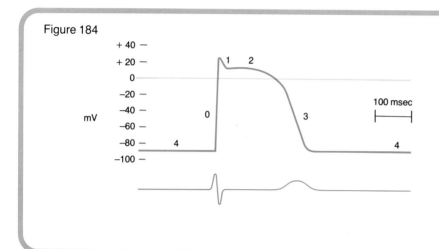

Figure 184

100 msec

mV

The action potential.
The resting membrane potential is about −90 mV. The onset of depolarisation (Phase 0) does not occur spontaneously but must be induced. This induced depolarisation (which gives rise to a "partial reverse polarisation" with the inside of the cell transiently becoming somewhat positive with respect to the outside) is inevitably followed spontaneously by the slow and complex process of repolarisation (Phases 2 and 3) before the resting potential (Phase 4) is restored.

The induction of Phase 0 of the action potential is produced by a sudden dramatic rise in the P_{Na} resulting from the opening of sodium channels in the membrane. This becomes transiently much larger than P_K or P_{Cl} and, under such conditions the Goldman equation simplifies to:

$$E \simeq -\frac{RT}{nF} \ln \frac{[Na^+]_o}{[Na^+]_i}$$

Insertion of known values into this equation produces a voltage of +46mV which is similar to that obtained by microelectrode recordings at the peak of Phase 0 of the action potential. Note that, although ions do flow across the membrane, the net ionic movement is very small and certainly insufficient to have a significant effect on the intracellular content of sodium ions. It is the change in ion **permeability** rather than the **ionic flux** or **change in ionic concentration** which induces the change in transmembrane voltage. Nevertheless a tiny number of sodium ions do enter the cell during depolarisation. During the recovery period complicated changes in permeabilities and fluxes of Na^+, K^+, Cl^- and Ca^{++} occur and the voltage is restored to the resting level. A minute net influx of Na^+ ions has occurred. This has to be rectified to prevent major long-term disturbances and there is a constant extrusion of sodium ions maintained by the **"sodium pump"** of the cell membrane which is metabolically active. This process is dependent upon the availability of ATP.

Propagated Action Potential

If an action potential is induced at one part of a cell membrane, it will inevitably spread to all other parts of that cell membrane and to the membranes of all cells with which it is in electrical continuity. The spread occurs because of the production of "battery conditions" (adjacent + and − charges) at the border zones between depolarised (peak Phase 0) and polarised (Phase 4) parts of the membrane (see Section 1, Figure 10, page 10). If a recording is made from a part of the cell distant from the point of initiation of the depolarisation, an action potential will be recorded after a suitable time has elapsed for transmission of the impulse. This is called the **propagated action potential.**

Threshold Potential

When a stimulus is applied to a cell which has a normal resting membrane potential, an action potential will ensue only if the stimulus is sufficient to raise (i.e. render less negative) the membrane potential at least to the critical level known as the **threshold potential.** Once this level (typically of the order of −60mV (Figure 185)) has been achieved the development of the action potential is inevitable.

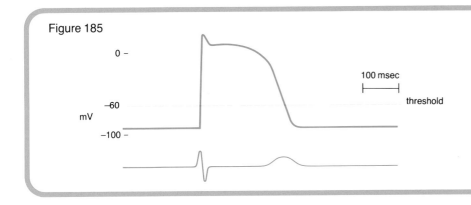

Figure 185

The threshold potential.
The interrupted line shows the threshold potential. An action potential follows when, and only when, the intracellular voltage is raised (rendered less negative) above the threshold level of approximately −60 mV.

Refractory Period

During the inscription of the action potential the cell becomes absolutely refractory, i.e. it cannot be activated again no matter how powerful the stimulus.

This **absolute refractory period** (ARP) begins when the transmembrane voltage has ascended to about −50mV and continues until the voltage falls again to approximately −55mV (Figure 186). (The level at which the absolute refractory period ends is similar to, but not identical to, the threshold level).

When the transmembrane voltage falls below approximately −55mV it becomes capable of being stimulated again (i.e. the sodium channels can be opened once more) though it will require a stronger stimulus than it did initially when the membrane voltage was −90mV. This responsive (but less responsive than normal) period of the membrane is called the **relative refractory period** (RRP).

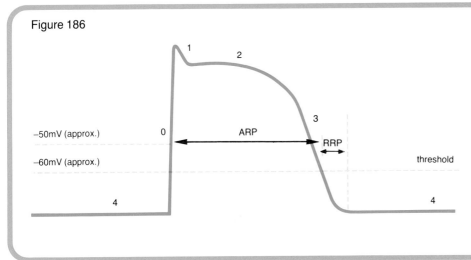

Figure 186

The refractory period.
The membrane becomes refractory once Phase 0 of the action potential ascends to approximately −50 mV. It remains **absolutely** refractory until Phase 3 of the action potential descends to approximately −55mV. From that point the membrane becomes **relatively relatively** refractory until the resting potential is restored. At this point, which indicates the commencement of Phase 4, the refractory period ends and the membrane becomes normally responsive once more.

Pacemaker Activity (Automaticity)

The most important feature which distinguishes pacemaker cells from myocardial cells is the absence of a "resting" (Phase 4) potential (Figure 187). In the case of pacemaker cells, Phase 4 is upsloping. The result of this is that the threshold potential is reached spontaneously and a spontaneous action potential results. Repolarisation then follows spontaneously and the whole cycle repeats spontaneously.

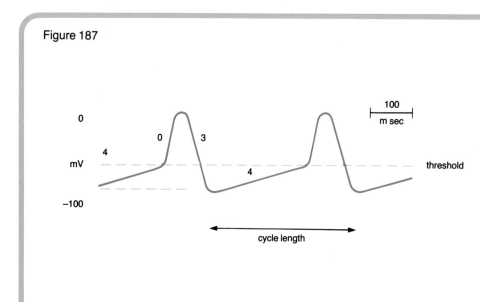

Figure 187

100 m sec

0

mV

−100

0   3

4

4

threshold

cycle length

The action potential of a pacemaker cell. Once the threshold level is reached spontaneous depolarisation (Phase 0) occurs and an action potential is produced. Phases 1 and 2 (as seen in the myocardial cells) are not apparent but Phase 3 repolarisation follows, restoring the maximum (most negative) diastolic potential from which the sloping Phase 4 again ensues giving rise to a further spontaneous action potential. The pacemaker cells thus have the property of rhythmicity or automaticity. The reciprocal of the time interval between identical points in consecutive cycles (i.e. the reciprocal of the cycle length) gives the discharge rate of the pacemaker.

Distribution of Pacemaker Tissue

Pacemaker activity (automaticity) is, in normal circumstances, confined to the tissues of the sino-atrial node, atrio-ventricular node, His bundle, right and left bundle branches and Purkinje network and the anatomy of this tissue has already been described (pages 342 to 344).

Intrinsic Rate of Pacemaker Tissue

Automaticity is a property common to all cells in the pacemaking and conducting tissue. Equally, all these cells are subject to influence by autonomic neural impulses and by changes in the circulating blood levels of catecholamines, P_{CO_2}, P_{O_2}, pH, blood temperature and other factors. Each cell has its own intrinsic discharge rate. The intrinsic rate of a cell is the rate at which the given cell would give rise to spontaneous depolarisations when perfused at normal physiological levels of P_{CO_2}, P_{O_2}, pH and temperature and when isolated from neural and humoral influences. The intrinsic pacing rate varies according to the location of the cell within the pacemaking and conducting tissue and also with the age of the subject. Thus the sino-atrial node may have an intrinsic discharge rate of 130-140 beats per minute at birth, may be 100-110 in youth and may fall to 70-80 in old age. At any given age the intrinsic discharge rate is highest in the SA node and progressively lower as one moves down the pacing system. Purkinje fibres may thus have a typical intrinsic discharge rate of 20 beats per minute.

Dominant Pacemaker

Since all the cells in the pacemaking and conducting tissue have the property of automaticity, any cell might be expected to give rise to spontaneous depolarisation. If this were to happen chaotic multifocal activity would be anticipated. However, since, in the normal heart, all excitable tissue is in electrical continuity with all other excitable tissue and since pacemaker cells, like other excitable cells, can **be depolarised** by an electrical stimulus arriving at that cell from elsewhere, the cell with the fastest discharge rate **at that moment** will, in normal circumstances, be the effective pacemaker at that time (Figure 188).

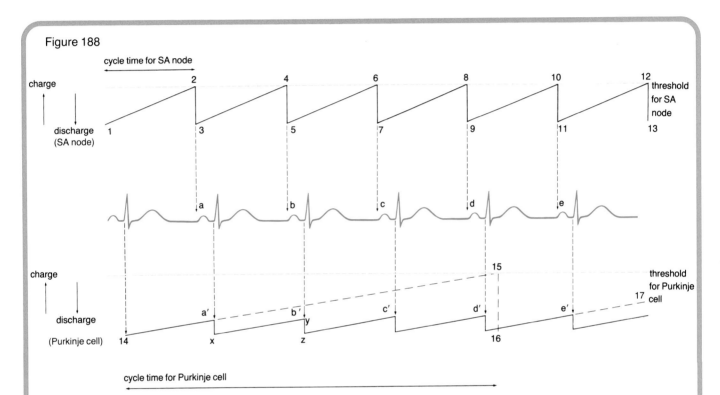

Figure 188

Suppression of subsidiary pacemakers by pacemaker tissue with higher intrinsic discharge rates

Sinus rhythm. The sinus rate is 60 beats/minute so that the cycle time for the sino-atrial node is one second. The upper ramp shows the charge/discharge cycle for the SA node. Thus the SA node charges from 1, reaches threshold at 2 and discharges, re-charges from 3 reaches threshold at 4 and discharges etc. SA nodal discharge (2-3; 4-5 etc) is followed by atrial myocardial depolarisation (indicated by the P waves which immediately follow lines a, b etc). The usual sequence of P, QRS, T then ensues with each cycle.
Consider the changes occurring in a Purkinje cell which has a cycle time of

4.2 sec (i.e. rate approximately 15 beats/min) and which commences its charging cycle (14) immediately after it has just been depolarised by the spread of the depolarising wave from the SA node, via the His bundle and bundle branches. If it were allowed to reach its threshold uninterrupted it would discharge at 15, start charging up again from 16 along and passing through 17 etc. This, however, does not occur. The SA nodal depolarisation 2-3 induces atrial myocardial depolarisation (a) and subsequently ventricular myocardial depolarisation. In the course of the latter (a') the depolarisation reaches

the Purkinje fibre which is still less than one quarter through its repolarisation time, causing it to be depolarised prematurely at x. Repolarisation of this Purkinje cell commences along xy only to be prematurely terminated again at yz. In this way a pacemaker with a faster discharge rate (i.e. shorter cycle time) will prematurely depolarise all pacemakers with slower discharge rates (longer cycle times) with which it is in electrical contact and the fastest pacemaker will become the effective pacemaker cell.

Electrophysiology of Rhythm Abnormalities

Control of the Basic Sinus Rate

The discharge rate of the SA node (as of any other pacemaker cell) depends upon the cycle length of its spontaneously repeating action potential (Figure 189a).

The discharge rate is increased whenever the cycle length duration is reduced. This can be achieved (Figure 189b) by:
1. increasing the slope of Phase 4 of the action potential, (Figure 189 b, (i))
2. decreasing (i.e. rendering more negative) the threshold potential, (Figure 189 b, (ii))
3. increasing (i.e. rendering less negative) the level of diastolic polarisation (DP), (Figure 189 b, (iii))
4. by a combination of the above factors.

These electrophysiological variations provide the mechanisms whereby the sinus rate is physiologically controlled. The most important of the mechanisms is variation in the slope of Phase 4. The slope of Phase 4 of the action potential is increased (and therefore the pacemaker firing rate is increased) by sympathetic nerve stimulation, infusion of noradrenaline or adrenaline, increased blood temperature, decreased blood pH, etc. The slope of Phase 4 (and consequently the pacemaker firing rate) is decreased by parasympathetic nerve stimulation, infusion of acetylcholine, decrease of blood temperature etc. In this way the SA node is able to modify the heart rate to respond to the varying metabolic needs of the body. **Sinus tachycardia, sinus bradycardia** and **sinus arrhythmia** are produced predominantly by modification in the Phase 4 slope of the cells of the SA node.

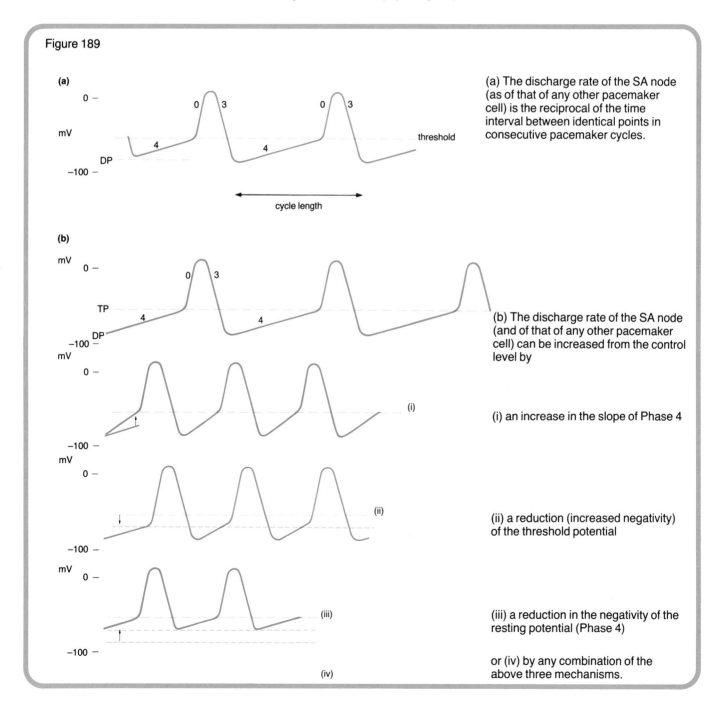

Figure 189

(a) The discharge rate of the SA node (as of that of any other pacemaker cell) is the reciprocal of the time interval between identical points in consecutive pacemaker cycles.

(b) The discharge rate of the SA node (and of that of any other pacemaker cell) can be increased from the control level by

(i) an increase in the slope of Phase 4

(ii) a reduction (increased negativity) of the threshold potential

(iii) a reduction in the negativity of the resting potential (Phase 4)

or (iv) by any combination of the above three mechanisms.

Impulse Formation from Ectopic Pacemaker Sites

As discussed earlier, the pacemaker which actually initiates a cardiac cycle is the one with the fastest discharge rate at that time, provided the pacemaker in question is in electrical continuity with all other excitable cells within the heart. In normal circumstances the sinus node fulfils these criteria.

Pacemaker activity may occur from ectopic sites as a result of the discharge of latent or subsidiary pacemakers. These are located in parts of the atria, the coronary sinus, the AV nodal (junctional) area, the His bundle, the bundle branches or the Purkinje network. Such sites may take over the pacing function in the heart for one or more

beats either as a result of speeding up of that pacemaker site (most commonly by increase in its rate of Phase 4 depolarisation) – in which case the beat is **premature** (i.e. occurred earlier than would have been anticipated on the basis of prior experience) – **or** it may occur because the existing pacemaker (usually the SA node) slows down to such a degree that a particular, subsidiary or latent pacemaker reaches threshold and depolarises first (without any change in its Phase 4 depolarisation rate). Such a beat is called an **escape** beat. Premature beats and escape beats are both ectopic. They both result from automaticity in the given pacemaker cell.

Premature Depolarisations (Premature Beats)

These occur when a subsidiary pacemaker reaches depolarisation threshold earlier than expected and before the next scheduled sinus node depolarisation (Figure 190). This can happen because of an increase in the Phase 4 slope (as shown in Figure190), because of a reduced (more negative) threshold potential, because of a less negative diastolic polarisation or because of a combination of these.

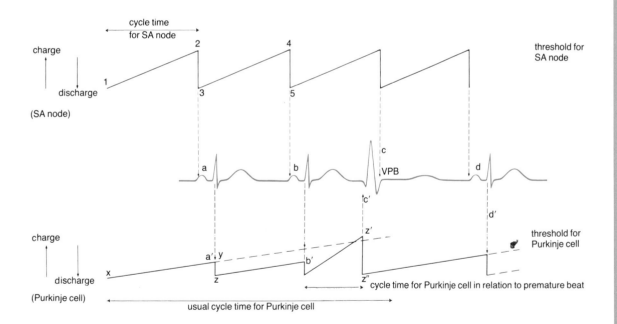

Figure 190 **A ventricular premature beat**

The electrocardiogram shows two sinus beats, a ventricular premature beat (VPB) and a further sinus beat. Activity of the SA nodal pacemaker is shown by the line 1,2,3,4,5 etc. Spontaneous activity of a Purkinje cell is shown as line xy. If this cell were not prematurely discharged by depolarisation spreading to the ventricles as a result of depolarisation spreading to the ventricles initiated at the SA node at a and b it would continue along the interrupted line extending from xy.

The first two beats are initiated by

sinus node depolarisation giving rise to atrial depolarisation (a, b) and then by conduction within the heart, to the first two (normal) QRS complexes. During the inscription of each of these QRS complexes the depolarisation reaches the Purkinje cell which is therefore prematurely depolarised (and "reset") at a' and b'. Something then happens to the Purkinje cell to cause it to reach threshold much sooner than usual (at z'). At this stage the sinus node has not yet reached threshold and no depolarisation wave is travelling through the heart. The

Purkinje cell is therefore able to depolarise the ventricular myocardium (c') and a ventricular premature beat (VPB) occurs. This depolarisation does not spread backwards through the AV node and therefore the SA node is not prematurely reset. The next P wave therefore occurs on schedule at c but is obscured by the QRS of the ventricular premature beat which occurs at the same time. The third QRS complex is both **ectopic** and **premature**. The next P wave at d is followed by a QRS as at a and b.

Escape Depolarisations (Escape Beats)

These occur either when the prevailing pacemaker ceases to depolarise or when its depolarisation is delayed, and the subsidiary pacemaker is allowed to achieve threshold without its depolarisation ramp being aborted as is usually the case when the prevailing pacemaker is functioning normally (Figure 191). This subsidiary pacemaker has then "escaped" from the normally dominant influence of the prevailing pacemaker and has exerted its standby function.

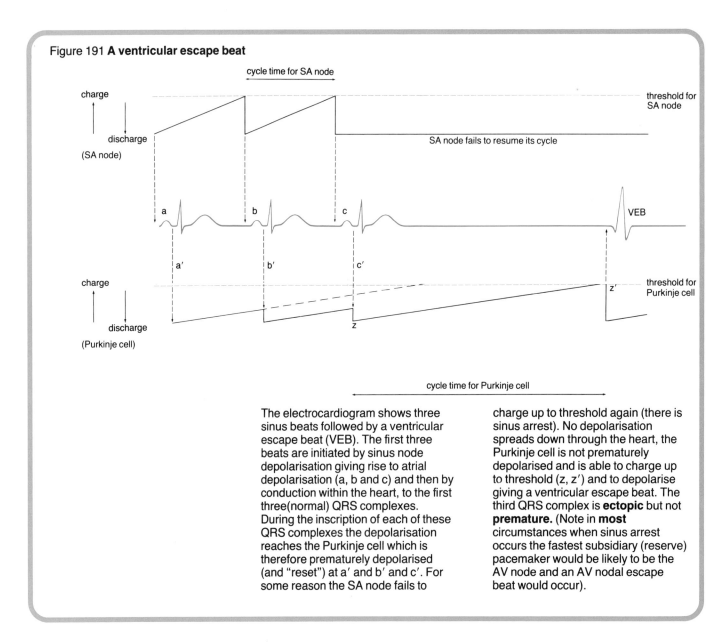

Figure 191 **A ventricular escape beat**

The electrocardiogram shows three sinus beats followed by a ventricular escape beat (VEB). The first three beats are initiated by sinus node depolarisation giving rise to atrial depolarisation (a, b and c) and then by conduction within the heart, to the first three (normal) QRS complexes. During the inscription of each of these QRS complexes the depolarisation reaches the Purkinje cell which is therefore prematurely depolarised (and "reset") at a′ and b′ and c′. For some reason the SA node fails to charge up to threshold again (there is sinus arrest). No depolarisation spreads down through the heart, the Purkinje cell is not prematurely depolarised and is able to charge up to threshold (z, z′) and to depolarise giving a ventricular escape beat. The third QRS complex is **ectopic** but not **premature.** (Note in **most** circumstances when sinus arrest occurs the fastest subsidiary (reserve) pacemaker would be likely to be the AV node and an AV nodal escape beat would occur).

Parasystolic Depolarisations (Parasystole)

These are depolarisations arising from subsidiary (ectopic) pacemakers which are "protected" from the influence of dominant (more rapid) pacemakers by **"entrance block"**. This term implies that the parasystolic focus is insulated from surrounding electrical events (classically parasystolic foci have been considered to be **completely** isolated from incoming depolarisation and thus to behave like a fixed rate (asynchronous) pacemaker but recent studies have indicated that the dominant cardiac rhythm can produce some modulation of the parasystolic discharge by speeding it up or slowing it down). Occasionally parasystolic foci may exhibit intermittent **"exit block"**, i.e. the impulse may intermittently fail to depolarise adjacent excitable myocardium. Figure 192 shows the mechanism of parasystole.

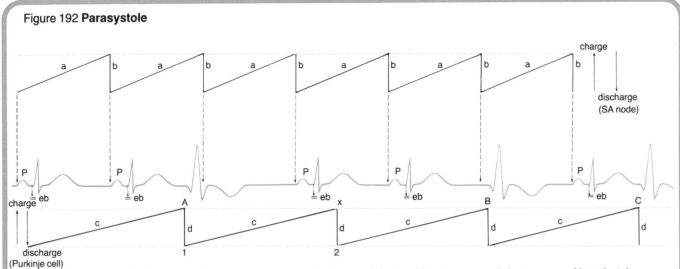

Figure 192 **Parasystole**

Sinus node repolarisation takes place repetitively at a and depolarisation takes place at b. Sinus depolarisation is followed by atrial myocardial depolarisation at P. Each P wave is followed in the normal way by a QRS complex. The QRS complex indicates ventricular myocardial depolarisation and normally all Purkinje cells would be depolarised during the QRS complex. However, if a parasystolic Purkinje cell focus is "protected" from the oncoming depolarisation wave by "entrance block" (eb) the Purkinje

cell can depolarise repetitively without any suppression from the sinus beats. The Purkinje cell will therefore repetitively repolarise at c and depolarise at d. When Purkinje cell depolarisation occurs between the onset of the QRS complex from the sinus-initiated beats and the end of the T wave of such beats, the ventricles are refractory (e.g. at x) and no ectopic beat is seen. When the Purkinje cell depolarisation occurs at times when the ventricles are not refractory (e.g. at A, B and C) an

ectopic beat occurs. Note that, in parasystole, the sinus mechanisms and the ectopic mechanisms are entirely independent and the coupling intervals between the "revealed" ectopic beats (A, B and C) and the respective preceding sinus beats are not constant. Note also that the time interval between consecutive recorded parasystolic beats is an integral multiple (in the case of A and B, a factor of two times and in the case of B and C a factor of one times) of the basic parasystolic interval (1-2).

Disorders of Impulse Conduction

Normal Conduction Velocities

The ability of heart muscle to conduct ("conductivity") is related to its rhythmicity (automaticity) and excitability.

Conduction velocities within the heart vary at different locations (Table 12).

Table 12

Location	Typical conduction velocity (mm/sec)
Atrial myocardium	800 – 1,000
AV node (AV junction)	200
His-Purkinje system	4,000
Ventricular myocardium	400

Decreased Conductivity

A depressed zone of conductivity in the conducting tissue may give rise to abnormal conduction in three possible ways:
1. Conduction of an impulse may fail completely at one point in the conducting system because of an anatomically sudden **decline in conductivity** at that point.
2. The cardiac impulse may actually pass through the depressed zone but may subsequently have a **slower than normal conduction velocity.**
3. Propagation of the impulse may be possible in one direction but not in the other (**unidirectional conduction**). If an

impulse arrives at two adjacent parallel zones, one of which has depressed conduction and one normal, the impulse may pass through the normally conducting area adjacent to the non-conducting area but may spend sufficient time passing parallel to the area of decreased conductivity for the latter to recover and permit the depolarisation wave to enter it and to spread both antegrade and retrograde. When this happens re-entry (circus movement) becomes a possibility.

Re-entry

This phenomenon, also known as circus movement, re-entrant excitation, reciprocal beating or echo beating, can only occur when there is unidirectional block.

Re-entry is an extremely important phenomenon which is probably the cause of most supraventricular and ventricular tachycardias, flutter and fibrillation. An understanding of the principles of re-entry is essential for an understanding of the modes of initiation and of management of many tachyarrhythmias (Figure 193).

Figure 193

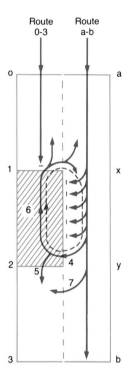

An oncoming impulse travels down two adjacent routes (a-b and 0-3). Route a-b has completely recovered from earlier depolarisations, route 0-3 has a segment (1-2) which has not yet recovered from the previous depolarisation. The impulse in route 0-3 therefore stops at 1. The impulse in route a-b continues normally along this route and also tries to enter the zone 1-2. It repeatedly finds this zone refractory until it reaches position 4 by which time the segment 1-2 has recovered and the impulse can enter. The impulse then travels in both directions (5 and 6) along the segment 1-2. The segment 2-3 will be depolarised by whichever impulse (5 or 7) arrives first. The impulse 6 will spread back into segment 0-1 and the potential for a repetitive loop (interrupted red line) exists. Conduction of the initial and all subsequent depolarisations along x-y must be sufficiently slow to allow time for segment 2-1 to recover if the re-entry mechanism is to recover. The cycle may then repeat.

Obviously the same effect can be achieved when there is a true unidirectional block (as opposed to a temporary unidirectional block due to prolonged refractoriness) in segment 1-2 (Figure 194).

Figure 194

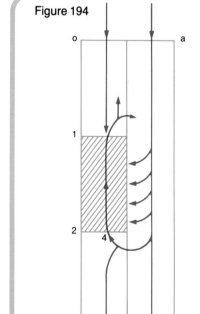

Impulse 0-1 stops at 1 because of unidirectional block. The impulse is able to enter segment 1-2 at 4. Segment 1-2 can conduct 2 → 1 but not 1 → 2. The potential for re-entry exists.

Effective "unidirectional block" is often an accidental consequence of the timing of the oncoming impulse and differences in refractory period between two parts of the conducting tissue or myocardium. Thus if an impulse travels down two adjacent parts of conducting or myocardial tissue (Figure 193), it may encounter tissue still refractory in one route. If so it will be unable to excite it. After passage down the non-refractory route the impulse may be able to re-enter the distal end of the now-recovered but formerly refractory tissue and set up a re-entry circus. Sufficient time must elapse during travel down the adjacent non-refractory tissue to permit the refractory tissue to recover. This means either that the length of recovered tissue must be considerable or the conduction slow. In practice (since really long segments of tissue are rarely available) this means slow conduction along x-y in Figure 193. This can easily be demonstrated. Let us assume a normal refractory period of 0.35 sec and a myocardial conduction velocity of 400 mm/sec. Then the length of myocardium required along a segment x-y to permit the re-entry phenomenon would be given by the length required for the conduction time to exceed the refractory period. The conduction time would have to be at least 0.35 sec and since:

$$\text{velocity} = \frac{\text{distance}}{\text{time}}$$

$$400 \ (\text{mm/sec}) = \frac{l \ (\text{mm})}{0.35 \ (\text{sec})} \quad \text{where } l \text{ is the length x-y}$$

It follows that
$$l = 140\text{mm}$$
$$= 14\text{cm}$$

If refractoriness is prolonged (say to 0.6 sec) an even longer strip would be needed (21 cm).

However, if the conduction velocity during x-y were severely reduced, re-entry could occur even in the presence of a prolonged refractory period. In some disease states conduction velocity in myocardium or Purkinje tissue can be as slow as 30 mm/sec. Then, even with a refractory period of 0.6 sec, a pathway of only 18mm would suffice and such a pathway could easily occur.

The requirements for re-entry are:

1. An available circuit.
2. Unequal excitability in the two parts of the circuit (one link of the circuit may show unidirectional block or may simply be refractory when the impulse arrives).
3. Slow conduction in the more responsive limb of the circuit.

Triggered Activity

This abnormal type of impulse formation is pacemaker activity arising from a cell or group of cells as an abnormal secondary depolarisation following a preceding impulse or series of impulses. The triggered activity is initiated by oscillatory "after potentials". These may occur **before** or **after** full repolarisation of the cell and are then known as **early** or **late** after depolarisations respectively (Figure 195).

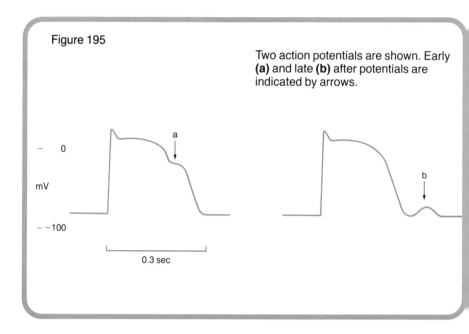

Figure 195

Two action potentials are shown. Early **(a)** and late **(b)** after potentials are indicated by arrows.

If an after depolarisation reaches threshold potential it may trigger another action potential, with a subsequent further after depolarisation and may therefore be self-perpetuating (Figure 196).

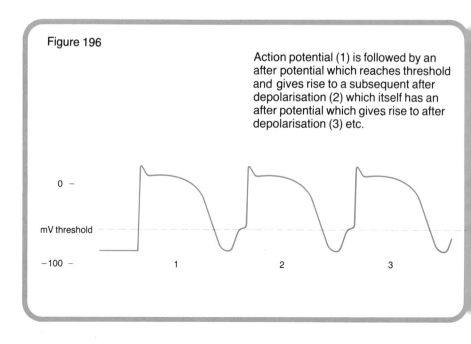

Figure 196

Action potential (1) is followed by an after potential which reaches threshold and gives rise to a subsequent after depolarisation (2) which itself has an after potential which gives rise to after depolarisation (3) etc.

Clinical Correlations with Electrophysiology

Although much is known about normal and abnormal electrophysiological mechanisms within the heart the correlation of these mechanisms with clinically recognisable arrhythmias is uncertain and at present is largely speculative. However, a possible association of clinical arrhythmias with electrophysiological mechanisms is given in Table 13.

Table 13 Probable Mechanisms of Common Arrhythmias

Rhythm	Probable mechanisms
1. Sinus tachycardia Sinus bradycardia Sinus arrhythmia	modulation of normal pacemaker activity by neuro-humoral autonomic influences
2. Atrial escape rhythm Junctional escape rhythm Ventricular escape rhythm	normal spontaneous automaticity occurring in the context of depressed activity at the SA node
Non-paroxysmal junctional tachycardia Idioventricular rhythm Parasystole	enhanced automaticity
3. First degree heart block Second degree heart block Third degree heart block Right bundle branch block* Left bundle branch block* Left anterior hemiblock* Left posterior hemiblock*	selective depression of conduction
4. Atrial flutter Atrial fibrillation† Paroxysmal atrial tachycardia Paroxysmal junctional tachycardia Reciprocating tachycardia of ventricular pre-excitation Paroxysmal ventricular tachycardia Ventricular fibrillation	re-entry
5. Digitalis-induced arrhythmia Hypokalaemia-induced arrhythmias Non-paroxysmal atrial tachycardia Arrhythmias in patients with mitral valve prolapse	may be due to **triggered** activity

* Not classified as arrhythmias since they do not disturb the ordered sequence of depolarisation of atrial and ventricular myocardium.

†In the case of atrial fibrillation, multiple localised re-entrant circuits within the atrial myocardium are postulated.

Note 1

2 and 5 are types of arrhythmia related to automaticity – 2 to spontaneous and 5 to triggered automaticity.

Note 2

3 and 4 are types of depressed conduction. 3 results in clinically apparent conduction problems but 4, whilst physiologically dependent on depressed conduction, manifests itself directly as a tachydysrhythmia.

Approach to Rhythm Analysis

The analysis of the cardiac rhythm presents considerably more difficulties than the morphological analysis of the electrocardiogram and no truly adequate systematic approach has yet been devised. It will, therefore, not be possible to produce a **simple** scheme for rhythm analysis which copes **comprehensively** with all possible arrhythmias. There must inevitably be a trade-off between the simplicity of the approach and the extent to which all possible arrhythmias are catered for. This is similar to the compromise required between sensitivity and specificity (see Section 2, page 108) in the electrocardiographic criteria for given abnormalities. The aim at this stage will be to make the approach as simple as possible and not to try to cover any complex or unusual rhythms. At a later stage (see pages 375-503) individual cardiac rhythms will be described and illustrated. Following these descriptions the reader will (hopefully) be better fitted to follow the slightly more complex approach to rhythm analysis given on pages 557 to 579.

Identification Data and Quality Control

It is essential to check the name, date and **time** (see Section 1, page 62) of the record. Often the electrocardiographic lead used will be a chest lead, but in other circumstances (and preferably always) the lead involved should be labelled. When a choice of lead is possible the choice should be made to ensure that the P waves are as clearly visible as possible. They are **not** (contrary to popular judgement) more important than QRS complexes in rhythm analysis, they are simply more often difficult to see. The chosen leads should show P waves and QRS complexes as clearly as possible and there is normally no difficulty with regard to the latter. In most cases a single (adequate) lead will serve to diagnose the cardiac rhythm but in difficult cases two or more leads may be required.

The record should be of good quality, free from baseline drift, AC interference and skeletal muscle tremor (though in emergency situations these aims may not always be achieved).

Determination of the Heart Rate

The "heart rate" is taken to be synonymous with the "ventricular rate". The heart rate is therefore determined by measuring the frequency of the QRS complexes. In clinical practice the number of pulses per unit time (typically measured over 15 seconds, 30 seconds or one minute) are usually counted but most ECG recordings involve records of a few seconds only and the heart rate is therefore assessed from the reciprocal of the time between consecutive QRS complexes (i.e. from the reciprocal of the R-R interval (Figure 197)).

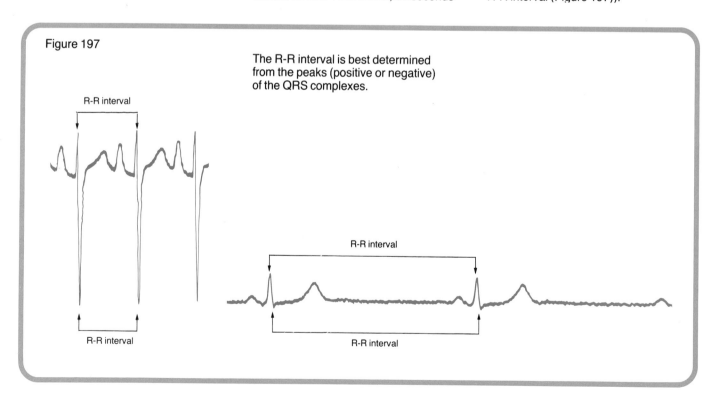

Figure 197

The R-R interval is best determined from the peaks (positive or negative) of the QRS complexes.

The R-R interval is the time interval between identical (as far as can be ascertained) points in consecutive QRS complexes. It is usually easier (Figure 197) to recognise peaks (positive or negative) in QRS complexes rather than the timing of onset. Since the number of R-R intervals per unit time gives the heart rate, the rate per minute is calculated as:

$$\frac{60 \text{ seconds}}{\text{R-R interval in seconds}}$$

The R-R interval is best measured with calipers and the caliper assessment then transferred to the ECG graticule. Alternatively the interval can be measured by making marks corresponding to each R wave on the edge of a straight piece of paper and then transferring this to the graticule. Each small ECG square (at normal paper speed) corresponds to 0.04 seconds and the greatest accuracy one can claim is a resolution of 0.01 seconds (though according to scientific principles one should not really claim accuracy more than 0.02 seconds – i.e. half the minimum measured resolution). More often, the R-R interval is measured in "small ECG squares" (rather than in seconds), i.e. in units of 0.04 seconds and the heart rate is then read as:

$$\frac{1500}{\text{Number of small squares in R-R interval}}$$

since there are 1500 small ECG squares per minute.

The heart rate determined in this way can be assessed from Table 14.

Table 14

Heart rate (per min)	Cycle time (number of 0.04 sec units – small ECG squares)	Cycle time (number of 0.2 sec units – large ECG squares)
300	5	1
250	6	
214	7	
187	8	
166	9	
150	10	2
136	11	
125	12	
115	13	
107	14	
100	15	3
93	16	
88	17	
83	18	
78	19	
75	20	4
71	21	
68	22	
65	23	
62	24	
60	25	5
57	26	
55	27	
52	28	
51	29	
50	30	6
48	31	
46	32	
45	33	
43	34	
42	35	7
41	36	
40	37	
39	38	
38	39	
37	40	
36	41	
35	42	
35	43	
34	44	
33	45	
32	46	
32	47	
31	48	
30	49	
30	50	

It is useful to remember the heart rates corresponding to R-R intervals involving an integral number of large ECG squares (Table 14). For example when there are three large ECG squares between consecutive QRS complexes the heart rate is 100, and when there are five such squares the heart rate is 60. **During tachycardias, therefore, there are fewer than three large ECG squares between consecutive QRS complexes and during bradycardias there are more than five large ECG squares between consecutive QRS complexes.**

An alternative method of measuring the heart rate is to use a ruler calibrated in heart rate units. Such a ruler has been prepared by the author and is illustrated in Figure 198.

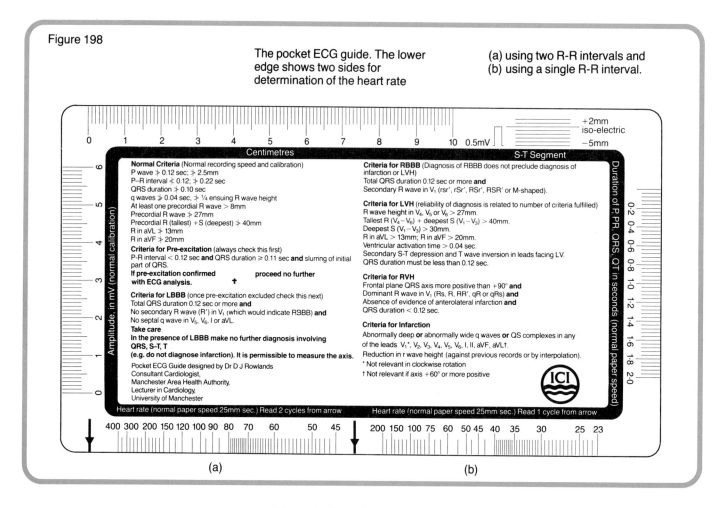

Figure 198

The pocket ECG guide. The lower edge shows two sides for determination of the heart rate (a) using two R-R intervals and (b) using a single R-R interval.

(a)   (b)

The scale shown in such rulers is simply an analogue version of the reciprocal of the R-R interval so that the heart rate can be read off directly. If two consecutive R-R intervals are used the accuracy achieved is doubled.

Many ECG rulers also provide a means of measuring the heart rate when the speed of the recording paper is twice normal. To record the ECG at twice the normal speed seems, to the author, to be a most unhelpful manoeuvre. The usual problem in rhythm interpretation is not in measuring the time interval between identifiable parts of the electrocardiogram, but in identifying parts of the electrocardiogram. This problem is increased, not diminished, by doubling the recording speed (Figure 199).

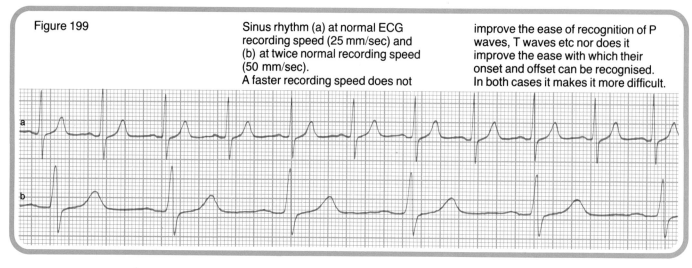

Figure 199

Sinus rhythm (a) at normal ECG recording speed (25 mm/sec) and (b) at twice normal recording speed (50 mm/sec). A faster recording speed does not improve the ease of recognition of P waves, T waves etc nor does it improve the ease with which their onset and offset can be recognised. In both cases it makes it more difficult.

Assessment of Regularity (or otherwise) of the Ventricular Rate

It should be noted that the methods described for assessing the heart rate are valid only if the rate is constant during the period of the recording. Otherwise different rates are obtained depending on the R-R interval of choice (Figure 200).

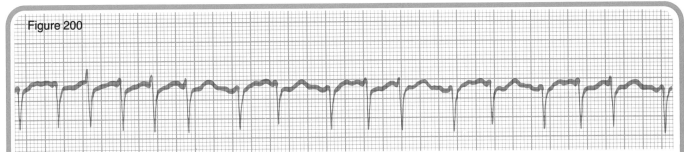

Figure 200

The heart rate (ventricular rate) is irregular. The use of one or two R-R intervals will therefore only give a rate appropriate to the R-R interval chosen or to the average of the two R-R intervals chosen. To obtain a reasonable estimate of the average heart rate the number of R-R intervals (not the number of QRS complexes because the number of QRS complexes is equal to the number of R-R intervals plus one) per 15 seconds should be multiplied by four to give the heart rate per minute (15 seconds is equal to 75 large ECG squares). It might be more convenient to assess the number of R-R intervals per 10, 6 or 5 seconds (50, 30 or 25 large ECG squares respectively) and to multiply respectively by 6, 10 or 12 to obtain the heart rate per minute. Reducing the sampling period naturally reduces the accuracy of the calculated mean heart rate.

A simple way to check the regularity or otherwise of the QRS complexes (if calipers are not available) is to apply a straight-edged piece of paper to the rhythm strip and make marks corresponding to each QRS complex (Figure 201). Subsequent lateral adjustment of the strip rapidly demonstrates whether the QRS rate is regular or not.

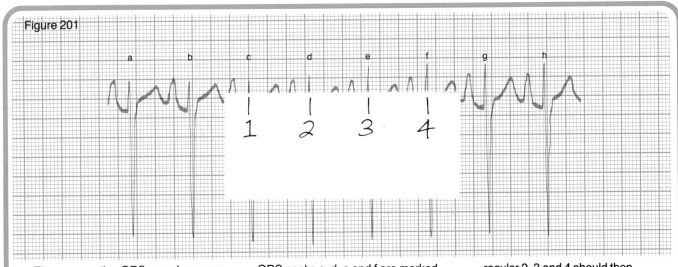

Figure 201

The consecutive QRS complexes are labelled a to h. A blank sheet of paper is placed on the ECG leaving the peaks of the QRS complexes visible. QRS peaks c, d, e and f are marked on the paper (here labelled 1 to 4). The paper is then slid along so that 1 aligns with d. If the heart rate is regular 2, 3 and 4 should then accurately align with e, f and g respectively. If not, the heart rate is irregular.

Assessment of the QRS Complexes

The Heart Rate. Tachycardias and Bradycardias

The most important feature of the QRS complexes, as far as the cardiac rhythm is concerned, is their frequency per minute (the heart rate). When the heart rate (ventricular rate) exceeds 100 beats per minute there is said to be a tachycardia.

Causes of Tachycardia

The causes of a tachycardia are given in Table 15.

Table 15 Causes of a Tachycardia

Sinus tachycardia

Atrial tachycardia

Atrial flutter

Atrial fibrillation

Junctional tachycardia

Ventricular tachycardia

When the heart rate is less than 60 beats per minute there is said to be a bradycardia.

Causes of Bradycardia

The causes of a bradycardia are given in Table 16.

Table 16 Causes of a Bradycardia

Depression of sino-atrial nodal function

Sinus bradycardia*

Junctional rhythm†

Depression of atrio-ventricular conduction

Blocked coupled atrial premature beats

Second degree heart block type I (Wenckebach phenomenon)

Second degree heart block type II (Mobitz type II block)

Third degree heart block

Atrial fibrillation with high degree of AV block #

* If the AV junctional area is not simultaneously depressed, the rhythm may be an "escape" (see page 352) junctional rhythm and the rate may or may not be less than 60 beats per minute.

† The presence of junctional rhythm implies that sino-atrial function is depressed, otherwise the AV junctional area would be depolarised by the cardiac impulse descending to it.

In the presence of atrial fibrillation, waves of depolarisation arrive at irregular intervals at the AV node and atrio-ventricular conduction malfunction cannot be classified as first degree, or second degree type I or type II but third degree block can be recognised (page 439). Defective atrio-ventricular conduction is indicated by the inappropriately slow and regular ventricular rate.

Regularity or Irregularity of the QRS (Ventricular) Rate

A second very important aspect of the QRS complexes in relation to arrhythmias is the regularity or otherwise of the QRS complexes i.e. the constancy or otherwise of the R-R interval.

Causes of Irregularity of the Ventricular Rate

These are given in Table 17.

Table 17   Causes of an Irregular Ventricular Rate

Irregularity of initiation of atrial myocardial depolarisation

  Sinus arrhythmia

  Intermittent sinus arrest

  Intermittent sino-atrial block

  Atrial premature beats

  Atrial paced beats (intermittent)

  Atrial fibrillation

Irregularity of atrio-ventricular conduction

  Second degree heart block type I (Wenckebach phenomenon)

  Second degree heart block type II (Mobitz type II block)

  Atrial tachycardia with varying AV block

  Atrial flutter with varying AV block

  Atrial fibrillation

Irregularity of initiation of ventricular depolarisation

  Junctional premature beats
  (atrial myocardial depolarisation is also irregular)

  Ventricular premature beats

  Ventricular paced beats (intermittent)

  Ventricular tachycardia (the irregularity of rate is minimal)

Fundamental change in cardiac rhythm during recording period e.g.:

  Sinus rhythm changing to atrial fibrillation

  Sinus rhythm changing to atrial tachycardia

  Sinus rhythm changing to atrial flutter

  Sinus mechanism remaining but complete heart block developing, etc.

**Duration of the QRS Complex
(QRS Width)**

A third important aspect of the QRS complexes in relation to cardiac rhythm analysis is the duration of the QRS complexes. This matter has already been seen to be of great importance in the morphological analysis of the electrocardiogram and this is one very important area where there is interaction between morphological and rhythm analysis of the ECG. The normal QRS does not exceed 0.10 seconds in duration (see Section 1, pages 39, 45, 68). **When the QRS duration is of normal width (0.10 sec) the cardiac cycle has been initiated by a** **supraventricular depolarisation** (i.e. the depolarisation of the ventricle was initiated at some point superior to the bifurcation of the His bundle). **Normality of the width of the QRS complex implies that the ventricular depolarisation has passed normally through the bundle of His, right and left bundle branches and Purkinje network before reaching the ventricular myocardium.** Depolarisation beginning superior to the bundle of His is said to be supraventricular (Table 18).

Table 18 Supraventricular Sites of Initiation of Depolarisation

Sino-atrial node
Atrial myocardium
Atrio-ventricular node

The QRS duration is usually normal when the depolarisation is initiated from supraventricular sites since the depolarising pathway to the ventricular myocardium is through the normal, rapidly conducting specialised tissue.

When an impulse arises from the ventricular myocardium inferior to the bifurcation of the His bundle (e.g. as in the case of a ventricular ectopic beat) the conduction pathway through the ventricular myocardium is necessarily abnormal (since it does not even start at the right place). Intraventricular conduction is slower and the QRS is therefore abnormally wide. The causes of abnormally wide QRS complexes are given in Table 19.

Table 19 Causes of Abnormally Wide° QRS Complexes

Supraventricular rhythms with intraventricular conduction abnormalities (i.e. morphological causes of wide QRS complexes)

Sinus rhythm

Sinus tachycardia

Sinus bradycardia

Sinus arrhythmia

Atrial tachycardia

Atrial flutter

Atrial fibrillation

Junctional rhythm

Junctional bradycardia

Junctional tachycardia

Atrial paced beats

> With right bundle branch block*,
>
> left bundle branch block*
>
> or with ventricular pre-excitation

Ventricular rhythms

Ventricular escape rhythms (e.g. in complete heart block)

Ventricular premature beats

Ventricular tachycardia

Idioventricular rhythm

Ventricular paced beats

° QRS complexes which are abnormally wide are often also abnormal in shape.

* Not infrequently a supraventricular tachycardia occurring in a subject without a pre-existing intraventricular conduction defect, may be associated with a transient (tachycardia-related) right (or less frequently left) bundle branch block if the tachycardia occurs at such a rate that the second atrial depolarisation wave spreads to the interventricular septum before the (usually) right (occasionally left) bundle branch has recovered from its period of refractoriness. This is called **aberrant intraventricular conduction, rate-related bundle branch block** or **functional bundle branch block** (see pages 403 to 407).

Assessment of the P Waves

Similar deductive processes (with some modification) can and should be applied to atrial myocardial depolarisation (i.e. to the P waves).

The Presence or Absence of P Waves

The first problem in rhythm analysis with respect to the P waves is whether or not they are recognisably present. The situations in which P waves may not be visible are given in Table 20.

Table 20 Conditions in which P Waves are not Visible

1. P waves not visible because they are not present

Sinus arrest

Sino-atrial block

Atrial flutter†

Atrial fibrillation*

2. P waves not visible because, although present, they are obscured for technical reasons

Poor recording

Sub-optimal choice of recording lead

Low voltage P waves (pericardial effusion, obese subjects etc)

3. P waves not visible because, although present, they are obscured by other parts of the ECG

P wave hidden in QRS

P wave hidden in S-T segment

P wave hidden in T wave

---

† Regular flutter waves may be visible
* Irregular fibrillation waves will usually be visible

Of those rhythms listed in section 1 of Table 20, sinus arrest and sino-atrial block are relatively uncommon and are usually transient. Their transient nature usually renders the interpretation clear. Atrial flutter is usually easily diagnosed by the presence of regular flutter waves (see pages 431 to 435). Atrial fibrillation is the commonest cause in the group listed in section 1 (Table 20). Irregular fibrillation waves are usually seen.

Of those situations listed in section 2 of Table 20 the first two items should be precluded by adequate techniques. The third item is a relatively uncommon cause

– if a 12-lead ECG is taken (or if an optimal lead is chosen) it is very rare in these circumstances not to be able to recognise a P wave.

The common problems and the greatest difficulties in recognising P waves usually arise because the P wave is, or might be, hidden in the QRS complex, the S-T segment or the T wave. It is therefore of the greatest importance to make a diligent search for the P waves by looking for any transient variation in form (with respect to the form in adjacent waves) of the QRS, S-T or T.

Determination of P Wave Rate

This is done in the same manner as for assessment of ventricular rate (heart rate).

Causes of a Rapid P Wave Rate

The causes of a rapid P wave rate are given in Table 21.

Table 21   Causes of a Rapid P Wave Rate*

Sinus tachycardia

Atrial tachycardia

Junctional tachycardia

Ventricular tachycardia with retrograde ventriculo-atrial conduction

*Atrial flutter is omitted since the flutter waves are not considered to be P waves.

Causes of a Slow P Wave Rate

The causes of a slow P wave rate are given in Table 22.

Table 22   Causes of a Slow P Wave Rate

Sinus bradycardia

Junctional rhythm

Intermittent sinus arrest

Intermittent sino-atrial block

Sino-atrial Wenckebach phenomenon

Regularity (or otherwise) of the P Wave Rate

This important feature should be checked for in the same way as for the regularity of the QRS rate (page 362 and Figure 201). Not only is this important for checking the basic regularity or otherwise of atrial myocardial depolarisation, but also it will often also reveal P waves which might otherwise be hidden but might be giving rise to minor but recognisable deformity of the S-T segment or T wave.

Causes of an Irregular P Wave Rate

These are given in Table 23.

Table 23   Causes of an Irregular P Wave Rate*

Sinus arrhythmia

Atrial premature beats

Atrial paced beats

Junctional premature beats

Ventricular premature beats with retrograde ventriculo-atrial conduction

Ventricular paced beats with retrograde ventriculo-atrial conduction

*Atrial fibrillation is omitted since the fibrillation waves are not considered to be P waves.

Abnormal Morphology of P Waves

One cannot recognise morphological abnormalities with the P waves as easily as one can morphological abnormalities of the QRS since the P wave is an altogether less definitive, predictable wave form.Slight changes in P wave morphology are not so easily recognised. In the case of P waves, abnormalities of **shape** are usually more easily recognised than abnormalities of width (though both are often present together).

Causes of abnormally shaped P waves are given in Table 24.

Table 24   Causes of Abnormally Shaped P Waves

Sinus rhythm with abnormal pathway of intra-atrial conduction (i.e. morphological causes of abnormal P waves)

    Sinus rhythm with atrial hypertrophy

    Sinus rhythm with atrial infarction

    Sinus rhythm with atrial ischaemia

Ectopic atrial rhythms

    Atrial premature beats

    Atrial escape beats

    Atrial paced beats

    Atrial tachycardia

    Junctional premature beats†

    Junctional escape beats†

    Junctional tachycardia†

    Junctional escape rhythm†

    Ventricular premature beats with retrograde ventriculo-atrial conduction

    Ventricular paced beats with retrograde ventriculo-atrial conduction

    Ventricular tachycardia with retrograde ventriculo-atrial conduction

---

† In these cases the P wave axis will be abnormal with negative P waves in Leads II, III and aVR.

The P Wave Axis

Determination of the frontal plane QRS axis was discussed in Section 1, pages 46 to 52. The same technique can be applied to the P waves to determine the mean frontal plane P wave axis (usually just simply known as "the P wave axis"). However, it is not usually necessary to determine the P wave axis with such care and precision. All that one usually needs to know about the P wave axis is whether it is approximately normal or is approximately 180° from normal. If atrial myocardial depolarisation is initiated from the sinus node (which is situated superiorly and to the right in the right atrium) the predominant direction available for atrial myocardial depolarisation will inevitably be downwards and to the left. The frontal P wave axis will therefore be close to +60° and the **P wave will be upright in Lead II.**

When atrial myocardial depolarisation is initiated from the AV junctional area the P wave vector will be reversed and is likely to be of the order of −120° and the **P wave will be inverted in Lead II.**

Knowledge of the actual position of the P wave axis is not necessary for rhythm analysis but recognition of a superiorly orientated vector (inverted P waves in aVF and II) points to a junctional origin for atrial myocardial depolarisation.

368

Assessment of the Relationship between P Waves and QRS Complexes

Although it is often possible to **infer** that a particular P wave precedes or follows a QRS, one can never be absolutely certain of this and the most important point initially is to determine whether or not the P waves and QRS complexes bear a **consistent** relationship to each other or whether any relationship or pattern can be recognised. Whenever a P wave is seen, if the time relationship between the P wave and the closest QRS is constant, it is likely that atrial and ventricular depolarisation are linked. The situations in which this occur are given in Table 25.

Table 25   Rhythms in which there is Atrio-ventricular Association

Sinus rhythm

Sinus tachycardia

Sinus bradycardia

Atrial premature beats (but only those which are conducted to the ventricles)

Atrial escape beats

Atrial paced beats which are conducted to the ventricle

Atrial tachycardia†

Atrial flutter#

Junctional premature beats (but only those which are conducted both to atria and to ventricles)

Junctional escape beats (but only those which are conducted both to atria and to ventricles)

Junctional tachycardia† (but only those which are conducted both to atria and to ventricles)

Junctional escape rhythms (but only those which are conducted both to atria and to ventricles)

Ventricular premature beats associated with retrograde ventriculo-atrial conduction

Ventricular escape beats associated with retrograde ventriculo-atrial conduction

Ventricular tachycardia associated with retrograde ventriculo-atrial conduction

Sinus rhythm with first degree heart block

---

† Sometimes only a proportion (typically 50%) of those depolarisations which reach the atria also reach the ventricles and are therefore associated. In this rhythm therefore, these may, for example, be alternating AV association and dissociation.
# The flutter waves (not strictly P waves) are associated intermittently.

Where there is no consistent relationship between P waves and QRS complexes there is said to be **atrio-ventricular dissociation.**

The causes of atrio-ventricular dissociation are shown in Table 26.

Table 26   Causes of Atrio-ventricular Dissociation

Defective atrio-ventricular conduction

　　Second degree heart block type I (Wenckebach phenomenon)†

　　Second degree heart block type II (Mobitz type II block)*

　　Third degree (complete) heart block

Premature ventricular activation

　　Junctional premature beats without retrograde atrial conduction

　　Junctional tachycardia without retrograde atrial conduction

　　Ventricular premature beats without retrograde ventriculo-atrial conduction

　　Ventricular paced beats without retrograde ventriculo-atrial conduction

　　Ventricular tachycardia without retrograde ventriculo-atrial conduction

---

† AV conduction is not strictly dissociated here but the association is not constant.

* Here there is intermittent AV dissociation

Necessary Steps in the Evaluation of the Cardiac Rhythm

The rhythm of the heart is the ordered sequence of depolarisation of the myocardium with respect to time (page 337). It follows that the true rhythm can only be deduced if the P waves are fully assessed, the QRS complexes are fully assessed and the relationships of P waves to QRS complexes are fully assessed. It should be noted that the S-T segments and T waves are irrelevant to the analysis of cardiac rhythm. Despite this irrelevance, the T waves should always be identified, whenever possible, so that they will not be confused with P waves. **In addition the morphology of consecutive T waves should be compared in case minor perturbations give the clue to the presence of partially obscured P waves.**

In this respect it is useful to recall the concept of the Q-T interval (see Section 2 pages 263 and 264). Every single QRS complex (whatever the rhythm, whatever the QRS morphology) will be followed by a T wave. No second QRS complex can be seen (from a single heart) until the repolarisation processes (S-T segment and T wave) are complete, or at least substantially complete. The T wave may not, however, always be readily visible. It may be small or be obscured by the succeeding QRS complex. It is important (from the point of view of rhythm analysis) to recognise the T waves only so that they are not confused with P waves. When the ventricular rate is slow (60 beats/min or less) the Q-T interval is likely to be of the order of 0.4 seconds and when it is rapid (100 beats/min or over) it is likely to be of the order of 0.3 seconds. It sometimes helps, therefore, when looking for T waves to remember that from the beginning of the QRS complex to the end of the T wave is likely to be approximately two large ECG squares when there is bradycardia and approximately one and half large ECG squares when there is tachycardia.

The basic approach to rhythm analysis therefore consists of the following:
1. Assess the QRS complexes
2. Assess the P waves
3. Assess the P/QRS relationships
4. Examine the T waves for clues relating to the P waves.

The approach to rhythm analysis will be considered more fully after the individual arrhythmias have been described.

The Normal Rhythm (Sinus Rhythm)

The normal rhythm of the heart is sinus rhythm with a regular rate of 60 to 100 beats per minute. The full implications of the unqualified statement "the heart is in sinus rhythm" were discussed on pages 337 to 341. Electrocardiographic criteria for sinus rhythm are given on page 338. They are reproduced in detail here.

Criteria for sinus rhythm

P waves must be present.
The P waves must have the morphology which is usual for the subject* and the lead.
The P wave axis must be normal.†
Each P wave must have the same morphology in a given lead.
The P wave rate must be constant.°
The P wave rate must not be outside the limits 60 to 100 beats per minute.††

There must be QRS complexes.
The QRS complex must have the morphology which is usual for the subject** and the lead.
The QRS rate must be constant.°

There must be one P wave to each QRS complex.
The P wave must be in front of each QRS complex.‡
The P-R interval must be normal.***
The P-R interval must be constant.

*When a subject has a morphological atrial abnormality (e.g. hypertrophy, ischaemia, infarction) the P wave size and shape may be abnormal but the morphological abnormality is not likely to change in the short-term and any short-term changes in shape indicate variation in the pathway of intra-atrial conduction and the most likely explanation for this is change in the site of initiation of depolarisation within the atrial myocardium (see page 368).

†Where a P wave has a different axis from normal, intra-atrial conduction has followed an atypical route and the atrial beat is probably ectopic. Minor (15° to 30°) variations in P wave axis are permissible in relation to respiratory movement.

°Defined as a variation in rate such that the difference between the maximum and minimum P-P intervals (expressed as a percentage of the minimum interval) is not more than 10% (see page 338). If there is one P wave to a QRS and the P-R interval is constant, then regularity of the P waves also implies regularity of the QRS complexes.
††Agreed arbitrary limits

**The same assumptions apply here as with abnormalities of the P wave. When a subject has a morphological QRS abnormality (e.g. left bundle branch block, right bundle branch block, left ventricular hypertrophy, right ventricular hypertrophy, myocardial infarction etc) the QRS will be abnormal but transient abnormalities of the QRS are likely to indicate ectopic depolarisation since the ventricular depolarisation has clearly followed a typical route. Sustained abnormalities of the QRS may, of course, indicate sustained arrhythmia.

***The normal P-R interval is between 0.12 and 0.22 seconds.

‡This can only be **inferred.** A P wave which appears before QRS number n + 1 has usually followed QRS number n and there is no **definitive** way of knowing which P wave is associated with which QRS. The inference is based on probability and this is dependent upon information obtained from preceding and succeeding cardiac cycles.

With very few exceptions (for example the placed beats) all of the examples shown in Sections 1 and 2 of this book shows sinus rhythm. Figure 202 shows sinus rhythm. The ECG lead is aVL. Since the subject has a mean frontal plane QRS axis of 0°, the QRS is dominantly upright in aVL (and would actually be maximal in I) and a qR type of QRS complex is seen (i.e. a left ventricular type of QRS). The P wave axis is +45° (a typical, normal figure) and therefore the P wave is upright but small in aVL (and would be maximal in II).

Figure 202   **Normal sinus rhythm. Lead aVL.**

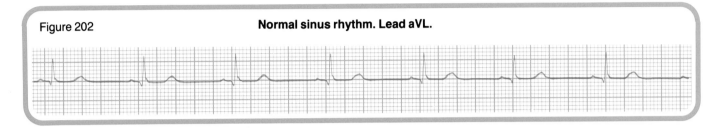

Figure 203 shows sinus rhythm. The lead is II. Since the frontal plane QRS axis is +60° the QRS is tall and upright (actually maximal) in this lead. Since the P wave axis is +45° the P wave is upright in this lead and is taller than it is in aVL (and is maximal in this lead).

Figure 203   **Normal sinus rhythm. Lead II.**

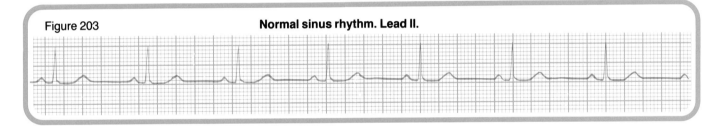

Figure 204 shows sinus rhythm recorded from Lead V_1. The subject is the same as in Figures 202 and 203. The P wave is biphasic (there is a tiny initial positive deflection followed by a slightly larger subsequent negative deflection) as is commonly found in V_1. The QRS is of the rS configuration (typical for normal QRS complexes in V_1).

Figure 204   **Normal sinus rhythm. Lead V_1.**

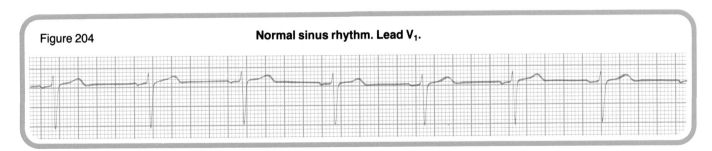

Despite the radically different appearances of the P waves and QRS complexes in these three leads aVL, II and V₁ (Figures 202, 203 and 204) all the criteria for normal sinus rhythm are fulfilled in each case.

If there is a morphological abnormality of the P wave, of the QRS complex or of both, the criteria for sinus rhythm will not be invalidated. Six examples will now be shown of records showing sinus rhythm with morphological abnormalities of the P waves or QRS complexes (Figures 205 to 210).

Figure 205

Lead V₁. The rhythm is sinus. All the criteria for sinus rhythm given on page 371 are fulfilled. The P waves are morphologically abnormal (dominant negative component) since the patient has left atrial hypertrophy. The P wave, however, has the morphology which is **usual for the subject** (since atrial hypertrophy is hardly likely to be intermittent!).

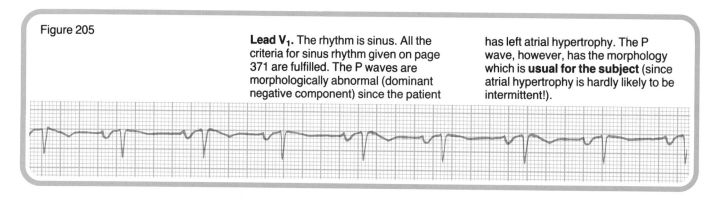

Figure 206

Lead V₁. The rhythm is sinus. All the criteria for sinus rhythm given on page 371 are fulfilled. The QRS complexes are morphologically abnormal (rSR′ in V₁) since the patient has right bundle branch block. The QRS morphology is that which is **usual for the subject.** (As will be shown later, QRS complexes of this type can occur when ventricular ectopic beats arise from the left ventricle. In this situation, however, the normal P-QRS relationship would be lost and QRS complexes other than those of the ventricular ectopic beat would be seen to be different and to reflect the "usual" QRS).

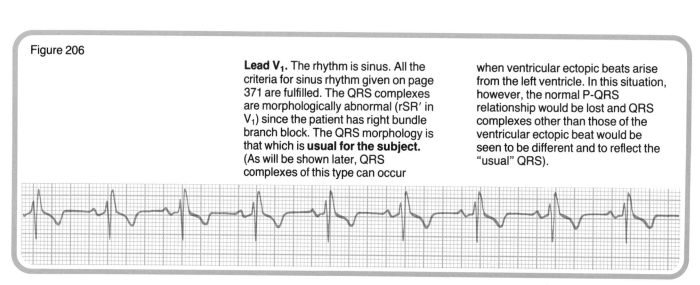

Figure 207

Lead V₁. The rhythm is sinus. All the criteria for sinus rhythm given on page 371 are fulfilled. The QRS complexes are morphologically abnormal (QS in V₁, total QRS duration prolonged) since the patient has left bundle branch block. The QRS morphology is that which is **usual for the subject.** The P waves are small and difficult to see. With a better choice of lead they become more obvious (Figure 208)

(as will be shown later QRS complexes of this type can occur when ventricular ectopic beats arise from the right ventricle. In this situation, however, the normal P-QRS relationship would be lost and QRS complexes other than those of the ventricular ectopic beat would be seen to be different and to reflect the "usual" QRS).

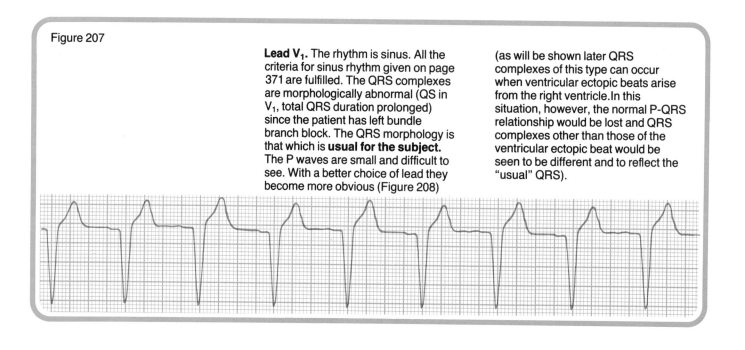

Figure 208

Lead II. The record is taken from the same subject as Figure 207. The record shows sinus rhythm in a patient with complete left bundle branch block. The full 12-lead record is shown in Section 1, Record 28, page 99.

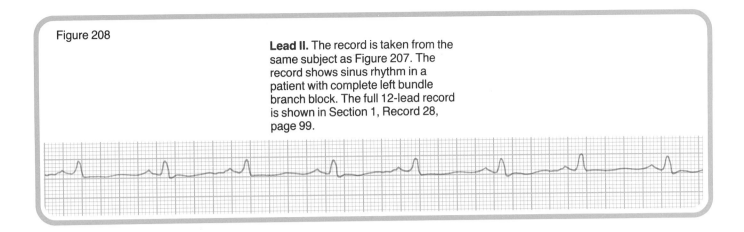

Figure 209

Lead II. The rhythm is best described as "sinus rhythm with ventricular pre-excitation". The P-R interval is abnormally short, there are delta waves and the QRS complexes are abnormally wide. Since the P-R interval is abnormal the rhythm cannot just be described as "sinus rhythm". For a typical 12-lead electrocardiogram in a case of ventricular pre-excitation see Section 2, Record 55, page 305.

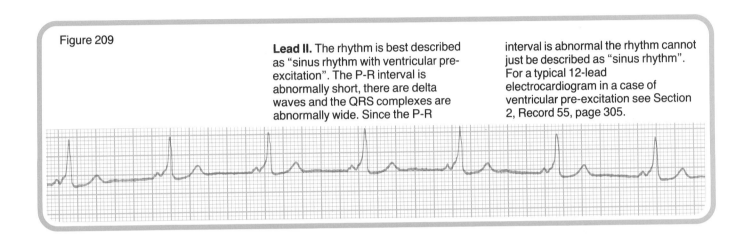

Figure 210

Lead V₂. The rhythm is sinus. The QRS complexes are abnormal (the patient has acute myocardial infarction). The QRS morphology is **usual for the subject during (and only during) the acute stage of myocardial infarction.** (When dealing with a changing appearance as during the evolutionary phase of the electrocardiogram in acute myocardial infarction, the use of the phrase "usual for the subject" is perhaps most problematical. The phrase is basically meant to imply that any deviation from normal appearances in the QRS is related to a morphological abnormality rather than to a change of cardiac rhythm).

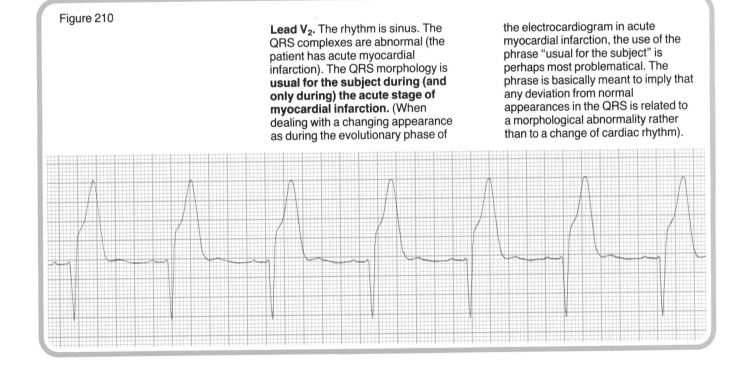

Classification of Arrhythmias

An arrhythmia is any cardiac rhythm other than straightforward (unqualified) sinus rhythm in which the heart rate is not outside the range of 60 to 100 beats per minute. The "diagnosis" of arrhythmias is thus by a process of exclusion. The definition of an arrhythmia contains arbitrary limits on rate. It follows that ventricular fibrillation on the one hand and sinus bradycardia at 59 beats per minute on the other hand, are both technically "arrhythmias" although the extent to which they diverge from the normal rhythm is clearly very different in the two cases.

Arrhythmias may therefore develop because of:
1. disturbances of impulse formation at the sino-atrial node
2. the development of premature ectopic depolarisation
3. the appearance of escape ectopic depolarisation
4. disturbances of conduction of a normally initiated depolarisation
5. combinations of the above.

This description forms a suitable basis for the classification of arrhythmias (Table 27).

Table 27 Classification of Arrhythmias

Disturbances of function at the sino-atrial node
Sinus tachycardia
Sinus bradycardia
Sinus arrhythmia
Sinus arrest

Premature ectopic rhythms
Atrial origin premature ectopic rhythms
    Atrial premature beats
    Atrial tachycardia
    Atrial flutter
    Atrial fibrillation
Junctional origin premature ectopic rhythms
    Junctional premature beats
    Junctional tachycardia
Ventricular origin premature ectopic rhythms
    Ventricular premature beats
    Ventricular tachycardia
    Ventricular fibrillation

Escape ectopic rhythms
Atrial escape beats
Atrial escape rhythm †
Junctional escape beats
Junctional escape rhythm †
Ventricular escape beats
Ventricular escape rhythm †

Conduction disturbances*
Sino-atrial Wenckebach**
Sino-atrial block (SA block)**
First degree atrio-ventricular block
Type I second degree atrio-ventricular block (Wenckebach phenomenon)
Type II second degree atrio-ventricular block (Mobitz block)
Third degree (complete) atrio-ventricular block

Combination of arrhythmias
Almost any combination of the above is possible.

---

† The term "escape rhythm" is used in preference to "escape beats" when the escape depolarisations are persistent rather than transient. In other respects the terms are identical.

*Conduction disturbances at the atrio-ventricular node, at the bundle of His or simultaneously blocking right and left bundle branches can be considered arrhythmias in the broader sense (though some authorities do not consider conduction disturbances under "arrhythmias" at all), but incomplete conduction problems below the His bundle (right bundle branch block, left bundle branch block, left anterior hemiblock, left posterior hemiblock, right bundle branch block with left anterior hemiblock, right bundle branch block with left posterior hemiblock) are not considered to be arrhythmias but are classified as intraventricular conduction disturbances.

** Sino-atrial Wenckebach is type I block at the SA node and sino-atrial block is type II block (see pages 485 to 491).

Premature Beats : Ectopic Beats

It is important clearly to understand the terms "premature" and "ectopic". **A premature beat** is one which occurs earlier than would be anticipated on the basis of the experience of preceding beats. Figure 211 shows one premature beat.

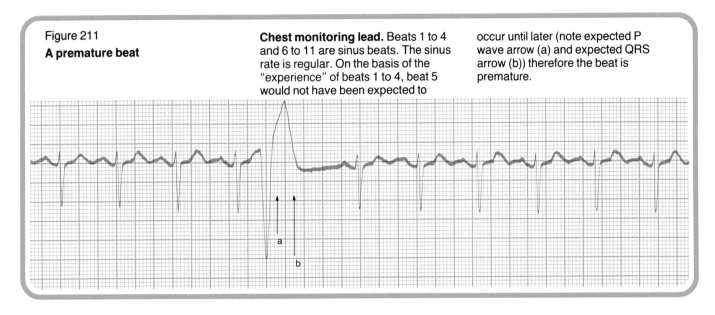

Figure 211
A premature beat

Chest monitoring lead. Beats 1 to 4 and 6 to 11 are sinus beats. The sinus rate is regular. On the basis of the "experience" of beats 1 to 4, beat 5 would not have been expected to occur until later (note expected P wave arrow (a) and expected QRS arrow (b)) therefore the beat is premature.

An ectopic beat is one which arises from any site other than the sino-atrial node. A beat is recognisably ectopic by virtue of several factors, one of which is a deviation from normal in the morphology of the depolarisation wave corresponding to the chamber (atria or ventricles) from which the ectopic beat originates. Thus atrial ectopic beats produce abnormally shaped P waves and ventricular ectopic beats produce abnormally shaped QRS complexes. The fifth beat in Figure 211 has a QRS complex which is **not usual for that subject** (based on the experience of the preceding beats). The fifth beat in Figure 211 is therefore ectopic (as well as premature).

Most premature beats are ectopic (premature sinus node depolarisation is the only non-ectopic premature beat and such depolarisations are very rare). Most ectopic beats are premature (if they are not premature they are usually suppressed as a result of prior depolarisation by a normal impulse). An ectopic beat which is not premature can only be an escape beat (see page 353). Such beats are not uncommon. They will occur when some subsidiary pacemaker (with a rate intrinsically slower than that of the SA node) "escapes" from the normal suppression induced by the spread of a depolarisation wave (initiated at the sino-atrial node) to the subsidiary pacemaker. This can only happen if the sinus node fails to depolarise or has its frequency of depolarisation reduced. Escape beats therefore occur only in the context of slow heart rates (i.e. bradycardias). Figure 212 shows the Venn diagram relationship between ectopic beats and premature beats.

Therefore, although the terms "ectopic" and "premature" are not synonymous the properties they describe are very frequently present simultaneously. It follows that it is often permissible to use either of the terms to describe the given beat.

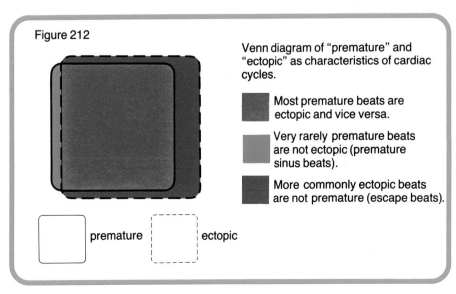

Figure 212

Venn diagram of "premature" and "ectopic" as characteristics of cardiac cycles.

Most premature beats are ectopic and vice versa.

Very rarely premature beats are not ectopic (premature sinus beats).

More commonly ectopic beats are not premature (escape beats).

premature ┆ ectopic

Disturbances of Impulse Formation at the Sino-atrial Node

Disturbances of impulse formation at the sino-atrial node include changes in rate (sinus tachycardia, sinus bradycardia, sinus arrhythmia) and defective sino-atrial node depolarisation (sinus arrest).

Sinus Bradycardia

The criteria for the diagnosis of this rhythm are simple. All the criteria for sinus rhythm are fulfilled except that the sinus rate is less than 60 beats per minute.

Criteria for sinus bradycardia

P waves must be present.
The P waves must have the morphology which is usual for the subject in the lead.*
The P wave axis must be normal.*
Each P wave must have the same morphology in a given lead.*
The P wave rate must be constant.*
The wave rate must be less than 60 beats per minute.†

There must be QRS complexes.

The QRS rate must be constant.*

There must be one P wave to each QRS complex.
The P wave must be in front of the QRS.*
The P-R interval must be normal.*
The P-R interval must be constant.*

†The criteria differ from sinus rhythm only in this respect
*See Footnotes on page 371

Examples of sinus bradycardia are shown in Figures 213 and 214.

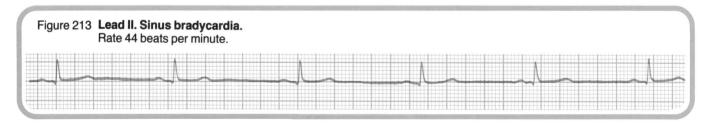

Figure 213 **Lead II. Sinus bradycardia.**
Rate 44 beats per minute.

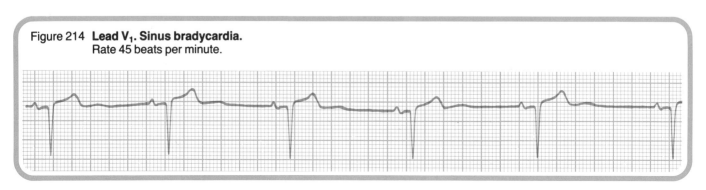

Figure 214 **Lead V₁. Sinus bradycardia.**
Rate 45 beats per minute.

Sinus Tachycardia

The criteria for the diagnosis of this rhythm are simple.

All the criteria for sinus rhythm are fulfilled except that the sinus rate is more than 100 beats per minute.

Criteria for sinus tachycardia

P waves
P waves must be present.

The P waves must have the morphology which is usual for the subject and the lead.*

The P wave axis must be normal.*

Each P wave must have the same morphology in a given lead.*

The P wave rate must be constant.*

The P wave rate must be greater than 100 beats per minute.†

QRS complexes
There must be QRS complexes.

The QRS complex must have the morphology which is usual for the subject* and the lead.

The QRS rate must be constant.*

P wave – QRS relationships
There must be one P wave to each QRS complex.

The P wave must be in front of the QRS.*

The P-R interval must be normal.*

The P-R interval must be constant.*

† The criteria differ from sinus rhythm only in this respect
*See Footnotes on page 371

Examples of sinus tachycardia are shown in Figures 215 and 216.

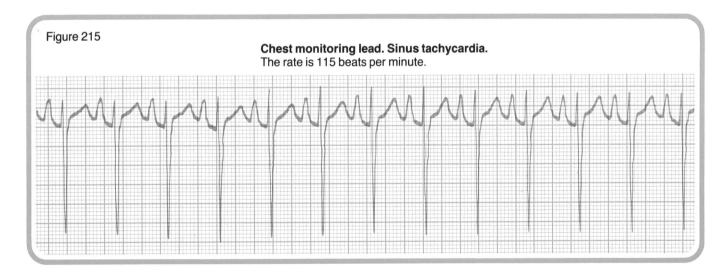

Figure 215

Chest monitoring lead. Sinus tachycardia.
The rate is 115 beats per minute.

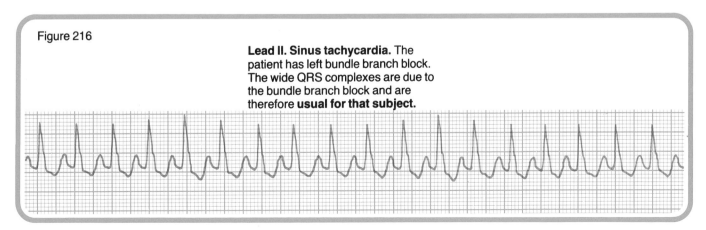

Figure 216

Lead II. Sinus tachycardia. The patient has left bundle branch block. The wide QRS complexes are due to the bundle branch block and are therefore **usual for that subject.**

The criteria for the diagnosis of sinus arrhythmia are simple. All the criteria for sinus rhythm are fulfilled except that the rate is not constant.

This variation is usually of the "concertina" type with cyclical increases and decreases (Figure 217).

Criteria for sinus arrhythmia

P waves
P waves must be present.
The P waves must have the morphology which is usual for the subject in the lead.*
The P wave axis must be normal.*
Each P wave must have the same morphology in a given lead.*
The P wave rate varies in cyclical fashion.†

QRS complexes
There must be QRS complexes.
The QRS complex must have the morphology which is usual for the subject* and the lead.
The QRS rate varies in a cyclical fashion.°†

P wave – QRS relationships
There must be one P wave to each QRS complex.
The P wave must be in front of the QRS.*
The P-R interval must be normal.*
The P-R interval must be constant.*

* See Footnotes on page 371
† The most typical form is a cyclical variation related to the respiratory cycle with an increase in the heart rate during inspiration and a decrease during expiration. The maximum sinus cycle length, minus the minimum sinus cycle length divided by the minimum sinus cycle length exceeds 10%. (An alternative definition states that the maximum sinus cycle length exceeds the minimum sinus cycle length by 120 milliseconds or more).
° If the P-R interval is constant the variation in QRS rate will match that in P wave rate.

Figure 217 shows an example of sinus arrhythmia. It is clear that all the criteria for sinus rhythm are fulfilled except for the lack of regularity of the P waves. Since the P-R interval is constant the QRS complexes display exactly the same irregularity as the P waves. The instantaneous R-R intervals and heart rates are given below the tracing in the figure.

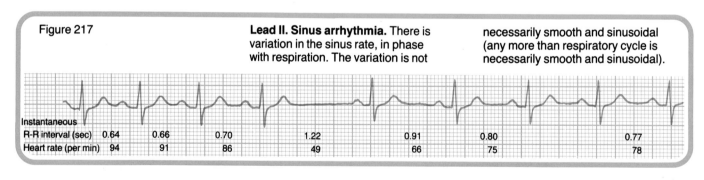

Figure 217

Lead II. Sinus arrhythmia. There is variation in the sinus rate, in phase with respiration. The variation is not necessarily smooth and sinusoidal (any more than respiratory cycle is necessarily smooth and sinusoidal).

Instantaneous R-R interval (sec)	0.64	0.66	0.70	1.22	0.91	0.80	0.77
Heart rate (per min)	94	91	86	49	66	75	78

Figure 218 is another example of sinus arrhythmia.

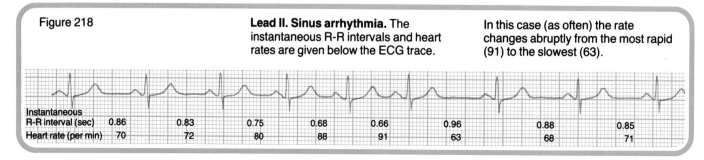

Figure 218

Lead II. Sinus arrhythmia. The instantaneous R-R intervals and heart rates are given below the ECG trace.

In this case (as often) the rate changes abruptly from the most rapid (91) to the slowest (63).

Instantaneous R-R interval (sec)	0.86	0.83	0.75	0.68	0.66	0.96	0.88	0.85
Heart rate (per min)	70	72	80	88	91	63	68	71

Sinus Arrest

In this arrhythmia there is a transient cessation of sinus node activity, usually just for a fraction of a second. The normal sinus activity usually then resumes though the problem will often recur after one or more beats. It is a relatively rare arrhythmia (contrast sinus tachycardia, sinus bradycardia and sinus arrhythmia which are common). The mechanism is shown in Figure 219.

Figure 219

Sinus arrest. The sinus node charges spontaneously to threshold for each of three consecutive beats (a to c) and normal sinus rhythm results (intervals ab and bc are equal). After the depolarisation c the sinus node is quiescent for an interval of time t and the cycle then resumes. There is therefore an unheralded, transient increase in the pause between successive sinus beats (cd – de). The duration of the sinus arrest (t) is easily deduced as de – cd (It is theoretically possible that there had been simply a slowing of the depolarisation process (Phase 4 of the action potential (page 349)) rather than sinus arrest, that is, that the sinus node manoeuvres are really described by a straight line joining fd rather than by fg and gd consecutively, but the end result on the ECG is the same and the appearance is known as sinus arrest). If the basic sinus rate is constant and sinus arrest does not occur in consecutive beats the interval de will equal the normal interval ab. It is important to note that the interval t will not (except by pure coincidence) equal the normal sinus interval ab.

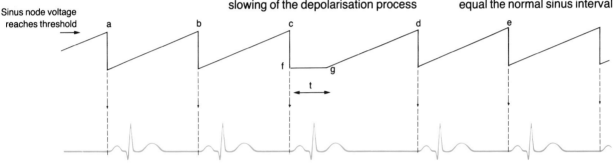

Sinus node voltage reaches threshold

a   b   c   d   e

f   g

t

Criteria for sinus arrest

P waves
P waves must be present.
The P waves must have the morphology which is usual for the subject and the lead.*
The P wave axis must be normal.*
Each P wave must have the same morphology in a given lead.
The P wave rate must be constant† except for the occasions when the sinus arrest occurs. During such an occasion or occasions the P wave rate transiently falls.‡
The wave rate must be less than 60 beats per minute.

QRS complexes
There must be QRS complexes.
The QRS complex must have the morphology which is usual for the subject* and the lead.
The QRS rate must be constant† except for the occasions when the sinus arrest occurs. During such an occasion or occasions the QRS rate transiently falls.‡°

P wave – QRS relationships
There must be one P wave to each QRS complex.
The P wave must be in front of the QRS.*
The P-R interval must be normal.*
The P-R interval must be constant.*

*See Footnotes on page 371
† The normal 10% variation in P wave rate is permitted.
‡ If sinus arrest should occur every alternate beat (extremely unlikely but possible) the appearances cannot be distinguished from sinus bradycardia. The distinction would be academic in any event since the consequences and management of the arrhythmia would be the same.
° If the P-R interval is constant the variation in QRS rate will match that in P wave rate.

An example of sinus arrest is seen in Figure 220.

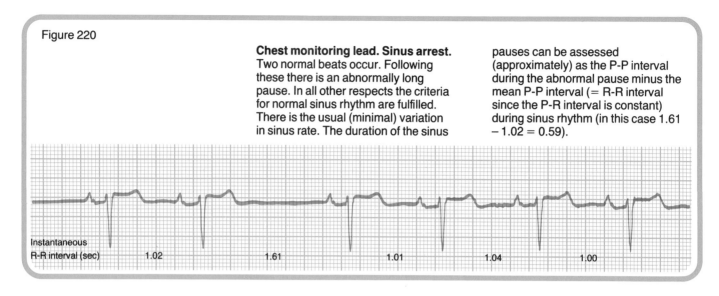

Figure 220

Chest monitoring lead. Sinus arrest. Two normal beats occur. Following these there is an abnormally long pause. In all other respects the criteria for normal sinus rhythm are fulfilled. There is the usual (minimal) variation in sinus rate. The duration of the sinus pauses can be assessed (approximately) as the P-P interval during the abnormal pause minus the mean P-P interval (= R-R interval since the P-R interval is constant) during sinus rhythm (in this case 1.61 − 1.02 = 0.59).

Instantaneous R-R interval (sec)   1.02   1.61   1.01   1.04   1.00

Sinus arrest, by definition, occurs only once before the next sinus beat is (or is not) resumed. If the sinus rate does not re-commence, spontaneous depolarisation then an escape rhythm would be anticipated. Figure 191 shows an example of sinus arrest with a ventricular escape beat.

Sinus arrest usually occurs on the background of sinus bradycardia. It is always a sign of sino-atrial disease. It is unlikely to be confused with sinus arrhythmia in view of the lack of any cyclical changes. Sinus arrhythmia is usually associated with a healthy sinus node.

Sino-atrial Block

In this arrhythmia there is no abnormality of sinus node depolarisation. Instead there is a (usually transient) failure of transmission of the depolarising impulse from the sinus node to the adjacent atrial myocardium.

The arrhythmia is, therefore, a conduction abnormality rather than a disturbance of function at the sino-atrial node and might properly be considered under "conduction disturbances" (see Table 27, page 375). Nevertheless because the electrocardiographic appearances are very similar to those of sinus arrest it is expedient to consider it here.

As a result there is complete failure of a P wave to appear and (unless there is a junctional escape beat (page 393) before the next anticipated P wave) a cycle suddenly appears which is twice the anticipated length (Figure 221).

Figure 221

Sino-atrial block. The sinus node charges spontaneously to threshold in an entirely normal fashion (a to f). On the first three and last two occasions (a to c, e and f) the depolarisation wave spreads successfully from the sino-atrial node to the atrial myocardium (interrupted, arrowed, vertical lines). On the fourth occasion (d) the depolarisation is not transmitted to the atrial myocardium. It follows that no P wave occurs. Unless there is a junctional or a ventricular escape beat (pages 389 to 393) no further myocardial depolarisation occurs until the atrial myocardium is depolarised again when a sino-atrial nodal depolarisation is transmitted to it. In sino-atrial block (which typically occurs for a single beat only) the interval ce is exactly twice the normal interval ab (assuming the basic sinus rate to be regular, i.e. intervals ab, bc and ef are equal).

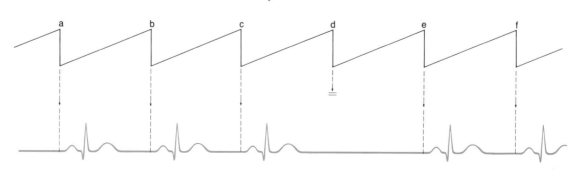

The typical appearance in sino-atrial block is therefore the transient doubling of the P-P interval (with doubling of the R-R interval unless there is a junctional or ventricular escape beat or variation in the P-R interval). An example is shown in Figure 222.

Figure 222

Chest monitoring lead. Sino-atrial block. The basic sinus rate (first three beats and last two beats) is not quite regular. The degree of irregularity is within acceptable limits for sinus rhythm. The interval between the fourth and fifth beats is approximately twice the average normal interval and the inference is that a sinus node depolarisation occurred between the fourth and fifth P waves but did not result in atrial myocardial depolarisation. The inference is based on the close approximation of the abnormal P-P interval (or R-R, since the P-R interval is constant) to an integral multiple (in this case, as is almost always so, twice the normal interval). This rhythm cannot, of course, be distinguished from a case of sinus arrest in which the period of arrest happens to equal the prevailing P-P interval.

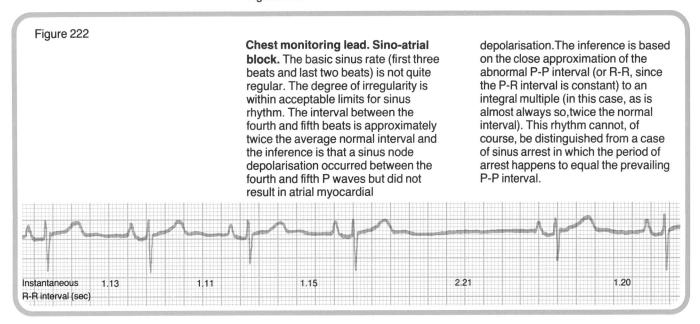

Instantaneous R-R interval (sec)

| 1.13 | 1.11 | 1.15 | 2.21 | 1.20 |

Criteria for sino-atrial block

The criteria for sinus rhythm are fulfilled except in relation to the (always transient*) SA block. In relation to the transient SA block the P-P interval is twice the normal P-P interval (and the R-R interval is twice the normal R-R interval).

If SA block occurs in two (or more) consecutive cycles the long pause will equal three (or more) normal intervals.

*If SA block is sustained there will be no sinus initiation of atrial depolarisation and an escape rhythm would be expected.

The only differences in the electrocardiographic appearances between sinus arrest and sino-atrial block is that in sino-atrial block the long pause is an integral multiple of (most often twice) the normal pause (for P waves and for QRS complexes) but in sinus arrest the long pause is not an integral multiple (except purely by chance). Compare Figure 220 (where the long pause is not an integral multiple of the basic pause) with Figure 222 (where the long pause is precisely twice that of the normal pause).

Causes of Disturbances of Impulse Formation at the Sino-atrial Node

Sinus Tachycardia

This may be due to increased sympathetic activity, decreased parasympathetic activity, non-autonomic influences or to a combination of all three (Table 28).

Table 28 Causes of Sinus Tachycardia

Increased sympathetic effect
Exercise
Emotion
Stress (including mental (e.g. anxiety) and physical (e.g. bleeding)).
Hypotension
Pain
Anaemia
Use of adrenergic drugs
Hypovolaemia
Congestive heart failure

Decreased parasympathetic effect
Atropine
Autonomic deficiency (e.g. Shy-Drager syndrome)

Non-autonomic influences
Pyrexia
Hyperthyroidism

Sinus Bradycardia

This may be caused by decreased sympathetic activity, increased parasympathetic activity, non-autonomic effects or a combination of all three (Table 29).

Table 29 Causes of Sinus Bradycardia

Increased parasympathetic effect
Vagotonic subjects
    Carotid sinus massage
    Valsalva manoeuvre
    Mueller manoeuvre
    Pain*
    Raised intracranial pressure
    Sleep

Decreased sympathetic effect
Use of beta-adrenergic blocking drugs

Non-autonomic influences
Hypothermia
Hypothyroidism
Obstructive jaundice
Sick sinus syndrome
Gram-negative sepsis
Mental depression

* The usual response to pain is increased sympathetic activity and tachycardia. Occasionally the vagal effect dominates and an inappropriate bradycardia may occur, for example, the subject may faint following venepuncture.

Sinus Arrhythmia

This occurs in a variety of situations. Most commonly it is found in normal subjects and the periodicity is related to that of the respiratory cycle. The causes of sinus arrhythmia are given in Table 30.

Table 30 Causes of Sinus Arrhythmia

Respiratory

Non-respiratory (sometimes the result of digitalis intoxication)

Ventriculo-phasic*

---

*This feature occurs when the ventricular rate is slow and some P-P intervals do not contain a QRS complex (the commonest example is complete heart block). Those P-P intervals which do contain a QRS complex are shorter than those which do not (the effect is probably an autonomic response to the change in ventricular stroke volume).

Sinus Arrest

This is always abnormal. A list of causes is given in Table 31.

Table 31 Causes of Sinus Arrest

Sinus node ischaemia

    Acute myocardial infarction

    Myocardial ischaemia

Non-ischaemic problems

    Degenerative fibrotic change

    Digitalis toxicity

    Overdosage with anti-arrhythmic drugs

Sino-atrial Block (Sino-atrial Exit Block)

This may occur as a result of vagal activity or of disease. A list of causes is given in Table 32.

Table 32 Causes of Sino-atrial Block

    Vagal stimulation

    Myocarditis

    Myocardial infarction

    Myocardial ischaemia

    Digitalis toxicity

Ectopic Arrhythmias

Ectopic beats were defined earlier (page 376) as beats arising from any site other than the sino-atrial node. An ectopic rhythm (which, by definition, is an arrhythmia and can therefore also be referred to as an "ectopic arrhythmia") is therefore simply a cardiac rhythm initiated from some site other than the sino-atrial node. The difference between an ectopic rhythm and an ectopic beat is simply that in the former case the arrhythmia is sustained to a greater or lesser extent without the interposition of non-ectopic (sinus-initiated) beats, whereas in the latter the rhythm disturbance is confined to a single beat. In the case, for example, of ventricular tachycardia with occasional capture beats (Figure 325) the predominant (sustained) rhythm is correctly described as a "rhythm" and the isolated perturbation of the rhythm as a beat. Difficulty with terminology (between "ectopic beats" and "ectopic tachycardia") will arise when there are just a few consecutive ectopic beats. These could be called a run of ectopic beats or a short burst of ectopic tachycardia. Arbitrary definitions therefore have to be agreed upon.

Definition of Tachycardia

The term "tachycardia" is used when the frequency of depolarisation of atria or ventricles exceeds 100 beats/ minute, i.e. when the interval between P or P′ waves or R or R′ waves is less than 0.6 sec (three large squares on the ECG graticule). This criterion is often exceeded for a single beat in relation to premature beats (thus the R-R′ or P-P′ interval of premature ventricular or atrial beats respectively will often be less than 0.6 sec) but the term "tachycardia" is not used in relation to isolated premature beats. A run of consecutive premature beats is usually required and the minimum criterion accepted is usually three consecutive premature beats.

In the case of ventricular tachycardia, for example, the Criteria Committee of the New York Heart Association requires the presence of three or more consecutive ventricular premature beats for the use of the term (ventricular) tachycardia. (Additional criteria are, of course, also required (page 469)). (In relation to rhythms involving a rate less than 100 beats/min the term "tachycardia" is applied, by common consent, if the intrinsic rate of the site of the rhythm is normally slow. Thus non-paroxysmal junctional tachycardia requires a rate in excess of only 60 beats/min (pages 441 and 458) and "slow ventricular tachycardia" a rate in excess of only 60 beats/min (pages 461 and 470)).

Origin of Ectopic Beats and Ectopic Tachycardias

Ectopic beats and ectopic tachycardias may arise from the atrial myocardium (possibly from specialised pacemaker cells within the atrial myocardium), from the atrio-ventricular junctional area or from the Purkinje network within the ventricles (atrial, junctional and ventricular ectopic rhythms respectively). **In considering the cardiac arrhythmias, therefore, it is advantageous to regard the heart as having (electrically speaking) two chambers rather than four. One "chamber"** (or, more strictly, one electrical entity) **consists of the atria and the other consists of the ventricles** (Figure 223).

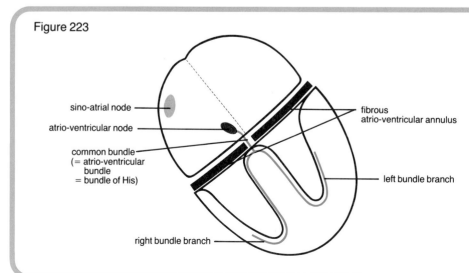

Figure 223

sino-atrial node

atrio-ventricular node

common bundle
(= atrio-ventricular bundle
= bundle of His)

right bundle branch

fibrous atrio-ventricular annulus

left bundle branch

In considering the cardiac rhythm it is best to regard the heart as having two electrical entities - "atria" and "ventricles". These two electrical entities are completely isolated from one another electrically save for the conduction pathway provided by the bundle of His. The atrio-ventricular fibrous annulus provides the insulation and is perforated by the bundle of His.

All-or-none Concepts of Atrial and Ventricular Depolarisation

Whenever depolarisation is initiated at some point within the atrial myocardium, that depolarisation will inevitably spread over the whole of the atrial myocardium since all parts of atrial myocardium are in electrical continuity with all other parts of atrial myocardium. (In some special situations the atrial myocardium may be depolarised from two or more sites simultaneously and a fusion beat (see page 476) might arise, but it will still be true that atrial depolarisation, whether initiated from one site or from two or more sites, will spread across the atrial myocardium in its entirety, assuming that all the atrial myocardium is viable).

The same principle holds true for the ventricular myocardium - once a depolarisation is initiated at one site within it it will, in normal circumstances, spread to all viable parts of the ventricular myocardium since all parts of the (right and left) ventricular myocardium are in electrical continuity with all other parts of the ventricular myocardium. (As with the atrial myocardium, fusion beats are possible if ventricular depolarisation is initiated from two or more sites before depolarisation from the first site has spread to involve the whole of the ventricular myocardium). In the case of atrial or ventricular myocardium it will occasionally happen that parts of the myocardium are "protected" from the oncoming depolarisation wave by "entrance block". In this way intra-atrial block or ventricular

parasystolic depolarisations (page 417) can occur.

Just as it is crucial to realise that all parts of atrial myocardium are in electrical continuity with all other parts of atrial myocardium and all parts of ventricular myocardium are in electrical continuity with all other parts of ventricular myocardium, it is absolutely crucial to realise that the atrial myocardium is only in electrical continuity with ventricular myocardium (and vice versa) via the specialised atrio-ventricular conducting tissue (Figure 223) which in normal subjects* consists of the common bundle (atrio-ventricular bundle, bundle of His). At all other points in the atrio-ventricular boundary there is complete electrical isolation of atrial from ventricular muscle. This electrical isolation is produced by fibrous atrio-ventricular annuli with their central fibrous body. The latter is perforated by the bundle of His on its way from the right atrium (where it leaves the distal end of the atrio-ventricular node) to the interventricular septum (where it divides into the right and left bundle branches).

* A small proportion of the population (about 0.1%) is born with additional routes of electrical communication between atria and ventricles (accessory pathways). Such pathways may give rise to ventricular pre-excitation (pages 212 to 219) and possibly to arrhythmias (pages 446 to 456).

Atrial Premature Ectopic Beats

Atrial ectopic beats are defined as beats in which the cardiac cycle is initiated by depolarisation at a site within the atria other than the SA node. Atrial premature beats are atrial ectopic beats in which the ectopic atrial depolarisation begins before the anticipated (from inspection of previous beats) onset of atrial myocardial depolarisation resulting from the expected sino-atrial depolarisation and its spread to the ventricular myocardium. Whether the

depolarisation occurs in myocardial tissue or in specialised cells within the atrial myocardium is uncertain (and in any event this may actually be a semantic difference). Once the depolarisation is initiated it will inevitably spread throughout the entire atrial myocardium (left and right) since all parts of the atrial myocardium are in electrical continuity with all other parts of the atrial myocardium (Figure 224).

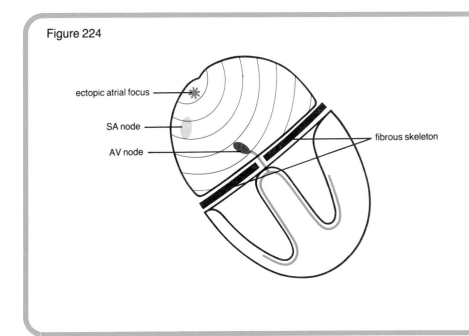

Figure 224

An ectopic atrial focus discharges high up in the right atrium. Depolarisation spreads from this focus in all directions (like ripples on a pond) to depolarise both atria. In so doing it gives rise to a P' wave. At the second ripple the depolarisation wave reaches the SA node and depolarises it. At the fifth ripple the depolarisation reaches the AV node and depolarisation will then spread down the common bundle, the right and left bundle branches, the His-Purkinje system and into the ventricular myocardium in exactly the same way as if a sinus beat had initiated AV nodal depolarisation. Since ventricular depolarisation and repolarisation proceed normally the QRS complex, S-T segment and T wave will be the same as in a sinus-initiated beat.

ectopic atrial focus

SA node

AV node

fibrous skeleton

Since the atria are depolarised from an abnormal site the P′ waves will differ in morphology from the sinus P waves. The QRS complexes will be the same as for the sinus-initiated beats (unless there is aberrant intraventricular conduction) (pages 403-407).

Non-premature Atrial Ectopic Beats ("Atrial Escape Beats")

An atrial ectopic beat may arise actively or passively. An active atrial ectopic beat arises because of enhanced pacemaker activity in the atria and is necessarily **premature**. A non-premature atrial pacemaker is normally itself prematurely discharged by the usual transmission of the depolarisation wave-form through the atrial myocardium, as shown for a Purkinje cell in Figure 188. A passive atrial ectopic beat arises precisely because the normal depolarisation does **not** reach the atrial myocardium so that an atrial myocardial cell **is** able to reach threshold and depolarise. Such atrial ectopic beats are **escape beats** and necessarily occur late. The P′ waves are abnormal since the pathway of atrial myocardial depolarisation is abnormal. The QRS complex, S-T segment and T wave of an atrial escape beat have the same form as for a sinus-initiated beat in that subject at that same time.

"Atrial Ectopic Beats"

In general usage "atrial ectopic beat" is held to imply an active beat (i.e. a premature atrial beat). Thus unless the term "escape" or some equivalent term is used, "ectopic" implies prematurity. Atrial escape beats are much less common than junctional or ventricular escape beats and the vast majority of atrial ectopic beats are premature. The **prematurity** of the beat is obvious from the ECG since the ectopic P wave (P′ wave) occurs earlier than would have been anticipated (on the basis of the behaviour of the previous P waves). The ectopic nature of the P′ wave is usually also apparent since the P′ wave has an unusual configuration (abnormal P′ wave shape and/or abnormal P′ wave axis). The P′ wave configuration differs from normal since atrial depolarisation starts from a site other than the sino-atrial node and therefore cannot follow the normal pathway through the atrial myocardium. Figure 225 shows an example of an atrial premature ectopic beat and Figure 226 an example of an atrial escape (ectopic) beat.

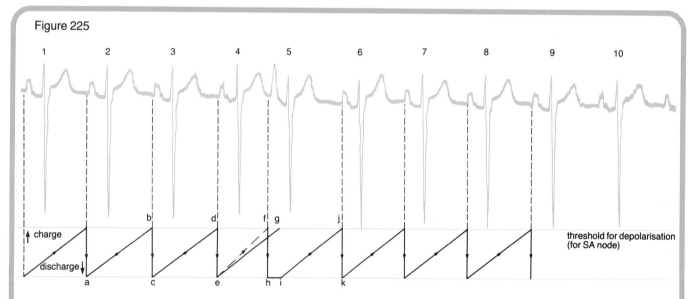

Figure 225

Chest monitoring lead.
Sinus rhythm with a single atrial premature ectopic beat.
Beats 1-4 and 6-10 are sinus beats. In these beats the P wave morphology is the usual one for that patient. (One has to be careful not to say that the P waves in these beats are normal for, of course, the patient could have left or right atrial hypertrophy in which case the beats which are "usual" for that patient would not be "normal"). The P′ wave of beat 5 has a shape significantly different from that of the P wave, indicating that the beat is ectopic. The P′ wave of beat 5 occurs earlier than the P wave which would have been anticipated as a result of inspecting beats 1-4, indicating that the beat is **premature**. The ectopic atrial depolarisation arises because the cell initiating the beat depolarises earlier than the sinus node (that is the slope of the ramp ef is greater than that of ab, cd or eg). The sinus node is (prematurely) depolarised by the P′ wave and is therefore re-set and the sinus node depolarisation "ramp" never reaches g. When the sinus node is prematurely depolarised from some external (to it) source it pauses briefly before starting its depolarisation "ramp" again. The onset of P′ indicates the time at which the first part of the atrial myocardium is depolarised. The time interval hi (time to re-setting of the SA node) indicates the travel time of this initial atrial depolarisation to the SA node plus the brief pause (referred to above) before the sinus node starts its ramp function again. The time interval fj is therefore slightly but significantly longer than the time interval bd. The interval hi can be calculated as fj−bd.

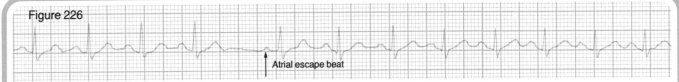

Figure 226

↑ Atrial escape beat

Lead II. Sinus rhythm with a single atrial escape ectopic beat. The first four beats show sinus rhythm with a rate of approximately 100/min. After the fourth beat there is a pause which is ended by an atrial ectopic beat. The beat is clearly ectopic since the P′ wave of the fifth beat has a different morphology from the P wave of the sinus beats. However, the beat is not premature, it is late. It is clear that when the anticipated sinus impulse fails to occur an ectopic site within the atrial myocardium "escapes" from its usual induced depolarisation (induced by the sinus node) and itself depolarises. Subsequently normal conduction down the AV node and intraventricular conducting pathways gives a normal QRS, S-T and T.

A premature, ectopic atrial depolarisation occurs earlier than anticipated (on the basis of one's knowledge of previous sinus beats) and spreads through the atrial myocardium using a route different from normal. This is necessarily so since the depolarisation starts in the "wrong" place. **The atrial depolarisation wave (P′ wave) is therefore premature and is different in morphology from the usual P wave.** The atrial depolarisation wave spreads across the myocardium of both atria like ripples on a pond (Figure 224) and inevitably depolarises (or prematurely re-sets) the AV node and the SA node. After arrival at the AV node **the depolarisation wave passes to the ventricles via the normal channels**. It follows that the QRS complex (and therefore the S-T segments and T waves) will have the same morphology as in sinus-initiated beats (in Figure 225 the QRS, S-T and T morphology of beat 5 is not significantly different from that of beats 1-4 and 6-10). The P′-R interval may be the same, longer or shorter than in the sinus beats. If the ectopic atrial site is closer to the AV node than is the sino-atrial node then the P′-R interval will be shorter, and if it is further away it will be longer. However, differences in the P-R interval related to differences in the site of origin of the ectopic P wave are likely to be small since it is travel time in the AV node which takes up most of the P-R interval in almost all circumstances, (in Figure 225 the P′-R interval of the atrial ectopic beat is marginally less than the P-R interval for the sinus beats in that subject at that time).

The time interval from the beginning of the ectopic (P′ wave) to the beginning of the next normal P wave is slightly longer than the usual P-P interval (the difference is shown as hk-ce in Figure 225). It follows that the interval between the beginning of the P waves of beats 5 and 6 is slightly greater than that of the corresponding interval between beats 1 and 2, 2 and 3 and 3 and 4. The interval between the QRS complexes of beats 5 and 6 will similarly be slightly longer than the interval between the QRS complexes 1 and 2, 2 and 3 and 3 and 4 unless there is a significant reduction in the P-R interval of beat 5.

The typical premature, ectopic atrial beat is recognisable by the features described. The much less common escape ectopic atrial beats have identical characteristics except that they are late rather than premature.

Criteria for atrial premature ectopic beats

1. The P′ wave occurs earlier than anticipated on the basis of observation of the preceding P-P intervals.

2. The P′ wave differs in morphology from the P wave* of the sinus beats.

3. The P′-R interval may be slightly longer or shorter than normal or can be entirely normal.

4. The QRS complex, S-T segment and T waves of the ectopic beats are similar to or identical to those of the normal sinus beats.†

5. The R-R interval (interval between consecutive QRS complexes) immediately after the ectopic beat is slightly longer than the interval of the sinus beats unless there is a substantial reduction in the P′-R interval of the ectopic beat. The increment in length is not sufficient to be "compensatory".

* The morphological difference can be slight. The P waves do not have such definitive shapes as QRS complexes and minor differences between P waves are less easy to spot than minor differences between QRS complexes.

† If the atrial ectopic beat is markedly premature the AV node may still be refractory (from the preceding sinus beat) when the depolarisation reaches it, in which case no QRS complex (and therefore no S-T segment and no T wave) will follow it, i.e. there will be a blocked atrial premature beat (page 400). If the AV node has recovered but part of the intraventricular conducting tissue is still refractory, the premature beat may be associated with functional (rate-related) bundle branch block and the QRS complexes, S-T segment and T waves will be modified correspondingly (pages 403 to 407).

** "Escape beats" typically occur in small numbers. When they persist, uninterrupted by the previously dominant rhythm, an "escape rhythm" (e.g. atrial escape rhythm) is said to be present.

Ventricular Premature Ectopic Beats

Ventricular ectopic beats are defined as beats in which the ventricular part of the cardiac cycle (and therefore the output from the heart, and therefore the pulse) is initiated by depolarisation of a cell situated below the termination of the bundle of His. Ventricular premature ectopic beats are ventricular ectopic beats in which the ectopic ventricular depolarisation begins before the anticipated (from inspection of previous beats) onset of ventricular myocardial depolarisation resulting from the expected sino-atrial discharge and its usual spread to the ventricular myocardium. Such a depolarisation could be initiated in the right or left bundle branches, in the Purkinje network or, in very abnormal circumstances, in the ventricular myocardium. In practice the vast majority of ventricular ectopic beats arise in the Purkinje network. Once the depolarisation is initiated at some point within the ventricles it will inevitably spread throughout the entire ventricular myocardium (Figure 227).

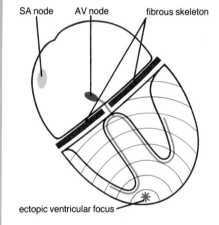

Figure 227

SA node   AV node   fibrous skeleton

ectopic ventricular focus

An ectopic ventricular focus discharges low down in the right ventricle. Depolarisation spreads from this focus in all directions (like ripples on a pond) to depolarise both ventricles. In so doing it gives rise to a QRS′ complex. Since ventricular depolarisation is inevitably followed by ventricular repolarisation, the QRS′ complex is followed by an S-T segment and a T wave. The depolarisation wave must spread in an abnormal pathway through the ventricular myocardium (since it starts in the "wrong" place). It follows that the QRS′ shape will be abnormal. In this example the QRS′ arises in the right ventricle, therefore right ventricular depolarisation occurs before left ventricular depolarisation and the interventricular septum will be depolarised from right to left. It follows that the QRS′ complex of a beat arising in the **right** ventricle will have a morphology similar to that of the QRS complex following a sinus beat when there is **left** bundle branch block. (Similarly when a beat arises in the **left** ventricle the right ventricle will depolarise late and the interventricular septum will depolarise from left to right. So the QRS′ complex of an ectopic beat arising in the **left** ventricle will have the shape of a QRS complex of **right** bundle branch block). Since depolarisation is abnormal, repolarisation will be abnormal and the S-T segment and T waves will be abnormal. The depolarisation wave will not usually travel backwards through the AV node (although it can sometimes do so) and it follows that atrial depolarisation does not usually occur in response to the ventricular ectopic beat.

Since the ventricles are depolarised from an abnormal site the QRS′ complexes will differ in morphology from the accompanying sinus-initiated beats. Usually the depolarisation fails to conduct backwards through the atrio-ventricular node and sinus-initiated depolarisation continues uninterrupted. Occasionally retrograde conduction does occur through the atrio-ventricular node in which a P wave will be seen after the QRS′ complex and it will have a polarity opposite to that of the sinus-initiated beats.

Non-premature Ventricular Ectopic Beats ("Ventricular Escape Beats")

A ventricular ectopic beat may arise actively or passively. An active ventricular ectopic beat arises because of enhanced pacemaker activity within the ventricles and is necessarily **premature**. A non-premature ventricular pacemaker is normally itself prematurely discharged by the usual transmission of the depolarisation waveform through the ventricular myocardium – as shown for a Purkinje cell in Figure 188. A passive ventricular ectopic beat arises precisely because the normal depolarisation wave does **not** reach the ventricular myocardium so that a Purkinje cell **is** able to reach threshold and depolarise. Such ventricular ectopic beats are **escape beats** and necessarily occur **late**. The form of the QRS complex, S-T segment and T wave depends on the location of the source of depolarisation within the ventricle (and on the condition of the ventricular myocardium) and the timing of the ventricular ectopic beat in relation to the preceding beat indicates whether the ectopic is an active or passive affair (Figure 229).

"Ventricular Ectopic Beats"

In general usage the term "ventricular ectopic beat" is held to imply an active ventricular beat, i.e. a ventricular premature beat rather than an escape beat. Thus, unless the term "escape" or some equivalent term is used "ectopic beat" infers also that the beat is premature (Figure 212, page 376).

The vast majority of ventricular ectopic beats are premature. The **prematurity** of the beat is obvious from the ECG since the ectopic QRS complex (QRS') occurs earlier than would have been anticipated by inspecting the preceding QRS complexes and does so despite the absence of any prematurity of the P wave and of any premature P' wave. The **ectopic** nature of the QRS complex is usually readily apparent from the fact that the configuration of the QRS' differs from that of the QRS although, as will be seen later, there is an alternative mechanism (apart from ectopic origin of the beat) which can result in differences in shape of the QRS complex). Figure 228 shows an example of a ventricular premature ectopic beat

and Figure 229 a ventricular escape ectopic beat. In both cases an abnormally-wide, abnormally-shaped QRS complex (a ventricular ectopic beat) interrupts the normal cardiac rhythm. However, in Figure 228 the ectopic QRS occurs earlier than expected and before the anticipated normal QRS has a chance to appear, whereas in Figure 229 it occurs late, and only after the expected normal QRS has failed to materialise.

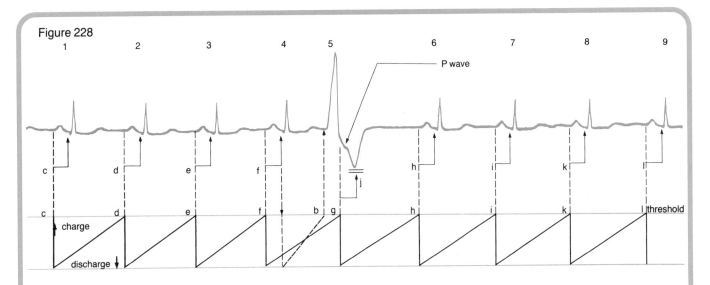

Figure 228

Beats 1-4, 6-9 are sinus beats. In these beats the P wave and QRS complex morphologies are the usual ones **for that subject.** (They are not necessarily normal since the patient might have left or right atrial hypertrophy, left or right bundle branch block, left or right ventricular hypertrophy, myocardial infarction or any other condition which can modify the P wave or the QRS complexes). Beat 5 is a premature ectopic ventricular beat. The QRS' of beat 5 is clearly different from that of the QRS complexes in the sinus beats indicating that the beat is **ectopic.** The QRS' of beat 5 occurs earlier than the QRS which would have been anticipated as a result of inspecting beats 1-4, indicating that the beat is **premature.** The ventricular ectopic beat arises because the cell initiating the beat depolarises earlier than the scheduled arrival of the depolarisation waves travelling to the ventricles as a result of the scheduled fifth sinus node depolarisation. In the four sinus

beats which precede this ectopic, sinus depolarisation occurs at c, d, e and f. At each of these points the "ramp" of the SA node reaches threshold and depolarises. This gives rise to the **P waves and after the usual P-R interval**, to the QRS complexes (this process is shown as the horizontal line followed by the vertical arrow). After f the next sinus node depolarisation occurs at g and would be expected to give rise to ventricular depolarisation at j. However, before this can occur the Purkinje cell depolarisation at b gives rise to the premature, ectopic QRS' of beat 5. Atrial depolarisation is initiated normally at g (and the P wave is seen to have normal timing, i.e. is half way between the P waves of beats 4 and 6), but when the depolarisation wave reaches the ventricles at j they are still refractory as a result of the premature depolarisation and no QRS complex follows the fifth P wave. The sixth to ninth sinus node and atrial depolarisations (h, i, k and l) are

followed by ventricular depolarisation in the usual way. It can be seen that the time interval between the P waves of beats 4 and 6 is exactly twice the interval between the P waves of beats 1-2 and 2-3 etc. The same will also apply to the time intervals between the QRS complexes of beats 4-6, i.e. it will be twice the time interval between the QRS complexes of beats 1-2 and 2-3 etc, provided there is no change in the P-R interval.
The pause between the ectopic beat (5) and the next normal beat (6) will be longer than the normal R-R interval by exactly the same amount as the interval between beats 4 and 5 is less than the normal R-R interval. The pause (5-6) is therefore said to be **compensatory.**
A demonstration of this important relationship will, of course, be possible only if the basic sinus rate is regular.
(The line ab shows the ramp for the Purkinje cell which produces the ventricular ectopic premature beat).

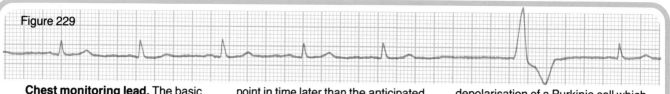

Figure 229

Chest monitoring lead. The basic rhythm is sinus with a rate of 70 beats/min. After the fifth sinus beat there is a long pause. No normal P wave or QRS complex is seen. At a point in time later than the anticipated sixth QRS complex an abnormally-wide, abnormally-shaped QRS complex is seen. This QRS is ectopic but not premature. It represents depolarisation of a Purkinje cell which has not been prematurely re-set (in the usual manner) by the normal oncoming depolarisation wave, i.e. it is a ventricular escape beat.

A premature ventricular beat (QRS') is usually followed by the next scheduled P wave. The P wave typically finds the ventricles still refractory from the QRS' and is therefore not followed by its own QRS (beat 5, Figure 228). No further QRS occurs until after the next scheduled P wave (beat 6, Figure 228). The result is that there is a longer than usual pause between a ventricular ectopic premature beat and the next sinus-initiated ventricular beat. The increment in the pause between 5 and 6 (Figure 228), above the control value, is exactly the same as the reduction in the pause between beats 4 and 5. Because of this the pause between beats 5 and 6 is said to be a "**compensatory pause**", i.e. the delay following beat 5 is exactly sufficient to compensate for the prematurity of beat 5 (Figure 228).

This feature is easily checked (providing the basic sinus rate is constant) by superimposing a piece of paper (or by using dividers) and marking out beats 1, 2 and 3, as shown in Figure 230.

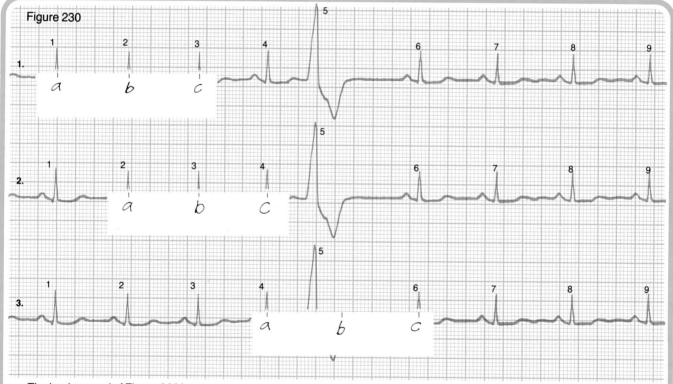

Figure 230

The basic record of Figure 228 is reproduced. To assess whether the pause following beat 5 is "compensatory" proceed as follows:
1. The basic heart rate (determined by R-R interval)
A piece of paper with a straight upper edge is applied over beats 1, 2 and 3 and the positions of the QRS complexes are marked – a, b, c. (Alternatively a pair of dividers is set to positions a-c.)

2. The regularity of the basic heart rate is confirmed
The paper is moved to the right to superimpose "a" on 2. The marks a, b and c should line up with beats 2, 3 and 4 if the basic rate of the P waves and the basic P-R intervals are constant. (Alternatively the dividers which were set at a-c should now precisely match the interval between beats 2 and 4).

3. The post-ectopic interval is checked to see if it is "compensatory'
Finally the paper is applied so that "a" lies opposite to beat 4. If c lies opposite to beat 6 the pause is truly compensatory. (Alternatively the dividers set at a-c should fit the gap between beats 4 and 6).
This test can only be applied if the sinus rate and P-R intervals are constant.

The typical premature, ectopic ventricular beat is recognisable by the features described. The much less common escape ectopic ventricular beats have identical characteristics except that they are late rather than premature. (Qualifications to these general features will be added later).

Criteria for ventricular premature ectopic beats

1. QRS′ complexes occur earlier than anticipated on the basis of the preceding R-R intervals.

2. The QRS′ complexes differ in morphology from the QRS complexes of sinus beats.* (In the majority of cases the QRS′ complex will be abnormally wide ($\geqslant 0.12$ sec)).**

3. The S-T segments and T waves of the ectopic beats are abnormal (since when depolarisation follows abnormal pathways repolarisation is likely also to be abnormal).

4. The P wave of the next scheduled sinus beat will usually occur with its normal anticipated timing and configuration since the premature ventricular depolarisation does not usually† spread back through the bundle of His and atrio-ventricular node to the atria and will therefore not usually give rise to premature depolarisation of the atrial myocardium or the sinus node.

5. The R-R interval immediately following the premature ectopic beat is longer than the usual R-R interval by the same amount as that by which the interval preceding the ectopic beat is shorter than usual. The pause following the premature ectopic beat will therefore be compensatory.‡

6. Ventricular ectopic beats arising in the **right** ventricle will have a **left** bundle branch block configuration and those arising in the **left** ventricle will have a **right** bundle branch block configuration.

Criteria for ventricular escape ectopic beats

1. There is a transient*** pause in the prevailing rhythm and this pause is ended by a QRS′ complex.

2, 3 and **6.** These criteria are the same as for those of ventricular premature ectopic beats.

* This difference can be slight but is usually very obvious – much more so than is the case with ectopic P waves since the QRS complexes are almost always larger and have much more readily identifiable shapes than the P waves.

** The only ventricular ectopic beats which give rise to QRS complexes of normal width will be those arising high up in the interventricular septum, i.e. in the fascicular area.

† Occasionally retrograde conduction will occur. In such cases premature P waves will follow the premature QRS′ complex. Since the atrial depolarisation starts from the AV nodal region it will predominantly spread upwards and in such a case the P wave will be inverted (see Figure 317) in leads in which it is usually upright (i.e. its axis will be abnormal).

‡ If the depolarisation process does spread backwards through the AV node and give rise to premature atrial depolarisation, the SA node will be re-set by the retrograde atrial depolarisation so that the post-ectopic pause cannot be precisely compensatory. In such a case the pause between the retrograde P wave and the next sinus P wave will resemble that found in an atrial premature beat in being slightly longer than the usual P-P interval and the overall pause between the QRS of the ectopic beat and the QRS of the next sinus-initiated beat will be more than "compensatory".

*** "Escape beats" typically occur in small numbers. When they persist uninterrupted by the previously dominant rhythm an "escape rhythm" (e.g. ventricular escape rhythm) is said to be present.

Junctional Premature Ectopic Beats

Junctional (atrio-ventricular junctional) ectopic beats are defined as beats in which the cardiac cycle is initiated by depolarisation at a site in the AV junctional area. Junctional premature ectopic beats are junctional ectopic beats in which the ectopic ventricular and atrial depolarisations begin before the anticipated (from inspection of previous beats) onsets of ventricular and atrial myocardial depolarisations resulting from the expected sino-atrial node discharge and its usual spread to the atrial and subsequently to the ventricular, myocardium. An ectopic impulse originating in the AV junctional area will spread in two directions simultaneously (Figure 231). Spread to the ventricles will be via a normal route and therefore the QRS, S-T and T will usually be normal (i.e. the usual for that subject). Spread to the atria will begin in an abnormal location and will follow an abnormal route and therefore the P waves will have an abnormal shape and axis.

Figure 231

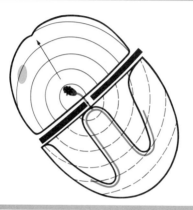

An ectopic focus arises in the AV node. Depolarisation spreads to the atria (i.e. in the opposite direction to normal) and to the ventricles (in the normal direction) simultaneously. At the fourth ripple the depolarisation wave reaches the SA node which will therefore be depolarised and "re-set" (refer to Figure 232, after beat 3 SA nodal depolarisation would be anticipated at f but the sinus node is prematurely discharged at h by the ectopic atrial depolarisation).

Non-premature Junctional Ectopic Beats ("Junctional Escape Beats")

Junctional ectopic beats may arise actively or passively. An active junctional ectopic beat arises because of enhanced pacemaker activity in the junctional region and is necessarily **premature**. A non-premature junctional pacemaker is normally itself prematurely discharged by the usual transmission of the depolarisation waveform through the junctional zone - in the same way as the Purkinje tissue is normally prevented from reaching its threshold potential (Figure 188). A passive junctional ectopic beat arises precisely because the normal depolarisation wave does **not** reach the junctional area so that a pacemaker cell at that site **is** able to reach threshold and depolarise. Such junctional beats are **escape beats** and necessarily occur later than the next anticipated beat. They commonly occur in the presence of depressed sino-atrial nodal function. The QRS complex, S-T segment and T wave of a junctional escape beat will have the same form as for a sinus-initiated beat in that subject at that time. Not infrequently, however, the junctional depolarisation fails to transmit retrogradely to the atria. In such a case no P wave appears. When (as is more common) retrograde spread to the atrial myocardium does occur, the P wave will typically be inverted since atrial depolarisation will occur in a reversed direction. The P wave, QRS complex, S-T segment and T wave of **premature** and of **escape** junctional beats will usually be identical unless the premature junctional beats are associated with aberrant intraventricular conduction (pages 403 to 407).

"Junctional Ectopic Beats"

In general usage the term "junctional ectopic beat" is held to imply an active junctional beat, i.e. a premature junctional beat. Thus, unless the term "escape", or some equivalent term, is used, "ectopic" beat implies prematurity.

The vast majority of junctional ectopic beats are premature. The **prematurity** of the beat is obvious from the ECG since the ectopic P wave (P' wave) and QRS occur earlier than would have been anticipated (on the basis of the behaviour of the previous P waves and QRS complexes). The **ectopic** nature of the P' wave is readily apparent since the direction of atrial myocardial depolarisation is away from the AV junction (arrow, Figure 231) and is in a direction almost exactly opposite to the normal pathway (The vector of the P' wave of a junctional beat is typically directed superiorly and to the subject's right, i.e. almost directly away from Lead II at about −120°). The P' wave is therefore inverted in relation to its normal direction in the given lead. The impulse spreads backwards to the atria but antegrade (and down normal pathways) to the ventricles so that the QRS complexes (and therefore the S-T segments and T waves) are normal. Figure 232 shows a junctional premature ectopic beat and Figure 233 shows a junctional escape ectopic beat.

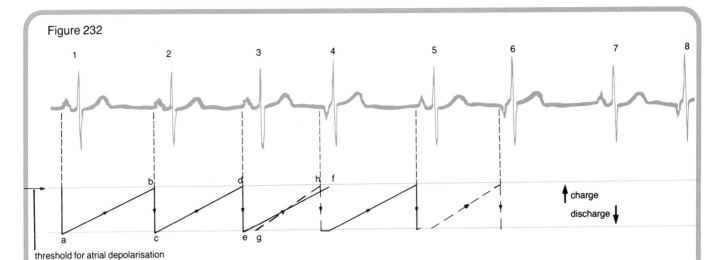

Figure 232

threshold for atrial depolarisation

charge ↑
discharge ↓

Beats 1, 2, 3, 5 and 7 are sinus beats. In these beats the P wave morphology is the usual for that patient. Beats 4, 6 and 8 are premature junctional ectopic beats. The P′ waves have shapes significantly different from those of the P waves, indicating that these beats are ectopic. The P′ waves are inverted indicating that the beats are arising in or close to the AV junctional area and are depolarising the atria predominantly in the direction opposite to normal. The P′ waves of beats 4, 6 and 8 all look the same indicating that the ectopic P waves are arising from the same site, i.e. that the ectopics are unifocal. The P′ wave of beat 4 occurs earlier than the P wave which would have been anticipated as a result of inspecting

beats 1-3, indicating that beat 4 is **premature**. By inference it can be seen that beats 6 and 7 are also premature. This latter can only be determined by inference since we do not have the benefit of two consecutive sinus beats immediately preceding these ectopic beats to tell us what the appropriate sinus pause is at that stage. However, it is likely to be similar to the sinus pause which obtained in relation to beats 1, 2 and 3. The ectopic atrial depolarisation arises since the cell initiating the beat depolarises earlier than the sinus node (i.e. the slope of ramp gh is greater than that of ramps ab, cd and ef). The ramp ef indicates the rate at which the sino-atrial node would reach threshold if left to do so without

being prematurely discharged by the junctional beat 4. Since the origin of the ectopic beat is (by definition, as it is a junctional beat) closer to the AV node than is the sinus node, the P′-R interval is slightly shorter than normal. The sinus node charges up along ramps ab, cd, ef etc. The junctional focus is depolarised by the oncoming wave from the sinus node at some point between the beginning of the P wave and the beginning of the QRS. The point cannot be recognised on the ECG. In relation to beat 4, junctional depolarisation is initiated at h and the depolarisation ramp of this beat probably starts in the approximate location designated as "g".

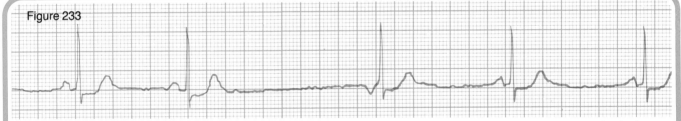

Figure 233

Chest monitoring lead. There is a basic sinus rhythm with a rate of 52* beats/min. The first two beats are sinus beats. After the second beat there is a long pause which is ended by a beat with an inverted P wave (indicating that atrial myocardial depolarisation takes place in a

reversed direction compared with normal) and a normal QRS, S-T segment and T wave (indicating that ventricular myocardial depolarisation takes place in the usual direction). A beat which initiates atrial depolarisation in retrograde fashion and ventricular depolarisation in

antegrade fashion must arise in the junctional area. It is ectopic, but it is not premature (compare Figure 232). In Figure 232 the junctional ectopic beats arise earlier than the next expected sinus beats and are premature. In this figure the junctional ectopic beats are late, escape beats.

The typical premature (ectopic) junctional beat has the features described. Junctional escape beats have identical characteristics except that they are late rather than premature. They are not uncommon.

* (Rate corresponding to the first R-R interval. After this the SA nodal activity is depressed (which is why the AV nodal (junctional) escape beat occurs). The SA nodal rate for the first two R-R intervals seen after the junctional escape beat is 42 beats/min).

Criteria for junctional premature ectopic beats

1. The P′ wave occurs earlier than anticipated on the basis of the preceding P-P interval.

2. The P′ wave differs in morphology from the P wave of the sinus beats, the most obvious difference being the complete change in polarity of the P′ waves so that the P′ wave direction in each lead is opposite to the normal P wave direction for that lead. Typically the P wave axis is in the region of − 120°.

3. The QRS, S-T and T waves of the ectopic beat are similar to or identical to those of normal sinus beats.‡

4. The P′-R interval tends to be slightly less than the usual P-R interval.†

5. The P′-R interval is frequently zero, i.e. the P′ wave is hidden in the QRS.

6. The R-R interval immediately after the ectopic beat tends to be slightly longer than the R-R interval of sinus beats. This increment in length is not sufficient to be compensatory.

The not uncommon junctional escape beats have identical characteristics except that they are late rather than premature.

Criteria for junctional escape ectopic beats

1. There is a transient* pause in the prevailing rhythm and this pause is ended by a beat which has a QRS complex similar to or identical with that in sinus rhythm. Either no P wave is visible or a reversed direction (for that lead) P wave is seen in front of, simultaneous with or following the QRS.

2–5. These criteria are the same as for those of junctional premature ectopic beats.

‡ If the atrial or junctional ectopic beat is markedly premature the AV node may still be refractory (from the preceding sinus beat) when the depolarisation reaches it, in which case no QRS complex (and therefore no S-T segment and no T wave) will follow it, i.e. there will be a blocked atrial premature beat (page 400). If the AV node has recovered but part of the interventricular conducting tissue is still refractory, the premature beat of atrial and junctional origin may be associated with functional (i.e. rate-related) bundle branch block and the QRS complexes, S-T segments and T waves will be modified accordingly (pages 403-405).

† Unless there is an additional process (e.g. disease in the distal part of the AV node) which independently lengthens the P-R interval.

* "Escape beats" typically occur in small numbers. When they persist, uninterrupted by the previously dominant rhythm, an "escape rhythm" (e.g. junctional escape rhythm) is said to be present.

It will be seen that there are striking similarities between atrial and junctional premature beats. The similarities and differences are given in Table 33.

Table 33

ECG feature	Atrial premature beat	Junctional premature beat
P-P′ (pre-ectopic interval)	Shorter than usual	Shorter than usual
P′-P (post-ectopic interval)	Longer than usual*	Longer than usual*
QRS, S-T, T wave	No change from the appearances in sinus beats‡	No change from the appearances in sinus beats‡
P′-R interval	May be normal, slightly prolonged, slightly shortened	Always slightly shortened† and is often zero (i.e. P′ wave is often hidden in the QRS)
P′ wave configuration	Different from usual (difference may be subtle)	Obvious differences from usual - reversed polarity in each lead.

* Not compensatory

‡ See Footnote ‡ on page 395

† See Footnote † on page 395

If an atrial ectopic impulse arises close to the sino-atrial node it will be difficult, or impossible, to distinguish it from a sinus node beat in terms of the P′ morphology, although its prematurity may be obvious. If an atrial ectopic impulse arises close to the atrio-ventricular node it will be difficult, or impossible, to distinguish it from an AV junctional beat, although again its prematurity may be obvious.

Supraventricular Beats and Supraventricular Rhythms

All beats which arise above the bifurcation of the bundle of His are referred to as **supraventricular** beats. Supraventricular **ectopic** beats include atrial and junctional ectopics. Supraventricular **premature** beats include sinus, atrial and junctional premature beats. Clearly, by definition, premature sinus beats are not ectopic. Supraventricular rhythms are rhythm-initiated at the SA node, atrial myocardium and AV junctional area. Supraventricular beats have abnormally-shaped P waves and usually have normal QRS complexes, S-T segments and T waves*.

Typical Appearances of Atrial, Junctional and Ventricular Premature Beats Compared

It is useful to compare the typical appearances of atrial, junctional and ventricular premature beats (Figure 234).

*Except as will be seen later, when there is aberrant intraventricular conduction (see pages 403 to 405).

Figure 234*

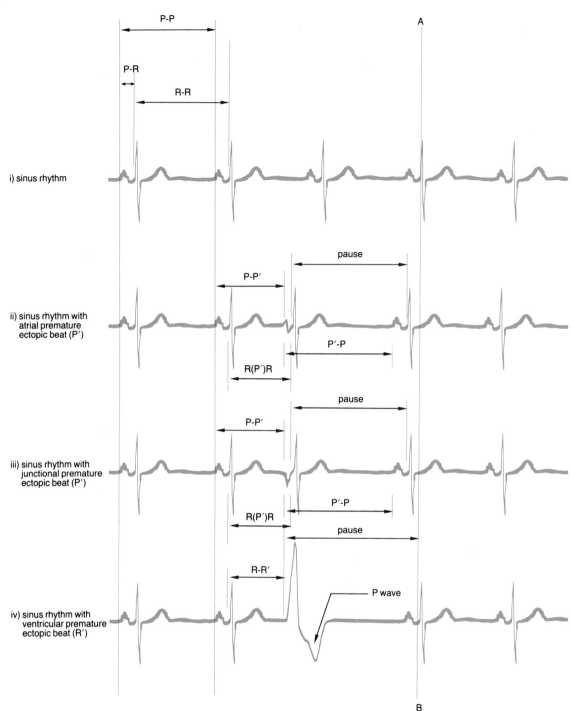

i) sinus rhythm

ii) sinus rhythm with atrial premature ectopic beat (P′)

iii) sinus rhythm with junctional premature ectopic beat (P′)

iv) sinus rhythm with ventricular premature ectopic beat (R′)

(i) Basic sinus rate is regular with a fixed P-P interval. In this case the P-R interval is constant so the R-R interval is regular and equal to the P-P interval. (This is not always true but this is the simplest case.)

(ii) and (iii) The prematurity of the atrial and junctional premature beats is indicated by the fact that P-P′ is less than P-P. The P′ waves of the atrial premature beats have different shapes from those of the sinus P waves. The P′ waves and the junctional premature beats have a polarity opposite to that of the sinus P waves. The P′-R interval is slightly less than the P-R interval.

The P′-R interval is slightly less than the P-R interval, indicating that the site of initiation of the atrial

depolarisation (i.e. of the premature beat) is closer (than the sinus node) to the AV node. The sinus node itself is prematurely depolarised by retrograde spread of the ectopic impulse. Whenever the sinus node is prematurely depolarised in this way there is always a slight pause (typically of the order of 0.1 to 0.2 sec) before it picks up again. It is this transient pause which makes the interval P′-P slightly greater than the interval P-P. This results in the fact that the interval between the R wave following the P′ wave and the R wave following the next normal P wave is slightly longer than the R-R interval which obtains during the sinus rhythm i.e. there is a pause. This pause, however, is not compensatory.

(iv) The prematurity of the ventricular premature beat is indicated by the fact that the R-R′ interval is less than the R-R interval. A P wave following the R′ wave is seen, occurring with normal timing (constant P-P interval) disturbing the down slope of the T wave. The ventricles are still refactory (from the ectopic beat) when the depolarisation wave from the P wave reaches them, so no QRS follows the P wave. The next QRS follows the next scheduled P wave and is "in step" (line AB) with the basic rhythm. Note that all three ectopic beats are followed by a pause which is longer than the R-R interval but that only in the case of **ventricular** premature ectopic beats is the pause compensatory.

Further Possible Features of Atrial, Junctional and Ventricular Premature Ectopic Beats

The fundamental aspects of atrial, junctional and ventricular premature beats have been covered. These aspects are the most easily recognisable and most commonly seen ones. However, additional features may be present. Unless recognised (when present) they may give rise to uncertainty and confusion.

Atrial Premature Ectopic Beats: Additional Features

Features to be considered here include variations in the P'-R interval, blocked (non-conducted) atrial premature beats, variations in the post-ectopic pause, unifocal or multifocal atrial premature ectopic beats, the frequency of the atrial premature beats and aberrant intraventricular conduction.

Variations in the P'-R interval

The P'-R interval in relation to atrial premature beats varies (as described on page 388) and it may be longer than, identical to or shorter than the P-R interval of the adjacent sinus beats. The features which determine the length of the P'-R interval with atrial ectopic (premature) beats are:

1. the proximity of the ectopic focus to the AV node,
2. the degree of prematurity of the ectopic atrial depolarisation,
3. the R-R interval of the beat preceding the ectopic, and obviously,
4. the condition of the AV node.

1. The closer the ectopic focus is to the AV node the shorter will be the P'-R interval (since the conduction distance of the atrial ectopic impulse to the AV node, and therefore the conduction time, will be less).
2. The more premature the ectopic P' wave the sooner the impulse will reach the AV node and the more likely it is that the AV node will be partially refractory with resultant prolongation of the AV nodal conduction time. As explained on page 485, the AV conduction time is the longest and most variable part of the P-R interval (other contributions to this interval include the atrial transmission time, bundle of His transmission time and time of transmission to the initial part of the left bundle). Markedly premature P' waves therefore tend to have longer P'-R intervals since the AV node is partially

refractory (Figure 235). If the P' wave is very premature the AV node may be **absolutely** refractory and may fail to conduct altogether. In this event the P' wave is not followed by a QRS complex and the atrial premature beat is "blocked" or "non-conducted" (Figure 236).

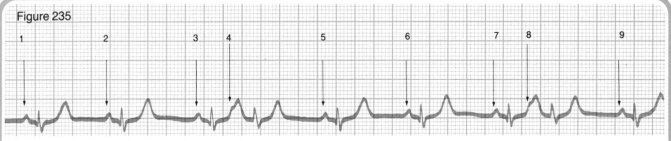

Figure 235

Chest monitoring lead. Sinus rhythm with atrial premature beats. P waves 1-3, 5-7 and 9 are of sinus origin. They are followed by normal P-R intervals. P waves 4 and 8 are atrial premature ectopic beats. Their prematurity is obvious from inspection of the timing of the first three P waves. The ectopic origin of the P' waves cannot be established with confidence since their morphology is obscured by the fact that they occur on the upstroke of the T wave (therefore it is possible (on the basis of P' wave timing and configuration) that they are sinus premature beats). The premature P' waves are followed by normal (for that subject) QRS complexes, S-T segments and T waves but even though the point at which the P' wave begins cannot be recognised with confidence, it is clear that the P'-R interval is longer than the P-R interval. It is clear that the AV node is partially refractory when it receives the depolarisation wave as premature as the P' wave 4 or 8.

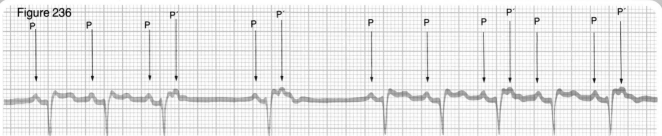

Figure 236

P P P P' P' P P P' P P P'

Chest monitoring lead. Sinus rhythm with frequent, blocked atrial premature beats. The basic rhythm is sinus rhythm with a rate of about 98 beats/min. The QRS complexes are wide with a slurred secondary r wave (i.e. there is right bundle branch block) and there is slight S-T segment elevation (the record was taken after acute myocardial infarction). The fourth, sixth, tenth and thirteenth P waves are atrial premature ectopic beats. Their prematurity is obvious from inspection of the first three consecutive P waves. Their ectopic origin is just apparent since the P′ waves can be seen to be morphologically different from the P waves. The P′ waves are not followed by QRS complexes (and therefore not by S-T segments or T waves) indicating that the P′ wave has reached some part of the atrio- ventricular conducting tissue whilst it was still refractory from the preceding beat. The likely site of this refractoriness is the AV node but it is also possible that it is the left bundle branch that has been found to be refractory (with no AV conduction possible if left bundle branch block (related to the prematurity of the P′ waves) is added to the pre-existing right bundle branch block).

3. The length of the R-R interval preceding the premature P′ wave also influences the P-R interval. This is because the longer the R-R interval of beat "n" the greater is the refractory period of all parts of the conducting tissue during the next beat,"n + 1". This might appear, at first sight, to be parodoxical since one might imagine that the longer the conduction tissue has to recover the less likely it would subsequently be to be refractory. However, it appears that the conducting tissue is made more responsive by an increase in the heart rate; the faster the rate (i.e. the greater the frequency of depolarisation) the more rapidly the conducting tissue recovers from each depolarisation. Presumably the factors which induce a tachycardia also facilitate recovery. In fact if this were not so significant increases in heart rate would become impossible. In view of this phenomenon of increasing refractoriness following longer R-R intervals (known as the **Ashman phenomenon**) atrial premature beats are likely to have prolonged P′-R intervals when they follow a longer R′-R interval than when they follow a shorter one (Figure 237).

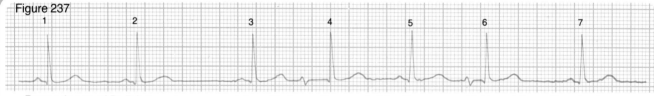

Figure 237

1 2 3 4 5 6 7

Dependence of P′-R interval on preceding R-R interval (Ashman phenomenon)
The basic rhythm is sinus but the sinus rate varies (sinus arrhythmia). The P-R interval of the sinus beat is normal. The fourth and sixth beats are premature (apparent by the early appearance of the P′ wave) and ectopic (apparent by the different morphology of the P′ wave) atrial beats. The coupling interval of the two ectopic beats is similar (i.e. the interval between the onset of the P wave of beat 3 and the onset of the P′ wave of beat 4 (which is the coupling interval of the first atrial premature beat) is similar to the time interval between the onset of the P wave of beat 5 and the onset of the P′ wave of beat 6) so the degree of prematurity of the beat is the same. The morphology of the P′ wave of beats 4 and 6 is similar so they are likely to arise in the same part of the atrial myocardium and are therefore likely to have similar atrial travel times. Despite these two features the P′-R intervals of beats 4 and 6 are different from each other and each is longer than the control P-R interval. Beat 4 follows a longer R-R interval (between beats 2 and 3) and has itself a longer P′-R interval (the Ashman phenomenon). Beat 6 follows a short R-R interval (between beats 4 and 5) and therefore has a shorter P′-R interval than that of beat 4 (but longer than that of sinus beats).

4. The length of the P′-R interval is also, of course, dependent upon the condition of the AV node. The length of the P-R interval (i.e.in a sinus beat) may itself be prolonged because of disease in the AV node. Sometimes a premature P wave will give rise to prolongation of the P-R interval which "reveals" a formerly occult problem in the AV node and in this situation a prolonged P′-R interval might be apparent even without undue prematurity of the atrial ectopic beat, without undue prolongation of the preceding R-R′ wave and without an undue distance between the site of origin of the premature beat and the AV node.

The prolongation of the P′-R interval following a long R-R interval is by no means a constant phenomenon. It is possible that, when present, it "reveals" an underlying occult problem in AV conduction through the nodes.

Blocked (non-conducted) atrial premature beats

These are usually the result of a degree of prematurity such that the atrial premature depolarisation spreads to the AV node before it has had time to recover. The degree of prematurity required before the AV node fails to conduct depends on the condition of the AV node. When it is healthy and is not under vagal suppression it probably requires an atrial coupling interval (P-P' interval) of about 0.4 sec or less. Blocked atrial premature beats may occur because of failure to conduct through the AV node or through the right and left bundle branches simultaneously. Examples of blocked atrial premature beats are seen in Figures 236 and 238.

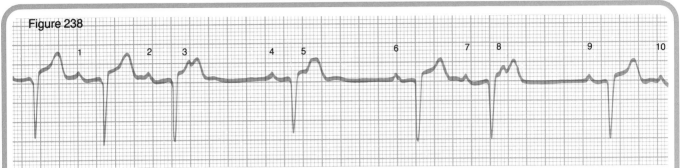

Figure 238

Chest monitoring lead.
Sinus rhythm and blocked atrial premature beats. The first two P waves (seen in association with the second and third QRS complexes) are of sinus origin and are associated with a slightly prolonged P-R interval (0.25 sec). The third P wave is an atrial premature, ectopic beat. Its prematurity is obvious from inspection of the first two P waves. Its ectopic origin cannot be established with confidence since its morphology is obscured by the fact that it occurs during the ascending part of the T wave, but it is more likely to be an atrial ectopic premature beat rather than a sinus premature beat since the latter are much less common. No QRS complex (and therefore no S-T segment and no T wave) follows the P' wave indicating that some part of the atrial ventricular conducting tissue is refractory when the depolarisation of the atrial ectopic beat reaches it. The P' wave is therefore blocked (non-conducted). The site of the block is likely to be the AV node (rather than the bundle of His or bilateral bundle branch refractoriness) and this view is strengthened by the initial long P-R interval – which is evidence of atrio-ventricular nodal conduction delay even with the sinus beats.

Variations in the post-ectopic pause

As discussed earlier, atrial premature ectopic beats usually propagate to the SA node and re-set it. This premature discharge of the SA node usually temporarily suppresses its rhythmicity so that the time interval between the ectopic P wave (P') and the next sinus P wave (P) tends to be just greater than the normal P-P interval for that subject at that time. If the P-R and P'-R intervals are the same it follows that the interval between the QRS complex which follows the P' wave and that following the next P wave is just greater than the usual R-R interval for that subject at that time (Figure 225). Very occasionally there may be retrograde sino-atrial block (i.e. atrio-sinal block) in which case the sino-atrial node is "protected" from the atrial ectopic beat. When this happens a full compensatory pause may occur, the sinus node is not re-set by the ectopic P wave, it discharges normally just after the ectopic P wave but finds the atria refractory and there is then a pause until the next scheduled P wave occurs to depolarise the atria and gives rise subsequently to ventricular depolarisation. This situation is, however, rare.

A full compensatory pause can also (again rarely) occur when the (ectopic) P' wave is only just premature (i.e. occurs just before the next anticipated P wave). In such a case sinus node depolarisation of the adjacent atrial myocardium and ectopic atrial depolarisation of atrial myocardium adjacent to the ectopic site occur simultaneously, giving an atrial fusion beat. Since the sinus node is not prematurely discharged, its sequence is not disturbed and the post-ectopic sinus beat is undisturbed in its timing. The pause is, therefore, compensatory but, just as the prematurity is minimal so the "pause" after the premature beat is only minimally (and to exactly the same extent) greater than normal.

Very rarely an atrial premature beat can be interpolated. This can only happen when (a) the sinus node is "protected" from the ectopically-induced atrial depolarisation wave by entrance block – so that its rhythmic activity is not disturbed, and **simultaneously** (b) the premature beat is so premature, or the basic rate is so slow, the atria have time to depolarise and repolarise (so as to be no longer refractory) before the next sinus depolarisation occurs(compare this with the much commoner ventricular interpolated beats, pages 411 and 412).

When there is an inappropriately long pause after an atrial ectopic beat before the next sinus beat, depression of function of the sino-atrial node should be suspected.

Unifocal or multifocal atrial ectopic beats

When several atrial ectopic beats are seen, whether they are unifocal or multifocal in origin is indicated by the uniformity or lack of uniformity (respectively) of the morphology of the P′ waves.

Figure 239a shows sinus rhythm with unifocal atrial ectopic beats and Figure 239b shows multifocal atrial ectopic beats.

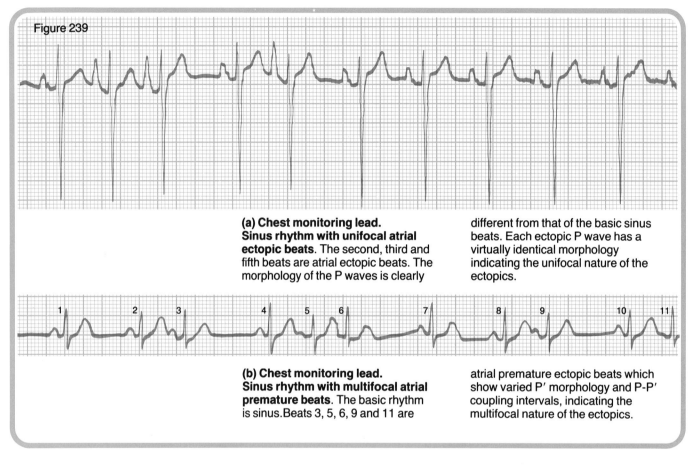

(a) Chest monitoring lead. Sinus rhythm with unifocal atrial ectopic beats. The second, third and fifth beats are atrial ectopic beats. The morphology of the P waves is clearly different from that of the basic sinus beats. Each ectopic P wave has a virtually identical morphology indicating the unifocal nature of the ectopics.

(b) Chest monitoring lead. Sinus rhythm with multifocal atrial premature beats. The basic rhythm is sinus. Beats 3, 5, 6, 9 and 11 are atrial premature ectopic beats which show varied P′ morphology and P-P′ coupling intervals, indicating the multifocal nature of the ectopics.

Wandering atrial pacemaker

This is simply the equivalent of multiple sites giving rise to atrial ectopic beats, the sites having a similar degree of prematurity so that no one site dominates the rhythm. The P′-P′ intervals tend to be relatively constant and the P wave morphology tends to vary. An example is shown in Figure 240.

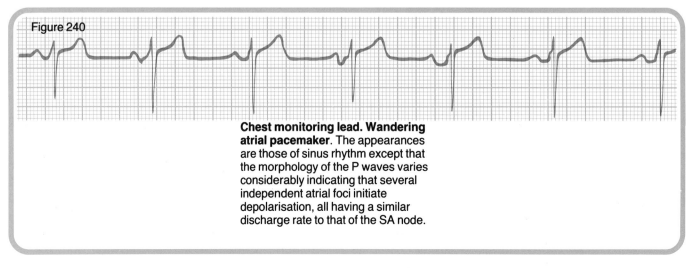

Chest monitoring lead. Wandering atrial pacemaker. The appearances are those of sinus rhythm except that the morphology of the P waves varies considerably indicating that several independent atrial foci initiate depolarisation, all having a similar discharge rate to that of the SA node.

Frequency of atrial premature ectopic beats

The frequency of atrial premature beats can be expressed in the terminology used. When such a beat occurs alternately with sinus beats the condition is referred to as "coupled atrial premature beats" or as "atrial coupling" or as "atrial bigeminy" (Figure 241).

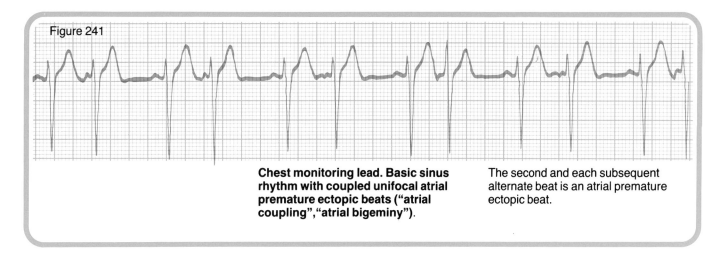

Figure 241

Chest monitoring lead. Basic sinus rhythm with coupled unifocal atrial premature ectopic beats ("atrial coupling","atrial bigeminy").

The second and each subsequent alternate beat is an atrial premature ectopic beat.

When the ectopic beats occur every third beat (two sinus beats to each atrial ectopic) the rhythm is sometimes referred to as "atrial trigeminy" (Figure 242).

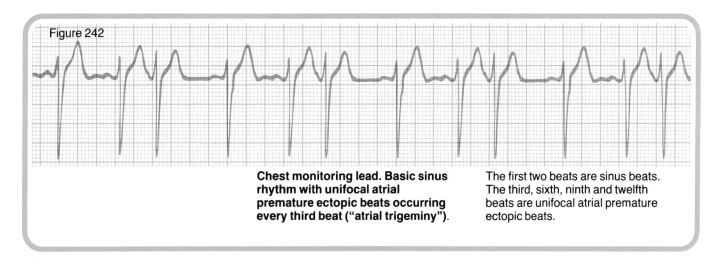

Figure 242

Chest monitoring lead. Basic sinus rhythm with unifocal atrial premature ectopic beats occurring every third beat ("atrial trigeminy").

The first two beats are sinus beats. The third, sixth, ninth and twelfth beats are unifocal atrial premature ectopic beats.

When three or more consecutive atrial premature beats occur (without any intervening sinus beat) a short run of **atrial tachycardia** is said to have occurred (Figure 243).

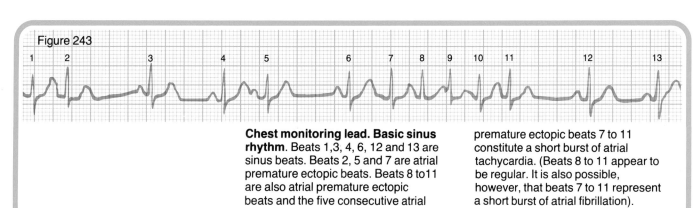

Figure 243

Chest monitoring lead. Basic sinus rhythm. Beats 1,3, 4, 6, 12 and 13 are sinus beats. Beats 2, 5 and 7 are atrial premature ectopic beats. Beats 8 to11 are also atrial premature ectopic beats and the five consecutive atrial

premature ectopic beats 7 to 11 constitute a short burst of atrial tachycardia. (Beats 8 to 11 appear to be regular. It is also possible, however, that beats 7 to 11 represent a short burst of atrial fibrillation).

Aberrant Intraventricular Conduction ("Rate-related Aberration").

The term "aberrant intraventricular conduction" is used when an alteration in the time interval between the arrival of successive supraventricularly-initiated beats at the ventricular conducting tissue results in a secondary alteration in the pathway of intraventricular conduction, with consequent changes in the QRS morphology. The term "rate-related aberration" may also be used. Most commonly, aberration occurs following a **premature** ventricular depolarisation initiated by a supraventricular mechanism ("acceleration-dependent aberrancy", "tachycardia-dependent

aberrancy") but occasionally it can occur because of **delayed** ventricular depolarisation initiated by a supraventricular stimulus ("deceleration-dependent aberrancy", "bradycardia-dependent aberrancy").

Acceleration-dependent Aberrancy ("Tachycardia-dependent Aberrancy")

Just as an atrial premature beat may find the AV node partially refractory so it may find part of the intraventricular conducting tissue (the right and left bundle branches, Purkinje network) refractory. The difference in terminology should be noted. The AV node may be **partially refractory** or completely refractory, the intraventricular conducting tissue may not. Either the intraventricular conducting tissue is refractory or it has recovered. However, it is possible for part of the intraventricular conducting tissue to be refractory when other parts have recovered. Thus right or left bundle branch block or partial ("incomplete") right (less frequently left) bundle branch block may occur.

In general the right bundle takes longer to recover than the left. An atrial premature beat can, therefore, with critical timing, arrive at the intraventricular conducting tissue to find that the right bundle is refractory although the left bundle has recovered (Figure 244).

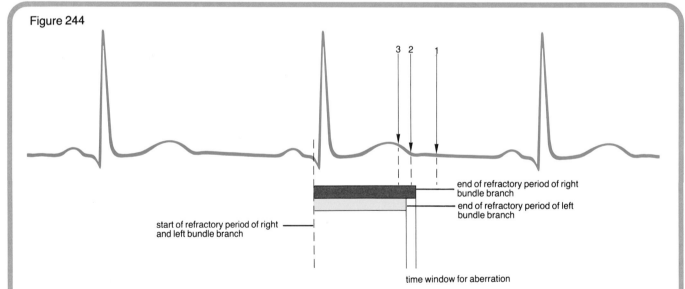

Figure 244

end of refractory period of right bundle branch
end of refractory period of left bundle branch
start of refractory period of right and left bundle branch
time window for aberration

Aberrant intraventricular conduction. The refractory period of each bundle branch begins with the first recognisable deflection of the QRS, when ventricular myocardial depolarisation can be seen to have started. The right bundle branch usually has a longer refractory period than the left. An atrial premature beat which reaches the bundle branches at 1 would find both branches fully recovered and normal intraventricular conduction would occur. This would give rise to a QRS following the atrial premature beat which would be

indistinguishable from the QRS of the sinus beat (the most commonly found situation). An atrial premature beat reaching the intraventricular conducting tissue at 3 would find both bundle branches completely refractory and would be blocked. No QRS complex at all would follow a P′ wave with such timing. An atrial premature beat reaching the bundle branches at 2 would find the left bundle fully recovered and the right bundle totally refractory. There would, therefore, be a QRS complex following such an atrial premature

beat and the QRS would have the right bundle branch block configuration. Such an occurrence does not indicate malfunction in the right bundle branch, merely that the ectopic beat is sufficiently premature to reach the right bundle during its normal refractory period. This phenomenon is called "functional bundle branch block", "rate-related bundle branch block" or "aberrant intraventricular conduction".

An example is shown in Figure 245a.

In a small proportion of cases (<10%) the refractory period of the left bundle may exceed that of the right (without disease or malfunction being present). In such a situation aberrant intraventricular conduction, if it is occurring, will be due to functional ("rate-related") left bundle branch block (Figure 245b).

Although acceleration-dependent left bundle branch block is less common than acceleration-dependent right bundle branch block it is important, for its presence can lead to confusion with ventricular ectopic rhythms. An example is shown in Figure 245b(i).

The length of the refractory periods of the left and right bundle branches are also dependent on the length of the preceding R-R interval (the Ashman phenomenon (page 399)) in exactly the same way as with the AV node. Since the refractory period of the right and left bundle branches elongate *pro rata* in association with a bradycardia, the absolute time difference between them also increases with reduction in the heart rate and therefore the "time window" in which an atrial premature beat could give rise to aberrant intraventricular conduction also increases (Figures 244 and 245a). Although each part of the intraventricular conducting tissue is either refractory or has recovered, varying degrees of right bundle branch block (i.e. varying degrees of aberrancy) may occur because a varying number of cells within the right bundle branch system has recovered. Figure 245a shows an example of two atrial premature beats associated with different degrees of aberrancy.

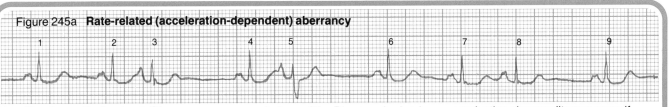

Figure 245a **Rate-related (acceleration-dependent) aberrancy**

Chest monitoring lead. Sinus rhythm with atrial premature beats which are associated with aberrant intraventricular conduction involving the right bundle branch. The basic sinus rate varies a little (see beats 6-9). Beats 3 and 5 are atrial premature ectopic beats (the P' waves can clearly be seen to be premature despite the uncertainty of the predicted R-R interval and the morphology of the P' waves is clearly abnormal). The P' wave of beat 3 is followed by a QRS which is slightly abnormal in its terminal portion. This is due to incomplete functional right bundle branch block ("aberration"). The P wave of beat 5 is followed by a QRS which shows more aberration (a greater degree of right bundle branch block) than the QRS of beat 3. A greater degree of intraventricular conduction abnormality can occur if the beat is more premature. Here, however, the degree of prematurity of beats 3 and 5 is similar. The difference is that beat 5 follows the longer R-R pause of interval 3-4 and it is therefore more likely, by the Ashman phenomenon (page 399), to show aberration.

Much less commonly aberration can occur because of a longer than usual pause between beats (deceleration-dependent aberrancy, Figure 245b).

Figure 245b **Rate-related (acceleration-dependent) aberrancy**

(i)

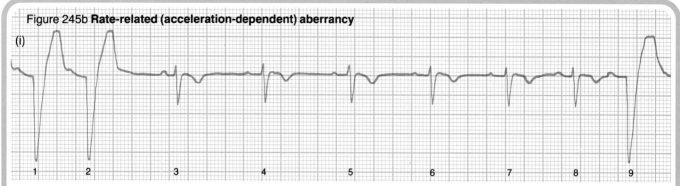

Chest monitoring lead. Sinus rhythm with acceleration-dependent aberrancy involving the left bundle branch.
(i) The first two beats show sinus beats with left bundle branch block. The P-P interval of these two beats is 0.58 sec. Since the P-R interval is constant the R-R interval is also 0.58 sec. Beats 3-8 show sinus rhythm with normal intraventricular conduction. In all of these beats the R-R interval is well in excess of 0.58 sec. Beat 9 follows beat 8 after an R-R interval of 0.58 sec and is associated with left bundle branch block. It appears that when the R-R interval is 0.59 sec or less intraventricular conduction occurs down the right bundle only i.e. that there is rate-related left bundle branch block. The P-R interval is the same during the beats with left bundle branch block as it is during the beats with normal intraventricular conduction.

(ii)

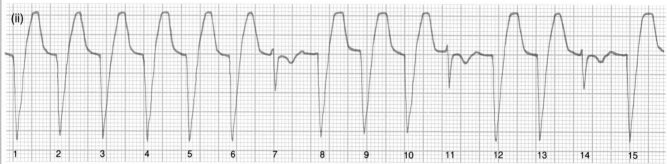

(ii) This record was taken from the same subject as (i) and the two records were made within minutes of each other. Beats 1-6 look like ventricular tachycardia (The complexes are abnormally wide and abnormally shaped, the rate is rapid and regular. It is difficult to see the P waves with confidence and therefore one cannot be sure whether or not there is association between the P waves and the QRS complexes). Beat 7 is clearly associated with normal intraventricular conduction and could conceivably be a capture beat (which would reinforce the diagnosis of ventricular tachycardia). Beat 8 could represent the start of ventricular tachycardia again, perhaps just happening to occur at a normal P-R interval following the P wave which can clearly be seen between beats 7 and 8. The same might be said of beats 12 and 15 but it would be a powerful coincidence if ventricular tachycardia* happened to be initiated at 8, 12 and 15, each time after a constant common normal P-R interval. The true explanation can be seen from record (iii) which is recorded during right-sided carotid sinus massage seconds after record (ii) was taken. (Superficial inspection might suggest that beats 7 and 11 are premature. This is an illusion because they are narrow and the other QRS complexes are not. The beginnings of beats 7 and 11 are not premature after the beginnings of beats 6 and 10 respectively).

Right carotid sinus massage

(iii)

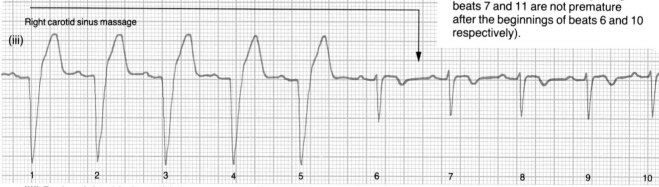

(iii) During right-sided carotid sinus massage.
The sinus rate is slow. Beats 1-5 clearly show sinus rhythm with left bundle branch block. The R-R interval is 0.74 sec. Beats 6-10 show sinus rhythm with normal intraventricular conduction. The R-R interval 5-6 is 0.81 sec. The P-R interval is constant during the record. The appearances are those of rate-related bundle branch block. The situation is complicated, however, since the R-R interval of 9-10 is 0.72 sec and on the basis of the experience of beats 1-5 one would have expected left bundle branch block. It is possible (i) that the minimum interval required to produce functional left bundle branch block is varying, (ii) that during beats 1-5 the induced vagal activity was prolonging the refractory period of the left bundle branch as well as slowing the sinus rate (vagal stimulation was terminated between beats 6 and 7), (iii) that there was "hysteresis" in the rate-related bundle branch block or (iv) that a combination of the above factors was operating.

*This term is not strictly applicable in relation to 12 since only two abnormal complexes are seen.

Deceleration-dependent aberrancy is much less common than acceleration-dependent aberrancy and aberration involving the left bundle branch is much less common than that involving the right bundle branch.

Deceleration-dependent Aberrancy ("Bradycardia-dependent Aberrancy")

The above-described variety of aberrancy is, strictly speaking, acceleration-dependent aberrancy although since it is far and away the commonest variety of aberrancy to be seen, it is often loosely termed "rate-related aberrancy". A much less common variety is deceleration-dependent aberrancy in which aberration follows an unusually-long cycle rather than an unusually-short one. The aberration may involve defective conduction or failure of conduction down the left bundle branch or down the right bundle branch. The problem, of course, is to be sure that it is not a ventricular escape beat which is being seen. Ventricular escape beats are rather commoner than deceleration-dependent aberrancy and in order to be sure that deceleration-dependent aberrancy has in fact occurred one needs to see two or more consecutive aberrant QRS complexes, each preceded by the same P-R interval (Figure 246a).

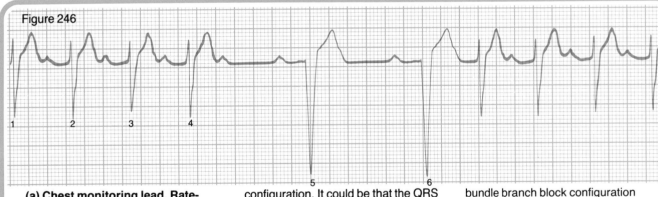

Figure 246

(a) Chest monitoring lead. Rate-related deceleration-dependent aberrancy.
The basic rhythm is sinus tachycardia with first degree heart block (P-R interval = 0.33 sec). After the fourth QRS there is failure of atrio-ventricular conduction for one beat but the next P wave is followed by a QRS (number 5) which has the same P-R interval as the first few beats but has a left bundle branch block configuration. It could be that the QRS number 5 is simply a ventricular escape beat but this is very unlikely since beat 6 (which also follows transient failure of atrio-ventricular conduction (there is a P wave deforming the downstroke of the T wave of beat 5)) has the same QRS, S-T and T morphology as beat 5 and has the same P-R interval. When (a) two or more consecutive QRS complexes have the (left or right) bundle branch block configuration **and** (b) each has followed a longer than usual R-R interval **and** (c) each has the same P-R interval (though it is not required that there should be the same P-R interval as during sinus rhythm) then it is likely that deceleration-dependent aberrancy is the mechanism. Contrast the situation in (b) and in Figure 245b(i).

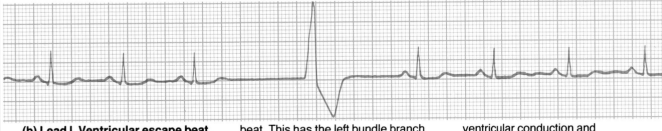

(b) Lead I. Ventricular escape beat.
The basic rhythm is sinus. After the first three beats there is a period of sinus arrest with a ventricular escape beat. This has the left bundle branch block configuration (as do beats 5 and 6 in (a)) but there is no P wave in front of the QRS so there is no atrio-ventricular conduction and deceleration-dependent aberrancy cannot be to blame.

Rate-related aberrancy of a given beat clearly depends on the proximity of that beat to the preceding beat (Figure 244) and on the size of the time window which represents the difference between the right and left bundle branch recovery (refractory) periods (Figure 244). Since this difference between the refractory periods of the two bundle branches bears a direct relation to the length of each refractory period (i.e. the longer the individual bundle branch refractory period the greater the absolute difference between the two – Figure 244) aberration in relation to beat R_n is more likely when the total refractory period of the preceding beat $R_{(n-1)}$ is long. (A long refractory period occurs in relation to any beat which follows a pause (the Ashman phenomenon)). Aberration is thus most likely to occur when a beat occurs early, following a beat which was itself preceded by a pause (i.e. if $R_{(n-2)}$ to $R_{(n-1)}$ is long (i.e. a pause) and $R_{(n-1)}$ to R_n is short (an early beat), R_n is likely to show aberration). The combination of a long pause followed by a short pause occurs most frequently in relation to atrial fibrillation and intermittent aberrant intraventricular conduction is most commonly seen in association with this rhythm (Figure 285). It may also occur in relation to supraventricular premature beats (Figure 245(a)) and in relation simply to an increase in supraventricular rate (e.g. in sinus tachycardia (Figure 245(b)) and supraventricular tachycardia). Since the refractory period of the right bundle branch is nearly always longer than that of the left bundle branch, aberrancy almost invariably means functional right bundle branch block (Figure 245(a)). Rarely it may involve functional left bundle branch block (Figure 245(b)).

Junctional Premature Beats : Additional Features

Essentially, the additional features of junctional premature beats are the same as those of atrial premature beats.

The P′-R interval

The length of the P′-R interval depends upon:
1. the degree of prematurity of the P′ wave,
2. the length of the preceding R-R interval,
3. the location of the ectopic focus within the AV junctional area (in the case of this latter variable, the variation in the P′-R interval depends on differences in AV nodal travel times (since different AV nodal travel distances are involved) rather than variations in atrial myocardial travel time as with atrial premature beats),
4. the condition of that part of the AV node which is distal to the focus of the premature beat.

Blocked (non-conducted) junctional premature beats

Blocked junctional ectopic beats are rare because part, at least, of the AV junctional area must no longer be refractory for the ectopic beat to occur. It is, of course, theoretically possible for an ectopic impulse to arise in the proximal part of the AV node at a time when the distal part is refractory; so, in theory at least, junctional ectopic beats could be blocked.

Variation in the post-ectopic pause

The principles involved here are essentially the same as those for atrial premature ectopic beats except that in respect of junctional premature ectopic beats it is much more frequently true that depolarisation does not transmit backwards to the atrial myocardium and therefore may not re-set the sino-atrial node.

Unifocal or multifocal junctional beats

These could theoretically occur but there would be no discernible difference in the P′ wave, since in each case the spread across the atria would be initiated in the AV junctional area. It is only possible to recognise such a phenomenon by variations in the P′-R interval (see Wandering junctional pacemaker).

Wandering junctional pacemaker

As with multifocal junctional premature beats this could only be recognised by variation in the P′-R interval during junctional rhythm. However, in the case of junctional premature ectopic beats the P′-R interval can be zero (P′ and R occur simultaneously) or can be negative (R occurs before P′) since ectopic impulses arising in the mid-AV node may reach the atrial myocardium (retrogradely) and the ventricular myocardium (antegradely) at the same time and those arising low down in the AV node may reach the ventricular myocardium before the atrial myocardium. It may also be that retrograde spread to the atrial myocardium is blocked and no P′ wave occurs.

Frequency of junctional premature beats

The terms "coupled junctional premature beats", "junctional coupling" and "junctional bigeminy" all refer to alternating sinus and junctional beats. Junctional beats occurring every third beat (two sinus beats to each junctional beat) could be called junctional trigeminy. When three or more junctional premature beats occur consecutively without any intervening sinus beat a short run of junctional tachycardia is said to have occurred.

Aberrant intraventricular conduction

This occurs with junctional premature beats in the same way as with atrial premature beats. This phenomenon can only occur if the premature junctional beat arrives at the level of the bundle branches at a time when one bundle branch (usually the left) has recovered and the other has not. When such a phenomenon occurs it is, in 90% of cases, the right bundle which is functionally blocked (and in 10% of cases the left bundle). In either case there is said to be aberrant intraventricular conduction.

Ventricular Ectopic Beats :
Additional Features

The coupling interval

The term "coupling interval" is only applied to ectopic beats which are premature (i.e. to active ectopic beats). The coupling interval of a ventricular ectopic, premature beat is the time interval between the onset of the premature QRS complex and the onset of the QRS complex which precedes it. The lower limit for the coupling interval is set by the refractory period for the ventricle following the ventricular depolarisation which precedes the ectopic. The upper limit will depend upon the time interval between the onset of consecutive QRS complexes in the underlying rhythm. Each of these variables will be related to the underlying heart rate (Figure 247).

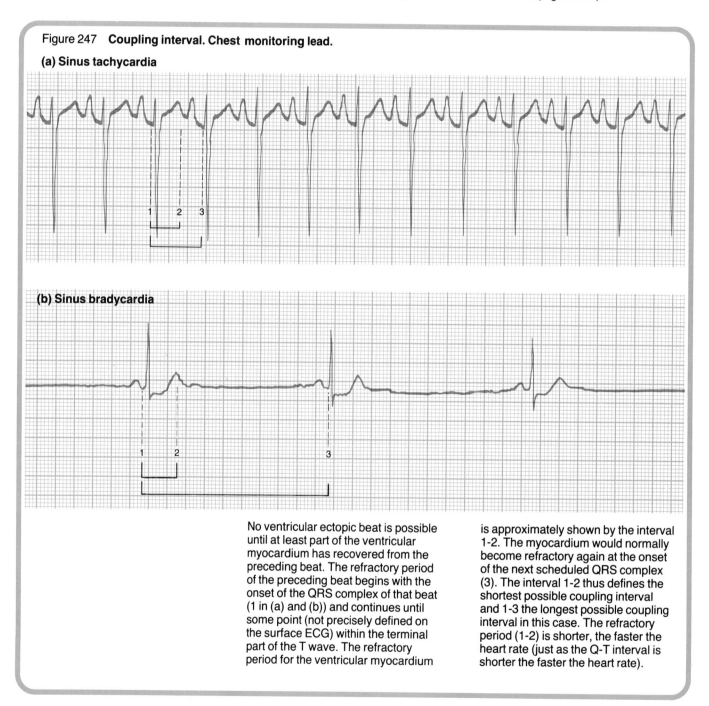

Figure 247   **Coupling interval. Chest monitoring lead.**

(a) Sinus tachycardia

(b) Sinus bradycardia

No ventricular ectopic beat is possible until at least part of the ventricular myocardium has recovered from the preceding beat. The refractory period of the preceding beat begins with the onset of the QRS complex of that beat (1 in (a) and (b)) and continues until some point (not precisely defined on the surface ECG) within the terminal part of the T wave. The refractory period for the ventricular myocardium is approximately shown by the interval 1-2. The myocardium would normally become refractory again at the onset of the next scheduled QRS complex (3). The interval 1-2 thus defines the shortest possible coupling interval and 1-3 the longest possible coupling interval in this case. The refractory period (1-2) is shorter, the faster the heart rate (just as the Q-T interval is shorter the faster the heart rate).

It is clear that for a ventricular ectopic beat to occur on the background of a rapid heart rate, the degree of prematurity must be great, i.e.it must occur soon after the preceding QRS. However, on the background of a bradycardia the degree of prematurity required is considerably less (Figure 248a and Figure 248b).

In the case of unifocal ventricular premature beats the coupling interval is usually constant (see Figure 254) where the time interval between the onset of the QRS of the normal beat and the onset of the QRS of the following ectopic beat is identical in relation to beats 2/3, 6/7 and 10/11). If, however, ectopic beats arise from different foci, then they have different coupling intervals. Figure 256 shows an example of two ventricular premature beats arising from different foci and having different coupling intervals.

Figure 248 **Chest monitoring lead.**

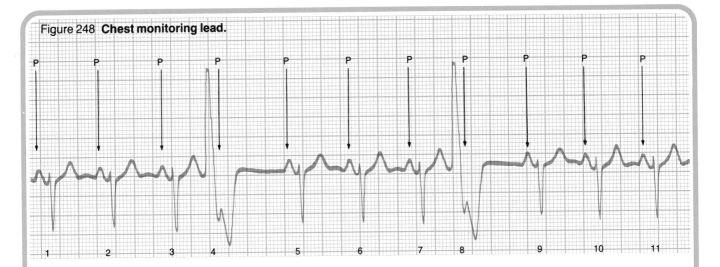

(a) Sinus rhythm with unifocal ventricular premature beats.
The sinus rate is just below 100 beats/min. The fourth and eighth beats are ventricular premature beats. They are premature because the QRS occurred earlier in beat 4 than anticipated from inspecting beats 1–3 and earlier in beat 8 than anticipated from inspecting beats 5–7. They are ventricular in origin since the QRS of beats 4 and 8 are abnormally wide and abnormally shaped, occur without a preceding P wave and are followed by a normal P wave occurring at precisely the time anticipated by inspecting the adjacent P waves. (There is therefore no retrograde conduction of the ventricular ectopic beat through the AV node). The time interval between QRS complexes 3 and 5 is exactly twice that between the QRS complexes of the sinus beats 1 and 2, 2 and 3 etc, i.e. the pause between 4 and 5 is truly compensatory. Beats 4 and 8 have identical morphologies and are likely to arise at the same site. They also have the same coupling interval (0.36 sec) and are therefore likely to arise on a re-entry basis (see later). This coupling interval is relatively short. In view of the background tachycardia any Purkinje cell attempting to depolarise with much less than this degree of prematurity (i.e. occurring appreciably later) would probably find the myocardium refractory from the next sinus-initiated beat.

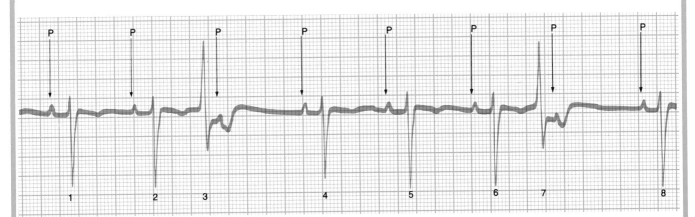

(b) Sinus rhythm with unifocal ventricular premature beats.
The sinus rate is just above 60 beats/min. The third and seventh beats are ventricular premature beats. They are premature beats because the QRS occurred earlier in each case than would be anticipated by inspecting the normal rhythm involved in beats 1 and 2 and beats 4, 5 and 6. They are ventricular in origin since the QRS of beats 3 and 7 are abnormally wide, are abnormally shaped, occur without a preceding P wave and are followed by a normal P wave occurring at precisely the time anticipated by inspecting the adjacent P waves. (There is therefore no retrograde conduction of the ventricular ectopic beat through the AV node). The time interval between the QRS complexes of beats 2 and 4 is exactly twice that between the normal QRS complexes of the sinus beats 1 and 2, 4 and 5, 5 and 6 etc, i.e. the pause between beats 3 and 4 and again between 7 and 8 is truly compensatory. Beats 3 and 7 have identical morphologies and are likely to arise at the same site. They also have the same coupling interval (0.56 sec) and they are therefore likely to arise on the basis of a re-entry mechanism (see later). It is possible for a beat with a long coupling interval like 0.56 sec to be premature only because the prevailing sinus rate is slow.

Interpolated ventricular premature ectopic beats

The compensatory pause which typically follows a ventricular premature ectopic beat occurs because the next sinus-initiated P wave occurring after the ventricular premature beat usually falls during the S-T segment or T wave of that beat so that the oncoming depolarisation wave from the next sinus beat finds the ventricles refractory (Figures 228, 230 and 248). If the sinus-initiated P wave following a ventricular premature beat does not result in spread of the depolarisation process to the ventricles until after they have recovered from the ventricular premature ectopic beat then ventricular depolarisation will follow and no pause will occur. This can happen either if there is sinus bradycardia (so that there is plenty of time for recovery of the ventricles from the ventricular ectopic beat before the next sinus-initiated beat is due) or because the ventricular premature beat is very premature (with the same result). Thus, for example, in relation to Figure 248b, if the sinus rate were appreciably slower then the P wave would occur well after the end of the T wave of the ventricular premature beat (3) and it would be followed by its own normal QRS. Likewise if the ventricular premature beat (3) occurred a little earlier than it does the same effect would occur without the need for a sinus bradycardia. Inspection of Figure 247 will reveal that a premature beat can only occur if ventricular depolarisation is initiated later than "2" and will only be interpolated if repolarisation following the ectopic beat is complete before "3". The opportunities for interpolation are clearly greater the slower the prevailing sinus rate.

An example of an intraventricular premature ectopic beat occurring on a background of bradycardia and being "interpolated" as a result of the slow background rate is shown in Figure 249.

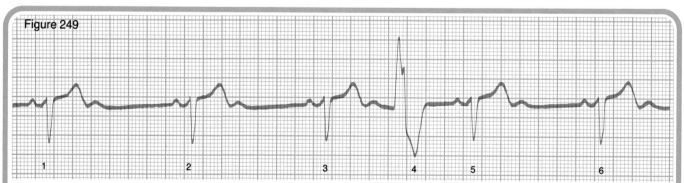

Figure 249

Chest monitoring lead. Sinus bradycardia with one interpolated ventricular premature ectopic beat.
The background rhythm is sinus bradycardia with a heart rate of approximately 40 beats/min (the rate varies slightly). The first three beats are sinus beats. A prominent U wave (pages 195, 227, 233 and 263) is seen after each T wave. After the third sinus beat there is a ventricular premature ectopic beat (beat 4). It is recognisably premature since the QRS' occurs recognisably earlier than the next anticipated QRS. It is recognisably ectopic in having an abnormal shape and width. No retrograde conduction of the depolarisation to the atria is seen (i.e. there is no inverted P wave following the QRS'). Repolarisation (S-T segment and T wave) following the QRS' is completed long before the next scheduled sinus beat (beat 5). The time interval between beats 3 and 5 is approximately (not precisely, since the sinus rate varies) the same as that between beats 1 and 2, 2 and 3 and 5 and 6 and beat 4 is therefore "interpolated".

An example of a ventricular premature beat occurring very early and being "interpolated" as a result of this marked prematurity is seen in Figure 250.

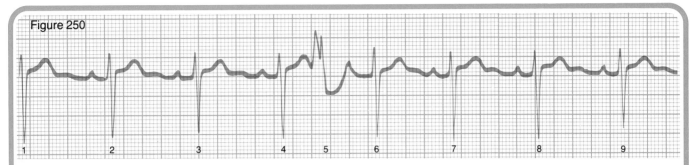

Figure 250

Chest monitoring lead. Sinus rhythm with a single interpolated ventricular premature ectopic beat. The first four beats are sinus beats. Just before the T wave of the fourth beat is complete, a ventricular premature ectopic beat occurs. This beat is markedly premature (it is an R-on-T ectopic – see Figure 251). The next sinus-initiated P wave occurs as anticipated and can be seen superimposed on the terminal part of the T wave of the ectopic beat (beat 5). This P wave is followed by a normal QRS. The interval 4-6 is approximately the same as the intervals 1-2, 2-3 and 3-4. The beat is interpolated between two normal sinus beats. It is interpolated because it is so premature that the ventricles have recovered (repolarised) from the ventricular premature beat before the next sinus beat is due. (Careful inspection reveals that the P-R interval of beat 6 is longer than that of beats 1-4. This indicates that depolarisation from beat 5 **did** spread retrogradely through (part at least) of the AV node causing a prolongation of the refractory period. This prolonged refractory period has "revealed" the otherwise occult retrograde conductions through the AV node. The occult retrograde conduction is said to be "concealed").

R-on-T ventricular ectopic premature beats

When the degree of prematurity of a ventricular premature ectopic beat is such that the R wave of the ectopic beat begins before the T wave of the preceding non-ectopic beat is completed, the premature beat is said to be of the "R-on-T" type. An example is shown in Figure 251.

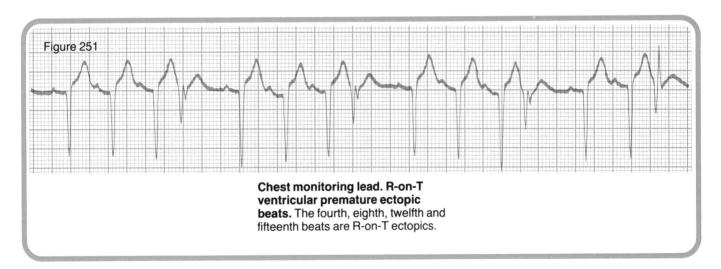

Figure 251

Chest monitoring lead. R-on-T ventricular premature ectopic beats. The fourth, eighth, twelfth and fifteenth beats are R-on-T ectopics.

R-on-T ectopics and the ventricular vulnerable period

An R-on-T ectopic is one in which the QRS complex ("R") of the premature beat occurs before the completion of the T wave of the preceding beat (Figure 251). During the terminal part of the T wave, part of the myocardium of the ventricle will have repolarised and will no longer be refractory, whereas other parts will still be refractory. The terminal part of the T wave is therefore referred to as the ventricular "vulnerable period" (Figure 252). Ventricular ectopic beats occurring during this period may give rise to ventricular tachycardia (see Figure 304) or even to ventricular fibrillation (see Record 78). Because of this, R-on-T ectopics occurring following acute myocardial infarction have been recognised as prognostically important and have been listed amongst the so-called "warning arrhythmias". However, about half of patients who develop ventricular tachycardia or fibrillation do so without "warning arrhythmias" and half of patients who do have warning arrhythmias do not develop ventricular fibrillation.

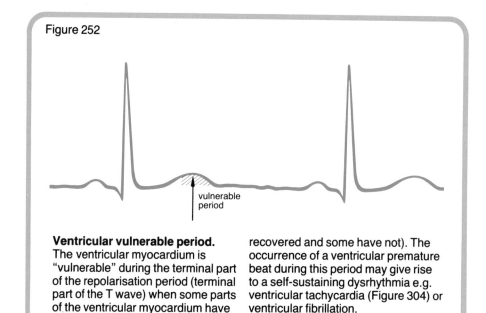

Figure 252

vulnerable
period

Ventricular vulnerable period.
The ventricular myocardium is
"vulnerable" during the terminal part
of the repolarisation period (terminal
part of the T wave) when some parts
of the ventricular myocardium have
recovered and some have not). The
occurrence of a ventricular premature
beat during this period may give rise
to a self-sustaining dysrhythmia e.g.
ventricular tachycardia (Figure 304) or
ventricular fibrillation.

Morphology of ventricular ectopic beats

Since ventricular ectopic beats arise within the Purkinje tissue of the ventricular myocardium the direction of spread of the depolarisation wave through the ventricular myocardium is necessarily abnormal. The depolarisation wave travels more slowly than normal and follows an abnormal route. Since the total travel time of the depolarisation wave is increased, the QRS duration is increased. Since the travel route is abnormal, the QRS morphology is abnormal. Since repolarisation is abnormal (because of the abnormality of depolarisation) the S-T segment and T waves are abnormal. The **duration** of the QRS complex of a ventricular ectopic beat is usually 0.12 sec or more. This is the same time criterion as for bundle branch block in which condition the pathway of intraventricular conduction is also abnormal. In the case of a supraventricular beat (sinus beat, atrial ectopic beat, atrial tachycardia, atrial flutter, junctional ectopic beats, junctional tachycardia etc) with bundle branch block and also in the case of a ventricular ectopic beat, one ventricle necessarily receives the depolarisation wave late, simply because the depolarisation wave does not travel via the normal (rapidly conducting) intraventricular conduction tissue pathways. In the case of an ectopic beat arising in the **right** ventricle, left ventricular depolarisation is necessarily delayed and contributes the **terminal part of the QRS complex.** This is exactly the same situation as that which obtains in relation to a supraventricular beat with **left** bundle branch block. Furthermore the interventricular septum is depolarised from left to right in the case of right bundle branch block and of left ventricular ectopic beats and the septum is depolarised from right to left in the case of left bundle branch block and of right ventricular ectopic beats. The direction of septal depolarisation determines the **initial part of the QRS.** Therefore a ventricular ectopic beat showing morphology for the QRS complexes, S-T segments and T waves identical to that anticipated in **left** bundle branch block must be arising in the **right** ventricle (including the right side of the interventricular septum) (Figure 253). Conversely a ventricular ectopic beat showing a **right** bundle branch block type of configuration must be arising in the **left** ventricle (including the left side of the interventricular septum).

Figure 253

(a) Leads V₁–V₆. Sinus tachycardia with right ventricular premature beats (the P waves indicate the presence of left atrial hypertrophy). The form of the ventricular premature beats is the same as that for left bundle branch block in a beat of supraventricular origin. (This short strip of recording does not provide sufficient information for one to be sure that the underlying rhythm is sinus tachycardia. This actually is the case, however, a short strip only being provided. There is a full compensatory pause after the ectopic beat).

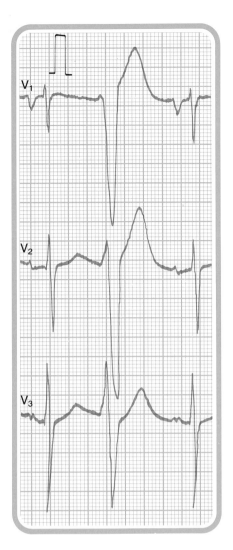
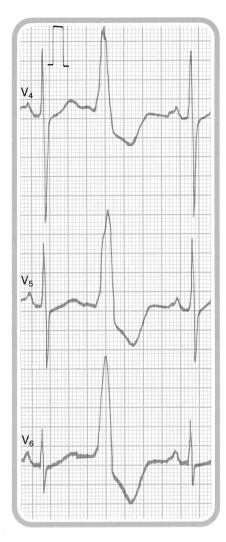

Figure 253

(b) Leads V₁–V₆. Sinus rhythm with left bundle branch block.

Note the similarity in the morphology of the QRS complexes of the ectopic beat in (b) with those of the sinus beats with left bundle branch block in (a).

Ventricular ectopic beats which have the QRS morphology of **left** bundle branch block arise from the **right** ventricle (including the right side of the interventricular septum).

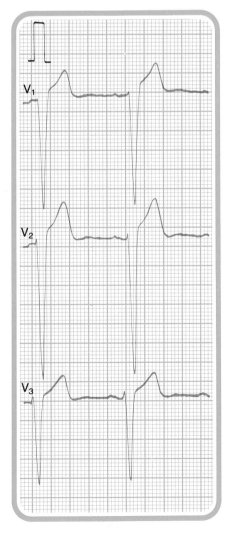
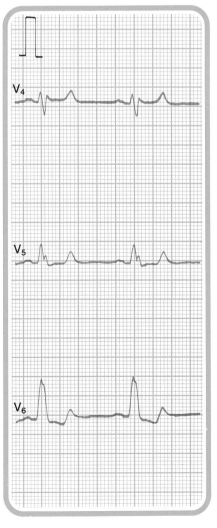

Uniform and multiform ("Unifocal and multifocal") ventricular premature ectopic beats

Ectopic beats which consistently arise from the same anatomical site (unifocal ectopics) will, in general, give rise to the same depolarisation configuration within the primary chamber (i.e. within the atria or within the ventricles). Thus unifocal atrial premature ectopic beats will give rise to abnormally shaped P waves in which the abnormality of shape is constant. Likewise unifocal ventricular premature ectopic beats give rise to abnormal QRS complexes with no significant variation in morphology amongst the shape of the ectopic QRS complexes. Figure 254 shows an example of unifocal ventricular premature ectopic beats. Figure 256 shows two ventricular premature ectopic beats arising from different foci. From the uniformity of morphology of the QRS complexes one can only conclude that the focus is in approximately the same area. For this reason most authorities have now adopted the terms "uniform" and "multiform" in preference to "unifocal" and "multifocal".

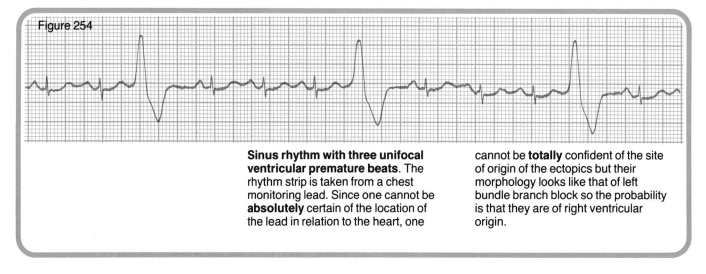

Figure 254

Sinus rhythm with three unifocal ventricular premature beats. The rhythm strip is taken from a chest monitoring lead. Since one cannot be **absolutely** certain of the location of the lead in relation to the heart, one cannot be **totally** confident of the site of origin of the ectopics but their morphology looks like that of left bundle branch block so the probability is that they are of right ventricular origin.

Frequency of ventricular ectopic beats

Ventricular ectopic beats are commonly observed to occur in what appears to be a haphazard fashion. The apparent frequency of ectopic beats is, of course, related to the time at which the record is taken and the duration of the recording period. A conventional 12-lead ECG will usually contain about 12 seconds of recording if a 3-channel machine is used or just over half a minute of recording if a single-channel recorder is used. If a single ectopic beat is recorded in a 12-lead record this could be the result of a chance capture of a rare event or could, if the record happens to be representative of the usual frequency of the events in that patient at that time, indicate the true frequency of occurrence of the ectopics*. Thus one ectopic occurring during a 30-second recording period could equate to almost 3,000 such ectopics per 24 hours or it could simply be the only ectopic which occurred. It is therefore extremely difficult to make any realistic assessment of the frequency of ectopic beats on the basis of a conventional 12-lead recording, although statistically it follows that in most cases when a ventricular ectopic beat is seen on a 12-lead record, the ectopic beats are very frequent. A 24-hour ambulatory ECG recording (see pages 542 to 552) provides a more realistic basis for such an assessment but even this technique gives only a modest time-sample. Nevertheless, when multiple ectopic beats are seen during a standard recording period it is clear that the frequency of their occurrence must be high. In respect of the kind of frequency of ectopics seen in Figure 254, these would certainly be regarded as "frequent" if the sample of ECG is typical of the frequency obtaining in that patient since three out of twelve beats were ventricular ectopics. They are most certainly "frequent" during that period of observation.

*Equally, of course, the record could have been taken when fewer than usual ectopics were occurring.

As in the case of atrial premature beats the terms "bigeminy" and "trigeminy" are sometimes used. **"Bigeminal rhythm", "bigeminy"** and **"coupling"** all refer to the presence of alternate, unifocal ectopic beats (usually, but not always, in the context of an underlying sinus rhythm) and the terms are applied to **ventricular** coupling in exactly the same way as they are to atrial coupling. Figure 255 shows an example of coupled ventricular premature beats.

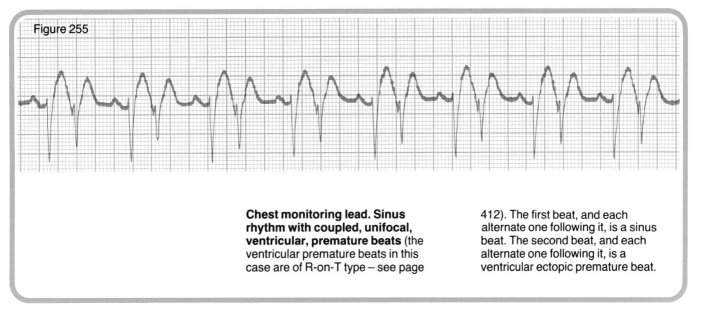

Figure 255

Chest monitoring lead. Sinus rhythm with coupled, unifocal, ventricular, premature beats (the ventricular premature beats in this case are of R-on-T type – see page 412). The first beat, and each alternate one following it, is a sinus beat. The second beat, and each alternate one following it, is a ventricular ectopic premature beat.

Self-perpetuation of ventricular premature ectopic beats

The initiation of a ventricular premature beat seems to be favoured by the occurrence of a long preceding cycle, i.e. a long R-R interval leading into the last normal QRS before the ectopic. Once a ventricular premature beat has occurred it will, of course, usually be followed by a compensatory pause (pages 390-392) which is, itself, a long R-R interval so that the normal QRS which occurs following a ventricular premature beat will itself be at the end of a long R-R interval (in this case an R′-R interval) and it follows that the next beat which follows this normal beat will be more likely to be an ectopic. In this way bigeminal rhythm (or coupling) tends to perpetuate itself (Figure 255). This phenomenon has been called "the rule of bigeminy".

Constancy of the coupling interval

In relation to a given subject at a given time, the coupling interval (R-R′ interval) of ventricular premature beats tends to be constant. (For example the coupling interval of the ventricular ectopic beats seen during the recording of V_1–V_3 in Figure 253a is the same as that seen later during the recording of V_4–V_6 in the same subject. Also the coupling interval of all three ventricular ectopic beats seen in Figure 254 is the same).

This constancy of the coupling interval is only seen in relation to **unifocal** ventricular premature ectopic beats.

This consistency of the coupling interval in relation to unifocal ventricular premature beats is thought to indicate that the premature beat is in some way linked to the normal beat which precedes it. This could be because of a re-entry mechanism or because of enhancement of sub-threshold activity. The concept of re-entry was discussed on page 355. In relation to the fixed coupling interval of unifocal ventricular premature beats the theory of their mechanism postulates that there is depression of conductivity within the myocardium in the area from which the ectopic beat arises. This area, with an adjacent area of normal refractoriness, gives rise to a re-entry circuit, similar to that shown in Figure 193 so that a second depolarisation (the ectopic beat) is triggered to follow the (pre-ectopic) normal beat. The coupling interval thus depends on the conduction velocity in the normal and abnormal myocardium and the length of the overall re-entrant circuit, but is likely to be constant for a given site of origin of the ectopic beat. An alternative theory to account for the usually fixed coupling interval for unifocal ventricular premature beats is that the impulse preceding the premature beats somehow results in enhancement of an adjacent sub-threshold focus which is thus constrained to depolarise before the next anticipated sinus beat.

The coupling interval will be variable if **either**
(a) there are multifocal ventricular premature ectopic beats (with differing local re-entry circuits)
or
(b) there is parasystole (see below).

An example of a rhythm strip showing two ventricular premature beats arising from different foci (and therefore having different QRS configurations) and having different coupling intervals is shown in Figure 256.

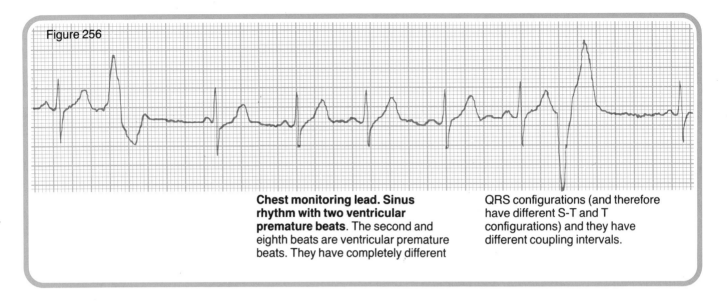

Chest monitoring lead. Sinus rhythm with two ventricular premature beats. The second and eighth beats are ventricular premature beats. They have completely different QRS configurations (and therefore have different S-T and T configurations) and they have different coupling intervals.

Parasystole

"Parasystole" describes a ventricular ectopic rhythm which is different from the usual form of ventricular ectopic activity both in its electrocardiographic manifestations and also in its probable mechanism. It is much less common than the usual form of ventricular ectopic beat. A parasystolic focus (usually in a Purkinje cell) can only express itself if it is "protected" from the spread of depolarisation which normally arrives at the Purkinje cell following spread from the sinus node, through the atrial myocardium, AV node, bundle branches and Purkinje network. Parasystole is a rare arrhythmia which behaves like a "protected" relatively slow idioventricular pacemaker. In normal circumstances all the idioventricular pacemakers are depolarised (before they can reach threshold themselves) by the oncoming activation wavefront, usually initiated by the sino-atrial node. If the sino-atrial node fails to depolarise within the time required for the AV node to re-cycle the AV node will usually depolarise (nodal or junctional escape) but if the AV node also fails to depolarise, an idioventricular escape beat will occur. If a given idioventricular focus is "protected" from the normal oncoming wavefront ("entrance block") it will depolarise at its own rate, independent of what is going on around it (Figure 192). It cannot, of course, initiate depolarisation of **adjacent** myocardium when the latter is refractory as a result of depolarisation from some other site. Thus a parasystolic depolarisation will give rise to a QRS, S-T and T wave of ventricular ectopic variety whenever it happens to occur between the end of a T wave and the beginning of the next QRS complex. It will still **itself** depolarise on schedule even when the adjacent myocardium is refractory (as between the onset of a QRS complex and the end of a T wave) but will not be apparent on the ECG – it will be "concealed". Parasystole is rare but even when present it is often missed for it will require a much longer rhythm strip than usual. The great clue to its presence is the **varied coupling interval to the preceding orthodromic QRS complex** despite constancy of the R′ morphology.

Most ventricular ectopic beats occur on a re-entry basis and have a fixed coupling interval to the preceding beat (R-R′ = constant – the time from the onset of the antecedent R wave to that of the ectopic R wave (R′) is constant). When this clue has been recognised it is sometimes (but not always – depending on how much of the rhythm trace is available) possible to assess the true periodicity of the parasystolic focus. The cycle length is always less than or equal to the minimum time interval between consecutive revealed parasystolic ectopic beats and each parasystolic interval will be an integral multiple of the fundamental cycle length. An example is shown in Figure 257.

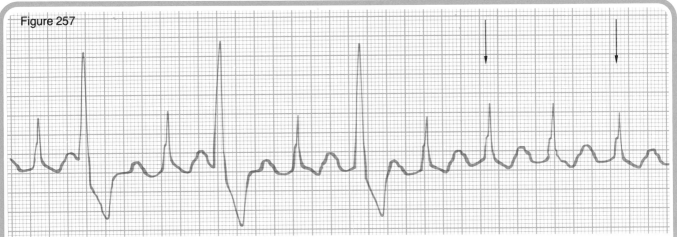

Figure 257

Chest monitoring lead. Sinus rhythm with ventricular parasystole. The sinus rate is approximately 90 beats/min. The beginning of each P wave merges with the end of each preceding T wave. Three ventricular premature beats are seen. They have identical morphology, indicating that they are unifocal ventricular ectopic beats but they do not have a constant coupling interval to the QRS complex of the preceding sinus beat. The varying coupling interval despite constant R′ wave morphology strongly suggests parasystole. This represents an independent ventricular focus depolarising at its own rate. It is "protected" by entrance block against the oncoming depolarisation re-setting it. The rate of the parasystolic focus is regular. The next two parasystolic ventricular ectopic beats would be anticipated at the times indicated by the arrows. They do not express themselves (i.e. are not visible) since the ventricles are discharged by the oncoming waveform (initiated originally from the sino-atrial node) before the parasystolic focus can fire. Only when the (independent) parasystolic focus lies outside the ventricular refractory period can an ectopic QRS complex be produced. The hallmark of the recognition of ventricular parasystole is the recognition of unifocal (i.e. constant morphology) QRS complexes which have a varying coupling interval to the preceding QRS. In this particular example three consecutive parasystolic ventricular discharges are seen so that the R′-R′ interval of the parasystolic focus is readily apparent. This is not always the case. Sometimes one is not able to record two consecutive parasystolic discharges. The parasystolic R′-R′ interval may have to be estimated by inspection of several intervals between consecutive parasystolic ectopics over quite a long period. The only common factor will be that the interval between two revealed parasystolic depolarisations will always be an integral multiple of the basic parasystolic interval. In this particular example the multiple is 1 but it may be any positive integer.

Not all examples of parasystole behave in this "ideal" manner. Minor degrees of modulation of the extrasystolic cycle length can occur, in which case the precise integral relationship between the basic parasystolic interval (extrasystolic cycle length) and the interval between revealed parasystolic depolarisations will not obtain.

Concealed retrograde conduction of ventricular premature ectopic beats

Although most ventricular premature ectopic beats do not conduct retrogradely to the atria, a sizeable minority do so. Such conduction is apparent only if it gives rise to subsequent retrograde (inverted) P waves or if it interferes with the next cycle. The latter phenomenon is most likely to occur with interpolated ventricular ectopic beats (page 411). Only if the ventricular ectopic is interpolated will the next sinus P wave be followed by a QRS and will there be a P-R interval from which one can assess if any process has taken place in the AV node to interfere with its normal recovery. A prolonged P-R interval in the beat immediately following an interpolated ventricular premature beat indicates that "concealed" retrograde conduction of the ventricular ectopic to the AV node did occur (see Figure 250).

The ECG in the Presence of a Heterotopic Heart

An even more unusual form of paraysytole occurs when the patient has two hearts, as in the heterotopic cardiac transplantation. Each heart may be in any given rhythm but the important point is that each is electrically isolated from the other. Figure 258 shows an example in which both hearts are in sinus rhythm. The atria are parasystolic with respect to each other, as are the ventricles.

Figure 258

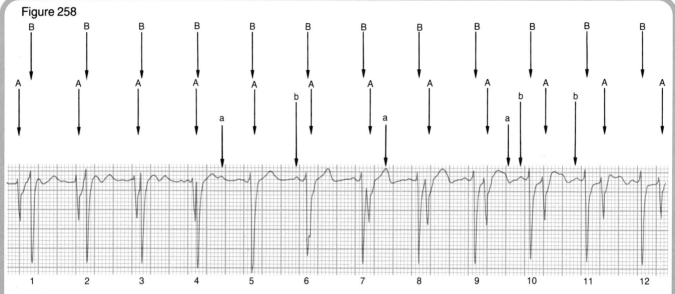

Lead V₁. Two hearts in one patient (heterotopic heart transplantation). The electrocardiogram is extremely complex.

The donor heart is the one producing the larger QRS complexes, labelled "B". This heart is in sinus rhythm with a normal P-R interval. Its P wave (b) can be seen clearly at 6, 10 and 11 when no other waves are interfering with its appearance. This heart is in sinus rhythm with a rate of 98 beats/min and a P-R interval of 0.12 sec.

It looks as though the S wave is rather too deep for normal in V₁ but no judgement can be made on this for the heart is not in a normal anatomical location and no adequate database yet exists for predicting the normal range of voltage in **individual** leads in heterotopically-transplanted hearts. The native heart is the one with the smaller QRS complexes labelled "A". Its P wave clearly seen at 4, can be seen to deform the peak of the T wave at 7 and deforms the downstroke of

the T wave at 9. This heart is in sinus rhythm with a P-R interval of approximately 0.32 (this can only be estimated approximately and is best seen as the interval a-A (beat 10)). The rate is 93 beats/min.

The two sets of QRS complexes are completely independent. When they coincide there is **summation** of the voltage. This is **not** fusion since the depolarisation pathways of the two sets of ventricular myocardium are totally discrete.

Ectopic Tachycardias

Ectopic tachycardias may arise from the atrial myocardium, from the AV junctional area or from the ventricular myocardium. In each case they may simply be thought of as a self-perpetuating ectopic beat from the appropriate site. The perpetuation of the depolarisation wave occurs because of a local re-entry circuit (see pages 355 and 356) or because of increased automaticity of the ectopic pacemaker.

The ectopic tachycardias are listed in Table 34.

Table 34	The ectopic tachycardias
Supraventricular origin	
Atrial origin	Atrial tachycardia
	Atrial flutter
	Atrial fibrillation*
Junctional origin	Junctional tachycardia
Ventricular origin	Ventricular tachycardia
	Ventricular fibrillation*

* These differ from the other tachycardias in that in each case the primary chamber involved (atria for atrial fibrillation, ventricles for ventricular fibrillation) shows chaotic depolarisation with no mechanical activity.

Supraventricular Tachycardias of Atrial Origin

ECG Features of Tachycardias of Atrial Origin

Atrial rate in tachycardias of atrial origin

In tachycardias of atrial origin the atrial rate (and therefore the P′ wave rate) will depend upon the conditions in the atria which initiate and sustain the tachycardia – i.e. either **increased automaticity of the ectopic pacemaker,** which both **initiates** and **sustains** the tachycardia, or the occurrence of a suitably timed **atrial premature beat** (which initiates the tachycardia) combined with a local **re-entry** mechanism (which **sustains** the tachycardia). The atrial cycle length is likely to be somewhere between 300 and 600 milliseconds and the atrial rate is therefore likely to be 200 to 100 per minute (rate per minute =

$$\frac{60}{\text{cycle length in seconds}}$$

).

Ventricular response in tachycardias of atrial origin

Since the disturbance of depolarisation at the atrium is the primary event, the atrial depolarisation rate is also the rate which reaches the AV node and the atrial rate must either equal the ventricular rate (if there is 1:1 atrio-ventricular conduction) or exceed it (if there is less than 1:1 atrio-ventricular conduction). Factors which determine the atrio-ventricular conduction are the **atrial cycle length** (i.e. effectively the **atrial rate)** and the **AV nodal refractory period.**

The AV nodal refractory period is normally of the order of about 0.3 sec but occasionally may be as short as 0.24 sec. This implies a maximum ventricular response rate to an atrial tachycardia of about 200 beats/min or, in occasional cases, up to 250 beats/min. When there is a more rapid ventricular rate than 200 beats/min in association with what is clearly a **supraventricular** tachycardia (i.e. the QRS complexes are narrow – of normal width) one should suspect the presence of an accessory AV conduction pathway and when the rate exceeds 250 beats/min the presence of such a pathway becomes highly likely. In most cases, however, the ventricular rate will be 200 beats/min or less. Factors which reduce the ventricular response to a given atrial rate will, in the absence of an anomalous AV connection, do so by increasing the AV nodal refractoriness (see Table 35).

Table 35 Ventricular rate in supraventricular tachycardia

Factors determining the ventricular rate in supraventricular tachycardia

Atrial rate
AV nodal refractory period
Presence of accessory pathway

Factors determining the ventricular rate in supraventricular* arrhythmias for a given atrial tachycardia rate and in the absence of any accessory pathway (i.e. factors affecting AV nodal refractory period)

Ischaemia Myocarditis Cardiomyopathy Rheumatic Fever Diphtheria Infiltrative diseases Surgery	Any of these conditions affecting the AV node may reduce the AV conduction ratio and slow the ventricular response.
Beta-blocking drugs Digitalis preparations Verapamil, diltiazem Amiodarone, sotalol, bretylium, Flecainide, lorcainide, encainide	Alone or in combination these drugs may depress AV nodal function and reduce the AV conduction ratio thereby slowing the ventricular response.
Increased vagal activity from carotid sinus massage, Valsalva manoeuvre, vomiting, action of digitalis etc	May cause a transient increase in AV nodal refractory period with a corresponding transient reduction in AV conduction ratio and therefore in ventricular rate.

* Theoretically one should also consider those factors which reduce the AV nodal refractory period and might increase the AV nodal conduction ratio, e.g. decreased vagal activity, increased sympathetic activity, sympathomimetic drugs etc. However, in the context of supraventricular tachycardia these factors are only very rarely significant in increasing the ventricular rate (unless they apply on the background of an already depressed ventricular rate resulting from other factors given in Table 35).

Wenckebach AV nodal block in relation to atrial tachycardias

The properties of the AV nodal tissue give rise (under certain conditions) to a phenomenon known as Wenckebach block. This phenomenon is by no means confined to the AV node but is most commonly seen at this location. The Wenckebach phenomenon at the AV node is characterised by a progressive lengthening of the AV nodal conduction time (shown on the ECG by a progressive lengthening of the P-R interval) until complete failure of AV conduction occurs (usually in respect only of a single atrial cycle, following which the P-R interval shortens suddenly, only to undergo further progressive prolongation until a complete failure of AV conduction occurs again and so on.

The Wenckebach phenomenon will be dealt with in more detail later (see pages 489 to 492). It tends to be most obvious in situations where there is disease of the AV node (e.g. ischaemia, acute rheumatic fever, diphtheria, myocarditis, etc) or in situations in which the atrial rate is inappropriately rapid for the degree of vagal and sympathetic activity obtaining (assuming no disease and no cardio-active drugs). Thus,

1. AV nodal Wenckebach phenomenon does not occur in the presence of normal sinus rhythm at a normal resting rate unless there is disease of the AV node,

2. AV nodal Wenckebach does not occur when the atrial rate is increased in situations in which vagal activity is diminished and/or sympathetic activity increased such as the sinus tachycardia of exercise, stress or disease,

3. AV nodal Wenckebach will occur (once the appropriate rate for the given AV node is achieved) during gradual increasing of the heart rate by atrial pacing in a recumbent subject. (In this situation, as opposed to that obtaining in the sinus tachycardia of exercise, stress or disease, sympathetic activity is not increased and parasympathetic activity is not diminished).

AV nodal Wenckebach occurs only relatively rarely in association with atrial tachycardia since there is usually reflexly-reduced parasympathetic and reflexly-increased sympathetic stimulation of the AV node in response to the atrial tachycardia*. **In most cases, therefore, the atrio-ventricular response in relation to atrial tachycardia will depend only upon (i) the atrial rate, and (ii) the total refractory period of the AV node.**

---

* When AV nodal Wenckebach occurs in association with atrial tachycardia, digitalis intoxication should be considered as a possible cause.

Atrio-ventricular conduction ratios in atrial tachycardias

It follows from the foregoing discussion that the atrio-ventricular conduction ratio obtaining in the presence of an atrial tachycardia will depend upon the interval between consecutive atrial depolarisation waves and the AV nodal refractory period. This is illustrated in Figures 259 and 260.

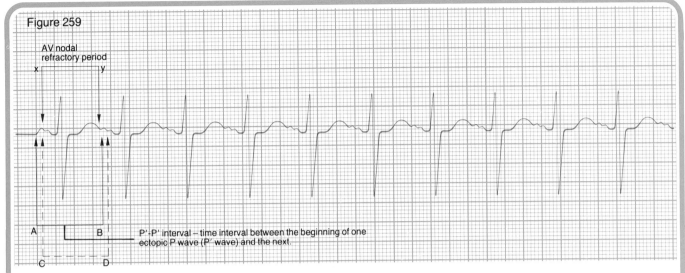

Atrial tachycardia with 1:1 conduction

The atrial cycle length is AB. At some point down the P′ wave (i.e. during atrial myocardial activation) the depolarisation wave reaches the AV node. This point cannot be recognised from the ECG. Assume it occurs at C. The time interval AC is the depolarisation travel time from the atrial ectopic site to the AV node and this will be the same for the next cycle (BD). Therefore AB = CD. If CD (and therefore if AB) is **greater** than the AV nodal refractory period (xy) there will be 1:1 AV conduction as shown here since the AV node will have recovered by the time the next ectopic atrial depolarisation arrives and accordingly will be able to conduct the impulse onwards.

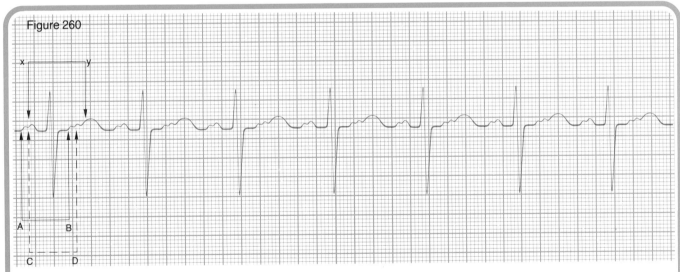

Atrial tachycardia with 2:1 AV block

The atrial cycle length is AB. At some point during the P′ wave (i.e. during atrial myocardial activation) the depolarisation wave reaches the AV node. This point cannot be recognised from the ECG. Assume it occurs at C. Then the time interval AC is the depolarisation travel time from the atrial ectopic site to the AV node and this will be the same for the next cycle (BD). Therefore AB = CD. If CD (and therefore if AB) is **less** than the AV nodal refractory period (xy) there will be failure of conduction of every second P′ wave and therefore there will be 2:1 AV conduction.

If the time interval between consecutive P′ waves is greater than the AV nodal refractory period, there will be 1:1 conduction. If this time interval is less than the AV nodal refractory period but is more than half that period (so that two P′-P intervals will exceed the AV nodal recovery (refractory) period) 2:1 atrio-ventricular conduction will occur. If the P′-P interval is less than the AV nodal refractory period and less than half the AV nodal refractory period but greater than one third of it (so that three P′-P intervals exceed the AV nodal recovery (refractory) period) 3:1 atrio-ventricular conduction will occur etc.

Thus most atrial tachycardias with atrial rates in the region of 180 to 200 or less will usually be associated with 1:1 AV conduction (unless AV nodal function is depressed by drugs or disease). Atrial tachycardias with more rapid atrial rates will usually show 2:1 AV block. The alternate blocked atrial beats in atrial tachycardia are analogous to blocked atrial premature beats, which occur if the atrial beats are very premature and such block does not indicate malfunction of the AV node.

P′ wave configuration in atrial tachycardia

The P′ wave configuration in atrial tachycardia usually differs from the P wave configuration in sinus rhythm (in exactly the same way as the P′ wave configuration in atrial ectopic beats differs from the P waves of sinus beats (page 387)). The closer the ectopic site to the sino-atrial node, the less obviously will the P′ wave differ from the P wave. In general the P′ waves of atrial tachycardia will tend to be upright in the inferior limb Leads II and aVF in contrast to the P′ waves of junctional tachycardia which tend to be inverted in these leads.

QRS configuration in atrial tachycardia

The QRS complexes during atrial tachycardia may show **the configuration usual for that patient** when the rhythm is sinus (and in so doing may be normal or abnormal), may show **functional right bundle branch block** or (rarely) may show **functional left bundle branch block.**

In general the development of atrial tachycardia does not result in any change in the QRS configuration. If the QRS is normal during sinus rhythm it will usually be normal during atrial tachycardia. If the QRS is abnormal during sinus rhythm (e.g. if the QRS complexes show left ventricular hypertrophy, right ventricular hypertrophy, left bundle branch block, right bundle branch block, changes of infarction, etc) then those same changes will be present during atrial tachycardia. This is exactly the same principle as described for sinus tachycardia (page 378 and Figures 215 and 216).

In certain situations **functional bundle branch block** (also known as **aberrant intraventricular conduction or rate-related bundle branch block**) may occur in association with atrial tachycardia in exactly the same way as described for atrial ectopic beats (page 403 and Figure 244). Thus if the time interval between the arrival of the depolarisation wave from the first ectopic P′ wave of an atrial tachycardia at the bundle branches and the arrival of a second such P′ wave is less than the recovery time of both bundle branches (or of the AV node or of the bundle of His) then the spread of the second depolarisation wave to the ventricles will be blocked.

The situation is similar to that described above in relation to conduction through the AV node – if the P′-P interval exceeds the refractory period of **both** bundle branches 1:1 conduction with normal* QRS complexes ensues. If the P′-P′ interval is less than the refractory period of both bundle branches but is greater than half the refractory period of both bundle branches (so that two P′-P′ intervals exceed the refractory period of both bundle branches) 2:1 atrio-ventricular block occurs (ventricular rate half the atrial rate) with normal* QRS complexes. A different situation arises if the P′ wave arrives at the bundle branches when one bundle branch has recovered and the other has not. If, for example, the P′-P′ interval exceeds the refractory period of the AV node and that of the left bundle branch but is less than that of the right bundle branch then there will be 1:1 conduction and functional right bundle branch block. Much less commonly the refractory period of the left bundle will be greater than that of the right bundle and in these circumstances functional left bundle branch block may be seen.

The terms "functional bundle branch block" and "aberrant intraventricular conduction" and "rate-related bundle branch block" are synonymous and do not imply the presence of disease in the bundle in question. The mechanism is illustrated in Figure 261.

* Unless there is pre-existing bundle branch block.

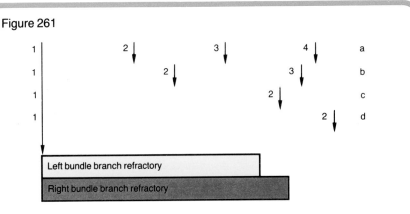

Figure 261

Left bundle branch refractory

Right bundle branch refractory

Influence of the frequency of depolarisation waves reaching the conducting tissue in determining the nature of the ventricular response.

Four different atrial depolarisation rates (a to d) are shown. In each case the first P′ wave (1) travels through the conducting tissue, depolarising the left and right bundles, and re-setting their refractory periods. In (a) the P′ rate is very rapid and the P′ waves 2 and 3 occur whilst both bundles are still refractory. Beats 2 and 3 are therefore completely blocked. Beat 4 finds both bundles recovered and there is therefore 3:1 atrio-ventricular block (i.e. three atrial beats (P′ waves) to each ventricular beat (QRS complex). In (b) the atrial rate is slower and the conduction tissue has recovered by beat 3. There is therefore 2:1 AV block. In (a) and (b) the QRS complexes are normal for each conducted beat. In (c) the rate is slower still. When the second beat reaches the left bundle this bundle has fully recovered but the right bundle is still refractory. Conduction therefore travels down the left bundle

alone and the QRS complex looks exactly like that in right bundle branch block. There is, in fact, nothing wrong with the right bundle, it simply has not had time to recover. The phenomenon is known as functional bundle branch block or as aberrant intraventricular conduction. With a slower rate still (d) each P′ wave finds that both bundles have recovered and there is 1:1 AV conduction without bundle branch block. It follows that with the most rapid rates there may be a high degree of atrio-ventricular block; with decreasing rates the degree of AV block gets less. Whether there is functional bundle branch block or not depends simply on whether any beat happens to arrive at the conducting tissue when one bundle has recovered and the other bundle has not. This is most likely to occur with a low degree of AV block. It most commonly occurs with 1:1 conduction but can occur with 2:1 conduction (if, for example, in situation (b) above the P′ wave 3 came a little earlier and fell within the refractory period of the right bundle branch).

Supraventricular Beats, Supraventricular Tachycardia

The term "supraventricular" used in relation to ectopic beats or ectopic tachycardias implies that the ectopic beat or tachycardia arises from some site above the bifurcation of the His bundle, i.e. in the His bundle itself, in the AV

node, in the atrial myocardium or in the sino-atrial node (page 396). Table 36 lists the ectopic rhythms and tachycardias included under the heading "supraventricular".

Table 36   Supraventricular arrhythmias

Anatomical origin of rhythm	Premature beats	Tachycardia
Sinus node	Sino-atrial premature beats (rare)	Sinus tachycardia Sinus node re-entrant tachycardia
Atrial myocardium	Atrial premature beats	Atrial tachycardia Atrial flutter Atrial fibrillation
AV junction	Junctional premature beats	Junctional tachycardia

The term "supraventricular" is used as a matter of convenience. Its use reflects the difficulty often experienced in distinguishing the anatomical origins of the rhythm. Whilst there are recognisable differences in general between the P waves from the three different anatomical origins of the rhythms (sino-atrial node, atrial myocardium, junctional area), the differences can be subtle or even unrecognisable. Thus while the P′ wave of an atrial premature beat is often recognisably different from the P wave of a sinus beat, the difference is less the closer the origin of the atrial ectopic beat to the sino-atrial node. Atrial premature beats arising from atrial myocardium close to the sino-atrial node will be virtually indistinguishable in terms of the morphology of the P wave from sinus beats. Similarly atrial premature beats arising close to the AV junction will be virtually indistinguishable in terms of the morphology of the P wave from junctional ectopic beats.

Sinus bradycardia, sinus arrhythmia and junctional bradycardia are all also "supraventricular", but the term finds its most frequent use in relation to ectopic beats and to tachycardias, as reflected in Table 36.

Furthermore, the term "supraventricular tachycardia" is not generally used in relation to sinus tachycardia, atrial flutter or atrial fibrillation (although each of these rhythms is clearly supraventricular in origin and each is clearly a tachycardia). In general it is used for atrial tachycardia or junctional tachycardia and its usefulness reflects the great difficulty often experienced in distinguishing between the two.

Terminology of Supraventricular Tachycardias

There are few areas of electrocardiography where the terminology is less universally agreed or more confusing. The problem essentially arises from the fact that supraventricular dysrhythmias are of interest to the electrophysiologist, the electrocardiographer and the clinician, and each imposes his own view-point on the terminology. Individual terms may be shared by all three categories of interested professional and the precise meaning of the term used may vary depending on which of the groups is using the term. Table 37 illustrates some of these terms.

Table 37 Descriptive terms used in relation to supraventricular tachycardias

Electrophysiological	Electrocardiographic	Clinical
Ectopic	Atrial	Paroxysmal
Re-entrant	Supraventricular	Repetitive
Reciprocating	Junctional	Sustained
Orthodromic	Tachycardia	Non-sustained
Antidromic	Flutter	Chronic
Slow-fast	Fibrillation	Persistent
Fast-slow	AVRT*	
Circus movement	AVNRT**	
Automatic		

From the electrocardiographic point of view (which, quite clearly, is the point of view which must be adopted in this text) the following are supraventricular tachycardias in the generic sense:

Sinus tachycardia
Atrial tachycardia
Atrial flutter
Atrial fibrillation
Junctional tachycardia

Each of these tachycardias will be rendered electrocardiographically more complex if there is also ventricular pre-excitation. Ventricular pre-excitation may, **coincidentally**, be present in any subject showing sinus tachycardia, atrial tachycardia, atrial flutter and atrial fibrillation. Ventricular pre-excitation is one of the **mechanisms** by which junctional tachycardia may occur (junctional tachycardia can occur because of re-entry within the atrio-ventricular node (AVNRT**) or because of re-entry between the atrio-ventricular nodal bundle on the one hand, and the pre-excitation pathway on the other hand (AVRT*) (i.e. the re-entrant loop may be entirely within the AV node or may involve the AV node bundle of His and the re-entrant pathway)).

When the term "supraventricular tachycardia" is used in a **specific** rather than a **generic** sense (i.e. when it is applied to a particular rhythm in a particular patient at a particular time) it is usually held to refer to atrial or junctional tachycardia with or without ventricular pre-excitation.

* Atrio-ventricular re-entrant tachycardia
** Atrio-ventricular nodal re-entrant tachycardia

There are three possible **sites** which can give rise to supraventricular tachycardias and there are two recognised **mechanisms** for the tachycardia in each case. The sites are the **sino-atrial node**, the **atrial myocardium** and the **atrio-ventricular node**. The mechanisms are **re-entry** and enhanced automaticity. The possible presence of an atrio-ventricular bypass tract (the anatomical substrate for ventricular pre-excitation) must also be considered. Figure 262 shows the anatomical substrate of the supraventricular tachycardias.

Figure 262

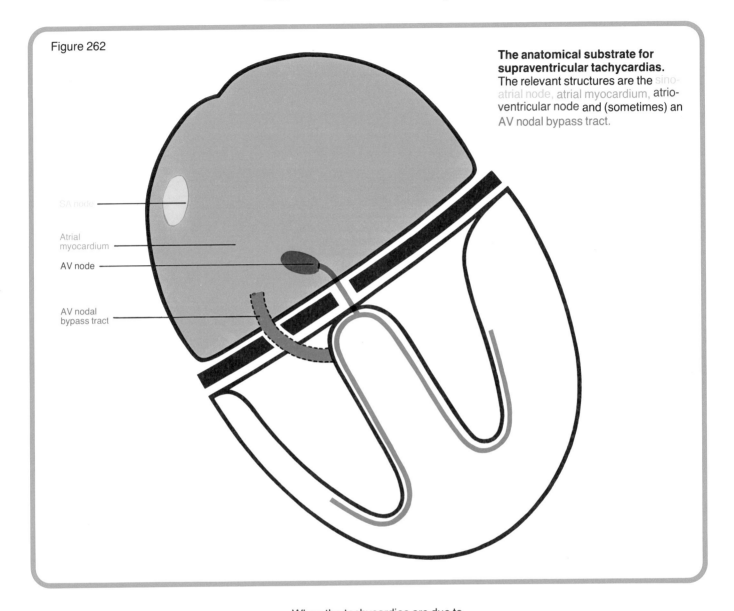

SA node

Atrial myocardium

AV node

AV nodal bypass tract

The anatomical substrate for supraventricular tachycardias. The relevant structures are the sino-atrial node, atrial myocardium, atrio-ventricular node and (sometimes) an AV nodal bypass tract.

When the tachycardias are due to the re-entry phenomenon a re-entrant loop for repetitive "circus" depolarisation is necessary. From this loop depolarisation is spread to adjacent myocardium. Four possible anatomical re-entrant loops in relation to supraventricular tachycardias are shown in Figure 263. The four sites are (i) the sino-atrial node itself, (ii) the atrial myocardium, (iii) the atrio-ventricular node and (iv) the atrio-ventricular node and bundle of His acting together with the atrio-ventricular bypass tract.

* Unless there is pre-existing bundle branch block and the re-entry cycle length is such as to produce aberrant intraventricular conduction (see page 427).

Figure 263 Possible sites for re-entrant supraventricular tachycardia.

a. Sino-atrial node re-entry. The re-entrant loop includes the sino-atrial node. The adjacent atrial myocardium will be depolarised from any part of the loop and this depolarisation will be initiated when depolarisation from the loop reaches an adjacent part of the atrial myocardium which is not in a refractory state. Depolarisation will then spread through the atrial myocardium in the normal way. When it reaches the atrio-ventricular node it will pass in the normal manner through the AV node, the His bundle and the bundle branches. The effective atrial rate could theoretically depend upon the duration of the circuit within the SA node or on the atrial myocardial refractory period. Since the latter is likely to be longer than the former it will, in practice, depend upon the latter.

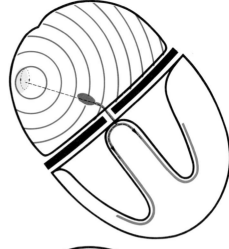

b. Atrial myocardial re-entry. The re-entrant loop is entirely within one portion of the atrial myocardium. The adjacent atrial myocardium will be depolarised from any part of the loop and this depolarisation will commence whenever depolarisation from the loop reaches an adjacent part of the atrial myocardium which is not in a refractory state. The depolarisation will then spread throughout the atrial myocardium in the normal way, giving rise to depolarisation in the atrio-ventricular node and to premature depolarisation (with re-setting) of the sino-atrial node. The depolarisation wave spreading through the atrio-ventricular node will subsequently travel down the bundle of His and the right and left bundle branches to activate the ventricles in the normal manner. Once more the effective atrial rate could theoretically depend upon the circulation time in the atrial loop or upon the atrial refractory period. In practice it is likely to depend upon the latter.

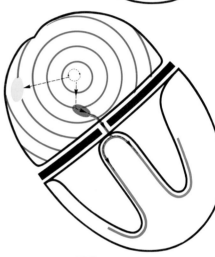

c. Atrio-ventricular nodal re-entry. The re-entrant loop is entirely within the atrio-ventricular node. The adjacent part of the atrial myocardium and the adjacent part of the bundle of His will be depolarised from any part of the loop and this depolarisation will commence whenever depolarisation of the loop reaches an adjacent part of the atrial myocardium and His bundle which are not in a refractory state. This initiation of atrial myocardial and His bundle depolarisation will not usually occur at exactly the same moment. When the depolarisation reaches the atrial myocardium it will spread through it in the normal manner and give rise to depolarisation (and premature re-setting) at the sino-atrial node. The depolarisation which travels down the His bundle will spread into the bundle branches and into the ventricular myocardium in the normal way*. Once more the effective atrial rate could theoretically depend upon the circulation time in the atrio-ventricular node or upon the atrial myocardial refractory period. In practice it is more likely to depend upon the latter.

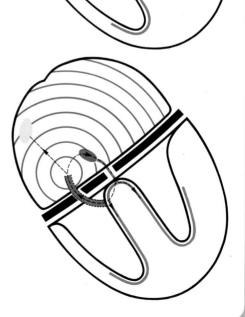

d. Junctional re-entry involving an AV nodal bypass tract. The re-entrant loop consists of the AV node, the common bundle, a small part of the myocardium within the interventricular septum, the AV nodal bypass tract and a small part of the atrial myocardium between the proximal end of the AV nodal bypass tract and the AV node itself. Conduction will usually be antegrade through the AV node and bundle of His and retrograde through the AV nodal bypass tract. Occasionally it will take place in the reverse direction. The atrial myocardial depolarisation will begin whenever depolarisation travelling up the AV nodal bypass tract reaches adjacent atrial myocardium which is not in a refractory state. Depolarisation will then spread over the whole of the atrial myocardium in the usual way, giving rise to depolarisation (and premature re-setting) of the sino-atrial node. Depolarisation travelling down the His bundle will give rise to ventricular myocardial depolarisation in the normal way. The atrial rate could depend either upon the circulation time of the re-entrant loop or on the atrial myocardial refractory period.

*See footnote page 426

Note that in all the four cases shown on page 427, ventricular myocardial depolarisation follows on travel of the depolarisation wave through the AV node, the bundle of His and the bundle branches. Unless, therefore, there is a primary abnormality of intraventricular conduction or an abnormality of the ventricular myocardium or there is aberrrant interventricular conduction, the QRS configuration will be expected to be normal and the frequency of ventricular depolarisation will depend upon that part of the atrio-ventricular conducting system (AV node, common bundle and proximal bundle branches) which has the longest refractory period and therefore the longest recovery time.

In practice this will usually mean the atrio-ventricular nodal refractory period. In the rare cases where an AV node/AV nodal bypass tract re-entrant loop is activated in the opposite direction (with antegrade conduction down the bypass tract and retrograde conduction through the AV node, i.e. antidromically) ventricular myocardial depolarisation may occur with much greater frequency since the refractory period of the AV nodal bypass tract is usually very much less than that of the AV node itself.

The above-described processes are all re-entry (circus loop) mechanisms. Re-entry is thought to be the electrophysiological mechanism of most tachycardias. Sometimes, however, their basic electrophysiological disturbance is an enhanced automaticity (increased spontaneous discharge rate) at the given site. Enhanced automaticity may occur at the sino-atrial node, at sites within the atrial myocardium or in the AV junctional area (to give supraventricular tachycardia).

As has been explained (page 419) atrial tachycardia is (whether it be due to re-entry or to enhanced automaticity), in effect, a self-perpetuating atrial premature beat. The state of tachycardia may be sustained by a re-entry mechanism or by the increased automaticity of an ectopic pacemaker site. The distinction between a series of atrial premature beats and a short burst of atrial tachycardia is arbitrary. A generally-accepted working definition is that three or more consecutive ectopic beats constitute a period of ectopic tachycardia. (Thus three consecutive atrial, junctional or ventricular premature beats (with no intervening beats of other origin) constitute the minimum criteria for short runs of atrial, junctional or ventricular tachycardia respectively).

Sino-atrial Nodal Re-entry

Sinus node re-entrant tachycardia is rare. An example is shown in Figure 264.

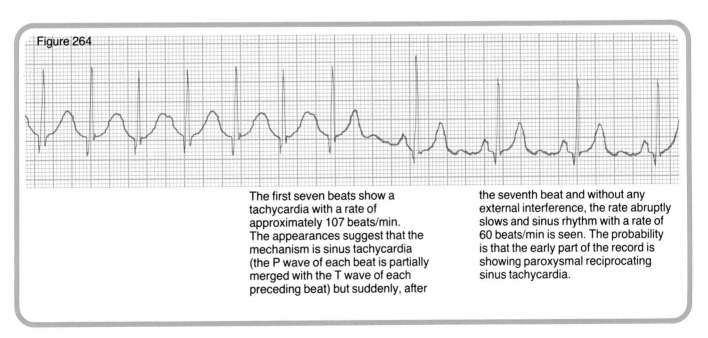

Figure 264

The first seven beats show a tachycardia with a rate of approximately 107 beats/min. The appearances suggest that the mechanism is sinus tachycardia (the P wave of each beat is partially merged with the T wave of each preceding beat) but suddenly, after the seventh beat and without any external interference, the rate abruptly slows and sinus rhythm with a rate of 60 beats/min is seen. The probability is that the early part of the record is showing paroxysmal reciprocating sinus tachycardia.

The P waves in the paroxysmal sinus tachycardia are not distinguishable from the P waves in sinus rhythm. A tachycardia of this type may stop spontaneously (as here) or may stop abruptly following carotid sinus massage. (In this respect it differs from the usual effect of carotid sinus massage on physiological sinus tachycardia which is gradual slowing with restoration of the rapid rate again once the carotid massage is released).

Atrial Tachycardia

Atrial tachycardia, by definition, "arises" from the atrial myocardium (whether by a local re-entry mechanism or by enhanced automaticity of an ectopic focus). The atrial depolarisation rate (P′ rate) depends on local conditions in the area giving rise to the tachycardia. The ventricular depolarisation rate (QRS rate) depends on the function of the AV node as discussed earlier. By definition, the QRS rate is equal to or less than the atrial rate. It will be equal to the atrial rate if the time interval between consecutive P′ waves is greater than the AV nodal refractory period and will be less than it if it is not.

ECG Features of Atrial Tachycardia

P′ morphology
This may or may not be recognisably different from the normal P wave morphology. (If the ectopic atrial site is close to the SA node the P′ wave will not be recognisably different from the P wave).

P′ rate
This will typically be in the range of 160-250 beats/min.

Relation of the P′ waves to the QRS complexes
This will depend on the time interval between adjacent P′ waves and the refractory period of the AV node (which is the part of the AV conducting tissue most likely to fail to conduct).

QRS configuration
The QRS configuration will typically be that which exists prior to the onset of the atrial tachycardia (whether normal or abnormal) but may differ from this because of aberrant intraventricular conduction (pages 403 to 405) in which case it will typically be that the changes of (functional) right, or occasionally left bundle branch block are added to the existing form of the QRS complex.

Regularity of the P′ waves
The P′ wave rate is usually constant, i.e. the P′ waves are usually regular.

Regularity of the QRS complexes
This depends on whether or not the conduction at the AV node is constant (1:1, 2:1, 3:1 atrio-ventricular conduction), or whether there are varying degrees of atrio-ventricular block.

Nature of the onset and termination of atrial tachycardia
This may give a firm clue as to the ECG mechanism but it is only rarely that one has the privilege of recording these events. The sudden increase in rate from a normal resting sinus rate to the atrial tachycardia rate, especially when the change follows an atrial premature beat, suggests a re-entrant tachycardia. Atrial tachycardia is most commonly initiated by an atrial premature beat in this way. For such an event to induce atrial tachycardia, the P′ wave has to occur during the **vulnerable period** of the atrial myocardium (Figure 265). If, as in the vast majority of cases, the **onset** of the atrial tachycardia is not recorded it may be impossible to distinguish atrial re-entrant tachycardia from atrial automatic tachycardia except that the atrial rate tends to be higher in the former.

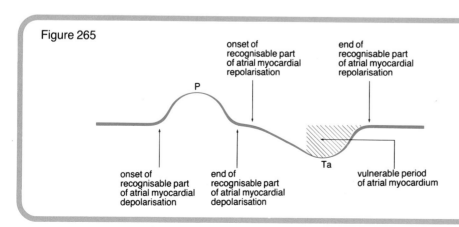

Figure 265

onset of recognisable part of atrial myocardial repolarisation

end of recognisable part of atrial myocardial repolarisation

P

Ta

onset of recognisable part of atrial myocardial depolarisation

end of recognisable part of atrial myocardial depolarisation

vulnerable period of atrial myocardium

Atrial myocardial vulnerable period
The atrial depolarisation wave is the P wave. The atrial repolarisation wave is the Ta wave. The atrial myocardium is "vulnerable" during the terminal part of the repolarisation period, when some parts of the atrial myocardium have recovered and some parts are still refractory. The myocardium may, in whole or in part, be refractory at this stage.

The term "vulnerable" indicates that an extra stimulus which at other times would be ineffective (if the myocardium is completely refractory) or would induce a single depolarisation (if the myocardium has completely recovered from the previous depolarisation) might, at this time result not only in a single contraction, but also in a repetitive cycle, i.e. in a tachycardia.

Figure 266 shows an example of atrial tachycardia.

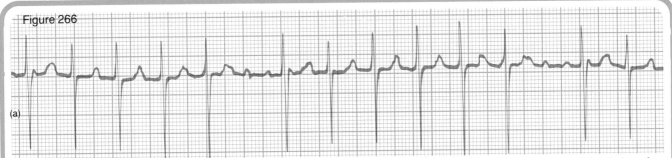

Figure 266

(a)

Atrial tachycardia.
Chest monitoring lead.

The QRS complexes are normal (i.e. the QRS duration lies within normal limits, i.e. ≯0.10 sec (see Section 1, page 40)). There is a rapid heart rate. In relation to the first five QRS complexes it is difficult to be sure of the presence of P waves or P′ waves. Narrow QRS complexes can be seen and T waves recognised. The ventricular rate is approximately 135 beats/min. It is clear, therefore, that there is a supraventricular tachycardia. The same situation obtains in relation to the ECG between the sixth and eleventh QRS complexes. Between the fifth and sixth QRS complexes the situation is clearly different. During this period P′ waves can be seen. When there is a break in the rhythm it is often rewarding to examine that part of the record carefully. If the timing of the P′ waves (revealed during this pause in the ventricular activity) is marked on a straight-edged piece of paper or cardboard (as was done in relation to the demonstration of a compensatory pause, page 391, Figure 230) the activity of the P′ waves can be extrapolated forwards and backwards (Figure 266b).

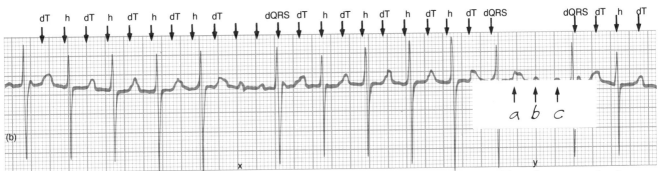

(b)

Extrapolation of the position of the P′ waves to other parts of the trace.

Whenever there is a break in the prevailing rhythm it is well worth while inspecting this part carefully. Such a break is seen at x and again at y. Inspection of the pause ("break") at y shows that three P waves can clearly be recognised, the first one is actually distorting the up-stroke of the T wave following the preceding QRS. The timing of these three beats should be marked on a piece of straight-edged paper in using the same technique as that for checking whether the QRS is regular or not (see Figure 201, page 362). The timing of these P waves is marked "a", "b" and "c". One should then look to see if the P wave timing has in fact remained constant throughout the record. This is done by sliding the straight-edged paper to the left so that arrow "c" is now superimposed on the P wave which was formerly labelled "a" and repeating this process until the location of all the P waves predicted to occur to the left of pause y (if the atrial rhythm was always that shown at pause y) are now seen. These positions are marked with vertical arrows. The process is also repeated to the right of pause y by moving arrow "a" onto the location of the P wave formerly labelled "c". In this way it can be seen that timing of the P waves shown at pause y fits in exactly with the timing of the P waves shown at pause x and this timing also remains constant throughout the whole record. P waves are seen with greater or lesser difficulty at various parts in the recording depending on what else is going on. P waves which (as shown by the arrows) have a timing synchronous with the QRS complexes are not seen but P waves can often be recognised by the variable deformation of the T wave which they induce.

Careful inspection of pauses in this way and subsequent extrapolation to left and right will often reveal the pattern of atrial depolarisation which in this record clearly is one of atrial tachycardia with a rate of approximately 300 beats/min. For the first five beats there is 2:1 AV block, during pause x there is 4:1 AV block, between pauses x and y there is 2:1 AV block and at pause y there is again transient 4:1 AV block. It can be seen that some of the P′ waves are hidden in the QRS complexes (h), some giving rise to deformation of the T waves (dT), and some are clearly deforming the QRS (dQRS).

The ventricular rate in this example varies as a result of variation in the atrio-ventricular conduction. In relation to beats 1-5 there is 2:1 AV block. This is **not** indicative of disease of the AV node. It is simply a result of the fact that the refractory period of the AV node exceeds the atrial cycle length. In this situation every other atrial beat finds the AV node refractory. After two atrial cycles the AV node has recovered so every alternate P′ wave is conducted. Between beats 5 and 6, 4:1 block occurs – perhaps because of fatigue of the AV node, perhaps because of additional vagal drive, perhaps because of ischaemia or perhaps because of a combination of these factors.

The rhythm is actually considerably more complex than has been described here. In addition to the 2:1 and 4:1 atrio-ventricular block there is Wenckebach atrio-ventricular conduction (see pages 489 to 492). This explains why pause x and pause y are not exactly twice the R-R intervals during 2:1 conduction and why the P′-R interval of conducted beats varies.

Atrial Flutter

Atrial flutter may be thought of as a special example of atrial tachycardia in which the atrial rate is between 250-350* beats/min and, in the majority of cases, is close to 300 beats/min. As a result of the duration of the flutter waves ("F waves") and their rapid rate there is no time for any isoelectric interval between consecutive F waves. Because of this the atrial activity gives rise to a "saw-tooth" pattern (Figure 267) of activity.

Figure 267

The atrial electrocardiogram in atrial flutter shows a saw-tooth pattern.

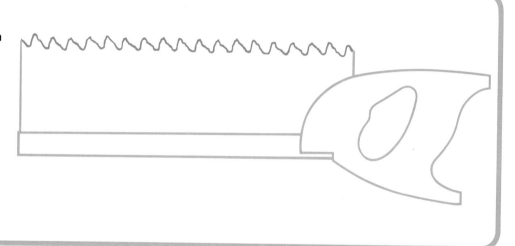

EGG Features of Atrial Flutter

P′ morphology
The P′ morphology is usually virtually that of a sine-wave – i.e. the "saw- tooth" pattern is produced.

P′ rate (atrial rate)
The atrial rate lies in the range of 250-350 beats/min, but is often very close to 300 beats/min.

Atrial regularity
The atrial rate in atrial flutter is usually constant for a given subject and is typically unaffected by carotid sinus massage.

Configuration of the flutter waves (F waves)
As indicated above, the direction of the F wave and the F wave rate, together with the atrial repolarisation wave (which is prominent in atrial flutter), result in the production of a sine-wave or saw-tooth pattern (Figure 268).

*The flutter rate may fall to 200 beats/min following treatment with drugs, for example, disopyramide and amiodarone. It may increase beyond 350 beats/min following treatment with digitalis.

431

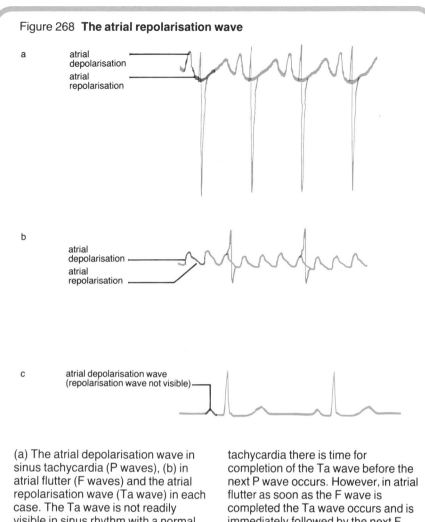

Figure 268 The atrial repolarisation wave

a   atrial depolarisation

     atrial repolarisation

b   atrial depolarisation

     atrial repolarisation

c   atrial depolarisation wave (repolarisation wave not visible)

(a) The atrial depolarisation wave in sinus tachycardia (P waves), (b) in atrial flutter (F waves) and the atrial repolarisation wave (Ta wave) in each case. The Ta wave is not readily visible in sinus rhythm with a normal resting rate (c) since it is small and brief and is generally obscured by the QRS complex which occurs at about the same time. In the presence of sinus tachycardia the Ta wave is increased in size (a). Even in sinus tachycardia there is time for completion of the Ta wave before the next P wave occurs. However, in atrial flutter as soon as the F wave is completed the Ta wave occurs and is immediately followed by the next F wave. This gives rise to the sinusoidal appearance of atrial depolarisation and repolarisation. The "sine-wave" or "saw-tooth" is not quite symmetrical.

The F waves tend to be largest in Leads II, III and aVF since the vector of the F wave tends to point inferiorly in the frontal plane. It should be remembered that leads at right angles to a given vector may show very little deflection in response to the given wave (Section I page 12). This is just as true in respect of F or P waves as it is in respect of QRS complexes. If, for example, the vector of the F wave is directed inferiorly it will be seen optimally in Lead aVF, will be very well seen in Leads II and III (which occupy the position 30° either side of aVF) but will be virtually invisible in Lead I (Figure 269).

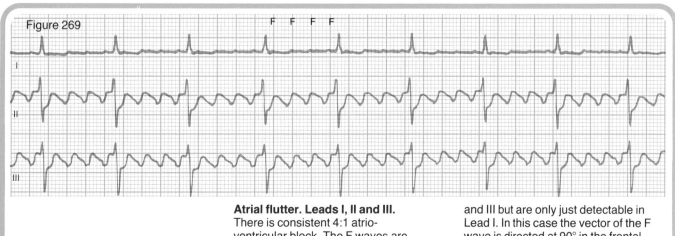

Figure 269

F   F   F   F

I

II

III

Atrial flutter. Leads I, II and III.
There is consistent 4:1 atrio-ventricular block. The F waves are easily visible in the inferior Leads II and III but are only just detectable in Lead I. In this case the vector of the F wave is directed at 90° in the frontal plane.

Ventricular rate

As in the case of all supraventricular tachycardias this depends on two things, (i) the atrial rate and (ii) the atrio-ventricular conduction. The refractory period of the normal AV node varies depending on the activity of the sympathetic or the parasympathetic nervous system (being decreased by sympathetic, and increased by parasympathetic activity) and is also modified by beta-blocking drugs, verapamil, calcium antagonists of the verapamil type and by digitalis preparations. In the absence of drug action or disease the AV junctional refractory period is typically of the order of 0.3 sec. If the atrial rate in flutter is 300 beats/min, the interval between consecutive atrial depolarisations will be 0.2 sec. In this situation every alternate flutter wave will be blocked and 2:1 AV block will occur (Figure 270).

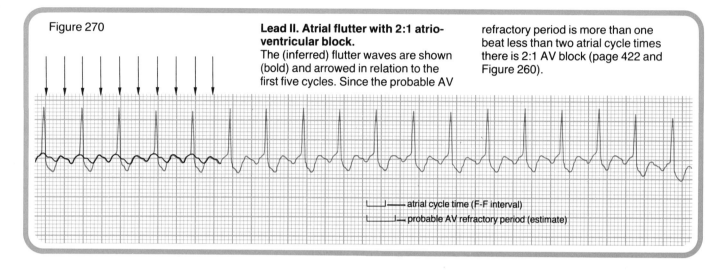

Figure 270

Lead II. Atrial flutter with 2:1 atrio-ventricular block.
The (inferred) flutter waves are shown (bold) and arrowed in relation to the first five cycles. Since the probable AV refractory period is more than one beat less than two atrial cycle times there is 2:1 AV block (page 422 and Figure 260).

atrial cycle time (F-F interval)
probable AV refractory period (estimate)

If the AV node is influenced by **disease** (e.g. ischaemia, diphtheria, acute rheumatic fever, myocarditis etc), **vagal activity** (e.g. during the response to carotid sinus massage) or **drugs** (e.g. digitalis preparations, beta-blocking drugs, calcium antagonists of the verapamil type) the degree of AV block may be substantially greater because of an increase in the AV nodal refractory period. In such a situation 3:1 or 4:1 AV block will typically occur (Figure 271).

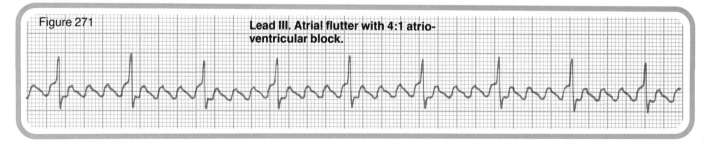

Figure 271

Lead III. Atrial flutter with 4:1 atrio-ventricular block.

The ventricular rate is usually an integral sub-division of the atrial rate. Thus, if the atrial rate is 300 beats/min, the ventricular rate will be 150, 100 or 75 depending on whether the AV block is 2:1, 3:1 or 4:1. Rarely the block will be 5:1, in which case the ventricular rate is 60 beats/min. The degree of AV block may vary even within a short time interval, and in this event the ventricular rate itself will be variable (Figure 272).

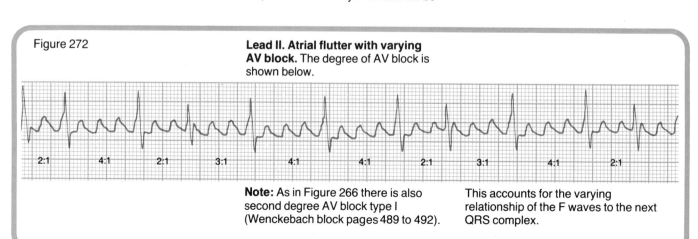

Figure 272

Lead II. Atrial flutter with varying AV block. The degree of AV block is shown below.

2:1   4:1   2:1   3:1   4:1   4:1   2:1   3:1   4:1   2:1

Note: As in Figure 266 there is also second degree AV block type I (Wenckebach block pages 489 to 492).

This accounts for the varying relationship of the F waves to the next QRS complex.

The refractory period of the AV node is of such a length as normally totally to preclude the possibility of 1:1 atrio-ventricular conduction during atrial flutter. However 1:1 atrio-ventricular conduction can occasionally occur and an example of this rare event is shown in Figure 273.

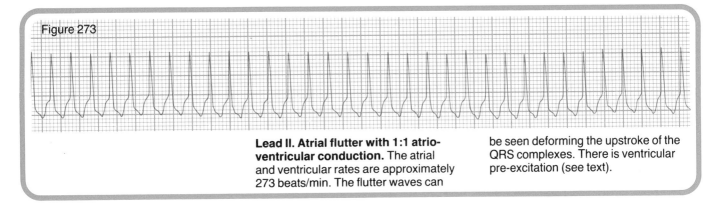

Figure 273

Lead II. Atrial flutter with 1:1 atrio-ventricular conduction. The atrial and ventricular rates are approximately 273 beats/min. The flutter waves can be seen deforming the upstroke of the QRS complexes. There is ventricular pre-excitation (see text).

When there is 1:1 atrio-ventricular conduction in association with atrial flutter or any supraventricular tachycardia with such a rapid atrial rate that the interval between consecutive atrial depolarisation waves is less than the AV nodal refractory period, it follows that there must be a rapidly conducting accessory pathway connecting atrial and ventricular myocardium (i.e. there must be ventricular pre-excitation). Figure 273 shows such an example. In a situation like this restoration of sinus rhythm usually reveals the pre-excitation pathway (Figure 274).

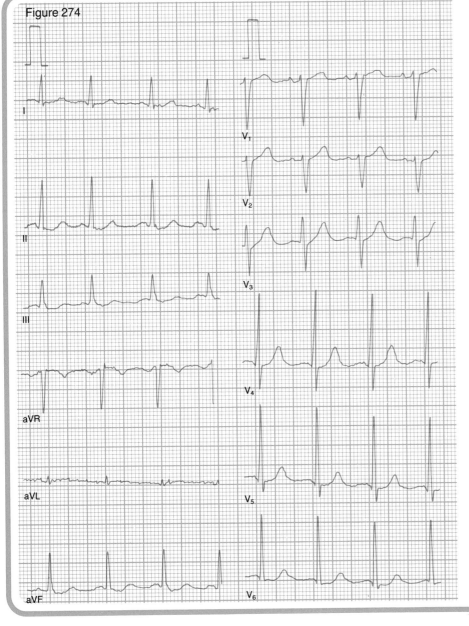

Figure 274

I

II

III

aVR

aVL

aVF

V₁

V₂

V₃

V₄

V₅

V₆

12-lead ECG showing the record obtained after the restoration of sinus rhythm in the patient whose records were shown as Figure 270 (atrial flutter with 2:1 atrio-ventricular block) and Figure 273 (atrial flutter with 1:1 atrio-ventricular block). It can be seen that there has been no significant change in the QRS configuration as seen in Lead II between any of these records. Superficial inspection of Figure 274 may lead to the conclusion that the record is within normal limits, but a more careful appraisal will reveal the short P-R interval (0.10 sec). This is well seen in V_1 and V_4. There is no delta wave. The patient has the Lown-Ganong-Levine syndrome (pages 447 and 448).

If there is complete atrio-ventricular block (i.e. complete heart block) the ventricular rate will be independent of the atrial rate and will generally be slow (Figure 275).

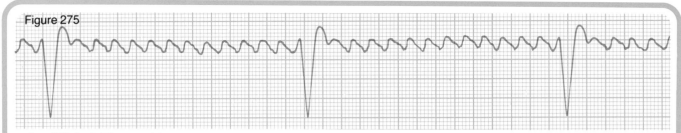

Figure 275

Lead III. Atrial flutter with complete heart block. The atrial rate is just under 300 beats/min. The QRS rate is very slow (approximately 30 beats/min). There is no consistent relationship between the flutter waves and the QRS complexes and there is complete atrio-ventricular block.

QRS morphology

The QRS complexes are usually unchanged by the onset of atrial flutter since the pathway of intraventricular conduction is unchanged. If the QRS is normal before the onset of atrial flutter it will usually remain normal, and if it is abnormal before the onset of atrial flutter it will usually retain the same abnormality. Figure 276 shows an example of atrial flutter with 2:1 atrio-ventricular block and complete right bundle branch block.

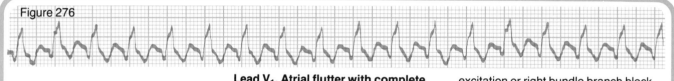

Figure 276

Lead V₁. Atrial flutter with complete right bundle branch block and 2:1 atrio-ventricular block. It is impossible from this record alone, to know whether there was pre-excitation or right bundle branch block existing before the onset of atrial flutter or whether aberrant intraventricular conduction has developed during the tachycardia.

If atrial flutter develops in a subject with normal intraventricular conduction and the flutter rate is such that alternate atrial depolarisation waves reach the right and left bundle branches at a time when the left bundle branch has recovered and the right bundle branch has not, then functional right bundle branch block (aberrant intraventricular conduction, rate-related bundle branch block) develops. Without the availability of an ECG recording preceding the onset of atrial flutter it is not possible to distinguish atrial flutter with functional right bundle branch block from atrial flutter with pre-existing right bundle branch block.

Criteria for atrial flutter

1. **Atrial rate** is regular.

2. **Atrial rate** is 250-350 beats/min (most commonly 300 beats/min).

3. **Atrial activity** will show the typical "saw-tooth" pattern in appropriate leads (typically II, aVF, V₁).

4. **QRS rate** is usually ½, ⅓ or ¼ of the atrial rate and may vary among these ratios.

In the presence of pre-excitation the ventricular rate may occasionally equal the atrial rate.

In the presence of complete heart block the ventricular rate may be very slow and independent of the atrial rate.

A QRS configuration is usually the same as that obtaining before the onset of atrial flutter. Occasionally the onset of atrial flutter may give rise to aberrant intraventricular conduction. This usually produces a QRS complex with the right bundle branch block configuration.

Atrial Fibrillation

Atrial fibrillation is a much more commonly seen arrhythmia than atrial flutter. The primary electrocardiographic abnormality in atrial fibrillation is the lack of co-ordinated atrial myocardial depolarisation. In all the supraventricular rhythms described so far, depolarisation is initiated at some point within the atrial myocardium and then spreads passively to the rest of the atrial myocardium in an orderly fashion. As a result, a P, P′ or F (flutter) wave is seen and the timing and frequency of atrial depolarisation can be recognised. In atrial fibrillation there is no co-ordinated atrial depolarisation. Instead multiple areas of atrial myocardium depolarise, in effect independently.

ECG Features of Atrial Fibrillation

Atrial depolarisation morphology

No P, P′ or F waves are visible. Instead an irregular baseline is seen, indicating continually varying atrial depolarisation. These irregular waves are called fibrillation (f) waves. Figure 277 shows an example of atrial fibrillation.

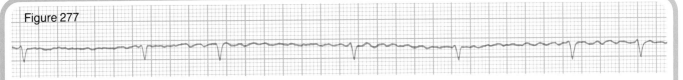

Figure 277

Lead V₁. Atrial fibrillation. There are no P or P′ waves. No regular F waves are seen. No co-ordinated atrial depolarisation of any kind is seen. The baseline is irregular, indicating the occurrence of numerous, localised depolarisation circuits in the atrial myocardium. None of these local circuits is sufficient to produce spread to the whole atrial myocardium to produce a co-ordinated depolarisation. As will be discussed later, the ventricular rate is irregular and the shape of the QRS complexes is usually unaffected by the onset of this rhythm.

Atrial depolarisation rate

Since there is no co-ordinated atrial myocardial depolarisation, the concept of "atrial depolarisation rate" is not strictly appropriate. Nevertheless it is useful to know the approximate rate at which depolarisation waves from the atrial myocardium reach the AV node. This rate is of the order of 600 beats/min or approximately twice that in atrial flutter. The range usually lies between 450 and 650 beats/min.

Ventricular rate

Untreated atrial fibrillation is usually associated with a rapid and irregular ventricular rate. Typically this lies within the range 120-200 beats/min. It is easy to understand why the ventricular rate is rapid in untreated atrial fibrillation, but it is less obvious why it is so irregular. The ventricular rate is rapid because the AV node is bombarded with impulses (depolarisation waves) at about 600 beats/min. The ventricular rate is therefore effectively set by the AV nodal refractory period. If the mechanism were as simple as this, one would expect very little variation in the ventricular rate (Figure 278).

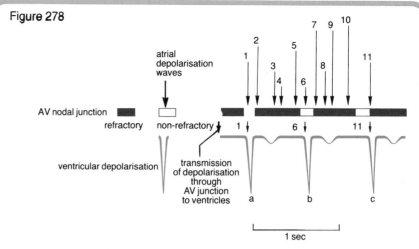

Figure 278

The ventricular response in atrial fibrillation. The diagram assumes that any atrial depolarisation wave reaching the AV node is capable of transmission through the node. (This concept is modified later, see Figure 279). If this simple behavioural model is representative of the true situation, the first beat to reach the AV node when it is non-refractory (1) will be transmitted and result in ventricular depolarisation giving a QRS complex (a). The AV node would then become refractory (its refractory period is shown here as 0.44 sec) and the first beat arriving at the AV node when it is again non-refractory will be transmitted through. Thus, not until the sixth atrial "beat" will a subsequent depolarisation spread to the ventricles. The cycle will then be repeated. The variation in R-R interval will then simply reflect the variation in "f" wave intervals which is likely to be small since 600 beats/min of such impulses reach the AV node. The mean variation in the R-R interval would, on the basis of this simple model, be expected to be only of the order of 0.1 sec.

Once a depolarisation wave reaches the AV node when the latter is non-refractory (1, Figure 278) it will pass through the AV node, spread to the ventricles and give rise to a QRS complex (a, Figure 278) which will inevitably be followed by its S-T segment and T wave. The AV node will then become refractory. The duration of the refractory period will depend on the health or sickness of the AV node, the existing sympathetic and parasympathetic drives to the node and the presence or absence of drugs which affect its function (digitalis preparations, beta-blocking drugs, calcium antagonists). In any given situation the refractory period is likely to be constant over a relatively short period of time so that the R-R interval in atrial fibrillation clearly should equal the AV nodal refractory period plus the time interval between the end of the refractory period and the arrival of the first depolarisation wave to occur after the refractory period (Figure 278). With an average atrial depolarisation rate of 600 beats/min (10 beats/sec) the average time interval between atrial depolarisation waves is likely to be about 0.1 sec. The R-R interval would then be expected to be equal to the AV nodal refractory period plus up to 0.1 sec. Thus if the AV nodal refractory period is 0.3 sec, the R-R interval would be expected to lie within the approximate range 0.3-0.4 sec. This is manifestly not the case in atrial fibrillation (see Figures 280 and 283). The deviation from the simple behavioural model occurs because of the phenomenon of **decremental conduction** at the AV node.

Decremental conduction and concealed conduction at the AV node

The term "decremental conduction" implies that the properties of the conducting tissue change along its length so that the action potential moving along the cell progressively loses its ability to excite the tissue ahead. In this way an excitatory process may "enter" tissue and yet be unable to self-propagate along the whole length of the tissue.

It appears that many of the impulses arriving at the atrio-ventricular node in atrial fibrillation behave in this way. They may enter the AV node but be unable to penetrate its full length. By activating the proximal part of the AV node they re-set the refractory period so that the "effective" refractory period (in the presence of atrial fibrillation) becomes significantly and variably longer than the single refractory period, which would obtain if single atrial depolarisations were presented to the AV node at varying time intervals. This electrocardiographic process by which depolarisation waves may be inferred to have entered the AV node but not to have emerged from it, is called **"concealed conduction"**. It is not directly apparent on the electrocardiogram but may be inferred because of the great variability of the R-R intervals (Figure 279).

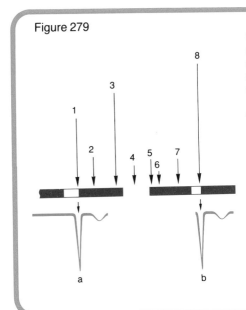

Figure 279

Concealed atrio-ventricular conduction due to decremental conduction of less powerful depolarisation waves reaching the atrio-ventricular node. Impulse 1 is "powerful" and travels right through the AV node. Impulses 2 and 3 find it refractory and do not enter. Impulse 4 is not powerful enough to enter. Impulse 5 is powerful enough to enter but not powerful enough to emerge. Impulses 6 and 7 find the AV node refractory because of the entry of impulse 5 (even though impulse 5 does not emerge from the AV node and give rise ultimately to a QRS complex). The next "powerful" waveform arising after the end of the AV nodal refractory period following the entry of impulse 5 passes through the AV node and gives rise to QRS(b). The time interval ab (the R-R interval) thus equals the AV nodal refractory period in relation to impulse 1, plus the time interval when the AV node is not refractory but no impulse is sufficiently powerful to penetrate it, plus the refractory period induced by partial depolarisation of the AV node in response to impulse 5, plus the period when the AV node is not refractory and just before impulse 8. The refractory period induced by impulse 5 can be less than the refractory period for a sinus-initiated beat. It is clear that the potential exists for very substantial variations in the interval ab and that the minimum interval that this can be is one single AV nodal refractory period.

Thus the ventricular rate in atrial fibrillation varies considerably (Figures 280 and 281). As explained above, one of the reasons for the great variability of the ventricular rate in atrial fibrillation is the occurrence of repeated episodes of a decremental conduction in the atrio-ventricular node. Though concealed conduction can be detected in other rhythms it is most commonly seen in association with atrial fibrillation and its sole expression in that rhythm is the variability of the ventricular rate. However, as explained on page 412, it can be seen in relation to ventricular premature beats which conduct backwards into the atrio-ventricular node and give rise to transient prolongation of the P-R interval in the next normal sinus beat following the ventricular ectopic (page 412 and Figure 250).

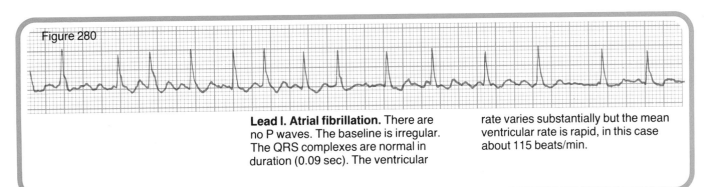

Figure 280

Lead I. Atrial fibrillation. There are no P waves. The baseline is irregular. The QRS complexes are normal in duration (0.09 sec). The ventricular rate varies substantially but the mean ventricular rate is rapid, in this case about 115 beats/min.

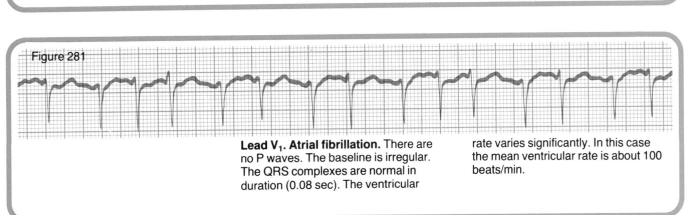

Figure 281

Lead V$_1$. Atrial fibrillation. There are no P waves. The baseline is irregular. The QRS complexes are normal in duration (0.08 sec). The ventricular rate varies significantly. In this case the mean ventricular rate is about 100 beats/min.

When atrial fibrillation is "treated" with digitalis (or with beta-blocking drugs or with calcium antagonists) the effective AV nodal refractory period is lengthened. Atrial activity is not significantly influenced but the ventricular rate falls (Figures 282 and 283).

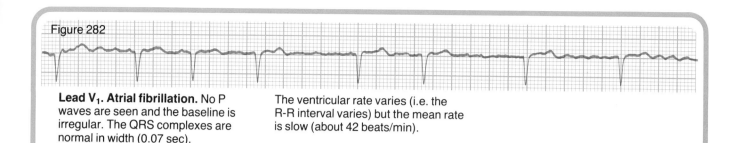

Figure 282

Lead V₁. Atrial fibrillation. No P waves are seen and the baseline is irregular. The QRS complexes are normal in width (0.07 sec).

The ventricular rate varies (i.e. the R-R interval varies) but the mean rate is slow (about 42 beats/min).

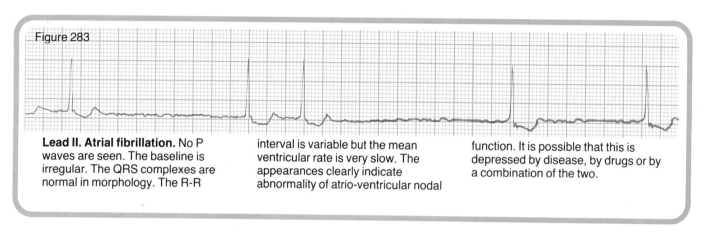

Figure 283

Lead II. Atrial fibrillation. No P waves are seen. The baseline is irregular. The QRS complexes are normal in morphology. The R-R interval is variable but the mean ventricular rate is very slow. The appearances clearly indicate abnormality of atrio-ventricular nodal function. It is possible that this is depressed by disease, by drugs or by a combination of the two.

QRS morphology

In general the QRS morphology is unchanged by the onset of atrial fibrillation. If the QRS complexes are normal before the onset of atrial fibrillation they usually remain normal afterwards. If they are abnormal before the onset of atrial fibrillation, the abnormality is usually unchanged. Figure 284 shows an example of atrial fibrillation with an abnormal QRS complex, the abnormality being present before the onset of atrial fibrillation.

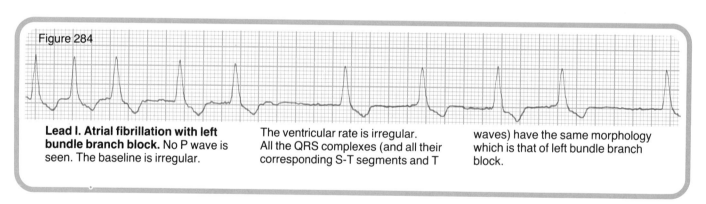

Figure 284

Lead I. Atrial fibrillation with left bundle branch block. No P wave is seen. The baseline is irregular. The ventricular rate is irregular. All the QRS complexes (and all their corresponding S-T segments and T waves) have the same morphology which is that of left bundle branch block.

Atrial fibrillation can also be associated with aberrant intraventricular conduction. Since the phenomenon of aberrant intraventricular conduction in relation to a given beat is dependent (a) on its proximity to the preceding beat (i.e. to the R-R interval preceding the beat) and (b) on the refractory period of the preceding beat (which in turn is related to the R-R interval of the beat before that) and since both of these functions (namely the R-R interval for a given beat and the refractory period of the preceding beat) are variable in atrial fibrillation, aberrant intraventricular conduction commonly occurs in this condition. Aberrant intraventricular conduction of beat 3 is more likely to occur when interval 2-3 is short and interval 1-2 is long (pages 403 to 405 and Figures 244 and 245). Consecutive long, then short intervals frequently occur by chance in atrial fibrillation which accounts for the fact that aberrant intraventricular conduction occurs from time to time in this arrhythmia. The longer the refractory period of a given beat the greater the difference between the refractory period of the right and of the left bundle branches and therefore the greater the time zone within which an impulse may find that the left bundle has recovered and the right bundle has not (Figure 244). A beat passing through the AV node in this time zone will show aberrant intraventricular conduction. The absolute size of this time zone will be greater in beats following a longer R-R interval.

In order to "find" this time zone the next beat must occur relatively early, so it follows that aberrant intraventricular conduction will most commonly be seen when there is a long pause followed by a shorter pause, and this situation obtains frequently during atrial fibrillation (Figure 285).

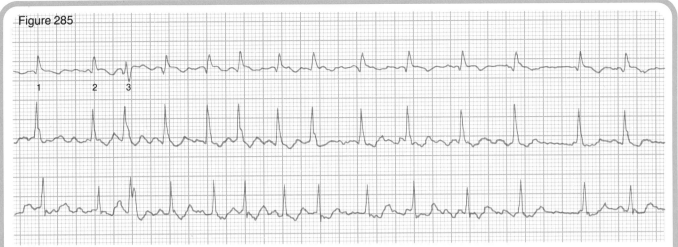

Figure 285

Leads I, II and III. Atrial fibrillation with a single example of aberrant intraventricular conduction.

The rhythm is clearly atrial fibrillation. No P waves are seen and the baseline is irregular. The ventricular rate is irregular. All the QRS complexes are similar to one another except for the third QRS complex. This shows aberrant intraventricular conduction. The R-R interval between QRS complexes 1 and 2 is long. As a result of this the refractory period of beat 2 will be longer than average. The refractory period of the right bundle branch will be longer than that of the left bundle branch and since the overall refractory period is longer than usual the absolute time gap between the end of recovery of the left bundle and the end of recovery of the right bundle (see Figure 244) will be greatest. There is therefore more chance of the next beat finding this time gap. For aberration to occur the next beat (beat 3) must be relatively close to beat 2. Whenever there is the combination of a long R-R interval followed by a short R-R interval in three consecutive beats which are all of supraventricular origin (like beats 1, 2 and 3 in this example) there is a distinct possibility of a third beat in this series showing aberration. Such a beat usually has the QRS waveform typical of right bundle branch block. It is, of course, not possible with confidence to distinguish aberrant intraventricular conduction occurring in the context of atrial fibrillation from a ventricular premature beat. It is merely that the circumstances (long interval 1, 2 followed by short interval 2, 3) makes it likely that aberration will occur and that the appearances of beat 3 (right bundle branch block type of configuration) make it a plausible explanation. Aberrancy becomes increasingly likely when, in a given period of observation, the extent of the deviation of the aberrant QRS (n) from the usual QRS correlates directly with the length of the pause (n-2) to (n-1) and inversely with the length of the pause (n-1) to n (see Figure 245a, page 404).

Criteria for atrial fibrillation

1. No P waves are seen.

2. No flutter waves are seen.

3. Atrial activity is either absent or is chaotic both in amplitude and in rate.

4. The QRS complexes have the form which is usual for the subject and the lead.*

5. The R-R interval is variable. During a given period of observation a maximum and a minimum R-R interval will be observed and within these extremes the R-R interval will be unpredictable.

* If the QRS is abnormal in morphology and/or width prior to the onset of atrial fibrillation then it will, of course, remain similarly abnormal subsequent to the onset of atrial fibrillation (Figure 284). In the presence of ventricular pre-excitation with conduction down the anomalous pathway the QRS complexes may be abnormally wide and associated with a delta wave (Figure 301).
When the interval $R_{(n-1)}$ to R_n is short and particularly if the interval $R_{(n-2)}$ to $R_{(n-1)}$ is long the QRS complex R_n may show aberrant intraventricular conduction (functional bundle block – right more commonly than the left) (Figure 285).
(Compare this with acceleration-dependant aberrancy; see page 407.)

Junctional Tachycardia

Junctional is a term used to describe a sustained supraventricular tachycardia arising in the atrio-ventricular junctional area. From an anatomical point of view the term includes† (i) low atrial re-entrant tachycardias (ii) atrio-ventricular nodal tachycardias, i.e. both non-paroxysmal, and re-entrant (the latter being known as atrio-ventricular nodal re-entrant tachycardia – AVNRT) (iii) atrio-ventricular re-entrant tachycardia (AVRT) involving an (accessory) atrio-ventricular nodal bypass tract and (iv) high fascicular tachycardia (page 466). Of these AVNRT and AVRT are far and away the commonest varieties. Whatever the anatomical origin, junctional tachycardia is an "active" rhythm, not an escape rhythm. The depolarisation process for each cardiac cycle begins in the atrio-ventricular junctional area and spreads antegradely to depolarise the ventricles and retrogradely to depolarise the atria (as in Figure 231). Each P wave and each QRS complex therefore has the characteristics associated with junctional premature beats. It follows that, as in the case of junctional premature beats, the P′ waves of junctional tachycardia are abnormal. They are most commonly negative in those leads in which sinus-initiated P waves are expected to be positive (e.g. Leads I, II, aVF and the precordial leads) and are positive in those leads in which sinus-initiated P waves are usually negative (e.g. aVR). Since the pathway of atrio-ventricular conduction is usually normal, the QRS complexes are usually normal. If there is pre-existing left or right bundle branch block, left or right ventricular hypertrophy, myocardial infarction, or any other condition giving rise to changes in the QRS complexes, then these changes will, of course, be present during the junctional tachycardia as during sinus rhythm, i.e. the QRS complexes will have that waveform which is usual for the particular patient (as in all supraventricular rhythms). However, QRS complexes which are normal during sinus-initiated rhythm may **become** abnormally wide during junctional tachycardia if the rate is such as to give rise to functional bundle branch block (aberrant intraventricular conduction (pages 403 to 405)). In cases where there is pre-excitation (pages 212 to 220 and 446 to 457) during sinus-initiated rhythm the QRS will be abnormal in shape and width but during re-entrant tachycardia activation travels retrogradely along the anomalous pathway and the QRS complexes **become** normal for the duration of the re-entrant tachycardia (Figure 297).

There are two clinically distinct types of junctional tachycardia: "non-paroxysmal" junctional tachycardia and "paroxysmal" (otherwise called "re-entrant") junctional tachycardia. Non-paroxysmal atrio-ventricular junctional tachycardia is due to a focal repetitive discharge from the AV junctional area, i.e. it is due to accelerated automatic discharge from the atrio-ventricular junctional zone. This rhythm is usually gradual in onset and is associated with a regular P wave rate in the range of 60-130 beats/min* and with identical QRS rates (unless there is an additional atrio-ventricular conduction problem). Paroxysmal atrio-ventricular junctional tachycardia is due to a local re-entry circuit in the AV junctional area. It is associated with a regular junctional discharge in the range of 150-250 beats/min. In common with other re-entrant arrhythmias its onset and offset are both usually abrupt. The non-paroxysmal type is rare and will involve one of three possible anatomical sites – the low atrial area, the AV node or the high fascicular region. The paroxysmal type is very common and may involve any of four anatomical sites, the low atrial area, the AV node, the high fascicular area and the circus pathway provided by the AV node and an anomalous atrio-ventricular communication together with the atrial myocardium between the proximal part of the anomalous pathway and the proximal part of the AV node and the ventricular myocardium between the distal part of the AV node and the distal part of the anomalous pathway (pages 448 to 450 and Figures 293 and 294). This latter type of paroxysmal tachycardia is known as atrio-ventricular re-entrant tachycardia (AVRT). The paroxysmal tachycardia which occurs because of a re-entrant mechanism within the atrio-ventricular node is known as atrio-ventricular nodal re-entrant tachycardia (AVNRT).

All three anatomical forms of non-paroxysmal junctional tachycardia are rare. Two forms (low atrial and high fascicular) of paroxysmal junctional tachycardia are rare and the other two are very common. Far and away the commonest forms of junctional tachycardia are AVNRT and AVRT. Both of these are re-entrant and therefore paroxysmal. AVNRT involves a re-entry mechanism entirely within the AV node whereas AVRT involves the AV node, an anomalous pathway and adjacent small areas of the upper interventricular septal myocardium – and the lower atrial myocardium.

Irrespective of the **mechanism** of the arrhythmia (i.e. paroxysmal, i.e. re-entrant or non-paroxysmal, i.e. enhanced automaticity) and irrespective of the **anatomical** site ((i) low atrial or (ii) AV nodal or (iii) high fascicular or (iv) low atrial plus AV nodal plus high septal plus low atrial for the paroxysmal variety and (i) to (iii) of the foregoing for the non-paroxysmal variety) the **fundamental** electrocardiographic appearances are similar (Figure 286).

†Not all authors define the term in this way. Indeed in most books on electrocardiography this term is not defined (and many other terms remain undefined!). Some authors appear to equate "junctional" with AV nodal.

*The term "tachycardia" is strictly applicable only when the depolarisation rate exceeds 100 beats/min. In the case of junctional tachycardia with rates of 80-100 beats/min, the term "tachycardia" is permitted by general consent since these rates are in excess of the rate of 60 beats/min and therefore constitute a "tachycardia" as far as the atrio-ventricular junctional depolarisation rate is concerned.

Figure 286

Paroxysmal and non-paroxysmal AV nodal tachycardia
a) AV junctional tachycardia due to re-entry within the AV node (paroxysmal junctional tachycardia). The ventricles depolarise in antegrade fashion and therefore the QRS complexes are of the form usual for that patient (i.e. they are normal except if there is pre-existing bundle branch block, pre-excitation or some other cause of QRS abnormality). The atrial myocardial depolarisation is retrograde and therefore the P waves have a reversed polarity (e.g. are negative in Lead II and positive in Lead aVR).

b) Atrio-ventricular junctional tachycardia due to enhanced automaticity (non-paroxysmal junctional tachycardia). The ventricular depolarisation proceeds in antegrade fashion exactly as in the paroxysmal variety. The atrial myocardial depolarisation proceeds in retrograde fashion exactly as in the paroxysmal variety. The overall appearances are similar to those in the paroxysmal variety except that the atrial and ventricular rates are very much less (the atrial rates being in the range of 60-130 beats/min as opposed to 150-250 beats/min).

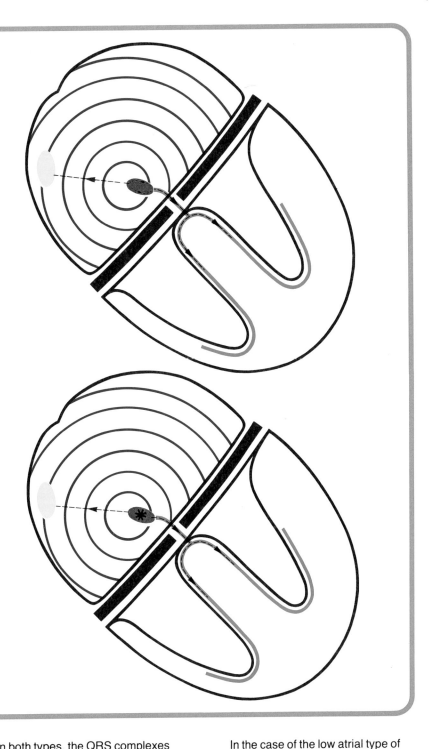

In both types, the QRS complexes are generally normal (i.e. usual for that subject) and the P waves are abnormal (and most commonly are reversed in polarity). The time interval between the P waves and the QRS complexes varies depending on the conducting pathway. Four possibilities exist as far as the relationship of the P waves to the QRS complexes is concerned: (i) **The atria and ventricles may be depolarised simultaneously** (in opposite directions and from the junctional zone in each case) in which case the inverted P′ waves will be hidden in the QRS complexes, (ii) **the atria may be depolarised after the ventricles** (in which case the inverted P′ waves will follow the normal QRS complexes, (iii) **the atria may be depolarised before the ventricles,** in which case the inverted P′ waves will precede the QRS complexes or (iv) **the atria may not be depolarised at all** since there may be retrograde block of atrial depolarisation.

In the case of the low atrial type of junctional tachycardia the P′ wave precedes the QRS (i.e. the P′-QRS interval is less than the QRS-P′ interval – Figure 288a). In the case of AVNRT the P′ wave is simultaneous with the QRS, most commonly being obscured by it (e.g. Figure 288d for the non-paroxysmal and Figures 289 and 290 for the paroxysmal type) or, occasionally, being visible as a deformation of the QRS (e.g. Figure 288b for the non-paroxysmal type). In the case of atrio-ventricular re-entrant tachycardia, which always involves an anomalous atrio-ventricular conduction pathway, the P′ wave follows the QRS, i.e. the P′-QRS interval exceeds the QRS-P′ interval (Figure 291).

Figure 287 shows an example of the uncommon variety of junctional tachycardia, "non-paroxysmal junctional tachycardia". In this particular case the depolarisation reaches the ventricles before the atria and inverted P' waves follow each QRS.

Figure 287

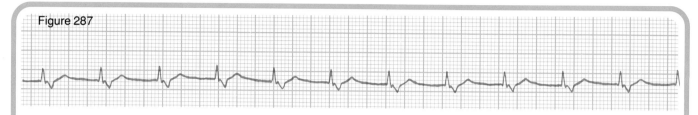

Lead II. Non-paroxysmal junctional tachycardia. The ventricular rate is 90 beats/min. The QRS complexes are of normal duration (not greater than 0.10 sec) and the ventricular activation is therefore of supraventricular origin. Negative P waves are seen (atrial depolarisation is being initiated in the AV junctional area and is travelling upwards and to the right giving negative P waves in Lead II). Since depolarisation from the AV node (the site of the rhythm in this case) reaches the ventricles before the atria, the QRS complexes occur before the P waves. The appearances are identical with those of "junctional rhythm" (see page 479) except that the rate is more rapid than in that rhythm and the appearances are also identical with those of paroxysmal junctional tachycardia except that the rate is much slower than in that rhythm.

The depolarisation sometimes reaches atria and ventricles simultaneously (in which case P' waves are buried in the QRS complexes) or before the ventricles (in which case the P' waves precede the QRS complexes) or there may be failure to conduct retrogradely to the AV node so that the atria may not depolarise at all or there may, very rarely, be independent sino-atrial node depolarisation (Figure 288).

Figure 288

Lead II. Non-paroxysmal junctional tachycardia. Varying relationship at the P' waves to QRS complexes.

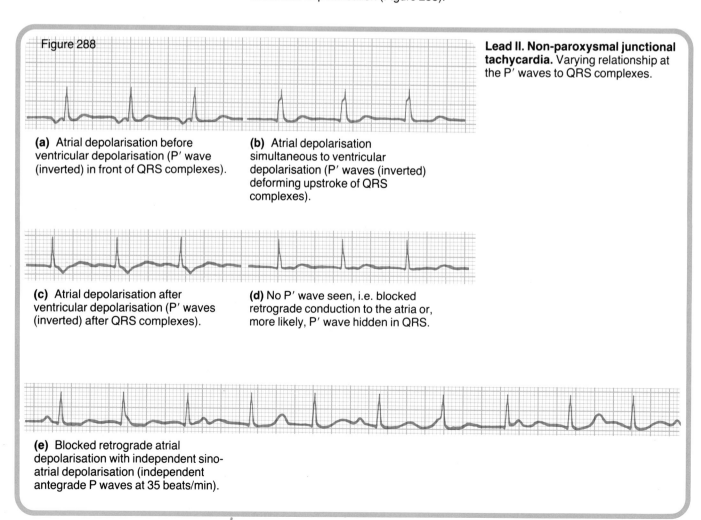

(a) Atrial depolarisation before ventricular depolarisation (P' wave (inverted) in front of QRS complexes).

(b) Atrial depolarisation simultaneous to ventricular depolarisation (P' waves (inverted) deforming upstroke of QRS complexes).

(c) Atrial depolarisation after ventricular depolarisation (P' waves (inverted) after QRS complexes).

(d) No P' wave seen, i.e. blocked retrograde conduction to the atria or, more likely, P' wave hidden in QRS.

(e) Blocked retrograde atrial depolarisation with independent sino-atrial depolarisation (independent antegrade P waves at 35 beats/min).

Atrio-ventricular Nodal Re-entrant Tachycardia (AVNRT)

Figure 289 shows an example of the much commoner variety of junctional tachycardia – "paroxysmal" (a clinical term) or "re-entrant" (an electrocardiographic term) form. The QRS complexes are normal, indicating the supraventricular origin of ventricular depolarisation. The ventricular rate is rapid (220 beats/min) and regular. No P waves can be identified. The appearances are typical of paroxysmal junctional tachycardia. It is probably AVNRT (see caption).

Figure 289

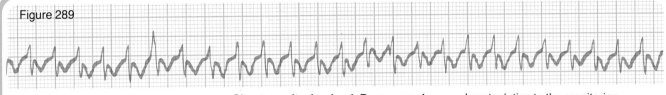

Chest monitoring lead. Paroxysmal (re-entrant) junctional tachycardia of the intra-AV nodal type, i.e. AVNRT. Ventricular rate 220 beats/min and regular. No P waves identified. QRS complexes are easily identified and are not abnormally wide. The T waves are easily seen. The slight variation in the form of the QRS complexes is probably related to slight changes in the position of the heart relative to the monitoring electrode as a result of respiratory movement. Since this supraventricular (narrow QRS) tachycardia has a rate of 150-250 beats/min (page 459) it is a **paroxysmal** supraventricular tachycardia. Since no P' waves can be seen it is likely to be intra-nodal, i.e. AVNRT.

In most cases of AVNRT the P wave is (i) hidden in the QRS (ii) absent or (iii) appears just at the end of the QRS. This is the usual "slow-fast" variety (page 446) and a typical example of this common form is seen in Figure 290a.

There is also a rare form of AVNRT (the "fast-slow" type) where the initial P wave occurs very late after the QRS. An example of this rare arrhythmia is shown in Fig 290b.

Figure 290

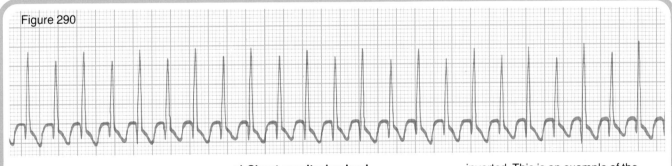

a) Chest monitoring lead. Paroxysmal (re-entrant) junctional tachycardia of the intra-AV nodal type, i.e. AVNRT. Ventricular rate 205 beats/min and regular. No P waves identified. QRS complexes are not abnormally wide. T waves are inverted. This is an example of the common variety of junctional tachycardia with the re-entrant pathway entirely within the AV node (i.e. AVNRT) and of the common "slow-fast" type (page 446).

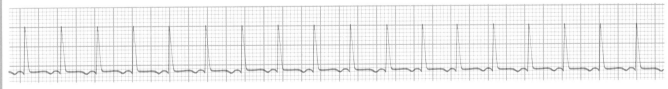

b) Ambulatory ECG recording. Paroxysmal (re-entrant) junctional tachycardia of the intra-AV nodal type (i.e. AVNRT but of the very uncommon "fast-slow" type). Ventricular rate 150 beats/min and regular. Inverted P waves are seen in front of the QRS complexes (i.e. QRS-P' interval exceeds P'-QRS interval). This is an example of the rare "fast-slow" type of AVNRT. The appearances are very similar to those seen in paroxysmal atrial tachycardia.

Atrio-ventricular Re-entrant Tachycardia (AVRT)

Figure 291 shows another example of junctional tachycardia. In this example retrograde activation of the atria is apparent after the QRS. The rhythm is therefore likely to be AVRT (with the concealed ventriculo-atrial accessory pathway which is usually present in such cases).

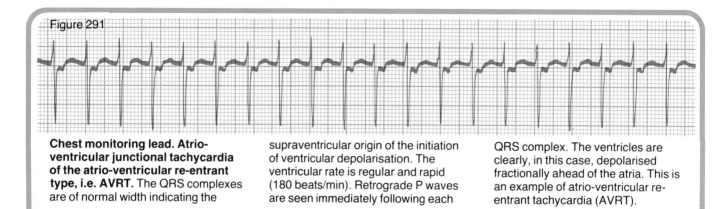

Figure 291

Chest monitoring lead. Atrio-ventricular junctional tachycardia of the atrio-ventricular re-entrant type, i.e. AVRT. The QRS complexes are of normal width indicating the supraventricular origin of the initiation of ventricular depolarisation. The ventricular rate is regular and rapid (180 beats/min). Retrograde P waves are seen immediately following each QRS complex. The ventricles are clearly, in this case, depolarised fractionally ahead of the atria. This is an example of atrio-ventricular re-entrant tachycardia (AVRT).

Electrophysiological Mechanism of AV Nodal Re-entrant Tachycardia

Re-entry mechanisms depend upon an activation circuit (circus movement – page 355). The re-entry phenomenon is dependent upon an anatomico-physiological substrate to permit spread of depolarisation in a continuous circuit. Within the atrio-ventricular node the anatomico-physiological substrate is thought to be produced by "longitudinal dissociation" within the node. Thus one side of the AV node has slowly-conducting cells which have a short refractory period (these cells constitute "α-pathways") and the other side has fast-conducting cells which have a longer refractory period (these cells constitute "ß-pathways"). When a premature beat enters the atrio-ventricular node it is more likely to be conducted by the α-(slow) cells since they have a shorter refractory period and are more likely to have recovered from the preceding beat. The fast (more slowly recovering) cells may well, however, have recovered by the time the depolarisation wave has reached the distal part in the AV node and in this way an atrial premature beat may initiate atrio-ventricular nodal re-entrant tachycardia (Figure 292).

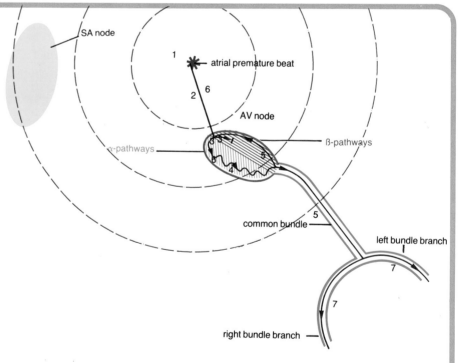

Figure 292

The mechanism of production of AV nodal re-entrant tachycardia by an atrial premature beat.

1. Spontaneous depolarisation occurs at some point within the atrial myocardium.

2. Depolarisation spreads in all directions within the atrial myocardium from the site of origin, but part of this depolarisation pathway travels towards and enters the atrio-ventricular node.

3. Depolarisation would be expected to travel down both sides of the atrio-ventricular node, but the ß-(fast) pathways are found to be refractory whilst the α-(slow) pathways have recovered from the previous depolarisation.

4. The depolarisation circuit therefore proceeds down the α-pathways only.

5. Depolarisation is able to spread down the common bundle and simultaneously retrogradely up through the ß-pathways which, by now, have recovered from their previous depolarisation.

6. Within the atrio-ventricular node the loop is completed and the impulse is able to spread both retrogradely to the atria and also antegradely once more through the α-pathways to initiate the next re-entrant beat.

7. The depolarisation which spreads down the common bundle goes on through the bundle branches and subsequently activates the ventricles.

The usual form of paroxysmal junctional tachycardia is initiated in this way by an atrial premature beat which enters the atrio-ventricular node, travels antegradely down the slow (α-) pathway to depolarise the ventricles and passes retrogradely up the fast (ß-) conducting pathway to give subsequent retrograde depolarisation of the atrial myocardium and to complete the re-entrant loop within the atrio-ventricular node. **This "slow-fast" variety is by far the commonest form of atrio-ventricular junctional tachycardia and in this variety the most usual electrocardiographic finding is that the retrograde P wave is completely hidden in the QRS complex and no P′ waves are therefore seen (as in Figures 289 and 290). Occasionally there may be delay in retrograde conduction to the atria and inverted P′ waves may be seen almost immediately after the QRS (as in Figure 291). Since the P′ waves are very close to the QRS this is still a "slow-fast" type.**

Less commonly still, the circuit within the atrio-ventricular node may be reversed and conduction may occur antegradely down the fast (ß-) pathway and retrogradely up the slow (α-)pathway. In this very unusual form of atrio-ventricular junctional tachycardia (the "fast-slow" variety) the ventricles will receive the depolarisation signal early and the atria will receive it late because of

slow conduction retrogradely through the slow pathway. This will result in a long delay between the QRS complex and the inverted P wave.

In the vast majority of atrio-ventricular junctional tachycardias there is either no P wave visible or the inverted P wave occurs immediately after the QRS.

Pre-excitation and Re-entrant Tachycardias

The term "pre-excitation" implies that some part of the myocardium receives the depolarisation wave earlier than would be anticipated. Strictly speaking, pre-excitation is said to occur **either** when the spread of atrial depolarisation reaches some part of the ventricular myocardium earlier than would be anticipated if the impulse travelled only by way of the normal atrio-ventricular conducting channels **or** when ventricular myocardial depolarisation spreads to the atrial myocardium earlier than would be anticipated if the impulse travelled (retrogradely) via the normal ventriculo-atrial conducting channels only. However, the term "pre-excitation" is most frequently used in relation to early excitation of part of the ventricular myocardium from spread of the atrial depolarisation wave. In such circumstances the use of the term "ventricular pre-excitation" eliminates one possible configuration.

Ventricular pre-excitation was discussed briefly in Section 2 (pages 212-220), where its impact on the morphological aspects of the electrocardiogram was discussed. Quite apart from its significance in modifying the morphological appearances on the 12-lead ECG (and giving rise to possible confusion with bundle branch block, infarction etc), ventricular pre-excitation is a very important anatomico-physiological substrate for arrhythmias for, together with the AV node, it provides

an anatomical pathway which supports a depolarisation circuit and by nature of the slow and fast conducting constituents of that pathway (slow in the AV node, fast in the anomalous connection) it provides a situation entirely analogous to that within the atrio-ventricular node itself (when "longitudinal dissociation" provides the substrate for tachycardias). A re-entrant tachycardia involving the AV node and an anomalous pathway (as well as small parts of adjacent atrial and ventricular myocardium) is known as an atrio-ventricular re-entrant tachycardia (AVRT).

**The Anatomy of Re-entrant
Tachycardias associated with
Ventricular Pre-excitation**

The commonest anatomical substrates for ventricular pre-excitation are shown in Figure 293.

These diagrams present simplified, idealized concepts. The anatomy of the accessory AV connections is uncertain and is the subject of controversy.

Figure 293 **The anatomical substrates for ventricular pre-excitation.**

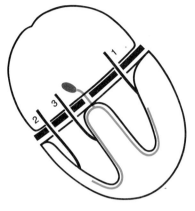

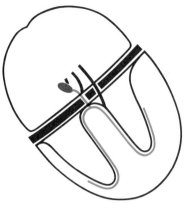

(a) The atrio-ventricular bypass tracts (often referred to as Kent bundles) which may be left-sided (1), right-sided (2) or septal (3). These pathways produce a short P-R interval, a delta wave and an abnormal QRS complex. (Wolff-Parkinson-White configuration).

(b) The atrio-nodal and atrio-Hisian bypass tracts connect the atrial myocardium with the AV node, with the bundle of His or with the bundle branches. The atrio-nodal bundle connections (James fibres) produce a short P-R interval and a normal QRS complex. (Lown-Ganong-Levine configuration). The atrio-Hisian fibres are known as Brechenmacher fibres.

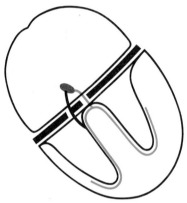

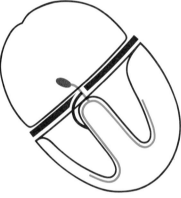

(c) The nodo-ventricular fibres (sometimes referred to as "Mahaim" fibres) connect the atrio-ventricular node to the ventricular myocardium. This produces a normal or short P-R interval and a fusion-beat type of QRS.

(d) The fasciculo-ventricular fibres pass from the His bundle to the ventricular myocardium. This produces a normal P-R interval and an abnormal QRS.

1. Atrio-ventricular Connections (Figure 293a)

The substrates for the commonest type of ventricular pre-excitation are the atrio-ventricular muscular connections. These are often referred to as the bundles of Kent. They are strands of ordinary cardiac muscle. Their presence produces (i) the typical short P-R interval (since the AV node is by-passed) and (ii) the typical delta wave and abnormal QRS complex (since the anomalous connection results in early activation of part of the ventricular myocardium). These aspects are discussed in Section 2, pages 212-219. The QRS complex is actually a fusion beat with activation both via the normal AV connection and via the bypass tract. These tracts can be found connecting the atrial and ventricular myocardium at any point and can be multiple, but they can conveniently be divided into left-sided, right-sided and septal connections (Figure 293a).

Left-sided connections produce type A pre-excitation. Premature activation occurs in the left ventricle and the QRS complexes are dominantly upright in the left-sided precordial leads.

Right-sided connections produce type B pre-excitation with premature activation of the right ventricle. They frequently give Q waves or QS complexes in II, III and aVF and they may mistakenly give the impression that there is inferior myocardial infarction.

The classification into type A and type B is, however, of limited usefulness. Type B pre-excitation gives inferior lead q wave, Q wave or QS complexes **only** if the anomalous connection is posteriorly located.

Many type A connections also give patterns in which the delta wave vector is superiorly orientated with resultant q wave, Q wave or QS complexes in the inferior leads.

2. Atrio-Hisian Connections (Figure 293b)

Fibres have been described connecting the atria with the bundle of His and with the proximal bundle branches. The fibres connecting atrial myocardium and AV node have been referred to as the James fibres and those connecting atria and the bundle of His as the Brechenmacher fibres. Their role in the aetiology of re-entrant arrhythmias is not absolutely clear, but the James fibres may be responsible for the Lown-Ganong-Levine syndrome with a short P-R interval and a normal QRS complex.

3. Nodo-ventricular Connections (Figure 293c)

These fibres pass from the distal part of the atrio-ventricular node to the ventricular myocardium. These fibres and the fasciculo-ventricular fibres (see below) are known as Mahaim fibres. These fibres are associated with a normal or short P-R interval (depending on how much travel occurs in the AV node before the bypass pathway emerges). The QRS complexes tend to be abnormal since they are usually fusion beats from the two activation pathways (His bundle and nodo-ventricular connections).

4. Fasciculo-ventricular Connections (Figure 293d)

These fibres are also known as Mahaim fibres. They pass from the common bundle to the ventricle. Their presence is associated with a normal P-R interval (since travel occurs normally through the AV node) and a constantly abnormal QRS complex (since ventricular activation is by fusion of activation from the normal and from the bypass pathways).

Each of the varieties of abnormal connections shown in Figure 293(a-d) provides an anatomical circuit capable of sustaining a re-entry mechanism. In the case of the atrio-ventricular connections (Figure 293a) and the atrio-Hisian connections (Figure 293b) an anatomico-physiological situation obtains similar to that of "longitudinal dissociation" in the atrio-ventricular node (page 445). The abnormal connection provides a pathway with rapid conduction velocity and a long refractory period and the atrio-ventricular node itself provides, in parallel, a slowly conducting pathway with a short refractory period.

The commonest variety of ventricular pre-excitation is seen in the Wolff-Parkinson-White syndrome. This syndrome requires the presence of one or more atrio-ventricular connections. In the presence of such a pathway a normal sinus beat results in the premature excitation of the ventricular myocardium because the pathway conducts more rapidly than the atrio-ventricular node (Figure 294). The ventricular myocardium is therefore "pre-excited" (see pages 212-220) giving rise to an abnormally-short P-R interval (less than 0.12 sec), an abnormally-wide QRS complex (greater than 0.11 sec) and a slurring of the initial part of the QRS complex (a delta wave). Strictly speaking, the term "Wolff-Parkinson-White syndrome" should only be applied when these electrocardiographic features are known to be present (at least for part of the time) **and** when there is a clinical history of paroxysmal tachycardia.

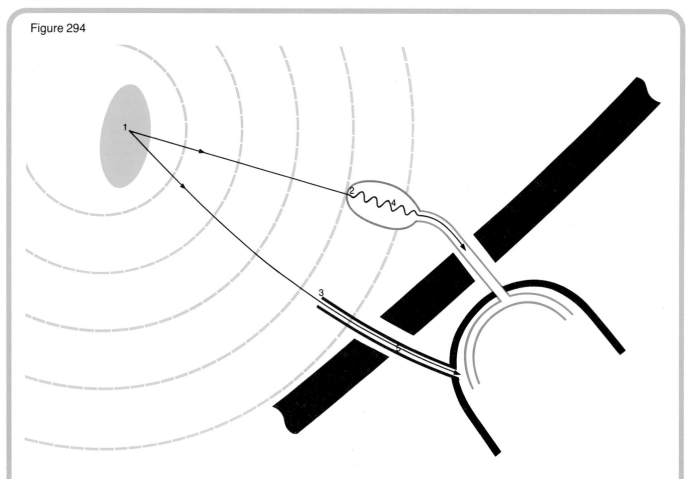

Figure 294

Ventricular pre-excitation.
Depolarisation is initiated at the sino-atrial node (1) and spreads normally through the atrial myocardium. Whether it reaches the AV node (2) or the bypass tract (3) first depends on the anatomical location of the latter. However, differences in the arrival time at these two points are small compared with differences between the very slow transmission through the AV node (4) and the very rapid transmission through the bypass tract (5). If transmission occurs through the bypass tract it is inevitable that ventricular myocardial depolarisation first occurs from this site. The presence of a bypass tract does not guarantee that depolarisation will travel down it. If depolarisation travels down the normal pathway only, the presence of the accessory pathway is "concealed".

Tachycardias in Association with Ventricular Pre-excitation

In precisely the same way as that within the atrio-ventricular node, the presence of a re-entry circuit with differential refractory periods gives rise to the potential for developing self-sustaining, re-entrant arrhythmias (Figure 295).

Note that the method by which an atrial premature beat initiates a re-entrant loop is entirely analogous to the way in which a re-entrant loop is initiated within the atrio-ventricular node itself (Figure 292). Note also that it is possible for a **ventricular** premature beat to travel retrogradely through the AV node (finding the accessory pathway refractory to retrograde travel) and to initiate a re-entrant loop in exactly the same way (but in the reverse direction). Some tachycardias are certainly initiated in this way.

Figure 295

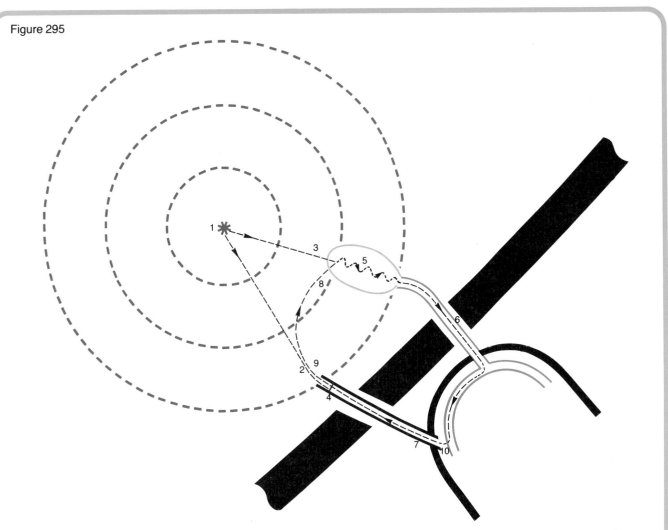

Mechanism by which an atrial premature beat may initiate re-entrant tachycardia in the presence of an anomalous atrio-ventricular conduction pathway. In the presence of sinus rhythm (not shown) the depolarisation wave travels down the AV node and down the accessory pathway as shown in Figure 294. An atrial premature beat (1) will give rise to atrial myocardial depolarisation which will spread to the accessory pathway (2) and to the AV node (3). If the beat is sufficiently premature it will find the accessory pathway refractory (4) but will be able to travel through the AV node (5), which has a shorter refractory period. It will travel down the His bundle (6) and gain entry to the distal end of the accessory pathway (7), which will have had time to recover. It will then travel retrogradely up this pathway and be able to re-enter the AV node (8). In this way a re-entrant loop will be established. Each time the activation wave enters atrial myocardium (9) atrial depolarisation will be initiated and each time it enters ventricular myocardium (10) ventricular depolarisation will be initiated.

Thus, in the presence of an anomalous atrio-ventricular bypass tract, when the subject is in sinus rhythm the ventricles are activated prematurely (i.e. are pre-excited) **by the bypass tract** (Figure 294) **and the P wave is of normal polarity, the P-R interval is short, the QRS complex is wide and has an initial delta wave** (see Section 2, page 212). However, **in the presence of an anomalous atrio-ventricular bypass tract during a re-entrant tachycardia atrio-ventricular conduction takes place via the atrio-ventricular node, the QRS complex is not abnormally wide** (unless there is some additional cause giving rise to an abnormal QRS) **and there is no delta wave. The appearances, therefore, look very similar to those in supraventricular tachycardia due to junctional re-entry. It may be very difficult indeed to tell these two arrhythmias apart. The best clue comes from the relationship between** the QRS complex and the P wave. **In most AV nodal re-entrant tachycardias the P wave is completely obscured by the simultaneous QRS complex** (Figure 290), **but occasionally an inverted P wave may be seen immediately after the QRS. In the case of a re-entrant tachycardia using an anomalous atrio-ventricular bypass tract, the inverted P wave is usually seen to occur rather later after the QRS and the time interval between the onset of the QRS and the onset of the retrograde P wave usually exceeds 0.07 sec** (Figure 296).

450

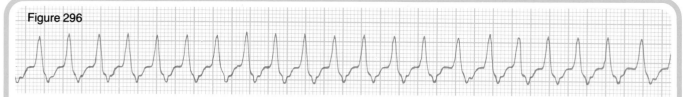

Figure 296

Lead II. Re-entrant tachycardia probably involving an AV nodal bypass tract. The ventricular rate is rapid (195 beats/min) and regular. The total QRS duration is at the upper end of the normal range (0.10 sec). Since the QRS complex is not abnormally wide there is no need to invoke the possibility of ventricular tachycardia (with retrograde conduction to the atria). Inverted P waves (travelling away from Lead II) are consistently seen after each QRS. The time interval from the onset of the QRS to the onset of the P waves is seen to be of the order of 0.12 sec and this long R-P interval suggests the presence of an atrio-ventricular bypass tract. Although the QRS complexes are not abnormally wide their width is at the upper end of the normal range and this is unusual in the more common "orthodromic" variety of re-entry mechanism associated with AV nodal bypass tracts. This suggests the possibility that the re-entrant circuit may, in this case, be antidromic, i.e. that it may be travelling antegradely through the bypass tract and retrogradely through the AV node. Without electrophysiological studies one cannot be certain of this. Note these appearances are very similar to those of the (very rare) "fast-slow" type of AV nodal re-entrant tachycardia.

Thus, persons with the Wolff-Parkinson-White syndrome, whilst in sinus rhythm, usually conduct from atria to ventricles via the atrio-ventricular bypass tract and manifest the typical ECG features of a short P-R interval, delta wave and widened QRS. However, during a paroxysm of tachycardia conduction usually takes place from atria to ventricles via the AV node **(orthodromic atrio-ventricular conduction)** with the bypass tract forming the return loop of the re-entrant circuit. This occurs because of the mechanism of initiation of the re-entrant tachycardia by atrial premature beats, as described on page 450 and in Figure 295. Thus, during the re-entrant tachycardia there is no delta wave and the QRS complex is not widened. Rarely, a re-entrant tachycardia may occur with **antidromic atrio-ventricular conduction** down the bypass tract and retrograde conduction through the AV node. In such a (relatively rare) situation, a paroxysmal tachycardia can occur in association with a delta wave and a wide QRS complex. However, such a mechanism for the tachycardia can only be **inferred** from the surface ECG (it can be confirmed by intracardiac electrophysiological studies) since a supraventricular tachycardia with orthodromic conduction down the AV node can also produce wide QRS complexes if the atrial rate is rapid enough to produce aberrant intraventricular conduction (pages 403 to 405).

The terms "orthodromic" and "antidromic" refer to the direction of conduction through the AV node during tachycardia. "Orthodromic" means atrio-ventricular conduction through the AV node and "antidromic" means ventriculo-atrial conduction through the AV node – in each case during a paroxysm of tachycardia.

Figure 297 shows an example of the electrocardiographic appearances in Lead II of a patient with the Wolff-Parkinson-White syndrome (a) when in sinus rhythm, and (b) when experiencing a paroxysm of "supraventricular"* tachycardia. The short P-R interval, delta wave and wide QRS (all indicating that atrio-ventricular depolarisation is proceeding by way of the anomalous atrio-ventricular pathway) are clearly seen during sinus rhythm, whereas during the re-entrant tachycardia the QRS is of normal width and has no delta wave.

* The term "supraventricular", whilst widely accepted in relation to episodes of re-entrant tachycardia in patients with ventricular pre-excitation, is, of course, not **strictly** accurate since a small area of the **ventricular** myocardium forms part of the re-entrant circuit (Figure 295 (10)). Electrophysiologists tend to use the term "atrio-ventricular" rather than "supraventricular".

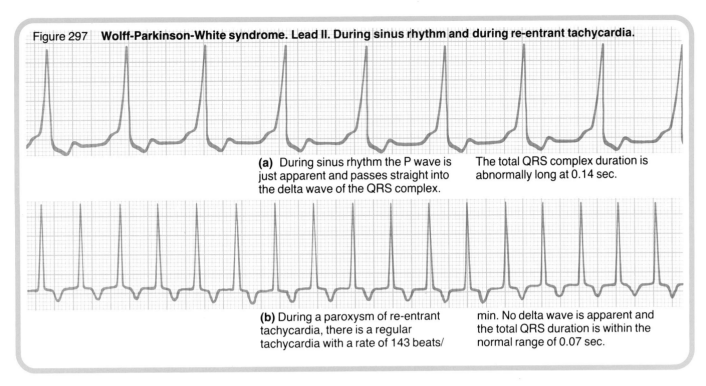

Figure 297   **Wolff-Parkinson-White syndrome. Lead II. During sinus rhythm and during re-entrant tachycardia.**

(a) During sinus rhythm the P wave is just apparent and passes straight into the delta wave of the QRS complex.

The total QRS complex duration is abnormally long at 0.14 sec.

(b) During a paroxysm of re-entrant tachycardia, there is a regular tachycardia with a rate of 143 beats/min. No delta wave is apparent and the total QRS duration is within the normal range of 0.07 sec.

Figure 298 shows a further example of re-entrant tachycardia in a patient with the Wolff-Parkinson-White syndrome. The ventricular rate is 140 beats/min and the QRS complexes are narrow. Retrograde P waves are seen after the QRS complex, just disturbing the upstroke of the T wave. The inverted wave following each QRS complex is probably partly a retrograde P wave and partly an inverted T wave. The P'-R interval is greater than the R-P' interval and the R-P' interval is substantially greater than 0.07 sec (it measures 0.16 sec) as is usually the case in re-entrant tachycardia involving an accessory pathway and with orthodromic conduction through the AV node.

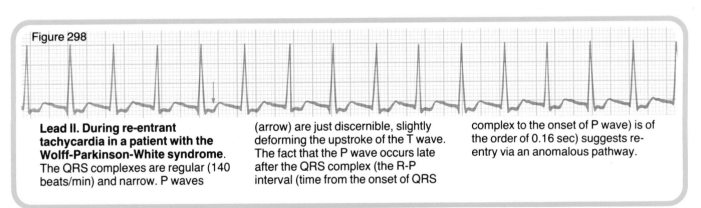

Figure 298

Lead II. During re-entrant tachycardia in a patient with the Wolff-Parkinson-White syndrome. The QRS complexes are regular (140 beats/min) and narrow. P waves (arrow) are just discernible, slightly deforming the upstroke of the T wave. The fact that the P wave occurs late after the QRS complex (the R-P interval (time from the onset of QRS complex to the onset of P wave) is of the order of 0.16 sec) suggests re-entry via an anomalous pathway.

The patterns described above (AV conduction down the anomalous pathway during sinus rhythm and down the normal AV pathway during re-entrant tachycardia) are the usual ones found in the Wolff-Parkinson-White syndrome, but both alternatives are possible. Thus (1) during sinus rhythm atrio-ventricular conduction may sometimes be down the normal AV pathway, and (2) during re-entrant tachycardia AV conduction may occur via the anomalous pathway. In the first of these two cases one will not be able to tell from the electrocardiogram that an anomalous pathway exists.
The presence of the anomalous pathway can be "revealed" in one of three ways:
1. The patient may vary the mode of atrio-ventricular conduction whilst in sinus rhythm – sometimes conducting normally and having no delta wave, wide QRS or short P-R interval, and sometimes conducting via the anomalous route and showing all of these features (Figure 299).
2. He (she) may have episodes of re-entrant tachycardia in which the retrograde P waves are seen following the QRS complexes and are separated from them by more than 70 milliseconds (Figure 298).
3. Electrophysiological studies (initiated because of the complaint of paroxysmal tachycardia) may demonstrate its presence.
The term "concealed" in relation to an accessory pathway means that is when the accessory pathway next conducts antegradely. In the event it is never apparent on the ECG during sinus rhythm or during re-entrant tachycardia. Its presence can be established by electrophysiological studies.

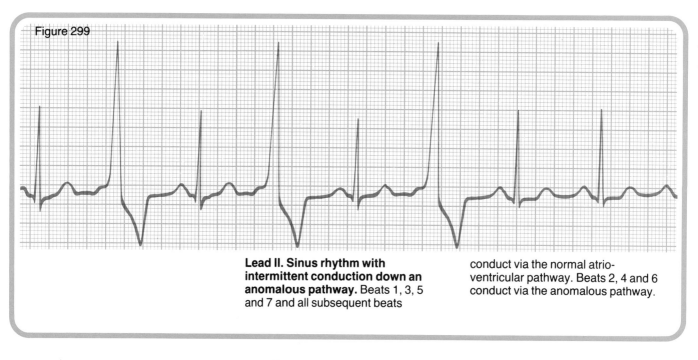

Figure 299

Lead II. Sinus rhythm with intermittent conduction down an anomalous pathway. Beats 1, 3, 5 and 7 and all subsequent beats conduct via the normal atrio-ventricular pathway. Beats 2, 4 and 6 conduct via the anomalous pathway.

Examples of re-entrant tachycardia with atrio-ventricular conduction via the anomalous pathway are rare and are almost entirely confined to situations where the rate of tachycardia is of the order of 200 beats/min or faster. This can be seen with atrial tachycardia or with atrial flutter. In Figure 300a there is sinus rhythm with atrio-ventricular conduction still down the anomalous pathway. In Figure 300b there is, in the same patient, re-entrant tachycardia with atrio-ventricular conduction still down the anomalous pathway. This is very unusual. It is, of course, not possible to be **certain** that this is the mechanism. An alternative explanation would be a re-entrant tachycardia with atrio-ventricular conduction via the normal pathway and with abnormal intraventricular conduction occurring because of the rapid ventricular rate (pages 403 to 405). However, the very close similarity of the morphology of the QRS complex in the same lead during sinus rhythm and during re-entrant tachycardia strongly supports the suggestion that the re-entrant wave travels from atria to ventricles via the anomalous pathway in just the same way as it does during sinus rhythm.

A similar but not entirely analogous situation (since it does not involve a re-entrant mechanism) can occur with atrial fibrillation (see page 454 and Figure 301).

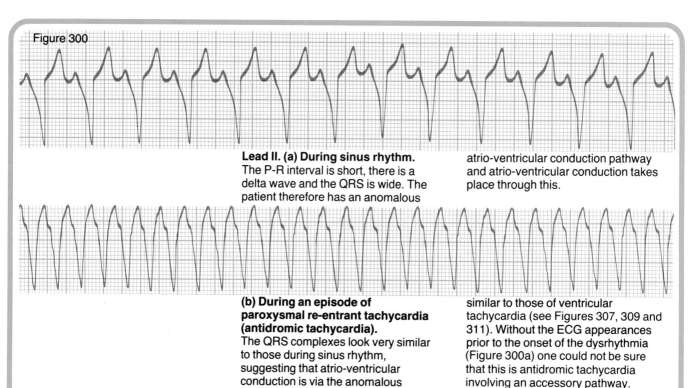

Figure 300

Lead II. (a) During sinus rhythm. The P-R interval is short, there is a delta wave and the QRS is wide. The patient therefore has an anomalous atrio-ventricular conduction pathway and atrio-ventricular conduction takes place through this.

(b) During an episode of paroxysmal re-entrant tachycardia (antidromic tachycardia). The QRS complexes look very similar to those during sinus rhythm, suggesting that atrio-ventricular conduction is via the anomalous pathway. The appearances are very similar to those of ventricular tachycardia (see Figures 307, 309 and 311). Without the ECG appearances prior to the onset of the dysrhythmia (Figure 300a) one could not be sure that this is antidromic tachycardia involving an accessory pathway.

Atrial Fibrillation in Association with Ventricular Pre-excitation

Atrial fibrillation in association with an anomalous atrio-ventricular pathway presents a special case, for the mechanism of atrial fibrillation is not a macro-re-entry route. It could be considered as multiple micro-re-entry routes or as multiple foci of activation; the effect is the same. The atrio-ventricular node and the anomalous pathway are both bombarded with multiple activation wavefronts. The refractory period of the AV node normally sets an upper limit to the ventricular rate of around 180-200 beats/min (page 436). Whilst inefficiently rapid, this ventricular rate is not usually intolerable unless there is severe underlying heart disease. **In the usual context of atrial fibrillation occurring in the presence of an anomalous atrio-ventricular pathway, this situation still obtains for the anomalous pathway, whilst able to conduct very rapidly, has a longer refractory period than the atrio-ventricular node. Antegrade conduction therefore usually takes place through the AV node and the presence of the anomalous pathway is irrelevant to the mechanism of the rhythm, to the ventricular rate and to the electrocardiographic appearances, which are simply those of atrial fibrillation (the electrocardiogram at the time gives no evidence of the existence of an anomalous pathway). Occasionally,** however, **the refractory period of the anomalous pathway may shorten abruptly in the presence of rapid sequential depolarisation from the atrial fibrillation and may become much shorter than that of the atrio-ventricular node. In such a situation atrio-ventricular conduction will then occur via the anomalous pathway, the QRS complexes will be wide and the ventricular rate will be very rapid** (Figure 301). Ventricular rates in excess of 300 beats/min can be achieved in this way. At such rates there is no time for ventricular filling and the cardiac output falls abruptly. **Sometimes in this situation the rapid ventricular response results in fragmentation of the ventricular depolarisation because not all parts of the intraventricular conduction pathway are able to conduct at the same rate. As a result repolarisation does not follow its usual ordered sequence and the abnormal depolarisation and repolarisation may result in ventricular fibrillation.** The combination of atrial fibrillation and the presence of an anomalous atrio-ventricular pathway is therefore a potentially lethal one.

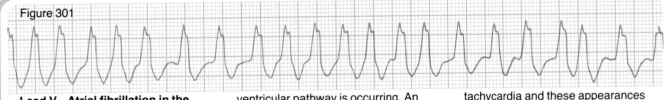

Figure 301

Lead V₁. Atrial fibrillation in the presence of a proven anomalous atrio-ventricular connection. No P waves are seen. The ventricular rate is very rapid (mean rate 220, peak rate 280 beats/min) and is irregular. The QRS complexes are wide. Atrial fibrillation with ventricular pre-excitation and atrio-ventricular conduction down the anomalous atrio-ventricular pathway is occurring. An alternative explanation could be atrial fibrillation occurring in association with right bundle branch block but this would be very unlikely since it would be highly improbable that the AV node and/or left bundle would be able to conduct impulses at this rate. ECGs of this type have often in the past been considered to indicate ventricular tachycardia and these appearances may be one reason for the relatively widespread (and generally incorrect) view that the ventricular rate may vary appreciably during ventricular tachycardia. (Variations in the R-R interval during ventricular tachycardia seldom exceed 40 msec.).

Functional or Organic Bundle Branch Block and the Wolff-Parkinson-White Syndrome

As with any supraventricular tachycardia, functional right (or occasionally left) bundle branch block may develop if the atrial depolarisation rate is appropriate. If the blocked bundle branch is on the same side as the anomalous bypass tract the tachycardia rate will fall immediately the bundle branch block develops. This is because the re-entrant circuit will be longer since the upper part of the interventricular septum will have to be traversed from one side to the other, and during this part of the travel the depolarisation wave will be travelling through slowly conducting myocardium. Thus in the case of functional **right** bundle branch block developing during a re-entrant tachycardia in a patient with a **right**-sided accessory pathway, the cycle length of the tachycardia will increase by about 50 milliseconds. With a **right**-sided accessory pathway the development of functional **left** bundle branch block would have no effect (Figure 302).

Thus if right bundle branch block develops **during** circus movement (re-entrant) tachycardia and if the R-R interval simultaneously lengthens by about 50 milliseconds the accessory pathway is located on the right. Likewise if left bundle branch block develops during circus movement tachycardia and if the R-R interval simultaneously lengthens by about 50 milliseconds the accessory pathway is located on the left. (It should be remembered that more than one accessory pathway may be present).

Figure 302   **Re-entrant tachycardia and bundle branch block.**

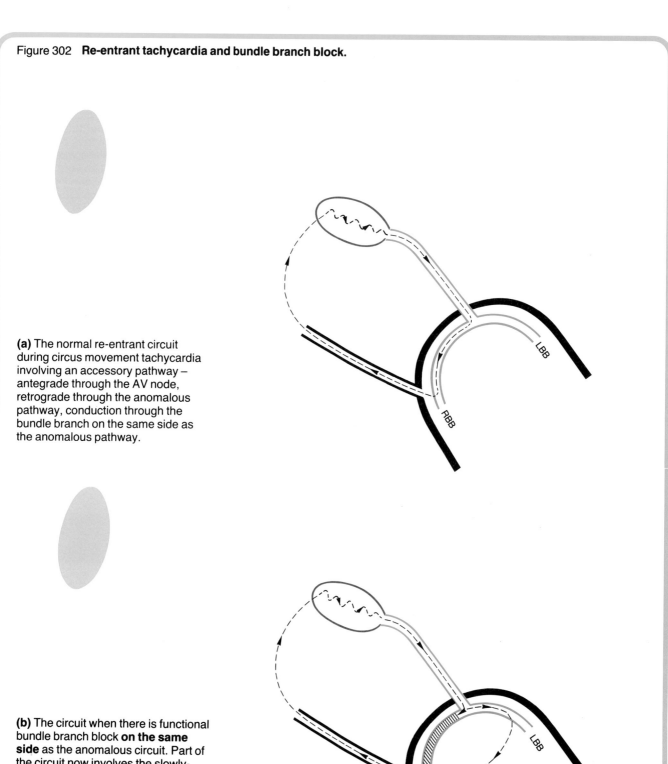

(a) The normal re-entrant circuit during circus movement tachycardia involving an accessory pathway – antegrade through the AV node, retrograde through the anomalous pathway, conduction through the bundle branch on the same side as the anomalous pathway.

(b) The circuit when there is functional bundle branch block **on the same side** as the anomalous circuit. Part of the circuit now involves the slowly-conducting myocardium between the left bundle branch and the right side of the interventricular septum. If there happened to be functional left bundle branch block instead of right bundle branch block the circuit would remain exactly as in (a).

Of course if there is **organic** bundle branch block on the same side as the re-entrant circuit the cycle length would be longer than in the absence of bundle branch block by the same amount but, unless the organic bundle branch block develops after a recording of the tachycardia in the absence of bundle branch block has obtained, this difference cannot be appreciated, since no **change** in the tachycardia rate is observed.

Relationship of Re-entrant Pathways and the ECG Appearances in Tachycardia Associated with the Wolff-Parkinson-White Syndrome

It will be seen from the foregoing discussion that the relationship is an exceedingly complex one. Some aspects of it are given in Table 38.

Table 38   Electrocardiographic Features of Tachycardias Associated with Pre-excitation

Atrial rhythm	Re-entrant circuit	AV conduction	IV conduction	VA conduction	P waves	P-R interval	R-P interval	Delta wave	QRS complexes	Tachycardia rate/min
Sinus	–	Anomalous AV pathway (WPW-type pre-excitation)	Abnormal	–	Normal	Short	–	Present	Wide	–
Sinus	–	AV node (normal)* His bundle	Normal	–	Normal	Normal	–	Absent	Normal	–
Re-entrant tachycardia (orthodromic)	Atria→ AV node→ His bundle→ bundle branch→ bypass tract→ atria	AV node + His bundle (Normal) [+]	Normal	Accessory pathway	Inverted (usually obscured)	–**	Usually[ø] 70 msec or more	Absent	Normal†	140-250
Re-entrant tachycardia (antidromic)††	Atria→ bypass tract→ bundle branch→ His bundle → AV node→ atria	AV bypass tract	Abnormal	His bundle[ε], AV node	Inverted (usually obscured)	–**	Usually[ø] 70 msec or more	Present	Wide	>200
Re-entrant tachycardia orthodromic with functional bundle branch block on same side as bypass tract	Atria→ AV node→ His bundle→ contralateral[øø] bundle branch→ intraventricular septum→ accessory pathway →atria	AV node, His bundle	Abnormal[+]	Accessory pathway	Inverted (usually obscured)	–**	Usually[ø] 100 msec or more	Absent	Wide[++]	125-210***
Atrial flutter or atrial fibrillation	Either (a) Atria→ AV node →His bundle→ bypass tract→ atria	AV node, His bundle	Normal	Accessory pathway	Absent (Flutter waves present)	–	–	Absent	Normal	100-250
	or (b) Atria→ accessory pathway→ His bundle→ AV node →atria	Accessory pathway	Abnormal	His bundle, AV node	Absent	–	–	Present	Wide	150-300 (atrial flutter) 150-600††† (atrial fibrillation)

* Concealed pre-excitation

** not applicable – ventricular activation before atria

*** slows because of travel through myocardium in upper part of IV septum (add 50msec to cycle length)

[ε] Antidromic

[ø] P waves often not visible

[øø] to bypass tract

[+] Orthodromic conduction (abnormal because of the BBB)

[++] Pre-existing or rate-related bundle branch block

† Unless there is pre-existing bundle branch block or aberrant intraventricular conduction

†† Rare

††† Ventricular rate may even be as high as 400 beats/min.

Electrocardiographic Features of Junctional Tachycardia

Ventricular (QRS) rate and regularity

In relation to junctional rhythm, the term "tachycardia" is generally agreed to indicate a rate more rapid than 60 beats/min (in relation to other areas of the heart "tachycardia" implies a rate greater than 100 beats/min). The rate is usually regular. In the non-paroxysmal variety the rate is typically in the range of 60-130 beats/min, and in the paroxysmal variety, 150-250 beats/min.

Atrial (P′) rate

This is usually the same as the ventricular rate, i.e. there is usually equally frequent conduction from the junctional origin to the ventricles and to the atria.

Relation between P waves and QRS complexes

The P′ waves may be in front of, simultaneously with or after the QRS complexes or may be entirely absent. Rarely, in association with junctional tachycardia with blocked retrograde conduction to the atria, there may be normal sinus node activation with independent (dissociated) P waves conducting antegradely through the atria but not spreading through the AV node. (Figure 288e).

P′ wave configuration

Atrial activation proceeds from the atrio-ventricular junctional zone to the atria and therefore the direction of atrial activation is opposite to the usual one and the P′ waves are typically inverted in Leads II, III and aVF. This is typically so in AVNRT, AVRT and fascicular tachycardia but need not be so in low atrial tachycardia.

QRS configuration

The QRS configuration will usually be the same as that which obtained before the onset of the tachycardia (i.e. the QRS complexes are normal for that patient). Thus in the absence of some primary cause for abnormality of the QRS complexes (e.g. right or left bundle branch block, right or left ventricular hypertrophy, myocardial infarction etc) the QRS complexes will be normal.

When the ventricular rate is sufficiently rapid to cause aberrant intraventricular conduction (pages 403 to 405) the QRS complexes may become abnormally wide and abnormally shaped in association with the onset of the tachycardia. In the case where there is ventricular pre-excitation during sinus-initiated rhythm (with QRS complexes which are abnormally wide and abnormally shaped) the QRS complexes will usually **become** normal with the onset of AVRT, since this usually involves retrograde conduction along the anomalous pathway (Figure 297).

Nature of onset and offset

Only rarely will a record be obtained showing the onset or offset of the tachycardia. Since it follows that the electrocardiographic features of the onset and offset are rarely seen, they cannot be relied upon to help with the diagnosis of the arrhythmia although they are certainly extremely helpful when they are seen. In the case of non-paroxysmal junctional tachycardia the increase in heart rate may be gradual. The initial event is sometimes, but not always, seen to be a junctional premature beat, but the junctional focus accelerates gradually to the rate of 60-130 beats/min. The offset of this arrhythmia may be sudden or gradual. The paroxysmal variety is always instantaneous in its onset – a junctional, an atrial or a ventricular premature beat is usually the event initiating a re-entry mechanism in the junctional area, giving rise immediately to the tachycardia rate which is then sustained. The offset is usually equally abrupt.

Criteria for Junctional Tachycardia

Numerous rhythms are involved under the heading "junctional tachycardia". These are as follows:

Non-paroxysmal junctional tachycardia (accelerated focus tachycardias)

Non-paroxysmal low atrial tachycardia

Non-paroxysmal nodal tachycardia

Non-paroxysmal fascicular tachycardia

Paroxysmal junctional tachycardia (re-entrant tachycardia)

Paroxysmal low atrial tachycardia

Paroxysmal atrio-ventricular nodal tachycardia (AVNRT)

Paroxysmal atrio-ventricular tachycardia (AVRT)

Paroxysmal fascicular tachycardia

Criteria common to the group will be given first, followed by criteria for the individual types.

Criteria for junctional tachycardia

1. The QRS rate is rapid.

2. The QRS rate is regular.

3. QRS complexes are the usual for that subject.†

4. P waves may be visible – in which case they are inverted compared with the usual orientation in the given lead.

5. The P waves, if present, may be in front of the QRS complex (with a short P-R interval) within the QRS complex or following the QRS complex. The P waves may be absent.*

† i.e. are normal unless some defect in intraventricular conduction antedates the onset of the arrhythmia or the ventricular rate is sufficiently rapid to induce aberrant intraventricular conduction. In the case where there is pre-excitation during sinus-initiated rhythm the QRS complexes become normal with the onset of AVRT. When there is orthodromic conduction round the re-entrant circuit (Figure 297) both remain abnormal with the onset of the AVRT if there is antidromic conduction round the re-entrant circuit (Figure 300).

* Rarely there is blocked retrograde conduction to the atria; normal sinus-initiated P waves may be seen independently.

Criteria for non-paroxysmal junctional tachycardia

1. The criteria 1-5 given for junctional tachycardia obtain.
2. The ventricular rate and atrial rate are the same at 60-130 beats/min.

Criteria for paroxysmal junctional tachycardia

1. The criteria 1-5 given for junctional tachycardia obtain.
2. The ventricular rate and the atrial rate are the same at 150-250 beats/min.

Criteria for the low atrial variety of junctional tachycardia

1. The criteria 1-4 given for junctional tachycardia obtain.
2. The atrial and ventricular rate are equal and are either 60-130 beats/min (non-paroxysmal variety) or 150-250 beats/min (paroxysmal variety).
3. The P′ wave precedes the QRS, i.e. the P′-QRS interval is less than the QRS-P′ interval.

Criteria for the atrio-ventricular nodal variety of junctional tachycardia

1. The criteria **1-4** given for junctional tachycardia obtain.

2. The atrial and ventricular rates are equal and are either 60-130 beats/min (non-paroxysmal variety) or 150-250 beats/min (paroxysmal variety, i.e. AVNRT).

3. Almost always the P' waves are hidden in the QRS (i.e. are invisible) or are seen in the terminal part of the QRS. In the very rare "fast-slow" form the P' waves may occur very late after the QRS, i.e. they precede the next QRS, i.e. the P'-QRS interval is less than the QRS'-P interval.

Criteria for the atrio-ventricular variety of junctional tachycardia – AVRT (of the orthodromic type)

1. The criteria **1-4** for junctional tachycardia obtain.

2. The atrial and ventricular rates are equal at 150-250 beats/min (this arrhythmia is always paroxysmal).

3. Typically the P' waves are seen after the QRS, i.e. the P'-QRS interval is greater than the QRS-P' interval.

Criteria for the atrio-ventricular variety of junctional tachycardia – AVRT (of the antidromic type)

1. Criteria **1-4** for junctional tachycardia obtain.*

2. The atrial and ventricular rates are equal at 150-250 beats/min (this arrhythmia is always paroxysmal).

3. The QRS complexes are abnormal and show the same appearances as during sinus rhythm with ventricular pre-excitation.*

4. The P waves are usually obscured and merge with the initial part of the QRS (Figure 300b).

Criteria for the high fascicular variety of junctional tachycardia

1. Criteria **1, 2, 4** and **5** for junctional tachycardia obtain.

2. The QRS complexes may be of the form usual for that subject but in most cases there is RBBB and LAH.†

3. The atrial and ventricular rates are equal and are 60-130 beats/min (non-paroxysmal variety) or 150-250 beats/min (paroxysmal variety).

* The QRS complexes are "normal for the subject" but show ventricular pre-excitation since the re-entrant pathway travels antegrade down the accessory pathway and retrograde through the AV node (i.e. the current is antidromic).

† In most cases right bundle branch block and left anterior hemiblock develop with the onset of the arrhythmia and clear when the arrhythmias cease.

459

Ventricular ectopic rhythms (ventricular ectopic beats, ventricular tachycardia) arise from activity in the specialised conducting tissue distal to the bifurcation of the His bundle or sometimes from the myocardium of the ventricles. The subsidiary pacemaker sites below the His bundle are normally suppressed by earlier depolarisation reaching them via normal conduction pathways following sinus node depolarisation (see page 349 and Figure 188). A ventricular premature beat occurs when, for example, a Purkinje cell reaches threshold earlier than the spread to it of the excitation wave from the sinus node (Figure 228). Such a beat is **ectopic** (because it arises from a site other than the sino-atrial node) and is premature (because it occurs earlier than anticipated). It is an active beat not an **escape** beat.

Ventricular tachycardia may develop from one of two mechanisms. The first results from an appropriately-timed ventricular premature beat reaching a circuit which permits a re-entrant loop to be established (page 355 and Figures 193 and 194). This is entirely analogous to the re-entrant loop found within the atrio-ventricular node in the AV nodal re-entrant tachycardia and within the AV node and bypass tract in re-entrant tachycardias associated with atrio-ventricular bypass tract.

The second mechanism is when enhanced automaticity is present in the ectopic ventricular site and repetitive firing occurs.

Whichever of the two mechanisms initiates the tachycardia the depolarisation necessarily begins at an ectopic site in the ventricular myocardium (Figure 303) and spreads to all parts of the ventricular myocardium. It will not **usually** spread back through the atrio-ventricular node to the atria so atrial depolarisation is **usually** initiated by the sinus node and proceeds independently (i.e. there is atrio-ventricular dissociation). The sinus rate will be slower than the ventricular rate.

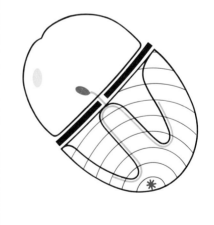

Figure 303

The mechanism of ventricular tachycardia. In the paroxysmal form a local re-entrant circuit initiates the depolarisation. In the non-paroxysmal form repetitive discharge occurs locally (in both cases represented by the asterisk). The depolarisation then spreads over the whole of the ventricular myocardium. The direction of spread is abnormal and therefore the QRS waveform is abnormally shaped. The spread is predominantly through myocardium and not through the rapidly conducting specialised conducting tissue and therefore the time taken for complete ventricular depolarisation is increased. Because of this latter feature the QRS complex is abnormally wide. If the depolarisation wave does not pass through the atrio-ventricular node there will be sinus-initiated atrial depolarisation proceeding independently.

The ECG of ventricular tachycardia induced by re-entry is effectively that of a self-perpetuating ventricular ectopic beat. It has an abrupt onset and offset. Ventricular tachycardia is defined by the Criteria Committee of the New York Heart Association as the occurrence of three or more ventricular premature beats in sequence separated by a fixed interval. The rate usually lies within the range of 140-250 beats/min and is approximately regular. Minor cycle length variations of the order of 0.01-0.02 sec occur (in contrast with the precisely regular supraventricular tachycardias).

Paroxysmal Ventricular Tachycardia

Ventricular tachycardia which begins abruptly, ends abruptly and is associated with a re-entrant mechanism, is sometimes called "paroxysmal" ventricular tachycardia.

Non-paroxysmal Ventricular Tachycardia, "Slow Ventricular Tachycardia", "Accelerated Idioventricular Rhythm"

The ECG of ventricular tachycardia induced by enhanced automaticity has a slower rate (typically 60*-130 beats/min) and has a gradual onset and offset. This rhythm is usually called "non-paroxysmal ventricular tachycardia", "accelerated idioventricular rhythm" or "slow ventricular tachycardia". This rhythm most commonly occurs in relation to acute myocardial infarction and tends to be benign.

Electrocardiographic Appearances of Ventricular Tachycardia

QRS rate

This usually lies within the range 150-250 beats/min for the **paroxysmal type** and 60-130 beats/min for the **non-paroxysmal type**. Minor variations in cycle length of the order of 0.01-0.02 sec may occur.

QRS configuration

The QRS complexes are abnormally shaped and are abnormally wide. They have a constant configuration apart from minor perturbations induced by the variably located superimposed P waves and by minor electrical axis shift occurring in association with respiratory movement. The mean frontal plane QRS axis is typically well outside the normal range of $-30°$ to $+90°$.

As in the case of ventricular ectopic beats, the configuration of the QRS complex gives a clue to the site of origin of the tachycardia. Thus ventricular tachycardia arising in the **left** ventricular myocardium gives rise to a **right** bundle branch block type of QRS complex with predominantly upright QRS complexes in the right precordial leads and significantly down-going QRS complexes in the left precordial leads. Conversely ventricular tachycardia arising from the **right** ventricle gives rise to a **left** bundle branch block type of QRS complex with dominantly negative QRS deflections in the right precordial leads and dominantly positive ones in the left precordial leads.

S-T segment and T waves

Analysis of the S-T segment and T waves plays no part in the estimation of cardiac rhythm (page 370) but it is worth remembering that the S-T segment and T waves are both usually deviated away from the direction of the QRS complex in ventricular tachycardia.

P waves

It may be difficult or impossible to see the P waves during ventricular tachycardia since they tend to be obscured by the much larger deflections (QRS, S-T and T). When visible, the most typical appearance is for the P wave rate to be regular and to be independent of the QRS. Occasionally, however, retrograde AV conduction (i.e. VA conduction) may occur and in this event inverted (for that lead) P waves will follow the QRS complexes.

The recognition of minor perturbations on the QRS waveform consistent with independent (superimposed) P waves is an important part of the recognition of ventricular tachycardia (Figure 307). The use of special leads (including oesophageal leads) may help in the recognition of the P waves.

---

*As in the case of non-paroxysmal junctional tachycardia (page 441) the use of the term "tachycardia" in relation to rates in the range 60 to 100 beats/min is permitted by general consent since these rates are clearly in excess of the normal idioventricular escape rates.

Relationship of P waves to QRS complexes

As indicated above, during ventricular tachycardia, there is typically no relationship between the QRS complexes and the P waves. This phenomenon of independence of P waves and QRS complexes is called **atrio-ventricular dissociation.*** In most cases of ventricular tachycardia the atrial mechanism is of sinus origin. Since the ventricular stroke output during ventricular tachycardia is less than in sinus rhythm, there tends to be a reflex sympathetic drive to the sino-atrial node and the sinus rate tends to be a little higher than it would be otherwise (Figure 308). If, for any reason, there is profound vagal activity then the sinus rate may, of course, be unduly slow. Sometimes during ventricular tachycardia depolarisation travels backwards from the ventricles, through the His bundle and AV node producing retrograde depolarisation of the atrial myocardium. It used to be thought that retrograde (ventriculo-atrial) conduction was very rare during ventricular tachycardia and that the recognition of a consistent relationship between P waves and QRS complexes (atrio-ventricular association) proved that a tachycardia was of supraventricular origin. Unfortunately, however, the occurrence of ventriculo-atrial conduction is not rare, and this fact has rendered more difficult the distinction between ventricular tachycardia and supraventricular tachycardia with aberration. In the supraventricular group of rhythms the relationship between the P waves (if visible) and the QRS complexes is constant (in ventricular tachycardia it will be variable if there is no ventriculo-atrial conduction but constant if ventriculo-atrial conduction does occur).

If the P waves are of sinus origin they will have the morphology which is usual for that patient. If the P wave occurs as a result of ventriculo-atrial activation it will be inverted. In either case, however, it will be unusual to be able to see much of the P wave morphology because of the dominance of the S-T segment and the T waves.

*Atrio-ventricular dissociation actually occurs in two situations:
1. in association with ventricular tachydysrhythmias when the ventricular depolarisation occurs without any prior depolarisation reaching the ventricle through the normal conducting pathways and when the ventricular rate is more rapid than the atrial rate but when there is no ventriculo-atrial (retrograde) spread of the depolarisation, and
2. in complete heart block when the activation wave fails to conduct through the normal atrio-ventricular conduction pathway and a ventricular escape rhythm occurs. In this situation the atrial rate exceeds the ventricular rate.

Onset and offset of ventricular tachycardia

Strictly speaking, there are two quite distinct electrocardiographic appearances (with very different clinical implications) which come under the heading of ventricular tachycardia. These two rhythms are known as **paroxysmal ventricular tachycardia** and **accelerated idioventricular rhythm.**

When the term "ventricular tachycardia" is used without qualification it is held to imply the paroxysmal, re-entrant variety.*

Paroxysmal ventricular tachycardia usually begins with a premature ventricular beat. This may be of the R-on-T type or may be a less premature ectopic.

In either event the onset is usually sudden and the peak rate of the tachycardia is achieved instantaneously since the arrhythmia results from the establishment of a re-entrant circuit. An example is shown in Figure 304.

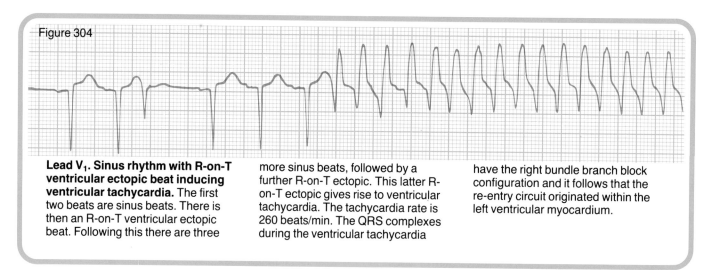

Figure 304

Lead V₁. Sinus rhythm with R-on-T ventricular ectopic beat inducing ventricular tachycardia. The first two beats are sinus beats. There is then an R-on-T ventricular ectopic beat. Following this there are three more sinus beats, followed by a further R-on-T ectopic. This latter R-on-T ectopic gives rise to ventricular tachycardia. The tachycardia rate is 260 beats/min. The QRS complexes during the ventricular tachycardia have the right bundle branch block configuration and it follows that the re-entry circuit originated within the left ventricular myocardium.

Just as a ventricular premature beat may initiate ventricular tachycardia by setting up a re-entrant circuit (in the same way as an atrial premature beat may initiate a supraventricular re-entrant tachycardia within the AV node or within the AV node and anomalous tract in the Wolff-Parkinson-White syndrome) so a ventricular premature beat, which, by chance has appropriate timing may stop a sustained ventricular tachycardia by inducing refractoriness in the re-entrant circuit just ahead of the oncoming depolarisation waveform, thereby breaking the re-entrant mechanism.

*The most important difference between paroxysmal ventricular tachycardia and accelerated idioventricular rhythm is the ventricular rate (typically 150-250 beats/min for the former and 60-130 beats/min for the latter). It is possible that some cases of paroxysmal ventricular tachycardia arise on the basis of mechanisms other than re-entry but this is uncertain.

**Accelerated Idioventricular Rhythm
(Slow Ventricular Tachycardia).**

This is not a re-entrant arrhythmia but occurs on the basis of enhanced automaticity. The tachycardia rate is much slower than in the paroxysmal variety and the tachycardia builds up slowly (Figure 305).

Figure 305   **Idioventricular rhythms**

(a) Mechanism of ventricular escape rhythm

The idioventricular pacemaker is normally suppressed by the SA node because of the higher rate of the latter (Figure 188, page 350). If the SA nodal discharge rate falls below the idioventricular rate the latter may "escape" from suppression by the SA node and give rise either to a single ventricular* escape beat or to sustained idioventricular rhythm (depending how long the reduction in the SA rate persists).

(b) Mechanism of accelerated idioventricular rhythm

The idioventricular pacemaker is normally suppressed by the SA node because of the higher rate of the latter (Figure 188, page 350). If the idioventricular rate increases to exceed the prevailing sinus rate the idioventricular pacemaker may become dominant either for a single ventricular premature beat or for sustained idioventricular rhythm.

(c) Ventricular escape rhythm

This is frequently transient and repetitive because the SA nodal rate may fluctuate.

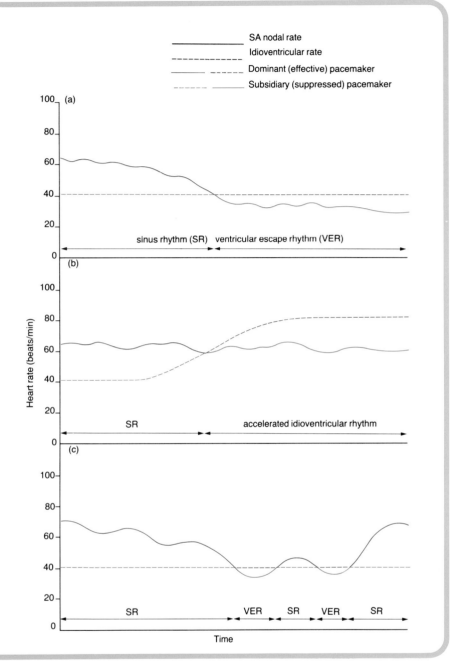

An example of ventricular escape rhythm consequent upon progressive slowing of the sinus rate (as in Figure 305a) is shown in Figure 306. An example of accelerated idioventricular rhythm (as in Figure 305b) is shown in Figure 307.

*More commonly, of course, the escape rhythm would be junctional (AV nodal). Failure of the AV node to provide the escape mechanism suggests that its intrinsic rate too is depressed.

464

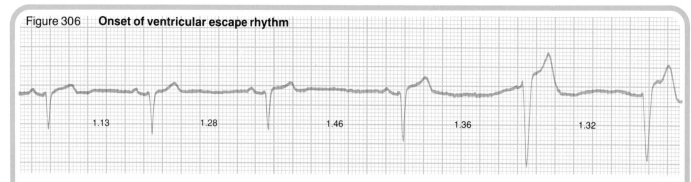

Figure 306   **Onset of ventricular escape rhythm**

1.13   1.28   1.46   1.36   1.32

Lead V₁. Onset of ventricular escape rhythm (the R-R intervals (in sec) are shown). The rhythm in this strip follows the pattern shown in Figure 305. The first three beats show sinus rhythm. The R-R intervals are lengthening (the sinus rate is progressively slowing). A ventricular escape rhythm appears in relation to

beats 4, 5 and 6. Beat 4 is a fusion beat in which the ventricles are predominantly depolarised as a result of the sinus-initiated beat but it is clear that the S wave is slightly deeper than in beats 1 to 3 owing to the influence of the ventricular escape beat with which the sinus beat is fused. Beats 5 and 6 are ventricular escape rhythm.

As is often the case, the R-R interval of **established** escape rhythm is less than that of the beat which **initiates** the escape rhythm. Thus interval 5-6 (which is representative of the intervals which continued over several minutes (not shown)) is less than that of interval 4-5.

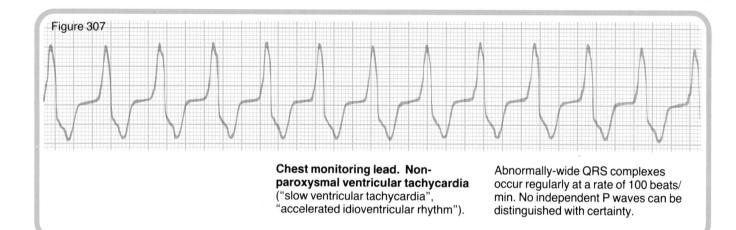

Figure 307

Chest monitoring lead. Non-paroxysmal ventricular tachycardia ("slow ventricular tachycardia", "accelerated idioventricular rhythm").

Abnormally-wide QRS complexes occur regularly at a rate of 100 beats/min. No independent P waves can be distinguished with certainty.

It is useful to compare Figures 304 and 324. Both show repetitive firing from an ectopic ventricular site. Figure 304 shows an example of paroxysmal ventricular tachycardia and Figure 324 shows an example of slow ventricular tachycardia. The former occurs on a re-entrant basis and the latter as a result of enhanced automaticity.

Paroxysmal Ventricular Tachycardia

Figure 308 shows an example of paroxysmal ventricular tachycardia. The QRS complexes are abnormally wide and the rate is 170 beats/min. P waves can be identified and are seen to be independent of the QRS complexes

(there is atrio-ventricular dissociation) and the rhythm is therefore clearly ventricular and not supraventricular with aberration (functional bundle branch block) or supraventricular with organic bundle branch block.

Figure 309 shows the termination of the ventricular tachycardia in the subject whose electrocardiogram was shown in Figure 308. The tachycardia in this case was terminated following the administration of lignocaine intravenously. Sinus rhythm is restored.

The sinus rate falls gradually as the reflex sympathetic drive falls. During the ventricular tachycardia independent P waves can be seen at 8, 7 (on top of the T wave), 6, 5, 4 (on top of the T wave) and 3 and are predictably observed at 9.

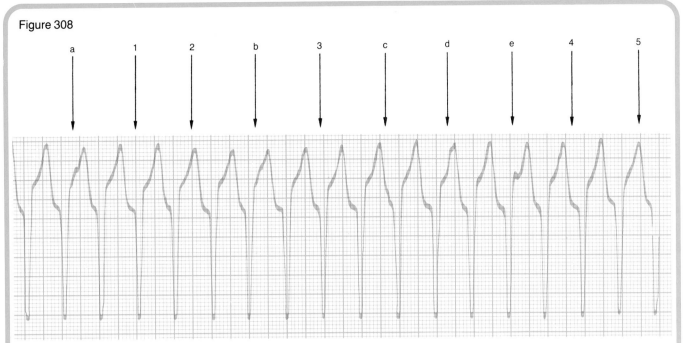

Figure 308

Chest monitoring lead. Ventricular tachycardia. The ventricular rate is rapid (170 beats/min) and regular. The QRS complexes are wide (0.11 sec). The rhythm could therefore be ventricular tachycardia or supraventricular tachycardia with aberrant intraventricular conduction ("functional", "rate-related" or "tachycardia-dependent" bundle branch block). Close inspection reveals perturbations on the waveform at a, b, c, d and e.

The perturbations are consistent with there being P waves superimposed on the ventricular waveform. If the rhythm were ventricular tachycardia one might well expect to find an independent sinus mechanism (since depolarisation frequently does not travel backwards through the AV node) and one would expect a modest increase in the sinus rate (a reflex response as a result of a reduced stroke volume coincident with the onset of ventricular tachycardia).

The P wave deflections at d and e are separated by a distance consistent with the expected cycle time of the sinus node and extrapolation to the left and right of this shows a consistent pattern with P wave perturbations visible at a, b, c, d and e and predictably obscured at 1, 2, 3, 4 and 5. The time interval between consecutive arrows is not quite constant implying slight variation in the sinus rate. This is not unusual.

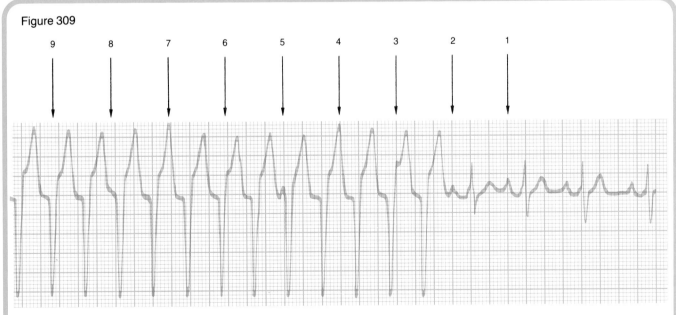

Figure 309

Chest monitoring lead. Ventricular tachycardia converted to sinus rhythm with intravenous lignocaine. Following the restoration of sinus rhythm the cardiac stroke volume will have improved and there will be therefore less sympathetic

drive. As a result of this the sinus rate falls slowly. The sinus interval 2-1 will be the one most closely related to that obtaining during the ventricular tachycardia and this interval can be extrapolated backwards from 1-9 to demonstrate the location of the P

waves. In this way independent P waves can actually be seen at 8, 7, 6, 5 and 3, P waves can be seen to be superimposed on the T waves at 7 and 4, and it can be seen that the P wave anticipated at 9 would be obscured by the QRS complex.

466

Figure 310a shows a further
example of ventricular tachycardia.
In this case the P waves are not
readily discernible.

Figure 310

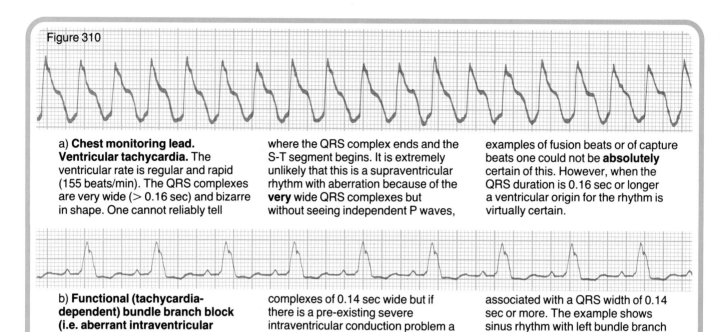

a) **Chest monitoring lead.
Ventricular tachycardia.** The
ventricular rate is regular and rapid
(155 beats/min). The QRS complexes
are very wide (> 0.16 sec) and bizarre
in shape. One cannot reliably tell
where the QRS complex ends and the
S-T segment begins. It is extremely
unlikely that this is a supraventricular
rhythm with aberration because of the
very wide QRS complexes but
without seeing independent P waves,
examples of fusion beats or of capture
beats one could not be **absolutely**
certain of this. However, when the
QRS duration is 0.16 sec or longer
a ventricular origin for the rhythm is
virtually certain.

b) **Functional (tachycardia-
dependent) bundle branch block
(i.e. aberrant intraventricular
conduction)** never produces QRS
complexes of 0.14 sec wide but if
there is a pre-existing severe
intraventricular conduction problem a
supraventricular rhythm may be
associated with a QRS width of 0.14
sec or more. The example shows
sinus rhythm with left bundle branch
block and a QRS duration of 0.20 sec.

Figure 311 shows the effect of DC
shock in the subject whose rhythm was
shown in Figure 310a. The resultant
rhythm is atrial fibrillation. Possibly this
was the atrial depolarisation mechanism
which obtained during the ventricular
tachycardia.

Figure 311

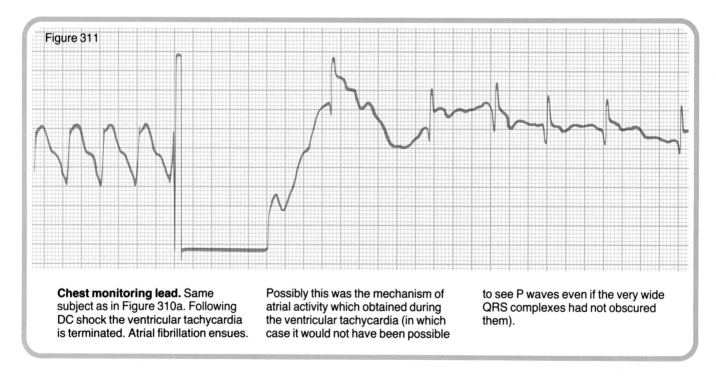

Chest monitoring lead. Same
subject as in Figure 310a. Following
DC shock the ventricular tachycardia
is terminated. Atrial fibrillation ensues.
Possibly this was the mechanism of
atrial activity which obtained during
the ventricular tachycardia (in which
case it would not have been possible
to see P waves even if the very wide
QRS complexes had not obscured
them).

Figure 312 shows a short burst of
ventricular tachycardia.

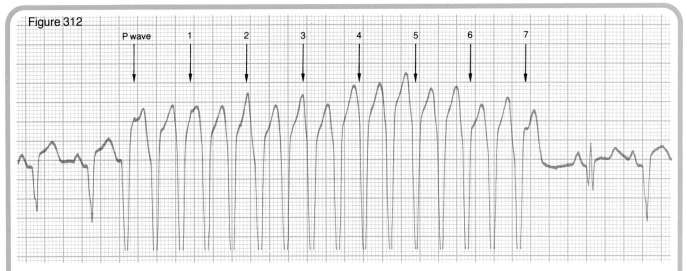

Figure 312

Chest monitoring lead. Burst of ventricular tachycardia. The first two beats are sinus beats. There then follows a run of abnormally-wide, abnormally-shaped QRS complexes (with minimal variation in the QRS morphology). Sinus rhythm returns spontaneously but the first sinus beat is conducted abnormally through the ventricles (possibly aberration or a fusion beat). The only P wave recognisable with confidence during the ventricular tachycardia is the first one to occur after the onset of the arrhythmia (arrowed) and it occurs at the same interval after the second P wave as the time interval between the first two P waves. If the anticipated timing of these first three P waves (two during sinus rhythm and one within the tachycardia) is extrapolated to the right (as in Figure 230) P waves can just be recognised at 1, 2 (on top of T), 3 (on top of T) and 7, and are predictably obscured at 4, 5 and 6.

When there is (as there usually is) failure of retrograde conduction via the AV node to the atria, and when there is continuation of sinus activation of the atria, the demonstration of atrio-ventricular dissociation (with a ventricular rate faster than the atrial rate) in association with a rapid, regular and abnormally-shaped and wide QRS complex proves that the rhythm is ventricular. However, when there is retrograde conduction to the atria the problem is not so clear. Figure 313 shows an example.

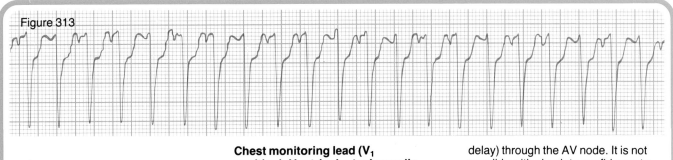

Figure 313

Chest monitoring lead (V₁ position). Ventricular tachycardia. The ventricular rate is regular at 190 beats/min and the QRS complexes are abnormally wide. Regular inverted P waves are seen occurring late after each QRS complex, probably indicating retrograde conduction (with delay) through the AV node. It is not possible with absolute confidence to be sure that this is not a supraventricular tachycardia with aberrant intraventricular conduction, but the probability is that it is ventricular tachycardia with retrograde conduction to the atria.

An example of repetitive, self-
limiting bursts of ventricular tachycardia
is shown in Figure 314.

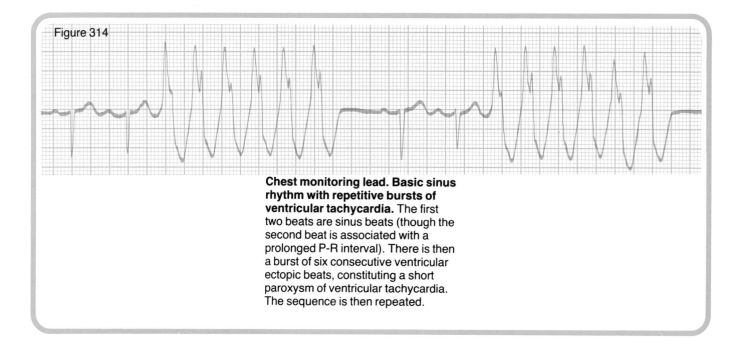

Figure 314

Chest monitoring lead. Basic sinus rhythm with repetitive bursts of ventricular tachycardia. The first two beats are sinus beats (though the second beat is associated with a prolonged P-R interval). There is then a burst of six consecutive ventricular ectopic beats, constituting a short paroxysm of ventricular tachycardia. The sequence is then repeated.

Criteria for ventricular tachycardia

ESSENTIAL CRITERIA (ALWAYS PRESENT):

1. **The QRS rate is 140-250 beats/min.**

2. **The QRS rate is regular or almost regular.***

3. **The QRS configuration is constant.****

4. **The QRS configuration is different from that which is usual for the subject and the lead when the rhythm is supraventricular.**†°

5. **The QRS axis is different from that which is usual for the subject when the rhythm is supraventricular.**††

6. **The QRS complexes are abnormally wide** (0.12 sec or more).[1]

CRITERIA NOT ALWAYS PRESENT BUT DIAGNOSTIC WHEN FOUND:

7. Atrio-ventricular dissociation is commonly[2] found in ventricular tachycardia and when present indicates a ventricular origin for the ectopic focus.

8. In the presence of atrio-ventricular dissociation if (as is usually but not always the case[3]) the atrial rhythm is sinus, occasional capture beats occur. This proves the ventricular origin of the main rhythm.

9. In the presence of atrio-ventricular dissociation if (as is usually but not always the case[3]) the atrial rhythm is sinus, occasional partial capture beats (i.e. fusion beats) may occur proving the ventricular origin of the main rhythm.

10. If the ventricular rate is consistently higher than the atrial rate (within the time window of observation) the rhythm is ventricular.

Criteria for accelerated idioventricular rhythm

1. The QRS rate is within the range 60-130 beats/min.

2. The QRS rate is regular or almost regular.*

3. The QRS configuration is constant.**

4. The QRS configuration is different from that which is usual for the subject and the lead when the rhythm is supraventricular.†

5. The QRS axis is different from that which is usual for the subject when the rhythm is supraventricular.††

6. The QRS complexes are abnormally wide (0.12 sec or more).

7. Sino-atrial activity is depressed (P waves usually absent, but occasionally seen occurring at a slower rate than the QRS complexes).

---

*Contrary to the frequently stated view, the QRS complexes in ventricular tachycardia are usually precisely regular. Minor irregularity with variations in R-R intervals of up to 0.04 sec can occur.

**In the presence of atrio-ventricular dissociation (which usually accompanies ventricular tachycardia) it may appear that there is intermittent slight variation in the configuration of the QRS complexes. This can occur because of the varying position of superimposed P waves distorting the QRS configuration.

° The one form of ventricular tachycardia associated with near-normal QRS morphology is fascicular tachycardia in which the ectopic focus is in or close to the His bundle.

† As with ventricular ectopic beats, so with ventricular tachycardia, the morphology of the QRS complexes is dependent on the origin of the ectopic impulse. Ventricular tachycardia arising in the **left** ventricular myocardium gives rise to QRS complexes resembling those in **right** bundle branch block and ventricular tachycardia arising in the right ventricular myocardium gives rise to QRS complexes resembling those in **left** bundle branch block.

†† The axis shift may be slight or may be dramatic. Whenever the axis is grossly abnormal (e.g. in the range −60° to −180° (travelling anti-clockwise from −60° to −180°)) a ventricular origin for the rhythm is highly likely.

[1] The wider the QRS complexes the more likely it is that the tachycardia is ventricular in origin. Pre-excitation, bundle branch block or aberrant intraventricular conduction may result in QRS complexes with a duration in the range of 0.12 to 0.14 sec but when the QRS is 0.16 sec or longer in duration a ventricular origin for the tachycardia is virtually certain. (An exception is shown in Figure 310b).

[2] Occasionally the retrograde activation of the atria occurs in association with each QRS in ventricular tachycardia (see Figure 312) in which case it may be impossible to distinguish the rhythm from supraventricular tachycardia with aberrant intraventricular conduction. Sometimes every alternate QRS will be followed by retrograde conduction to the atria. In this case the ventricular origin is certain (since there are two QRS complexes to each P wave and this can only happen with a ventricular origin rhythm). In both cases (i.e. when there is 1:1 or 2:1 ventriculo-atrial conduction) the atria would be activated retrogradely and the P waves would have reversed (compared with the usual) polarity in every lead.

[3] There is no reason why, during ventricular tachycardia, the atrial rhythm should not be any of the possible ones (sinus rhythm, sinus tachycardia, sinus bradycardia, sinus arrhythmia, atrial tachycardia, atrial flutter, atrial fibrillation etc), however, in most cases the atrial rhythm will be sinus.

Torsade de pointes (Polymorphic Ventricular Tachycardia)

An unusual, polymorphic form of ventricular tachycardia is sometimes known as "torsade de pointes".*
An example is shown in Figure 315. The rhythm looks like a ventricular tachycardia in that there are rapid, almost regular, abnormally-wide and abnormally-shaped QRS complexes but the difference in appearance from the usual one for ventricular tachycardia is that the form of the QRS complexes changes. There is a rhythmic shifting of the cardiac axis so that the QRS complexes appear tall for a few beats and then shorter. The name "torsade de pointes" means "twisting of the points". The arrhythmia is frequently self-limiting and repeats for 5-10 sec at a time.
It usually arises on the background of a prolonged Q-T interval and may be **induced** by anti-arrhythmic drugs.

Figure 315

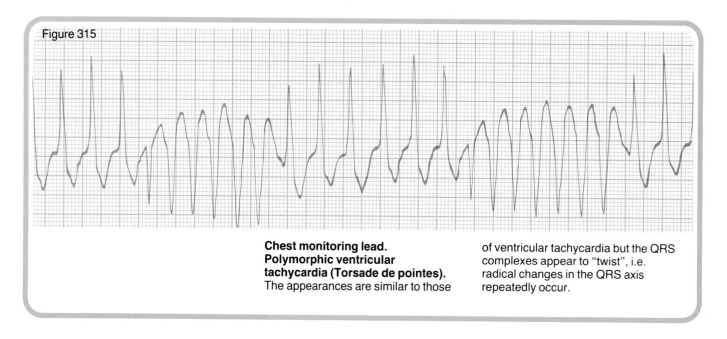

Chest monitoring lead. Polymorphic ventricular tachycardia (Torsade de pointes). The appearances are similar to those of ventricular tachycardia but the QRS complexes appear to "twist", i.e. radical changes in the QRS axis repeatedly occur.

Criteria for Torsade de pointes

1. The QRS rate is rapid (typically between 200-250 beats/min).

2. The amplitude of the QRS complexes within the given lead frequently changes in a sinusoidal fashion.

3. The ventricular tachydysrhythmia may be self-limiting but repetitive with cycle times for the periods of the arrhythmia and for the periods of normality of several seconds.

Feature commonly found in between the episodes of Torsade de pointes.

1. Prolongation of the Q-T interval.

* French. Torsader = to twist. Torsade = a twisted fringe. Pointe = a point.

Fascicular Tachycardia

This is a relatively uncommon form of tachycardia in which the ectopic site is in or close to the His bundle. Ventricular activation therefore follows near-normal pathways but in the majority of cases the onset of fascicular tachycardia is accompanied by the development of right bundle branch block and left anterior hemiblock, thus the QRS complexes are often abnormally wide and abnormally shaped but are not bizarre (as in ventricular tachycardia) and have the typical RBBB plus LAH configurations (pages 139 and 140). As far as the QRS complexes are concerned, therefore, the appearances are those of a supraventricular tachycardia. The ventricular origin of the tachycardia can only be determined from the surface ECG if one or more of the following features can be recognised: (i) fusion beats, (ii) capture beats, (iii) atrio-ventricular dissociation, (iv) ventricular rate greater than atrial rate.

Ventricular Flutter

This is an extremely severe, usually pre-fatal arrhythmia which resembles ventricular tachycardia in that there are abnormally-shaped, abnormally-wide QRS complexes with a rate in the region of 180-250 beats/min. It differs in appearance from ventricular tachycardia in that the QRS waveform is more amorphous and is virtually unchanged when viewed upside down. The QRS complexes are very bizarre and it is impossible to tell when the QRS ends and the S-T segments or T waves begin. An example is shown in Figure 316.

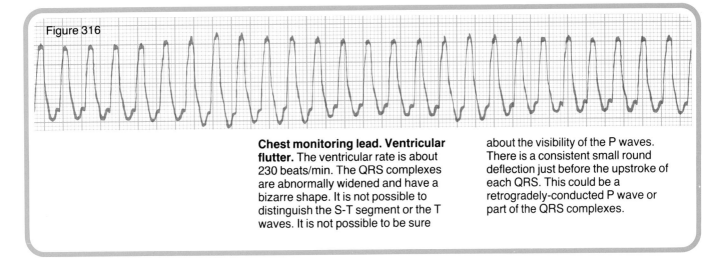

Figure 316

Chest monitoring lead. Ventricular flutter. The ventricular rate is about 230 beats/min. The QRS complexes are abnormally widened and have a bizarre shape. It is not possible to distinguish the S-T segment or the T waves. It is not possible to be sure about the visibility of the P waves. There is a consistent small round deflection just before the upstroke of each QRS. This could be a retrogradely-conducted P wave or part of the QRS complexes.

Another example of ventricular flutter is seen in Figure 317. This example is unusual in that it looks as though there is retrograde activation of the atria, with constant, inverted P waves after each QRS complex. Although such retrograde conduction is uncommon the record is, in all other respects, typical of ventricular flutter.

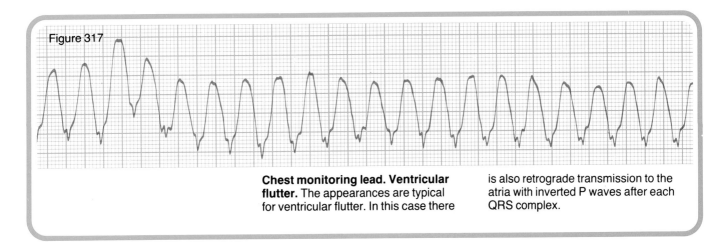

Figure 317

Chest monitoring lead. Ventricular flutter. The appearances are typical for ventricular flutter. In this case there is also retrograde transmission to the atria with inverted P waves after each QRS complex.

Criteria for ventricular flutter

1. The QRS rate is rapid (180-250 beats/min).

2. The QRS rate is regular.

3. The QRS configuration is constant.

4. The QRS configuration is different from that which is usual for the subject and the lead when the rhythm is supraventricular.

5. The QRS complexes are virtually symmetrical.*

6. The QRS axis is different from that which is usual for the subject when the rhythm is supraventricular.

7. The QRS complexes are abnormally wide (>0.12 sec).

8. The atrial activity is usually obscured by the QRS complexes but may be present and independent of the QRS complexes or may bear a consistent relationship to the QRS complexes, being retrogradely conducted and following the QRS.**

* Appear similar if turned upside down.
** Figure 317.

Ventricular Fibrillation

This rhythm represents the terminal stage in the breakdown of an "organised sequence of depolarisation of the myocardium" (the definition of the cardiac rhythm, page 337). During ventricular fibrillation small areas of ventricular myocardium depolarise randomly without any co-ordination with neighbouring areas. The resulting electrocardiogram is extremely erratic. When large groups of fibres happen to depolarise simultaneously a large deflection resembling a ventricular ectopic beat may occur, but at other times the amplitude of the ECG may be extremely small. The appearances of the QRS complexes in ventricular fibrillation are very similar to those of the P waves in atrial fibrillation except that they are much larger. No S-T segment or T waves are recognisable. Two examples are shown in Figure 318.

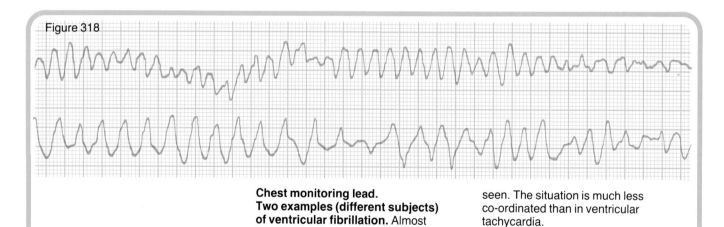

Figure 318

Chest monitoring lead. Two examples (different subjects) of ventricular fibrillation. Almost totally chaotic electrical activity is seen. The situation is much less co-ordinated than in ventricular tachycardia.

Figure 319 shows a most unusual record. It is a complete 12-lead recording of ventricular fibrillation and no malpractice suit followed! The patient was already connected to the automatic, 3-channel, 12-lead recorder when ventricular fibrillation developed. The technician pressed the auto-record button immediately before resuscitative measures were instituted. The patient recovered and left hospital with no detectable neurological deficit (It is not recommended that 12-lead records should be obtained once ventricular fibrillation has been diagnosed!).

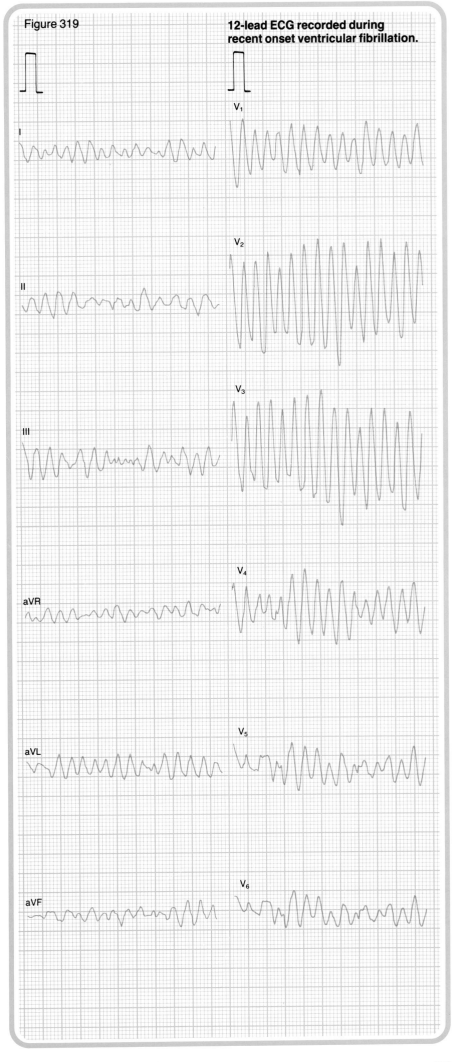

Figure 319

12-lead ECG recorded during
recent onset ventricular fibrillation.

474

During the process of dying from heart disease the rhythm may alternate between ventricular fibrillation and ventricular asystole (the atria may also be asystolic or may depolarise normally).

Ventricular fibrillation and asystole are indistinguishable clinically. Each is associated with complete cessation of cardiac output. The rhythm may alternate for hours after clinical death (Figure 320).

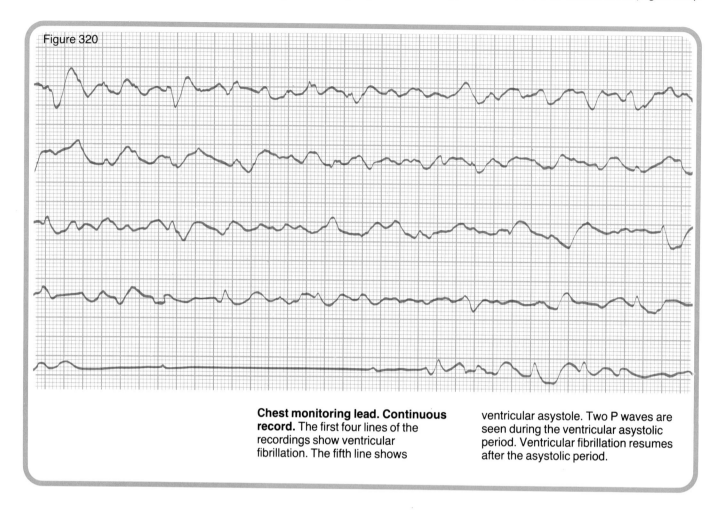

Figure 320

Chest monitoring lead. Continuous record. The first four lines of the recordings show ventricular fibrillation. The fifth line shows ventricular asystole. Two P waves are seen during the ventricular asystolic period. Ventricular fibrillation resumes after the asystolic period.

Criteria for ventricular fibrillation

1. The "QRS" morphology is continuously variable and unpredictable (in amplitude, duration and frequency). No true QRS complexes can be identified.

2. Atrial activity may be present or absent but even if present it is almost completely obscured by the QRS complexes.

Ventricular Asystole

This term is self-explanatory: there is no ventricular depolarisation for an inappropriately long period. If no QRS complexes are visible at all the ECG is either a straight line or a straight line interrupted by P waves (Figures 321a and 321b).

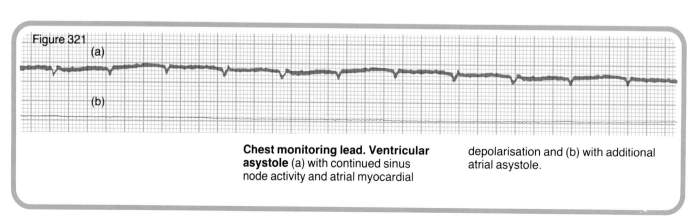

Figure 321
(a)
(b)

Chest monitoring lead. Ventricular asystole (a) with continued sinus node activity and atrial myocardial depolarisation and (b) with additional atrial asystole.

475

"Ventricular asystole" can also be present for an inappropriately long period even though some ventricular activity is apparent, as shown in Figure 322. It is likely that clinical death has already occurred in the situation.

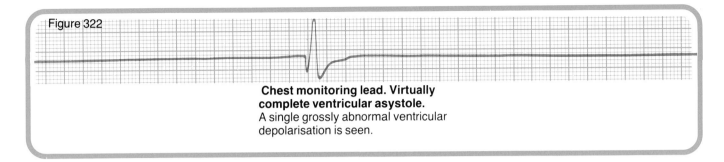

Figure 322

Chest monitoring lead. Virtually complete ventricular asystole. A single grossly abnormal ventricular depolarisation is seen.

The inappropriately long* ventricular asystole, seen in Figure 322, indicates extensive left ventricular damage as demonstrated by the single grossly abnormal and very wide QRS complex. Inappropriately long ventricular asystole can also occur in the presence of extensive disease confined to the conducting tissue without any involvement of the contractile myocardium. Such a situation commonly occurs in the "sick sinus syndrome" (the "brady-tachy syndrome") in which disease of the sino-atrial node leads to intermittent prolonged sinus node and atrial myocardial asystole and when, as sometimes, but not always happens, similar malfunction is present in the AV node, His bundle or Purkinje tissue (Figure 323).

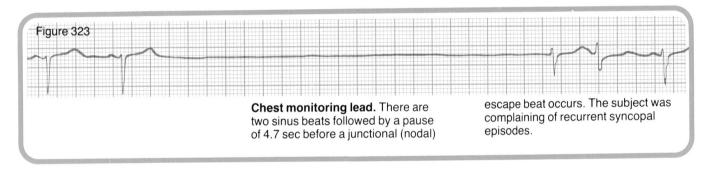

Figure 323

Chest monitoring lead. There are two sinus beats followed by a pause of 4.7 sec before a junctional (nodal) escape beat occurs. The subject was complaining of recurrent syncopal episodes.

Fusion Beats

A **fusion beat** is a beat in which the depolarisation of the ventricle (or of the atria) is induced simultaneously from two separate sites. In either case (atrial fusion beats or ventricular fusion beats), a second activation waveform initiates depolarisation of part of the myocardium (of atria or of ventricles) before an antecedent depolarisation (in atria or ventricles) has completed its spread. Thus with atrial fusion beats the atria are activated from two different sites and with ventricular fusion beats the ventricles are activated from two different sites. In each case the contours of the fusion waveform are intermediate in shape between the two independent waves which have fused, though the later the second wave occurs after the onset of the activation by the first wave the closer the appearances of the wave (P or QRS) will lie to the morphology associated with the first wavefront. Since P waves are relatively amorphous it is quite difficult to demonstrate fusion (except with atrial pacemakers) but it is rather easier in the case of QRS complexes. One of the most common situations for fusion beats to be seen is during ventricular pacing when the ventricle may be depolarised both spontaneously and simultaneously from the pacemaker. The QRS morphology then has a shape intermediate between that typical for a ventricular pacing beat and that typical for ventricular ectopics (see Figure 369, page 520). Figure 324 shows an example of ventricular fusion beats. **When occasional fusion beats occur during a period of wide QRS complex tachycardia, it is very likely that the tachycardia is ventricular in origin since it is more likely that a supraventricular beat will be conducted to the ventricles at the same time as the spontaneous QRS complex occurs from the ventricular tachycardia than that a separate ectopic ventricular focus could depolarise during sustained ventricular tachycardia** (see Figure 325).

* Technically this is a necessary part of the definitions since even during sinus rhythm the ventricle is **normally** asystolic (this period of asystole is called "diastole!) between the end of the T wave and the beginning of the next QRS, and this period can, of course, be quite long in association with profound bradycardias.

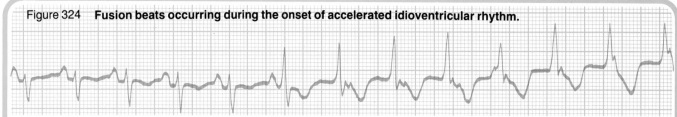

Figure 324 Fusion beats occurring during the onset of accelerated idioventricular rhythm.

The basic rhythm is sinus and the first five beats are straightforward sinus beats. Then an accelerated idio-ventricular rhythm (slow ventricular tachycardia) becomes apparent and there is progressive change in the waveform of the QRS complexes as an increasing proportion of each succeeding QRS complex occurs as a result of the idioventricular depolarisation. Initially (to the left of the trace) ventricular depolarisation occurs via the normal route, in the mid-portion the QRS complexes are fusion beats and ultimately the QRS complexes are totally those of the idioventricular pacemaker. (Compare Figure 305b).

Capture Beats

A "capture beat" is a conducted beat occurring at a time when the rhythm immediately preceding the beat in question shows AV dissociation. Atrio-ventricular dissociation means that the atria and ventricles are depolarising independently. Atrio-ventricular dissociation occurs in complete heart block (when the P wave rate is higher than the ventricular rate) and in ventricular tachycardia (when the QRS rate is greater than the P wave rate). **The recognition of occasional** capture beats during a period of wide QRS complex tachycardia powerfully points towards a ventricular origin for the tachycardia since their presence implies that the AV junctional area is not refractory and is able to conduct to the ventricles (if the wide QRS complex tachycardia were due to supraventricular tachycardia with functional or pre-existing bundle branch block, the AV junction would be refractory between adjacent conducted beats). Figure 325 shows an example.

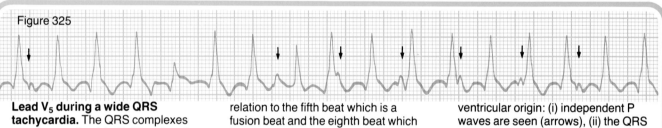

Figure 325

Lead V$_5$ during a wide QRS tachycardia. The QRS complexes are abnormally wide (0.16 sec) and occur at an abnormal rate (142/min). The QRS rate is regular except in relation to the fifth beat which is a fusion beat and the eighth beat which is a capture beat. The record has many features which clearly point to a wide QRS complex tachycardia of ventricular origin: (i) independent P waves are seen (arrows), (ii) the QRS width is appreciably increased (0.16 sec), (iii) a capture beat is seen, (iv) a fusion beat is seen.

Escape Mechanisms

The majority of the ectopic rhythms discussed so far have been "active" rhythms in which depolarisation at the ectopic site occurs prematurely. Escape rhythms, on the other hand, represent the late depolarisation of latent pacemakers consequent upon the failure of the normal "higher" pacemaker to suppress the ectopic pacemaker site. As explained on page 353 escape depolarisation occurs when the rate of the higher pacemaker falls. In general there is a "hierarchy" of instrinsic rates for given pacemaker sites and in descending order of intrinsic rate with hierarchy it reads as follows:

Sino-atrial node
(atrial myocardium)

Atrio-ventricular node
↓ } junctional area
His bundle

Bundle branches
Purkinje network } ventricular area
ventricular myocardium

Any pacemaker subsidiary to the sinus node may give rise to an escape beat (a single beat like a single premature beat) or an escape rhythm (a sustained rhythm). Thus atrial, junctional and ventricular escape rhythms may occur. An escape beat or the individual beats of an escape rhythm will have the morphological characteristics associated with an ectopic beat or an ectopic rhythm from the same site (escape beats are ectopic but not premature).

Escape Beats

Isolated or occasional escape beats tend to occur whenever the sinus rate falls sufficiently and their presence merely manifests the "stand-by" role of the subsidiary pacemaker site (see pages 353, 387, 389 and 393 and Figures 191, 226, 229 and 233).

It is inevitable that the commonest escape beats to be seen will be junctional escape beats since the pacemakers in the junctional area have the second fastest intrinsic discharge rate (after the sino-atrial node) and "lower" pacemakers will only give escape beats if the AV nodal pacemaker is depressed as well as the sino-atrial pacemaker. Figure 326 shows an example of junctional escape beats and Figure 327 of ventricular escape beats.

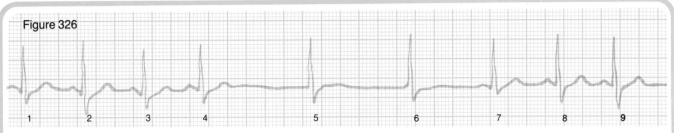

Figure 326

Ambulatory recording. Chest monitoring lead. Junctional escape beats. The first four beats show sinus rhythm. Sino-atrial function then appears depressed.

Beat 5 is a junctional escape beat. It is exactly like a junctional premature beat except that it is not premature. Junctional escape beats and junctional premature beats are equally ectopic. Beat 6 is a further junctional escape beat. Subsequently sinus rhythm returns.

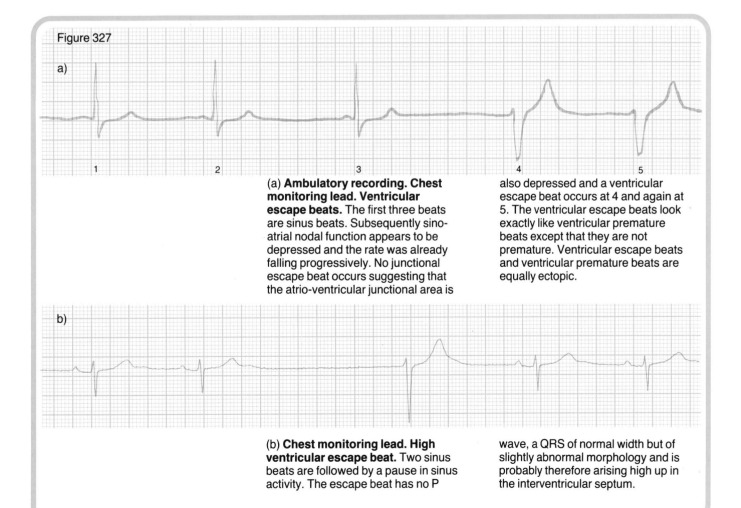

Figure 327

a)

(a) **Ambulatory recording. Chest monitoring lead. Ventricular escape beats.** The first three beats are sinus beats. Subsequently sino-atrial nodal function appears to be depressed and the rate was already falling progressively. No junctional escape beat occurs suggesting that the atrio-ventricular junctional area is also depressed and a ventricular escape beat occurs at 4 and again at 5. The ventricular escape beats look exactly like ventricular premature beats except that they are not premature. Ventricular escape beats and ventricular premature beats are equally ectopic.

b)

(b) **Chest monitoring lead. High ventricular escape beat.** Two sinus beats are followed by a pause in sinus activity. The escape beat has no P wave, a QRS of normal width but of slightly abnormal morphology and is probably therefore arising high up in the interventricular septum.

Escape Rhythms

As escape rhythm is simply a repeated escape beat. The commonest escape rhythm is junctional rhythm ("nodal" rhythm). If sino-atrial function is depressed for a period of time then, in the absence of similar depression of the atrio-ventricular nodal function, there will be a regular junctional escape rhythm.

Junctional Escape Rhythm ("Junctional Rhythm", "Nodal Rhythm")

Junctional rhythm is a regular, slow rhythm of junctional origin. The morphology of the beats in this rhythm will be exactly the same as those of a junctional premature beat (i.e.the QRS complexes, S-T segments and T waves will be of the usual form for that subject). The P wave may be absent, inverted and after the QRS, inverted and before the QRS or inverted and during the QRS complex (Figure 328).

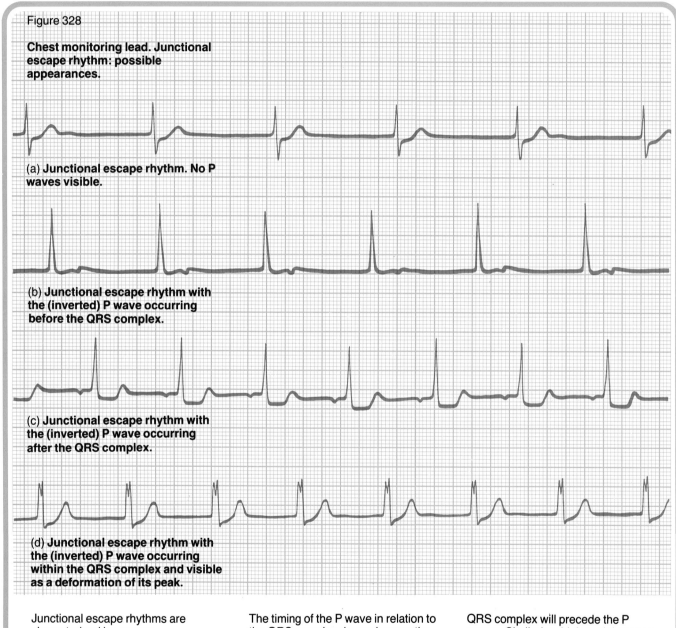

Figure 328

Chest monitoring lead. Junctional escape rhythm: possible appearances.

(a) **Junctional escape rhythm. No P waves visible.**

(b) **Junctional escape rhythm with the (inverted) P wave occurring before the QRS complex.**

(c) **Junctional escape rhythm with the (inverted) P wave occurring after the QRS complex.**

(d) **Junctional escape rhythm with the (inverted) P wave occurring within the QRS complex and visible as a deformation of its peak.**

Junctional escape rhythms are characterized by narrow (supraventricularly-originating) QRS complexes, usually occurring at a relatively slow rate and either associated with absence of P waves (failure of retrograde conduction to the atria) or with inverted P waves (atrial conduction occurs in a direction which is the reverse of normal) which can occur before, during or after the QRS complex.

The timing of the P wave in relation to the QRS complex depends upon the location of initiation of depolarisation within the AV node and upon the relative conduction velocity in antegrade and retrograde directions. Thus, for example, an impulse originating low down in the AV node is likely to reach the ventricles by antegrade conduction before it reaches the atria by retrograde conduction and in this situation the QRS complex will precede the P waves. Similarly a high-nodal escape rhythm will have P waves in front of the QRS and a mid-nodal escape rhythm may result in simultaneous P waves and QRS complexes. Whatever the site of initiation of depolarisation within the AV node there may be failure of retrograde conduction to the atria.

Criteria for junctional escape rhythms*

1. The QRS complexes have the morphology which is usual for that subject in that lead.**

2. The QRS complexes are of normal width (0.10 sec or less).**

3. The escape interval† is usually 1.5 sec or more. The escape rate† is typically 40 beats/min or less.

4. Atrial activity is either absent or is present just before, within or just after the QRS complex (as in Figure 288) but if the atrial activity is present the P waves have a polarity opposite that for sinus P waves in that given lead.

* Junctional escape rhythm is also known as "junctional rhythm" or as "nodal rhythm".

** In the presence of pre-existing intraventricular conduction abnormalities the QRS complexes may be abnormal in morphology and duration. In the presence of aberrant intraventricular conduction they may be transiently abnormal in shape and duration but aberrant intraventricular conduction is very rare in association with the slow rate with which junctional escape rhythm is usually associated.

† The term "escape interval" is used in respect of "escape beats" (see note * page 481). The term "escape rate" is used in respect of "escape rhythm" (see note * page 481).

Ventricular Escape Rhythm

The commonest situation in which ventricular escape rhythm occurs is complete heart block (page 501) when none of the atrial myocardial depolarisations are successfully transmitted to the ventricles. Occasionally, in the presence of simultaneous depression of sino-atrial nodal and atrio-ventricular nodal function there may be a ventricular escape rhythm (Figure 329).

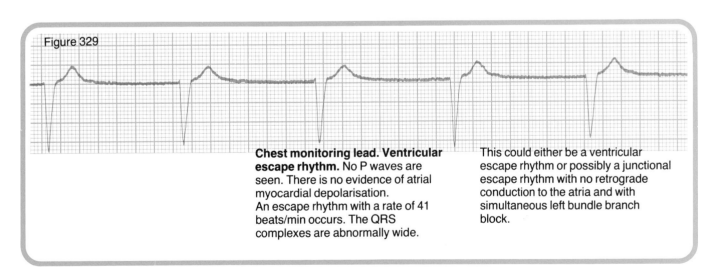

Figure 329

Chest monitoring lead. Ventricular escape rhythm. No P waves are seen. There is no evidence of atrial myocardial depolarisation. An escape rhythm with a rate of 41 beats/min occurs. The QRS complexes are abnormally wide.

This could either be a ventricular escape rhythm or possibly a junctional escape rhythm with no retrograde conduction to the atria and with simultaneous left bundle branch block.

* Where the escape mechanism is transient (Figures 326 and 327) the term "escape beat" is used. Where the escape mechanism rhythm is sustained (Figures 328 and 329), the term "escape rhythm" is used.

** The term "escape interval" is used in respect of "escape beats" (see note * above). The term "escape rate" is used in respect of "escape rhythm" (see note * above).

† e.g. Figures 229 and 327.

*** e.g. sinus arrest, sino-atrial block.

†† Transiently in second degree atrio-ventricular block or consistently in complete heart block.

Echo Beats

An echo beat (also known as a "reciprocal beat") is defined as a ventricular depolarisation initiated by a retrogradely-induced atrial depolarisation which itself followed an antegrade ventricular depolarisation. Echo beats are probably generated by a special form of re-entry mechanism and they almost always occur in association with junctional escape beats, junctional premature beats or junctional tachycardia. Occasionally they may be induced by ventricular premature beats arising high in the interventricular septum close to the junctional area. The junctional beat activates the ventricle antegradely (giving rise to a normal QRS complex), the activity travels to the atria retrogradely and arrives late (giving a late inverted P wave) and the P wave is able to re-cross the atrio-ventricular node (antegrade this time) to give rise to a further (normal) QRS. The phenomenon requires longitudinal dissociation of the AV node as discussed for atrio-ventricular nodal re-entrant tachycardia.

Thus one "side" of the AV node is considered to be refractory initially and retrograde transmission to the atria takes place through the other "side". By the time this activation wave has reached the atrial myocardium the formerly refractory side of the AV node has recovered and antegrade transmission is once more possible. An example is shown in Figure 330.

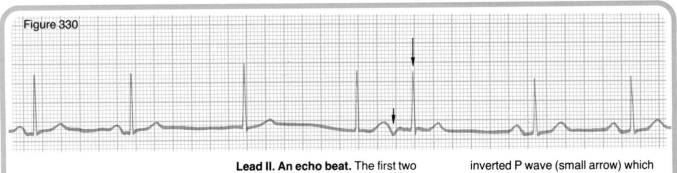

Figure 330

Lead II. An echo beat. The first two beats are sinus beats. The third and fourth beats are junctional escape beats. After the fourth beat (the second junctional beat) there is a late inverted P wave (small arrow) which triggers off a reciprocal (echo) ventricular beat (large arrow). Thereafter sinus rhythm returns.

The Sick Sinus Syndrome

Although this is a clinical rather than an electrocardiographic term, it is worthy of inclusion here in view of its relevance to escape rhythms. It refers to the combination of spontaneous (usually repetitive) depression of sino-atrial nodal activity, sometimes with similar depression of atrio-ventricular nodal activity and sometimes with sino-atrial block. There are frequently also episodes of supraventricular tachydysrhythmias (atrial tachycardia, atrial flutter, atrial fibrillation). An example of an ambulatory electrocardiographic recording in such a case is shown in Figure 331.

Figure 331

Chest lead. Ambulatory monitoring (see pages 542 to 552). The record (a) – (c) is continuous.

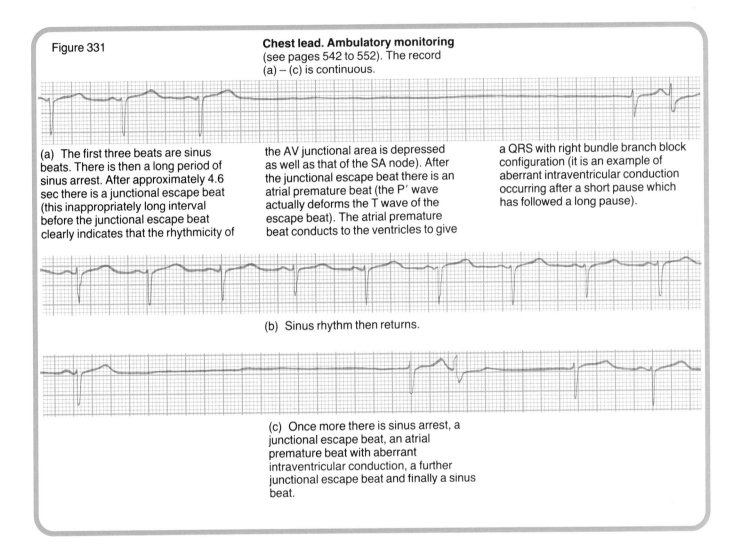

(a) The first three beats are sinus beats. There is then a long period of sinus arrest. After approximately 4.6 sec there is a junctional escape beat (this inappropriately long interval before the junctional escape beat clearly indicates that the rhythmicity of the AV junctional area is depressed as well as that of the SA node). After the junctional escape beat there is an atrial premature beat (the P′ wave actually deforms the T wave of the escape beat). The atrial premature beat conducts to the ventricles to give a QRS with right bundle branch block configuration (it is an example of aberrant intraventricular conduction occurring after a short pause which has followed a long pause).

(b) Sinus rhythm then returns.

(c) Once more there is sinus arrest, a junctional escape beat, an atrial premature beat with aberrant intraventricular conduction, a further junctional escape beat and finally a sinus beat.

Carotid Sinus Hypersensitivity

Suppression of sinus node function, sometimes with an ectopic escape rhythm, can occur in response to accidental or deliberate pressure on the carotid sinus area in those subjects who are unusually sensitive to this form of stimulation. Figure 332 shows an example of sinus node arrest during right-sided carotid sinus massage in a patient in sinus rhythm, complaining of syncopal episodes. No nodal escape beat occurs indicating that the carotid sinus massage has caused suppression of the atrio-ventricular nodal pacemaker as well as of the sino-atrial node. Sinus rhythm returns when the carotid massage ceases.

Figure 332

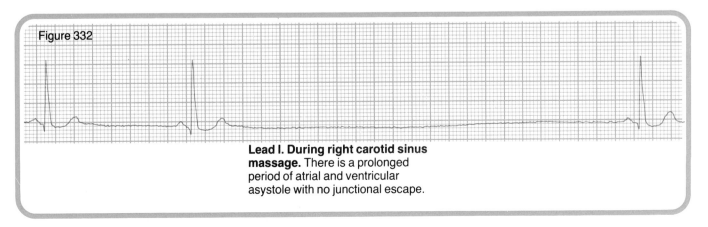

Lead I. During right carotid sinus massage. There is a prolonged period of atrial and ventricular asystole with no junctional escape.

Conduction Disturbances

The conduction disturbances form a discrete group of rhythm disturbances in which the basic fault is malfunction of one or more of the mechanisms involved in the conduction of the cardiac impulse from its site of initiation. The commonest and most important of the conduction disturbances are those involving the atrio-ventricular conducting mechanism. It will be recalled (page 385) that the atria are totally isolated electrically from the ventricles (by the fibrous atrio-ventricular ring) except for that electrical communication which depends on the atrio-ventricular node and its continuation, the His bundle. Those disturbances of conduction which are dependent upon the presence of anomalous atrio-ventricular communications (ventricular pre-excitation) are not usually included under "conduction disturbances" and defects of intraventricular conduction (right bundle branch block, left bundle branch block, left anterior hemiblock, left posterior hemiblock, diffuse intraventricular block) are usually considered as conduction disturbances, but since they are disturbances only of the **intraventricular** conduction they are not usually classified as "arrhythmias". Wenckebach type of malfunction of the **sino-atrial** node is usually classified under the same heading ("conduction disturbances") as the similar but much more common Wenckebach type of malfunction at the atrio-ventricular node. **In practical terms, the vast majority of problems of conduction relate to problems of atrio-ventricular conduction, which is often loosely referred to as "heart block".**

Heart Block

This term is used to describe an impairment of conduction (transient or permanent) at the atrio-ventricular junction. The block may occur because of impairment of function:
1. at the atrio-ventricular node
2. in the His bundle
3. in both bundle branches (simultaneously)
4. in any combination of the preceding three sites (Figure 333).

Heart block is categorised into three levels (or degrees) of disturbance – first degree heart block, second degree heart block and third degree ("complete") heart block. In **first degree heart block** each and every depolarisation of atrial myocardium reaching the atrio-ventricular node is transmitted to the ventricles and there is **one QRS complex to each P wave. In third degree ("complete") heart block** each and every supraventricular depolarisation reaching the atrio-ventricular node fails to be transmittted to the ventricular myocardium and the **QRS complexes are totally independent of the P waves. In second degree heart block** some atrial depolarisations are conducted to the ventricles and some are not, therefore **some P waves give rise to an ensuing QRS complex and some do not.** From this last definition it will be clear that a great range of possible electrocardiographic appearances can lie within the definition of second degree heart block for, strictly speaking, it could be that a single atrial depolarisation out of thousands **failed** to conduct to the ventricles or, conversely, that a single beat out of thousands **succeeded** in being conducted to the ventricles – each of these extreme possibilities would lie within the definition of second degree atrio-ventricular block. In practice this does not actually present a problem since any description given of the cardiac rhythm can refer only to that rhythm which obtained during the period of observation (i.e. during the "time window") and most electrocardiographic observations are made in respect of a relatively short time zone. Even if a long period is studied, for example during ambulatory electrocardiography, conclusions are usually made and expressed in relation to short time zones. In addition, second degree heart block nearly always involves more conducted beats than blocked beats or, occasionally, equal numbers of conducted and blocked beats and only rarely more blocked than conducted beats.

When the term "heart block" is used without qualification as to location it refers to atrio-ventricular block, and when it is used without qualification as to degree it is commonly held to refer to complete heart block.

Although, as indicated above, "heart block" refers predominantly to malfunction of the atrio-ventricular conducting mechanism, the same concepts are applicable to block ("conduction block") between the sino-atrial node and the atrial myocardium (sino-atrial block), within the atria (intra-atrial block) or within the ventricles (intra-ventricular block). Block may occur at any point in the conducting pathway within the heart. The important zones which are potential sites of block are given in Table 39.

Table 39 Possible sites for conduction block

Location	Descriptive term
Junction of sinus node and atrial myocardium	Sino-atrial block
Within the atria	Intra-atrial block
Atrio-ventricular junctional area	Atrio-ventricular block, ("heart block")*
Within the ventricles	Intra-ventricular block

    By far the most important type of heart block is block in the atrio-ventricular junctional area. This will be discussed first.

* When the term "heart block" is used without qualification as to its location, it **always** refers to atrio-ventricular block. When there is no qualification as to degree it **often** refers to complete heart block.

Figure 333

Anatomical site of heart block.
This can be at the atrio-ventricular node alone, in the His bundle alone, in the right and left bundle branches (simultaneously) alone or in any combination of these three.

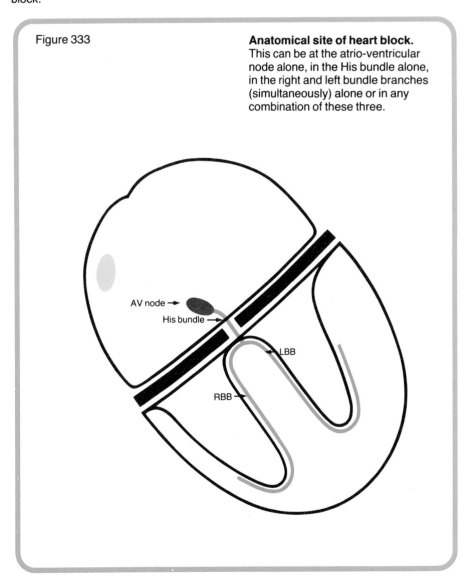

AV node →
His bundle →
LBB
RBB →

    Heart block needs to be distinguished from "interference" in which a disturbance of conduction at a given location occurs because there is functional (physiological) refractoriness at the location resulting from the recent excitation by a preceding depolarisation. Interference may occur at any site that block can occur.

Constituent Parts of the P-R Interval

The P-R interval is a measure of the total transmission time from the beginning of atrial myocardial depolarisation to the beginning of ventricular myocardial depolarisation (see Figure 179a, page 339). It therefore reflects the sum of:

1. transmission time from the atrial myocardium adjacent to the sino-atrial node (this is what gives rise to the first part of the P wave) to the atrio-ventricular node via the shortest route,
    plus

2. atrio-ventricular nodal transmission time,
    plus

3. bundle of His transmission time,
    plus

4. transmission into the proximal part of the left bundle from which position ventricular myocardial depolarisation first commences (Figure 334).

Figure 334 **The P-R interval**

During sinus rhythm depolarisation is initiated from the sino-atrial node and spreads out from this site in all directions through the atrial myocardium. When that part of the myocardium adjacent to the AV node is depolarised the P wave starts. The P wave finishes when the last part of the atrial myocardium is depolarised. At some point during atrial myocardial depolarisation (and therefore at some point during the P wave) depolarisation reaches the atrio-ventricular node. This point is not recognisable on the surface ECG. The depolarisation spreads slowly through the atrio-ventricular node and then rapidly down the His bundle and bundle branches. As soon as the depolarisation "emerges" from the upper part of the left bundle branch into the ventricular myocardium (in the upper part of the interventricular septum) the QRS complex begins and the P-R interval is ended.

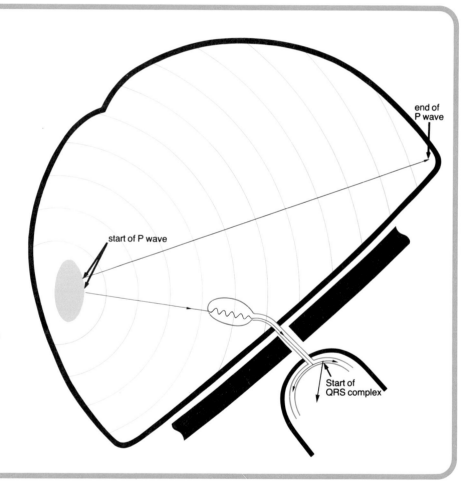

end of P wave

start of P wave

Start of QRS complex

Thus the P-R interval is a composite measurement. The largest single part of the P-R interval is the AV nodal transmission time since the conduction velocity through the AV node is relatively slow. AV nodal transmission time is also the most variable constituent of the P-R interval. The P-R interval is therefore often used as an approximate measure of AV nodal function even though it never actually measures that particular variable itself. Since, however, that variable is the single largest constituent of the P-R interval and is also the most variable constituent of the P-R interval, the use of the P-R interval to assess AV nodal function is not unreasonable.

It is possible (by invasive investigation (His bundle electrocardiography) but not from the surface ECG) to separate out the various components of the P-R interval. An example of the kind of information provided by such His bundle electrocardiography is shown in Figure 335. By this technique it is possible to measure the intra-atrial transmission time, the intra-nodal transmission time and the "His-Purkinje" transmission time.

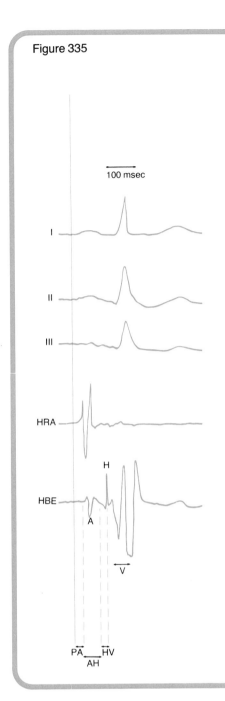

Figure 335

100 msec

I

II

III

HRA

HBE

H

A

V

PA̅ ̅HV
AH

His bundle electrocardiography.
Surface Leads I, II and III are shown
(the recording speed is faster than in
conventional electrocardiography).
Atrial myocardial depolarisation is
deemed to commence at the time
when the first deflection of the P wave
in any lead is recognisable. "HRA"
refers to a high right atrial cavity
recording (from an intra-atrial
electrode). "HBE" refers to the His
bundle electrocardiogram. This shows
low right atrial activity (A), His bundle
activity (H) and activity in the upper
part of the interventricular septum (V).
The PA interval represents the time
interval between initial atrial
depolarisation (adjacent to the sino-
atrial node) and low right atrial
depolarisation and therefore
approximately represents the time
between depolarisation leaving the
sino-atrial node and that arriving at
the atrio-ventricular node. The AH
interval represents atrio-ventricular
nodal conduction time. This is the
largest (and most variable) part of the
total P-R interval. The HV interval
represents the time between the
arrival of the depolarisation wave at
the His bundle (after emerging from
the atrio-ventricular node) to the
emergence of the impulse from the
upper part of the left bundle into the
interventricular septum.

Normal values* for the
electrophysiologically-recognisable
subdivisions of the P-R interval are as
follows:

Intra-atrial travel time
— PA interval   10–45 msec

Atrio-ventricular nodal
conduction time
— AH interval   55-130 msec

His/upper septal conduction
time ("His-Purkinje")
— HV interval   30-55 msec

The total P-R interval is 0.12-0.20
sec, i.e. 120-200 msec.

*Published data from different centres
give slightly varied results but the values
given here are representative of typical
measurements.

First Degree Atrio-ventricular Block

The functional abnormality in first degree atrio-ventricular block is that, although each atrial myocardial depolarisation is transmitted to the ventricles, each is transmitted with delay and this delay is recognisable as a constant prolongation of the P-R interval.

ECG Features of First Degree Atrio-ventricular Block

P waves

These have the form which is usual for the subject at the given time.

P-R interval

This is defined as the time interval from the onset of the P wave to the onset of the QRS complex (whether the latter begins with a q wave or an R wave, see Section 2, page 212) and the normal P-R interval does not lie outside the limits 0.12 to 0.20 sec. (Note: an abnormally short P-R interval is defined as 0.11 sec or less (see Section 2, page 215). As pointed out on page 215 the limit of resolution of time measurements on the electrocardiogram recorded at normal speed is considered to be one quarter of one small square on the recording paper, i.e. 0.01 sec. It follows that no points are considered to exist between 0.11 and 0.12. Therefore the phrases "less than 0.12" and "0.11 or less" are considered to be synonymous).

First degree heart block is defined as a constant, prolonged (i.e. greater than 0.20 sec, i.e. 0.21 sec or longer) P-R interval. Usually the degree of prolongation is modest (typically in the range 0.21 to 0.4 sec) but occasionally values of up to 1 sec may occur. Figure 336 shows an example of first degree heart block with a P-R interval of 0.32 sec.

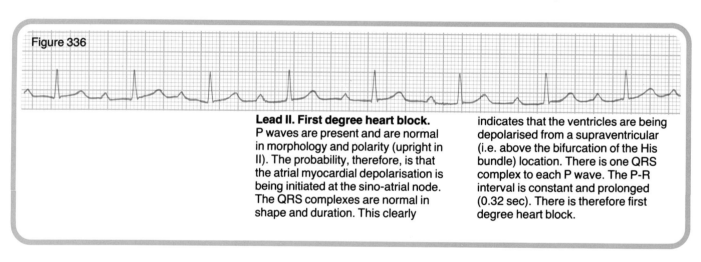

Lead II. First degree heart block. P waves are present and are normal in morphology and polarity (upright in II). The probability, therefore, is that the atrial myocardial depolarisation is being initiated at the sino-atrial node. The QRS complexes are normal in shape and duration. This clearly indicates that the ventricles are being depolarised from a supraventricular (i.e. above the bifurcation of the His bundle) location. There is one QRS complex to each P wave. The P-R interval is constant and prolonged (0.32 sec). There is therefore first degree heart block.

Figure 337 shows an example of an unusual degree of prolongation of the P-R interval (0.92 sec) in association with sinus bradycardia.

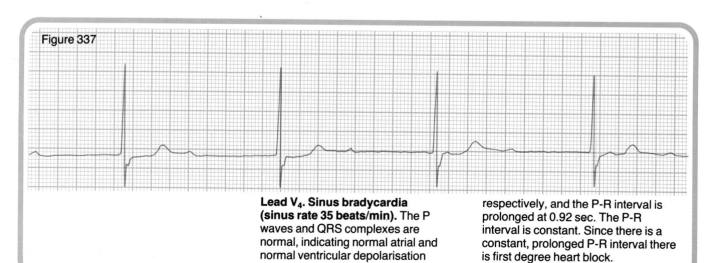

Lead V₄. Sinus bradycardia (sinus rate 35 beats/min). The P waves and QRS complexes are normal, indicating normal atrial and normal ventricular depolarisation respectively, and the P-R interval is prolonged at 0.92 sec. The P-R interval is constant. Since there is a constant, prolonged P-R interval there is first degree heart block.

First degree heart block may occur irrespective of whether the sinus rate is normal (Figure 336) or abnormally slow (Figure 337) or rapid (Figure 338).

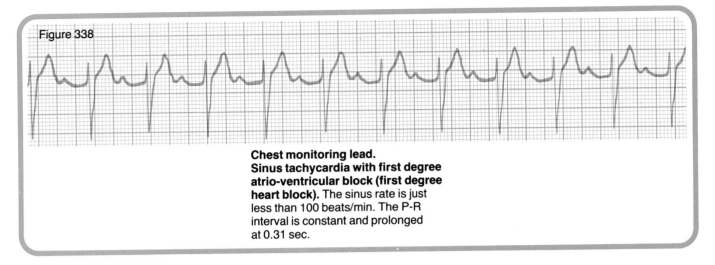

Figure 338

**Chest monitoring lead.
Sinus tachycardia with first degree atrio-ventricular block (first degree heart block).** The sinus rate is just less than 100 beats/min. The P-R interval is constant and prolonged at 0.31 sec.

The sino-atrial and atrio-ventricular nodes are both under vagal control. Vagal activity decreases the SA nodal discharge frequency. It also decreases AV nodal discharge frequency (but this is often not apparent since the sinus node is still likely to be the dominant pacemaker when both the SA and AV nodes are depressed by vagal activity) and in addition it increases conduction delay in the atrio-ventricular node. When a prolonged P-R interval (first degree heart block) is associated with profound sinus bradycardia there is a suggestion of vagal activity and both the sinus node rate and the atrio-ventricular conduction velocity may increase following the administration of atropine. However, when a prolonged P-R interval is associated with sinus tachycardia it is intrinsically unlikely that the vagus is involved since **selective** vagal activity on the atrio-ventricular node is not possible in intact man.

QRS complexes
These have the form that is usual for the subject at the time. They may be normal, show ventricular hypertrophy, bundle branch block, infarction etc.

Atrio-ventricular conduction ratio
In first degree heart block this is unity. Each P wave is associated with one QRS complex.

R-R interval
Since the P-R interval is constant the R-R interval equals the P-P interval. Thus if the sinus rate is regular the P wave rate is regular.

Criteria for first degree heart block

1. There must be P waves.

2. There must be QRS complexes

3. The P waves must have a morphology and an axis usual for the subject.†

4. The QRS complexes must have a morphology and an axis usual for the subject at the time.††

5. There must be one P wave to each QRS complex.

6. The P-R interval must be constant.

7. The P-R interval must be prolonged (i.e. ≥0.21 sec).*

† In the presence of a morphological abnormality of the atria, the P wave shape may well be abnormal and the P wave axis minimally abnormal (see footnote to Criteria table on page 371). When the P wave axis is at 180° to the usual normal (i.e. is about − 120°) a junctional origin for atrial depolarisation is likely.

†† In the presence of (a) a pre-existing morphological abnormality (including bundle branch block, hypertrophy, ventricular pre-excitation) or (b) rate-related aberrancy (pages 403 to 407) the QRS complexes will be abnormal.

* ≥0.21 sec is equivalent to >0.20 sec since the limit of time resolution is held to be 0.01 sec (page 487).

Second Degree Atrio-ventricular Block

As indicated earlier in this section, the feature common to all types and levels of second degree atrio-ventricular block is that some atrial depolarisations do transmit through the atrio-ventricular conducting tissue to give rise subsequently to QRS complexes and some do not. For a diagnosis of second degree atrio-ventricular block to be made there must be more P waves than QRS complexes within the period of observation in respect of which the diagnosis of second degree block is made, although the difference between the number of P waves and the number of QRS complexes is usually small. The ratio between the number of P waves

and the number of QRS complexes may typically be 2:1, 3:2, 4:3, 5:4, 3:1 or n:n-1 (in the latter case only an occasional beat is dropped).

There are two types and varying levels of second degree atrio-ventricular block. The two types are called "type I block" (also known as the "Wenckebach phenomenon" and as "Möbitz type I block") and "type II block" (also known as "Möbitz type II block" or sometimes, loosely, as "Möbitz block") . Type I block is much commoner than type II.* Type I block typically results from conduction problems in the AV node and type II block from problems below the AV node.

Type I Second Degree Atrio-ventricular Block (Wenckebach Second Degree Block, Möbitz Type I Second Degree Block)

This condition is usually recognised in the context of normal background sinus activation of the atria and there is a progressive prolongation of the P-R interval (with each successive beat) until

one P wave fails to be followed by a QRS complex. Following this dropped beat the P-R interval usually shortens abruptly and the cycle starts all over again. Figure 339 shows an example.

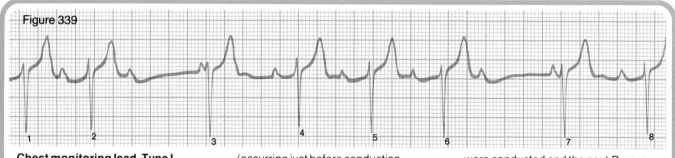

Figure 339

Chest monitoring lead. Type I second degree atrio-ventricular block ("Wenckebach block", "the Wenckebach phenomenon", "Möbitz type I second degree atrio-ventricular block"). The third QRS could be a sinus-initiated beat, but the P-R interval is very short. It is likely that the P wave is of sinus origin but the QRS may be a nodal escape beat

(occurring just before conduction through the A-V node). The fourth, fifth and sixth QRS complexes are all sinus-initiated with gradual prolongation of the P-R interval from one beat to the next. The P wave after the sixth QRS complex is not conducted (no QRS complex follows it). At this point second degree atrio-ventricular block can be diagnosed since beats 3-6

were conducted and the next P wave is not. Subsequently (beat 7) there is conduction with a short P-R interval which begins to lengthen again at 8. In retrospect it is clear that beats 1 and 2 are also part of a Wenckebach process with failure of atrio-ventricular conduction of the P wave following beats 2. Beats 3-7 show 5:4 conduction, i.e. 5 P waves to 4 QRS complexes.

* Second degree atrio-ventricular block was first described in 1899 by Wenckebach. The description referred to what is now called "type I block". In 1924 Möbitz described the two types of second

degree atrio-ventricular block as type I and type II. Type I second degree atrio-ventricular block is the same as that described by Wenckebach.

ECG Features of Type I Second Degree Atrio-ventricular Block

P waves

These have the form usual for the subject at the time. Typically there will be regular sinus rhythm P waves which are morphologically normal except in the presence of atrial hypertrophy, atrial infarction etc.

P-R interval

Within any series of beats demonstrating type I second degree atrio-ventricular block, the initial P-R interval will be normal or prolonged but the P-R interval of each succeeding conducted beat then becomes progressively longer until a single P wave fails to be followed by a QRS complex (i.e. there is transient failure of atrio-ventricular conduction). The cycle then recommences with the same P-R interval as the first beat in the series.

QRS complexes

These have the form usual for the subject at the time. Their timing depends on the behaviour of the atrio-ventricular conduction (i.e. the length of the P-R interval or the failure to conduct).

Atrio-ventricular conduction ratio

This is typically "n:(n-1)" where "n" is usually 3, 4 or 5 (i.e. typical AV conduction ratios are 5:4, 4:3; 3:2).

Characteristic behaviour of the R-R intervals in AV nodal Wenckebach block

Although type I atrio-ventricular block is associated with progressively **increasing** P-R intervals (until the dropped beat occurs) there is also, inevitably, a progressive **decrease** in the R-R intervals (if the basic sinus rate is regular). This is because, although the P-R interval increases, it increases by progressively diminishing amounts. Thus in Figure 339, R-R interval 3-4 exceeds that of 4-5, which in turn (just) exceeds

that of interval 5-6. The phenomenon (which at first sight often seems paradoxical to the student) is illustrated in Figure 340. A typical sequence of R-R intervals in type I atrio-ventricular block, as shown in Figure 340, would be 0.96, 0.92, 0.88, 1.24, 0.96, 0.92, 0.88, 1.24 etc. This sequence of gradually reducing R-R intervals followed by a sudden prolongation for a single beat is typical of type I block.

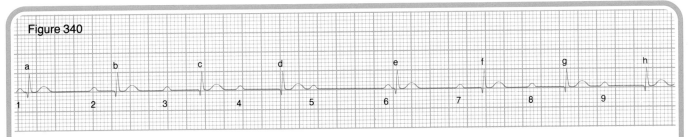

Figure 340

The Wenckebach phenomenon: behaviour of the R-R intervals.
The P waves (1-9) are absolutely regular. P waves 1-4 are followed by QRS complexes a-d respectively. P wave 5 is not followed by a QRS. P waves 6-9 are followed by QRS complexes e-h respectively. Consider P waves 1-5. The respective P-R intervals are given as follows:

1-a = 0.12)
2-b = 0.28)   difference = 0.16
3-c = 0.40   difference = 0.12
4-d = 0.48   difference = 0.08
5-not followed by QRS

Thus, although each P-R interval is longer than its predecessor, the **increment** in P-R intervals progressively falls so that the R-R interval progressively **decreases.**
The R-R intervals in this example are given as follows:

Interval a-b	=	(P-P interval)	+	(interval 2-b)	−	(interval 1-a)
	=	0.8	+	0.28	−	0.12
	=	0.96				

Interval b-c	=	(P-P interval)	+	(interval 3-c)	−	(interval 2-b)
	=	0.8	+	0.4	−	0.28
	=	0.92				

Interval c-d	=	(P-P interval)	+	(interval 4-d)	−	(interval 3-c)
	=	0.8	+	0.48	−	0.4
	=	0.88				

The interval d-e is, of course, much longer than the others but is less than two cycle lengths:

Interval d-e	=	2 x (P-P interval)	+	(interval 6-e)	−	(interval 4-d)
	=	1.6	+	0.12	−	0.48
	=	1.24				

The duration of two sinus intervals = 1.6 sec.
Thus a typical sequence of R-R intervals in type I block is: 0.96, 0.92, 0.88, 1.24, 0.96, 0.92, 0.88, 1.24 etc.

If the basic sinus rate is not constant the typical progressive decrease in the R-R interval in association with type I second degree atrio-ventricular block can be disturbed. An example is shown in Figure 341.

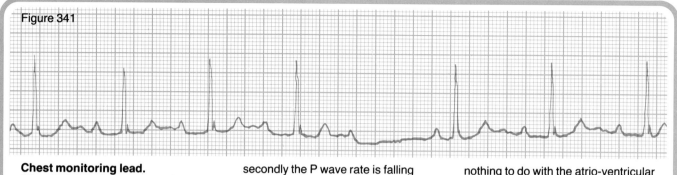

Figure 341

Chest monitoring lead. Wenckebach phenomenon (type I second degree atrio-ventricular block). This figure shows two unusual features, first the ratio of P waves to conducted beats is 5:4 (ratios of 4:3 and 3:2 are much commoner) and secondly the P wave rate is falling gradually so that the second P-P interval is slightly longer than the first and the third is slightly longer than the second. This progressive increase in the P-P interval (which is due to the falling sinus rate and is absolutely nothing to do with the atrio-ventricular conduction problem) just compensates for the expected progressive shortening of the R-R intervals which actually remain approximately constant until the dropped beat occurs.

Ratio of P waves to QRS complexes in type I second degree atrio-ventricular block

As has already been explained, the diagnosis of second degree atrio-ventricular block requires that some atrial depolarisations be conducted to the ventricles and that some are not. The proportion of "dropped" beats varies from one patient to another and, for a given patient, from time to time. The atrio-ventricular ratios involved are typically 3:2, 4:3 or 5:4. Other ratios are much less common. The mid-portion of Figure 339 shows a ratio of 5:4 (starting with beat 3 and ending before beat 7 there are five P waves and four QRS complexes). Figure 341 also shows an example of 5:4 conduction. 2:1 conduction can also occur but can only be diagnosed with confidence as a Wenckebach type block if there is evidence of typical Wenckebach in other parts of the record (Figure 343).

Figure 342 shows sinus rhythm with AV nodal Wenckebach and a conduction ratio of 3:2.

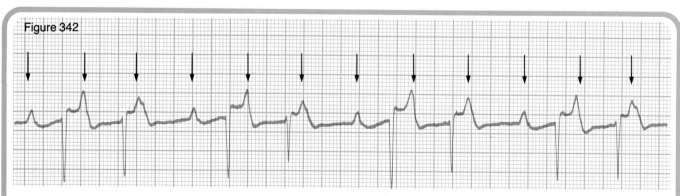

Figure 342

Chest monitoring lead. Sinus rhythm with a regular P wave rate. All P waves are arrowed. The first P wave has a P-R interval of 0.38 sec. The second P wave has a P-R interval of 0.46 sec. The third P wave fails to conduct to the ventricles. The fourth P wave has a P-R interval of 0.38 sec and the cycle of progressive conduction failure is repeated.

Figure 343 shows sinus rhythm with
AV nodal Wenckebach block and a
conduction ratio of 2:1 in parts and 3:2
in parts.

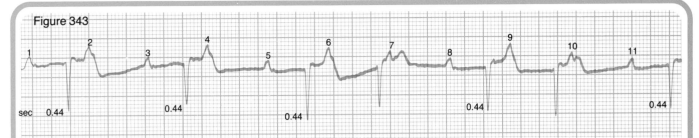

Figure 343

sec 0.44   0.44   0.44   0.44   0.44

Chest monitoring lead. Taken from the same patient as Figure 342. Regular P waves (numbered) are seen throughout. The first P-R interval is 0.44 sec. The second P wave fails to conduct. The third, fifth, eighth and eleventh P waves all have a P-R interval of 0.44 sec. This is too constant to be coincidental and indicates that there is atrio-ventricular

conduction of the P waves 1, 3, 5, 8 and 11. The second and fourth P waves fail to conduct but as some P waves are conducting and some are not there is clearly secondary atrio-ventricular block (but in relation to P waves 1-5 it is not possible to tell whether this is type I or type II). In relation to P waves 5-11 there is clearly 3:2 Wenckebach. It is only

because one can easily recognise 3:2 Wenckebach (type I second degree atrio-ventricular block) in relation to these P waves 5-11 and because the P-R interval of P waves 1 and 3 is the same as the P-R interval of P waves 5, 8 and 11 that one can be sure that there is Wenckebach block in relation to P waves 1-4.

Criteria for type I second degree atrio-ventricular block

1. There must be P waves.

2. There must be QRS complexes.

3. The P waves must have a morphology and an axis usual for the subject.†

4. The QRS complexes must have a morphology and an axis usual for the subject at the time.††

5. There must be progressive prolongation of the P-R interval with each succeeding beat until one P wave occurs without a QRS (i.e. there is a dropped beat). There will be "n" P waves to "(n-1)" QRS complexes, where "n" is a small positive integer.*

6. The longest P-R interval is the one immediately before the dropped beat. The shortest P-R interval is the one associated with the first conducted beat after the dropped beat.** The P-R intervals before the blocked beat increase and do so by progressively decreasing amounts so that the consecutive R-R intervals before the blocked beat actually progressively shorten.

† See footnote † to Criteria table page 488.

†† See footnote †† to Criteria table page 488.

* Typically "n" is 3, 4 or 5 (or variable within this range). Where n=2, there is 2:1 AV block. This can be type I or type II block (see pages 496 and 497).

** The P-R interval of the first conducted beat after the dropped beat is usually normal (Figures 339, 340 and 341) but may be prolonged (Figures 342 and 343).

Type I second degree block may occur anywhere in the heart but the description which has been given so far refers to the electrocardiographic appearances in association with type I second degree block at the **atrio-ventricular junctional area.**

Type II Second Degree Atrio-ventricular Block

This is much less common than type I second degree atrio-ventricular block. As indicated earlier, the criterion for the diagnosis of second degree atrio-ventricular block is that during the period of observation, some atrial depolarisations are transmitted to the ventricles and some are not. In the case of type II second degree atrio-ventricular block the dropped beats occur without any prior "warning" change in the P-R interval of the preceding beats. The beats preceding the dropped beat have a constant P-R interval (whether it be normal or prolonged). The P waves (in the presence of sinus-initiated atrial depolarisation) have the form which is usual for that patient and the QRS complexes also have the form which is usual for that patient. An example of type II second degree atrio-ventricular block is shown in Figure 344.

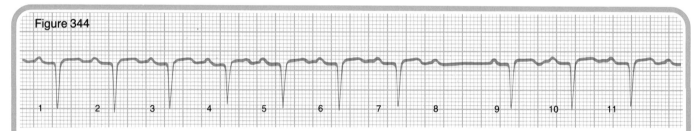

Figure 344

Chest monitoring lead. Sinus rhythm with first degree atrio-ventricular block and type II second degree atrio-ventricular block. The first seven beats show sinus rhythm with a slightly prolonged P-R interval (0.24 sec). The P-R interval is constant. (Since the P-R interval is constant and prolonged there is first degree heart block). The P waves are within normal limits.

The QRS complexes are of normal width. (The QRS complexes could be normal if this is a V_1 location of the recording electrode or could be associated with an anterior infarction if the recording comes from further to the left (with respect to the patient) in the precordial series, but in either case, their normal width indicates the supraventricular initiation of ventricular myocardial

depolarisation). The eighth P wave is not followed by a QRS complex. The ninth, tenth and eleventh P waves are followed by QRS complexes in the normal way, with a constant, prolonged P-R interval. This intermittent failure to conduct to the ventricles, without any prior prolongation of the P-R interval is typical of type II second degree atrio-ventricular block.

Another example of type II second degree atrio-ventricular block, this time with concomitant left bundle branch block, is shown in Figure 345.

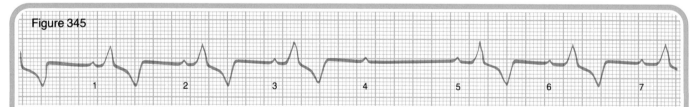

Figure 345

Chest monitoring lead. Sinus rhythm with left bundle branch block and type II second degree atrio-ventricular block. In relation to the first three cardiac cycles the P-R interval is normal at 0.16 sec. The QRS complexes are wide (there is left

bundle branch block). The S-T, T segments are abnormal because of the intraventricular conduction disturbance. The fourth P wave is not conducted to the ventricles. The fifth, sixth and seventh P waves are conducted like the first three.

Since some (in fact most) beats are conducted and one is not, there is second degree atrio-ventricular block. Since there is no warning prolongation of the P-R interval the second degree block is of the type II variety.

ECG Features of Type II Second Degree Atrio-ventricular Block

Failure of atrio-ventricular conduction
The cardinal feature is intermittent failure of conduction of the atrial activation to the ventricles, i.e. intermittently a P wave is not followed by a QRS complex.

P waves
The P waves have the form which is usual for the subject.†

P-R interval
Usually this is normal, but if there is also pre-existing first degree heart block the P-R interval will be prolonged. In either event, however, the **P-R interval will be constant.**

QRS complexes
The QRS complexes have the form which is usual for the subject.†† If the QRS complex is of normal duration then when failure of atrio-ventricular conduction occurs it could happen in the His bundle or simultaneously in the right and left bundle branches (much less frequently it could have occurred in the atrio-ventricular node). If there is **right** bundle branch block in association with the conducted beats, then the type II block may indicate transient failure of conduction in the **left** bundle branch and vice versa. Thus in the example in Figure 345, there was pre-existing left bundle branch block and the type II block indicates transient additional failure of conduction in the right bundle branch or transient failure of conduction in the His bundle (in the latter case the pre-existing left bundle branch block would not be partially responsible for the AV conduction failure).

Atrio-ventricular conduction ratio
There are "n" P waves to "(n-1)" QRS complexes (where n is a positive integer* which may range from 3 up to a very large number). The relation of "n" P waves to "(n-1)" QRS complexes indicates that only occasional atrial beats are blocked.

R-R interval
The R-R interval of the conducted beats is the same as the P-P interval (since the P-R interval is constant). If there is regular sinus rhythm the P-P intervals and therefore the R-R intervals are constant. The R-R interval which brackets a non-conducted P wave is twice the normal R-R interval (assuming regular sinus rhythm). The R-R interval of the blocked beat is never more than twice the normal R-R interval for if two or more P waves fail to conduct consecutively (i.e. there is 3:1 AV block or a higher degree still) then "high-grade" block (by definition) is present (see pages 499 and 500).

---

† See footnote † to Criteria table page 488.

†† See footnote †† to Criteria table page 488.

* Where "n"=2, there is 2:1 AV block. This can be type I or type II block (see pages 496 and 497).

Criteria for type II second degree atrio-ventricular block

1. There must be P waves.

2. There must be QRS complexes.

3. The P waves must have a morphology and an axis usual for the subject.†

4. The QRS complexes must have a morphology and an axis usual for the subject at the time.††

5. The P-R interval of conducted beats may be normal or long. Within the period of observation one P wave is not followed by a QRS complex. There must be no change in the P-R interval before the transient failure of atrio-ventricular conduction. There will be "n" P waves to "(n-1)" QRS complexes for each example of transient type II block. "n" will be 3 or more.*

6. Although failure of AV conduction may occur more than once within the period of observation, failure of conduction is not seen in relation to two or more **consecutive** P waves.

7. The P-R interval must be constant for all conducted beats (i.e. for each P wave followed by a QRS complex).

8. The QRS complexes after the transient AV conduction failure have the same morphology as those preceding it.

† See footnote † to Criteria table page 488.

†† See footnote †† to Criteria table page 488. Not uncommonly in relation to type II block, the QRS complexes of conducted beats may show bundle branch block.

* "n" will typically be much larger than 3. Where "n" = 2 there is 2:1 AV block. This can be type I or type II block (see pages 496 and 497).

2:1 Atrio-ventricular Block

This is a particular variety of second degree AV block in which the "n" of the atrio-ventricular conduction ratio: "n" to "(n-1)" has the value 2. When there are two P waves to each QRS complex and the underlying atrial rhythm is sinus,†

Abnormal 2:1 atrio-ventricular† block refers to the alternate failure of conduction of the atrial activation process to the ventricles when the P-P interval is such that the conducting tissue in the atrio-ventricular node and in the

If there are coupled atrial premature beats then the sinus beats will usually be conducted to the ventricles and the coupled atrial premature beats (if sufficiently premature) may not. This condition will sometimes simulate 2:1 atrio-ventricular block but is quite distinct from it (compare Figures 350 and 351 with Figures 346, 347 and 348).

Figure 346 shows an example of 2:1 atrio-ventricular block.

2:1 atrio-ventricular block is said to be present. This is obviously a variety of second degree block since some beats (half of them) are conducted and some are not. It can occur at the AV node (type I) or below the AV node (type II).

bundle branches would be expected to have recovered excitability between one beat and the next. If the rhythm is sinus there should always be 1:1 atrio-ventricular conduction no matter what the sinus rate.†*

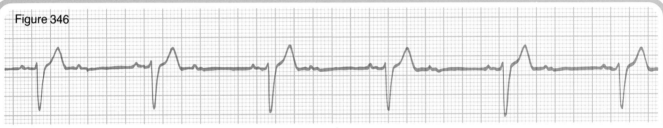

Figure 346

Chest monitoring lead. Basic sinus rhythm with 2:1 atrio-ventricular block. The atrial (of sinus origin) rate is approximately 96 beats/min. The P waves are biphasic (indicating some intra-atrial conduction abnormality) but the morphology is the usual one for that subject and is constant. Every alternate P wave is conducted (i.e. is followed by a QRS complex) and every alternate one fails to conduct (i.e. is not followed by a QRS complex). The conducted beats have a constant normal P-R interval of 0.18 sec. The conducted beats have a total QRS duration which is slightly prolonged (0.12 sec) indicating the presence of an intraventricular conduction problem. This is probably left bundle branch block. Since there is left bundle branch block in association with the conducted beats the probability is that failure of conduction occurs on the basis of intermittent failure in the right bundle branch (i.e. this is probably a type II block) but it could occur because of intermittent failure in the atrio-ventricular node (more likely to be a type I response and in this event the pre-existing left bundle branch block would be coincidental) or it could occur because of intermittent failure of conduction at the His bundle (this is usually a type II block and again in this event the pre-existing left bundle branch block would be incidental to the mechanism but possibly related in terms of the aetiology).

†If the atrial rhythm is atrial tachycardia, 2:1 atrio-ventricular block will often occur and this does not imply an abnormality of atrio-ventricular conduction. This block will occur when the P-P interval falls within the refractory period of any part of the conducting pathway between the atrial aspect of the AV node and the bifurcation of the bundle of His (see page 422). In this situation 2:1 atrio-ventricular block occurs as a manifestation of **normal** function of the conducting tissues (if the P-P interval falls within the refractory period of one but not of both bundle branches, then functional bundle branch block (aberrant intraventricular conduction) will occur. This is again a manifestation of **normal** function of the AV conducting tissue).

*If a person at rest and not under the influence of atropine is paced artificially from the atrial myocardium at increasing rates, then atrio-ventricular block will occur at a rate which, in the normal subject, would be something of the order of 150 beats/min. This does not occur on exercise during sinus tachycardia for there is withdrawal of vagal activity and augmentation of sympathetic activity during exercise and both of these processes facilitate conduction at the atrio-ventricular node. If the resting subject is given atropine and then is atrially paced at increasing rates, atrio-ventricular block either does not occur or occurs only at a higher rate. In these artificial situations of atrial pacing the atrio-ventricular block is almost invariably of the type I variety and indicates a **normal** response of the atrio-ventricular node.

Figure 347 shows another example
of 2:1 atrio-ventricular block.

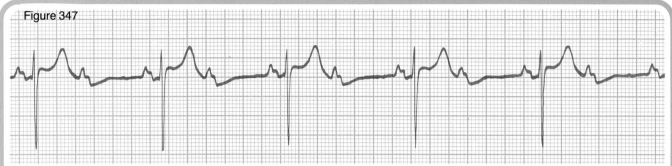

Figure 347

Chest monitoring lead. Basic sinus rhythm with 2:1 atrio-ventricular block. The P waves have an abnormal but constant morphology. The P waves are known to be upright in Lead II and the rhythm is of sinus origin. Alternate P waves conduct to the ventricles with a normal, constant P-R interval. The QRS complexes are normal in shape and duration indicating that there is normal intraventricular conduction. It is impossible, from the record, to tell whether the intermittent conduction failure is at the AV node (and therefore is probably type I block) or is at the His bundle or occurs bilaterally at both bundle branches (and therefore is probably type II block).

Figure 348 shows a further example
of 2:1 atrio-ventricular block.

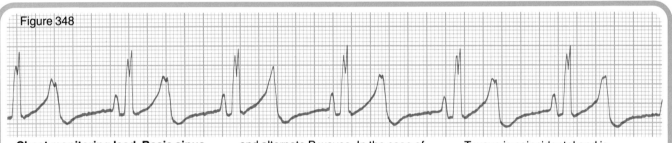

Figure 348

Chest monitoring lead. Basic sinus rhythm with 2:1 atrio-ventricular block. At first sight this might be mistaken for sinus rhythm but in fact every alternate P wave sits on top of the T wave of the preceding beat. The slight variation which occurs in the sinus rate reveals slight shifts in the relative position of the T waves and alternate P waves. In the case of the T wave following the third QRS complex the P wave sits precisely on top of the peak of the T wave and gives a pointed, apparently monophasic, T wave. In the remaining cases the blocked P waves do not sit precisely on top of the T waves. This occurrence of the P wave on top of the T wave is coincidental and is dependent simply on the fact that the P-P interval happens to be approximately equal to the P-R interval plus the time interval from the onset of the QRS complex to the peak of the T wave.

2:1 atrio-ventricular block is unquestionably "second degree" since some beats are conducted and others are not. However, it is often possible to say whether the second degree block is of the type I or the type II variety. When the QRS complexes of the conducted beats are clearly wide (i.e. when there is bundle branch block **during** atrio-ventricular conduction) the **probability** (but not the **certainty)** is that when AV block occurs it is because of failure of conduction in the contralateral bundle branch and that the conduction disturbance is probably of the type II variety. **If, in the presence of 2:1 atrio-ventricular block, the intraventricular conduction is normal in association with beats which are conducted from atria to ventricles,** no prediction can be made about whether the conduction disturbance is of the type I or type II variety. Occasionally prolonged observation may indicate that at times the conduction ratio changes from being 2:1 to being 3:2 and if such an observation can be made then the nature of the 2:1 conduction can be predicted. If 3:2 (or 4:3 or 5:4 etc) atrio-ventricular block can be observed and is associated with a prolongation of the P-R interval before the dropped beat, then the atrio-ventricular conduction problem is of the type I variety. If 3:2 (or 4:3 or 5:4 etc) conduction occurs transiently without any change in the P-R interval, then it is virtually certain that the block is of the type II variety whereas if 3:2 (or 4:3 or 5:4 etc) conduction occurs with progressive prolongation of the P-R interval before the transient failure of AV conduction, it is virtually certain that the adjacent examples of 2:1 AV block are of the type I variety.

Figure 349 shows an example of 2:1 atrio-ventricular block of type I. During the 2:1 AV block no conclusion can be made about whether it is type I or type II but following the return of 1:1 conduction it can be seen that there is a progressive prolongation of the P-R interval.

Subsequent to this, in this particular recording 2:1 atrio-ventricular block returned, though this is not shown in the figure, and the progressive prolongation of the P-R interval clearly indicated that the block was of the type I variety.

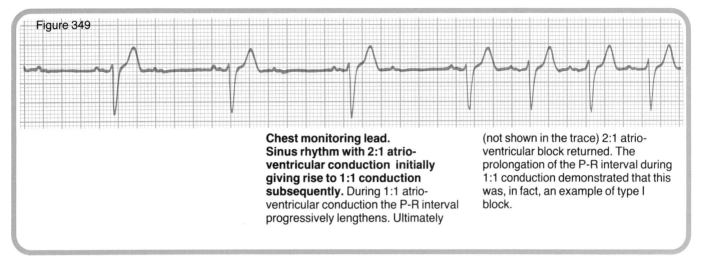

Figure 349

Chest monitoring lead. Sinus rhythm with 2:1 atrio-ventricular conduction initially giving rise to 1:1 conduction subsequently. During 1:1 atrio-ventricular conduction the P-R interval progressively lengthens. Ultimately (not shown in the trace) 2:1 atrio-ventricular block returned. The prolongation of the P-R interval during 1:1 conduction demonstrated that this was, in fact, an example of type I block.

Differential Diagnosis of Second Degree Atrio-ventricular Block

It is important to remember that two conditions may occasionally be confused with second degree atrio-ventricular block. The first is **coupled atrial premature beats** in which the atrial premature beats occur at such a time that when the depolarisation waveform reaches the AV conducting tissue the latter is refractory so that the atrial premature beats are blocked. The clue to the correct diagnosis here is given either by the fact that the atrial premature beats have an abnormal morphology compared with the sinus beats (i.e. the premature beats are ectopic as well as premature) or by the fact that the P-P′ interval (interval between the sinus beat and the atrial ectopic beat) is significantly less than the P′-P interval (interval between the atrial ectopic beat and the next sinus beat) (see Figure 350).

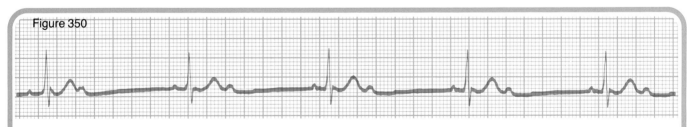

Figure 350

Chest monitoring lead. Sinus rhythm with coupled, blocked atrial premature beats. The first beat is a sinus beat. The second P wave is seen immediately after the first T wave. The morphology of the second P wave is different from that of the first P wave. It is ectopic. It is also premature. These premature ectopic atrial beats fail to conduct the ventricles. Superficially the situation resembles 2:1 atrio-ventricular block. It is, in fact, 2:1 atrio-ventricular block in one sense but the prematurity of the ectopic P waves is partly or totally the cause of the conduction failure (see page 400) and the rhythm should certainly not be described as 2:1 atrio-ventricular block. It is fundamentally sinus rhythm with blocked premature atrial ectopic beats. The clues to the correct diagnosis are (i) the morphological differences between P′ and P waves and (ii) the fact that the P-P′ interval is less than the P′-P interval.

Figure 351 shows a further example of blocked atrial premature beats. This time it occurs on the background of first degree heart block.

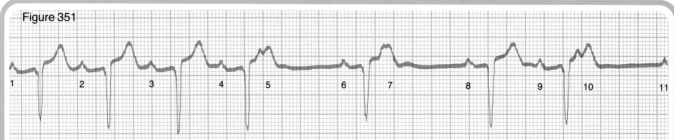

Figure 351

Chest monitoring lead. First degree heart block with subsequent blocked atrial premature beats. The first four beats show sinus rhythm with first degree heart block (P-R interval = 0.30 sec). The P-R interval is constant. The fifth P wave occurs prematurely and is seen disturbing the upstroke of the S-T segment. This P wave fails to conduct to the ventricles. As is usually the case with atrial premature beats the interval between the ectopic P wave and the next sinus P wave (the P'-P interval) is longer than the pre-existing P-P interval and there is then a pause before the next sinus beat. This sinus beat (6) has a shorter P-R interval than that of preceding beats (possibly because the atrio-ventricular node has had rather more time to recover since it was last required to conduct). The QRS complex associated with this beat is also followed by a premature ectopic P wave (7) disturbing the upstroke of the T wave. Again there is a long P'-P interval and the next P wave (8) is followed by a normal P-R interval. The QRS complex after the eighth P wave is not followed by an atrial premature beat but is followed by a sinus-initiated P wave in the same way as occurred during the first four beats. The P-R interval once more is long (as with the first four beats) and the QRS complex following this (ninth) P wave is once more followed by an atrial premature beat (10) disturbing the upstroke of the T wave. Following this there is a long interval before the next scheduled P wave. In relation to the fourth to sixth QRS complexes (fourth to eighth P waves) there are two P waves to each QRS complex and this might superficially look like 2:1 atrio-ventricular block but analysis of the events occurring before and after this period clearly reveals that the fundamental problem is that of blocked atrial premature beats.

The second situation which may cause confusion is **sinus bradycardia.** Superficial inspection of Figure 348 could lead to a conclusion that the rhythm is sinus bradycardia until it is realised that there are twice as many P waves visible as is apparent at first sight, and that every alternate P wave is sitting on top of a T wave. Sometimes the reverse problem may occur and true sinus bradycardia may be misconstrued as indicating 2:1 atrio-ventricular block. This is only likely to occur when there is a prominent U wave following the T wave and the U wave is thought to be a second P wave. The morphology of the U wave will usually be very different from that of the P waves and careful examination of this will reveal the correct situation. It should also be noted that (except by pure coincidence) the interval between the beginning of the P wave and the beginning of the U wave should not be the same as the interval between the beginning of the U wave and the beginning of the next P wave.

High-grade (or "Advanced") Atrio-ventricular Block

High-grade atrio-ventricular block is defined as second degree block (i.e. some beats are conducted and some are not) **in which the atrio-ventricular conduction ratio is 3:1 or higher.** The electrocardiographic differentiation from complete heart block (see later) depends upon the fact that in high-grade atrio-ventricular block some beats are conducted, as demonstrated by the fact that a repeatable constant P-R interval can be demonstrated for those P waves which immediately precede a QRS complex. The conduction ratios associated with high-grade block may be 3:1, 4:1, 5:1 or 6:1. It is uncommon for higher ratios to occur and the "even" ones (4:1, 6:1 etc) are said to be commoner than the "odd" ones. Figure 352 shows an example of high-grade second degree atrio-ventricular block.

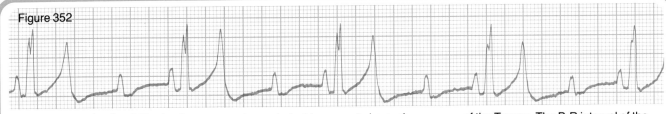

Figure 352

Chest monitoring lead. Basic sinus rhythm with high-grade atrio-ventricular block. The record shows consistent 3:1 atrio-ventricular conduction ratios. The record is taken from the same patient as that of Figure 348. As in the earlier figure the sinus rate just happens to be such that the P-P interval exactly equals the sum of the P-R interval and the interval from the beginning of the QRS complex to the peak of the T wave. As a result of this the P wave following each conducted beat falls on the peak of the T wave. The P-R interval of the conducted beats (i.e. those beats from which a P wave is followed by a QRS complex) is absolutely constant at 0.14 sec.

Figure 353 shows varying high-grade and 2:1 atrio-ventricular block.

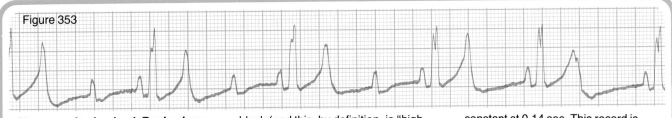

Figure 353

Chest monitoring lead. Basic sinus rhythm with second degree atrio-ventricular block. In the first part of the record there is 3:1 atrio-ventricular block (and this, by definition, is "high-grade") and in the latter part there is 2:1 AV block. In relation to each conducted beat the P-R interval is constant at 0.14 sec. This record is taken from the same patient as those shown in Figures 348 and 352.

High-grade atrio-ventricular block may be of type I or type II but more commonly is of the type II variety (occurring in the His bundle or in the bundle branches). Since during the high-grade atrio-ventricular block itself there are (by definition) no **consecutive** conducted beats, it is impossible to say whether or not there is any prolongation of the P-R interval in relation to conducted beats and therefore it is not absolutely possible to categorise the rhythm as type I or type II. If two consecutive conducted beats do occur in part of the record and the P-R interval is constant in those beats, then when the AV block occurs (in the following beat) it is of the type II variety.

Criteria for high-grade atrio-ventricular block

1. There must be P waves.

2. There must be QRS complexes.

3. The P waves must have a morphology and an axis usual for the subject.†

4. The QRS complexes must have a morphology and an axis usual for the subject and the lead at the time.††

5. Some P waves are followed by QRS complexes and some are not.

6. The atrio-ventricular conduction ratio is 3:1 or higher.*

7. The P-R interval of beats in which a QRS complex follows a P wave may be normal or long but must be constant.

† See footnote † to Criteria table page 488.

†† See footnote †† to Criteria table page 488.

* The AV conduction ratio must be "n":1 where "n" is a positive integer not less than 3 and may be variable. Since the P-R interval of conducted beats is constant the R-R interval is "n" times the P-P interval.

Third Degree Atrio-ventricular Block ("Complete Heart Block", "Complete Atrio-ventricular Block")

In this condition there is total failure of atrio-ventricular conduction. Ventricular depolarisation occurs only by virtue of ventricular escape beats and the atrial and ventricular depolarisations are completely independent (there is atrio-ventricular dissociation). The atria may, of course, be depolarised by any mechanism (sinus rhythm, atrial tachycardia, atrial fibrillation, atrial flutter) but the arrhythmia is best understood in the context of the simplest situation which is when atrial depolarisation is initiated by the sino-atrial node. In this event the P waves occur at a regular rate. The QRS complexes (which are all ventricular escape beats) usually also occur at a regular rate – the rate in question being appropriate to the ventricular escape pacemaker which is operative. Unless there is some additional depression of the sino-atrial node the atrial rate will be faster than the ventricular rate. The QRS complexes will most commonly be abnormally shaped and abnormally wide (if the ventricular escape pacemaker is situated below the bifurcation of the His bundle in the bundle branches or in the Purkinje network), but occasionally may have a morphology which is usual for the patient (if the ventricular escape pacemaker is situated above the bifurcation of the His bundle (ensuring that intraventricular conduction is initiated in a normal direction)).

Figure 354 shows an example of third degree atrio-ventricular block.

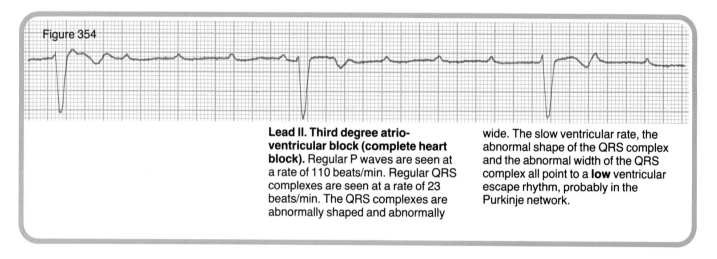

Lead II. Third degree atrio-ventricular block (complete heart block). Regular P waves are seen at a rate of 110 beats/min. Regular QRS complexes are seen at a rate of 23 beats/min. The QRS complexes are abnormally shaped and abnormally wide. The slow ventricular rate, the abnormal shape of the QRS complex and the abnormal width of the QRS complex all point to a **low** ventricular escape rhythm, probably in the Purkinje network.

Figure 355 shows a further example of third degree atrio-ventricular block.

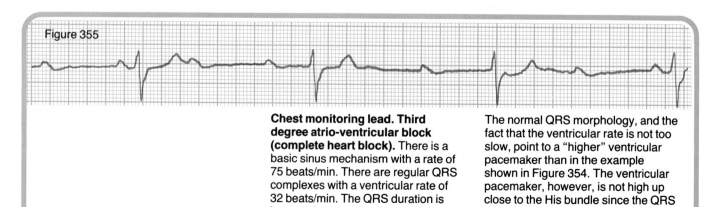

Chest monitoring lead. Third degree atrio-ventricular block (complete heart block). There is a basic sinus mechanism with a rate of 75 beats/min. There are regular QRS complexes with a ventricular rate of 32 beats/min. The QRS duration is beyond the normal range at 0.12 sec. The normal QRS morphology, and the fact that the ventricular rate is not too slow, point to a "higher" ventricular pacemaker than in the example shown in Figure 354. The ventricular pacemaker, however, is not high up close to the His bundle since the QRS duration is prolonged.

Figure 356 shows an example of congenital complete heart block. The electrocardiographic features are the same as those of acquired heart block except that the QRS complexes tend to be relatively normal in shape and duration and that the ventricular escape rate tends to be faster than in the acquired form.

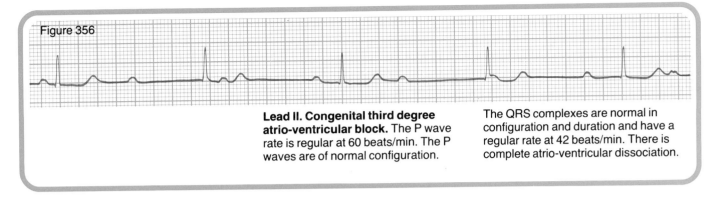

Figure 356

Lead II. Congenital third degree atrio-ventricular block. The P wave rate is regular at 60 beats/min. The P waves are of normal configuration. The QRS complexes are normal in configuration and duration and have a regular rate at 42 beats/min. There is complete atrio-ventricular dissociation.

The occurrence of narrow QRS complexes and a relatively rapid (40 to 60 beats/ min) QRS rate can also, however, occur in acquired heart block. Figure 357 is an example.

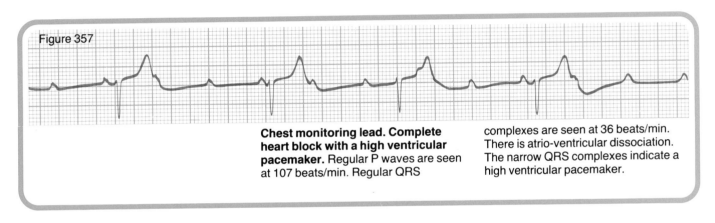

Figure 357

Chest monitoring lead. Complete heart block with a high ventricular pacemaker. Regular P waves are seen at 107 beats/min. Regular QRS complexes are seen at 36 beats/min. There is atrio-ventricular dissociation. The narrow QRS complexes indicate a high ventricular pacemaker.

ECG Features of Third Degree Atrio-ventricular Block

Relationship between atrial and ventricular activity

There is no relationship between atrial and ventricular activity, i.e. there is atrio-ventricular dissociation. The ventricular rate is lower than the atrial rate. The ventricular rhythm is an escape rhythm.

P waves

In most cases the atrial depolarisation will be of sinus origin. In this situation the P waves will have the configuration which is usual for that subject (e.g. a patient with normal atria will have normal P waves and one with left atrial hypertrophy will have biphasic or bifid P waves), the P wave rate will be regular and the P wave rate will tend to be slightly faster than the usual resting sinus rate (simply because, in the presence of complete heart block and a slow ventricular rate the cardiac output will be less than it would otherwise be and there may well be reflex sympathetic activity); sinus rates of around 90-110 beats/min are common in this situation. There is, of course, no reason why the atrial activation mechanism should not be other than of sinus origin and it is perfectly possible to see examples of atrial tachycardia, atrial flutter, atrial fibrillation and atrial premature beats in association with complete heart block. Whatever the atrial mechanism the ventricular activation is independent of it and is at a slower rate.

P-R interval

This term is meaningless in the context of complete heart block since, by definition there is no significant relationship between the P waves and the QRS complexes. Many of the P waves are not followed by QRS complexes and when a P wave is followed by a QRS complex the relationship between the two is pure chance (there is atrio-ventricular dissociation) and the P-R interval may range from zero (i.e. the P waves and QRS complexes happen to be simultaneous) to just less than the P-P interval (when the P-R interval reaches the P-P interval P waves and QRS complexes become simultaneous again and the P-R interval returns once more to zero).

QRS complexes

Ventricular activity is independent of atrial activity. Ventricular activity can, therefore, only occur as a result of a **ventricular escape rhythm.**
The anatomical location of the escape rhythm will **depend on** the location of the block and will **determine** the form of the QRS. If there is block in the AV node or in the proximal part of the His bundle a low His bundle escape mechanism may occur. If the block is below the His bundle bifurcation or extends down to such a level a low ventricular escape mechanism can occur.

In the case of a low His bundle escape rhythm the QRS complex will be of normal width and morphology and the rate will be relatively high (e.g. 50-60 beats/min). In the case of a low ventricular escape mechanism the QRS complexes will be abnormally wide and abnormally shaped and the rate will be lower (e.g. 20-40 beats/min).

AV conduction ratio

By definition no conducted beats occur and the AV conduction ratio is infinite.

R-R interval

Ventricular depolarisation depends on the ventricular escape mechanism. The R-R interval is typically regular (though it may be irregular if more than one escape focus is active – and in this case the morphology of the QRS complexes may also vary).
The ventricular rate may typically range from 20 per minute (in the case of a low Purkinje escape focus) to 60 or more per minute (in the case of a His bundle escape focus).

Variations in P-P interval (ventriculo-phasic sinus arrhythmia)

When the atrial activity is of sinus origin the P waves are usually regular. However, there can be phasic sinus arrhythmia in the presence of complete heart block just as there can in the presence of normal atrio-ventricular conduction. The rhythm is then simply sinus arrhythmia with complete heart block. However, there is also an unusual form of variation in the sino-atrial depolarisation rate called "ventriculo-phasic sinus arrhythmia". This variation is said to occur in 30% of cases of complete heart block, but in the Author's experience the incidence is much less than this. The essence of this "arrhythmia" is that P-P intervals which include a QRS complex are shorter than those which do not. An example is shown in Figure 358.

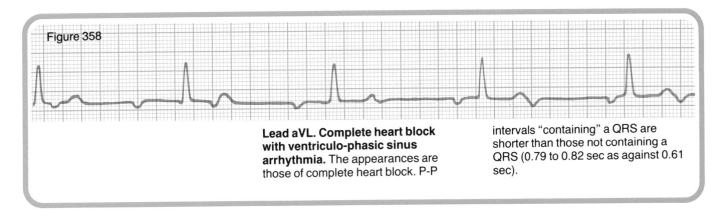

Lead aVL. Complete heart block with ventriculo-phasic sinus arrhythmia. The appearances are those of complete heart block. P-P intervals "containing" a QRS are shorter than those not containing a QRS (0.79 to 0.82 sec as against 0.61 sec).

This can be contrasted with the more usual appearance when the sinus node shows no detectable variation in rate in relation to the QRS complexes (Figure 359).

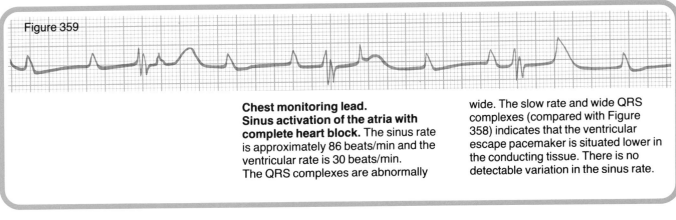

Chest monitoring lead. Sinus activation of the atria with complete heart block. The sinus rate is approximately 86 beats/min and the ventricular rate is 30 beats/min. The QRS complexes are abnormally wide. The slow rate and wide QRS complexes (compared with Figure 358) indicates that the ventricular escape pacemaker is situated lower in the conducting tissue. There is no detectable variation in the sinus rate.

The mechanism of ventriculo-phasic sinus arrhythmia is unknown. It has been postulated that ventricular contraction reflexly (via baro-receptors) induces transient increases in the sinus rate via the sympathetic nervous system. This explanation is highly speculative. Variation in sinus rate during complete heart block is of no significance.

Criteria for third degree ("complete") atrio-ventricular block

1. No consistent or meaningful relationship between atrial and ventricular activity can be recognised.

2. The QRS complexes may be normal in shape, duration and axis* but more often are abnormal in shape, duration and axis.†

3. The form of the QRS complexes is usually constant.**

4. The QRS rate is usually constant†† and lies within the range of 15-70 beats/min.†††

5. Any form of atrial activity may be seen, or there may be no atrial activity.***

* In the case of the uncommon high septal or His bundle escape mechanism.

† In the case of the common low ventricular escape mechanism.

** The form of the QRS complexes may vary if the active escape site varies or two or more escape sites are active simultaneously.

†† If the ventricular escape site varies (4, above) the rate will vary.

††† With a high septal or His bundle escape mechanism the rate will be in the region of 60 beats/min. In the case of a low ventricular escape mechanism the rate will usually be in the region of 20-30 beats/min.

*** Most commonly the atrial activity will be sinus-initiated. Typically the sinus rate will be rapid (90-120 beats/min) and constant. Occasionally ventriculo-phasic arrhythmia (page 503) will be seen.

Anatomical Site of Heart Block

Third Degree Atrio-ventricular Block ("Complete Heart Block")

Third degree atrio-ventricular block may occur because of:

1. complete failure of conduction through the atrio-ventricular node

or

2. complete failure of conduction through the His bundle

or

3. complete failure of conduction through the right and left bundle branches simultaneously (see Figure 333).

Second Degree Atrio-ventricular Block

Second degree atrio-ventricular block may occur because of:

1. partial (i.e. intermittent) failure of conduction at the atrio-ventricular node

or

2. partial (i.e. intermittent) failure of conduction at the bundle of His

or

3. simultaneous partial (simultaneously intermittent) failure of conduction in both bundle branches (a relatively uncommon occurrence)

or

4. partial (intermittent) failure of conduction in one bundle branch in the presence of pre-existing complete (persistent) failure of conduction in the contralateral bundle branch.

Type I second degree atrio-ventricular block

The atrio-ventricular node is the site of the vast majority of type I second degree atrio-ventricular block.* Electrophysiological studies indicate that type I block can occasionally occur below the atrio-ventricular node (i.e. in the His bundles or bundle branches) but examples of this are very rare.

Type II second degree atrio-ventricular block

Either the His bundle or the bundle branches is the site of the vast majority of type II second degree atrio-ventricular block. Again electrophysiological studies do indicate that type II block can be seen in the atrio-ventricular node but examples are very few. Effectively, therefore, type I block indicates an AV nodal disturbance and type II block an infranodal disturbance.

2:1 Atrio-ventricular Block

This represents a special case which can be type I or type II. It can therefore occur because of malfunction at the AV node or below this site (in the bundle of His or simultaneously in both bundle branches). Analysis of the ECG during sustained 2:1 atrio-ventricular block does not permit the distinction to be made. If, however, periods of 2:1 block are interrupted by periods of 3:2, 4:3 or higher proportions of conducted beats, then the distinction can usually be made by inference for during such periods the P-R interval of the conducted beats is either incremental (in which case type I block is present) or fixed (in which case type II block can be presumed).

High-grade Atrio-ventricular Block

This is usually indicative of infranodal disease (i.e. the disturbance in conduction is in the bundle of His or the bundle branches).

---

* Type I block may be physiological or pathological. As stated in the text (page 496) type I block will normally occur during incremental atrial pacing (and typically when a rate of 150-160 beats/min is achieved) if the subject does not receive atropine and it is known to occur spontaneously in trained athletes after exertion. It may, of course, also occur as a result of disease of the atrio-ventricular node. It is recognisably pathological when it is present despite the absence of a sufficiently rapid atrial depolarisation rate to make it inevitable. (This rate depends on the age of the subject but in adults it tends to be in the range 130-150 beats/min).

505

First Degree Atrio-ventricular Block

First degree heart block is almost always due to conduction delay in the atrio-ventricular node. Relatively rarely, first degree atrio-ventricular block with normal QRS complexes may be shown electrophysiologically to be the result of intra-His conduction delay, but such examples are very uncommon.

A summary of the anatomical sites of the ECG appearances in the various types of atrio-ventricular block is given in Table 40.

Conduction Disturbances other than at Atrio-ventricular Level

This chapter has concentrated on disturbances of **atrio-ventricular** conduction mechanisms. Other conduction disturbances (which are dealt with elsewhere in this text) include:

Sino-atrial block (see pages 381 and 382)

Intra-atrial block (see below)

Intraventricular block (i.e. right bundle branch block, left bundle branch block, left anterior hemiblock, left posterior hemiblock, parietal block (see pages 110-143)

Intra-atrial block

Intra-atrial block gives rise to an abnormal P wave configuration in the same way that intraventricular block gives rise to an abnormal QRS configuration (e.g. bundle branch block). Intra-atrial block is difficult to distinguish from other causes of changes in the P wave morphology (e.g. left atrial hypertrophy and right atrial hypertrophy) and is of no practical significance.

Table 40 Atrio-ventricular block

Designation	ECG criteria	Frequency	Usual anatomical site of lesion
First degree	Constant, prolonged P-R interval. The QRS complex has the usual form for that subject and will tend to be normal unless there is a prior abnormality of intraventricular conduction.	Common	Atrio-ventricular node
Second degree type I (Wenckebach)	Progressive prolongation of P-R interval in successive beats until transient atrio-ventricular block for one beat occurs followed by initial restoration of the P-R interval and further successive prolongation until a dropped beat occurs again.	Common	Atrio-ventricular node
type II (Möbitz type II)	Transient AV block (one beat at a time) in the absence of prior P-R interval prolongation. The QRS complexes will have the form which is usual for that subject. They will be normal unless there is a pre-existing defect of intraventricular conduction.	Uncommon	His bundle, bundle branches
2:1 type I }* 2:1 type II	Alternate P waves conduct and alternate P waves fail to conduct (therefore there is no possibility of observing a change in the P-R interval). The QRS complexes will have the form which is usual for that subject. They will therefore usually be normal unless there is a pre-existing defect of intraventricular conduction.	Relatively common	*{ AV node His bundle and bundle branches
High grade (usually type II but can be type I)	Two or more P waves fail to conduct for each P wave which does conduct (AV conduction ratio is 3:1 or greater). The P-R interval of the conducted beats is constant.	Relatively uncommon	His bundle, bundle branches
Third degree type I	P waves will have the usual form for the subject. QRS complexes may also have the usual form for the subject (if there is a high ventricular escape pacemaker situated above the bifurcation of the bundle of His. In this event the ventricular escape rate will tend to be relatively rapid and of the order of 50-60 beats/min). More commonly the QRS complexes will be abnormally wide and abnormally shaped and the escape rate will be substantially less (in the region of 20-40 beats/min). In this event the ventricular escape pacemaker is situated low down in the ventricles and probably in the Purkinje network.	Common	AV node (a)
type II	as for **Third Degree** type I (above)	Common	His bundle (b) or both divisions (left anterior and left posterior) of the left bundle together with the right bundle branch (c) or combinations of (b) and (c) (above) sufficient to interrupt the atrio-ventricular pathway.
type I and II combined	as for **Third Degree** type I (above)	Common	(a) + (b) or (a) + (c) (above)

*These two cannot be distinguished from the surface ECG during 2:1 conduction

Pacemaker Electrocardiography

Artificial cardiac pacemakers are, of course, effectively devices for delivering a brief electrical stimulus to part of the heart to induce depolarisation at the chosen site. Both the electrical stimulus and the resulting local depolarisation are readily visible on the electrocardiogram. Analysis of the stimulus artefact, the resulting atrial and/or ventricular myocardial depolarisation and the relationship of the stimulus artefact and myocardial depolarisation to preceding and to succeeding spontaneous or pacemaker-induced cardiac cycles, forms the essence of analysis of pacemaker electrocardiograms. This is actually an exceedingly complex and difficult field and it is constantly evolving as pacemaker technology develops. For these reasons and because numerous specialised books have been written on the subject (and will continually have to be updated), only fundamental essentials of the subject will be considered and no attempt will be made to be comprehensive.

Fundamental Aspects of the Pacemaker Electrocardiogram

The Stimulus Artefact ("Pacemaker Spike")

Pulses delivered to the myocardium by artificial cardiac pacemakers are of relatively large voltage and relatively brief duration. To gain a correct perspective of the amplitude and duration of the stimulus artefact it should be observed that the calibration signal seen at the top left hand side of Figure 1 (Section 1, page 4) represents (at normal gain on the ECG amplifier) 1 millivolt and has a duration of 120 msec (0.12 sec). A typical pacemaker stimulus delivers about 5 volts to the myocardium and results in a surface-recorded pacemaker artefact of about 200mV (i.e. 200 times longer than the calibration signal). Conventional electrocardiographic recorders cannot adequately cope with such a rapid signal or with such a large signal as the pacemaker stimulus artefact. The artefact is therefore very incompletely and inadequately displayed on conventional electrocardiographic records and where detailed analysis of the stimulus artefact is required (as in pacemaker follow-up and management) oscilloscopic (or equivalent) recording is required. However, for the purpose of analysing pacemaker function with the conventional ECG recorder, the mere recognition of the presence of the stimulus artefact is usually sufficient.

The Myocardial Response: Ventricular Myocardium

When a pacing stimulus is applied to the ventricular myocardium, if the stimulus is sufficiently strong to "capture" the myocardium (i.e. to give rise to a local action potential) the locally-induced depolarisation will spread to all parts of the myocardium which are in electrical continuity with the site at which the depolarisation was initiated. The typical location for the tip of a ventricular pacing electrode is in the apex of the right ventricle. Depolarisation of the ventricles induced by such an electrode is, in effect, a ventricular ectopic beat and will have all the electrocardiographic characteristics of such a beat. Thus the ventricular depolarisation wave has approximately the same form as the QRS complexes of a ventricular ectopic beat. Since the ventricular myocardial depolarisation is initiated in the **right** ventricle the ventricular myocardial response has the form of a right ventricular ectopic beat (i.e. resembles left bundle branch block (page 414)). Since the apex of the right ventricle is inferior with respect to most of the ventricular myocardium, the ventricular depolarisation wave is superiorly orientated and the frontal plane QRS axis of the ventricular depolarisation wave (QRS complex) tends to be in the region of −75 to −90°.

Figure 360a shows the typical shape of a pacemaker stimulus artefact. Figure 360b shows the pacemaker spike immediately followed by a ventricular response. The pacing stimulus is extremely brief. The ECG recorder only captures the terminal, descending part of the stimulus artefact. The induced QRS is wide and abnormally shaped. The ventricular depolarisation (QRS) is induced by the pacemaker stimulus. Ventricular repolarisation (the T wave) inevitably occurs following the depolarisation.

Figure 360

The pacemaker stimulus and the ventricular response

a) The typical configuration of the pacing stimulus as seen on an oscilloscope. The voltage rises virtually instantaneously. There is a slow decay over about 5 msec and the voltage then falls abruptly. To display such a waveform the recorder would have to have a frequency response two orders of magnitude greater than that possessed by the conventional electrocardiograph and would have to accept higher voltages than these machines can manage. On a conventional electrocardiographic recorder only the terminal part of the decay of voltage would be detected (shown thickened on this diagram).

b) The typical appearances of a pacing stimulus and ventricular response as seen on a conventional electrocardiograph. The upstroke of the pacing stimulus is not seen – there is merely a break in the trace. The first part of the stimulus artefact to be shown is the terminal part of its decay (see (a) above). This leads straight into an abnormally-wide, abnormally-shaped QRS complex (with consequent abnormally-shaped S-T segment and T wave).

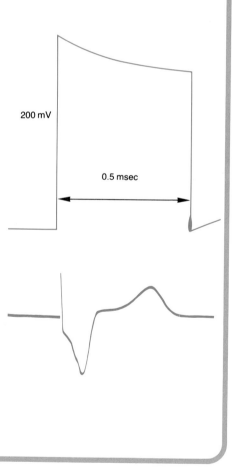

200 mV

0.5 msec

An example of ventricular pacing is shown in Figure 361. The pacing stimulus is apparent in each lead. The pacing-induced QRS complexes have the same morphology as in left bundle branch block and the mean frontal plane QRS axis is −75° (an "abnormal" degree of left axis deviation but actually entirely appropriate for ventricular pacing from the apex of the right ventricle).

Figure 361

12-lead electrocardiogram. Ventricular pacing.

In each lead the **pacing stimulus** (pacemaker spike) is visible as a fine vertical line at the beginning of each QRS complex. The deflection shown is only a tiny part of the pacemaker spike since the electrocardiograph cannot cope with the speed or amplitude of the voltage change induced by the pacing stimulus. Even though only the slowest part of the pacing stimulus is shown it is still the fastest deflection recorded (i.e. it contains higher frequency components than any other part of the recorded electrocardiogram). Following each pacing stimulus there is a QRS complex. It is clear, therefore, that each pacing stimulus "captures" (i.e. results in the adjacent depolarisation of) the ventricular myocardium. Ventricular myocardial depolarisation is therefore ectopic and the induced QRS complexes have the characteristics of ventricular ectopic beats. Since ventricular depolarisation is initiated in the right ventricle it has the characteristics of a right ventricular ectopic beat, i.e. the QRS complexes have the morphology of left bundle branch block (page 414). The QRS complexes are therefore abnormally wide (0.12 sec or longer) and do not display initial q waves in leads facing the left ventricle (as in left bundle branch block, Section 2, page 124). Further, since the pacemaker electrode tip is normally situated at the apex of the right ventricle (virtually the most inferior position of the ventricular endocardium) the predominant direction of ventricular myocardial depolarisation is from inferior to superior. As a result the mean frontal plane QRS axis is directed superiorly (usually in the region of −75 to −90°).

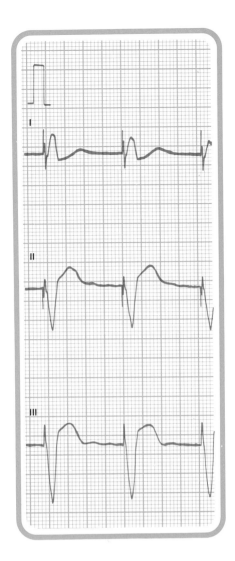
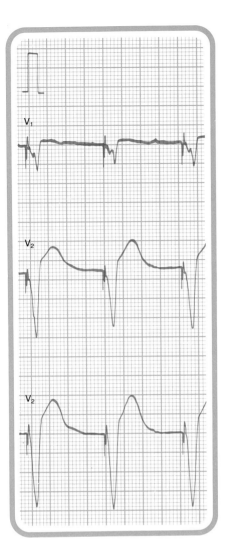
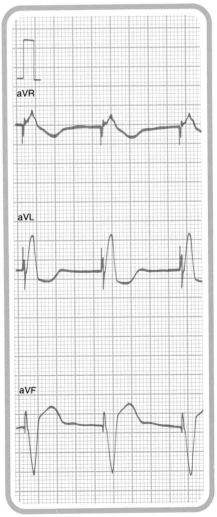
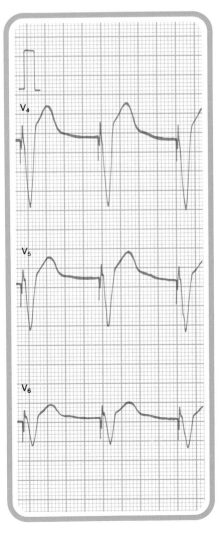

The Myocardial Response: Atrial Myocardium

If the pacemaker electrode is applied to the atrial rather than to the ventricular myocardium each pacing spike initiates, and is immediately followed by, an ectopic atrial depolarisation. If the pacing electrode is situated in the right atrium the resulting P waves will, of course, have the same morphology as the P waves of right atrial ectopic beats. Since the morphology of the P waves is rather nondescript (compared with that of the QRS complexes) it is often difficult or impossible to be sure of the precise site of origin of atrial myocardial depolarisation from the shape of the P waves. (In the case of atrial beats of junctional origin it is, of course, easy to recognise negative P waves in the inferior limb leads (page 393)). Figure 362 shows an example of atrial pacing. Each pacing spike is followed by a P wave. A normal QRS follows after a P-R interval of 0.22 sec. The normal (i.e. in shape and width) QRS complex indicates that ventricular myocardial depolarisation is consistently being induced from a site above the bifurcation of the His bundle and it is likely that it has been initiated as a result of the spread of atrial myocardial depolarisation (itself initiated by the pacing stimulus in the right atrium) to the atrio-ventricular node and through it to the His bundle.

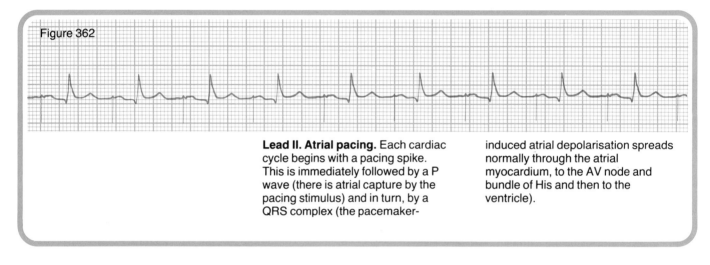

Figure 362

Lead II. Atrial pacing. Each cardiac cycle begins with a pacing spike. This is immediately followed by a P wave (there is atrial capture by the pacing stimulus) and in turn, by a QRS complex (the pacemaker-induced atrial depolarisation spreads normally through the atrial myocardium, to the AV node and bundle of His and then to the ventricle).

Pacemaker Sensing of Ventricular (Non-pacemaker-induced) Myocardial Depolarisation

The earliest pacemakers were very simple devices which applied a depolarising stimulus to the myocardium at a regular rate, taking no account of the presence or absence of any spontaneous depolarisations. These "fixed rate", or "asynchronous" pacemakers have become obsolete.

The next important development was that of the "demand" pacemaker. This device permits the recognition of spontaneous depolarisation and the subsequent inhibition of the artificial pacing stimulus for defined intervals of time following such recognition. In the case of ventricular demand units, spontaneous ventricular depolarisation is recognised by the pacemaker unit (the spontaneous voltage being sensed via the same wire electrode which is used for pacemaker stimulation). When such a spontaneous depolarisation is recognised the pacemaker unit is inhibited for a defined period (called the "escape interval"). If a further spontaneous voltage is recognised during this period the inhibition is initiated once more and the escape interval of inhibition is recommenced.

The mode of functioning of a
demand ventricular pacemaker is shown
in Figure 363.

Figure 363   Ventricular demand pacing: basic features

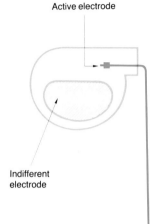

Active electrode

Indifferent
electrode

a) The pacemaker unit contains all the control electronics. The pacing electrode is a single-wire connection from the pacing unit to the apex of the right ventricle. The electrode is covered with insulating material except at its point of connection to the pacemaker unit ("active electrode") and at its tip in the right ventricle. A circuit (current path) is formed as follows: active electrode, pacemaker wire, pacemaker tip, right ventricular myocardium, body fluids between right ventricular myocardium and the

indifferent electrode, indifferent electrode, pacemaker electronics, active electrode. In this geometrically complex circuit the current density is greatest at the pacing electrode tip within the right ventricle. It is this differential current density which guarantees that right ventricular depolarisation is induced but that chest-wall muscle depolarisation is not. Stimulation and sensing are carried respectively from and to the pacemaker unit via the pacing electrode.

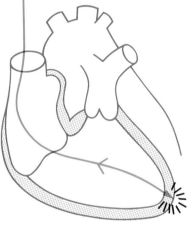

Ventricular
pacemaker
output
escape
interval

(VOEI)

Ventricular
pacing
interval

b) During any rhythm in which QRS complexes are generated and recognised by the pacemaker electronics, the recognition of the QRS complex induces resetting of the pacemaker ventricular output escape interval (VOEI). No pacemaker stimulus occurs until one complete escape interval has elapsed following the last recognised QRS complex. The first five beats in the illustration are sinus beats. The interval between consecutive QRS complexes during this period is less than the escape interval and no pacing stimulus occurs. After the fifth QRS complex there is a longer pause. When no

QRS is recognised within the defined (for that particular pacemaker unit) "pacemaker escape interval", the pacemaker unit will deliver a pacing stimulus. This is immediately followed by a pacemaker-induced QRS complex. Like a ventricular ectopic beat, it is abnormally wide and abnormally shaped and is followed by an abnormal S-T segment and an abnormal T wave. The QRS complex, S-T segment and T wave have the configurations appropriate to left bundle branch block since the beat is, in effect, a (pacemaker-induced) right ventricular ectopic beat (see page 510). Since no spontaneous QRS

follows the sixth beat before the completion of the automatic pacing interval, a further paced beat follows. In this case (as is often so) the pacemaker escape interval is longer than the automatic pacing interval. This phenomenon (which is totally dependent on the form of the pacemaker circuitry or programming) is called "hysteresis". Its purpose is to allow spontaneous sinus rhythm (which is haemodynamically preferable to ventricular pacing) to be maintained at a lower rate than the standby pacing rate.

Ventricular demand pacing permits only (a) **sensing** ventricular activity (supraventricularly-initiated QRS complexes or ventricularly-initiated QRS complexes) and (b) **stimulation** of the ventricular myocardium if no QRS has been sensed within the ventricular output escape interval. Examples of the possible behaviour of such a system are shown in Figure 364.

Figure 364   **Ventricular demand pacing: some examples of behaviour**

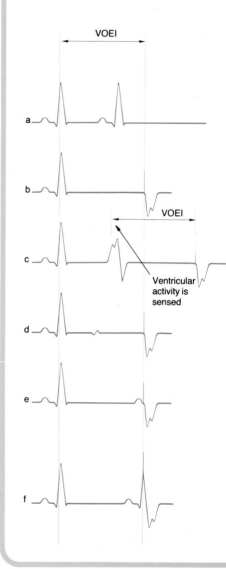

a) R-R interval is less than the ventricular output escape interval (VOEI) therefore ventricular pacing is inhibited. (No pacing spikes, no myocardium paced).

b) No spontaneous QRS complex occurs within the VOEI. A ventricular pacing spike is thus "released" and this is followed by ventricular depolarisation. (No ventricular sensing, ventricular pacing spike, ventricular response).

c) A ventricular premature beat occurs within the VOEI. This interval is therefore re-set. Since no further ventricular activity occurs within this re-set VOEI a pacing stimulus occurs followed by ventricular capture. (Ventricular sensing, ventricular spike, ventricular capture).

d) An atrial premature beat occurs within the VOEI. This cannot be sensed by the pacemaker. It is not conducted to the ventricles and no QRS complex occurs within the VOEI. Inevitably, therefore, a ventricular pacing spike is "released" and is followed by an induced QRS. If the atrial premature beat had been conducted to the ventricles it would have been recognised by the pacemaker and the VOEI would have been re-set.

e) A P wave occurs before the end of the VOEI but then cannot be sensed by the pacemaker. There may well have been a QRS to follow the P wave but the end of the VOEI occurs soon after the P wave (and before the QRS could possibly appear). A ventricular pacing spike occurs at the end of the VOEI and is followed by ventricular capture. (No ventricular sensing, ventricular pacing spike, ventricular capture).

f) As in (e) a P wave occurs within the VOEI, but in this case it occurs sufficiently early for conduction to proceed to the ventricles. The beginnings of a normal QRS are initiated. Within the early part of this QRS the VOEI terminates and a ventricular pacing spike occurs (i.e. the pacing spike is "released" before ventricular sensing is achieved). The QRS is a fusion beat, partly initiated spontaneously and partly pacemaker-induced.

Atrial Demand Pacing

If the pacing electrode is in contact with atrial myocardium rather than with ventricular myocardium, an entirely analogous set of circumstances will obtain. If asynchronous (fixed rate) atrial pacing (i.e. with no sensing of spontaneous P waves) is utilised, regular atrial pacing will occur. The pacing stimulus will compete with the sino-atrial node for capture of the atrial myocardium. As in the case of asynchronous ventricular pacing (fixed rate ventricular pacing) so in the case of asynchronous atrial pacing (fixed rate atrial pacing) this mode of pacing is obsolete. If the pacemaker unit has sensing capability then atrial demand (atrial synchronous) pacing will occur. Figure 365 shows the mode of operation of atrial demand pacing.

Figure 365 **Atrial demand pacing: basic features**

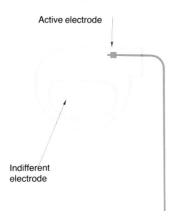

Active electrode

Indifferent electrode

a) The pacemaker unit contains all the control electronics. The pacing electrode is a single-wire connection from the pacing unit to the right atrial appendage. The electrode is covered with insulating material except at its point of connection with a pacemaker unit ("active electrode") and at the tip in the right atrial appendage. A circuit (current path) is formed as follows: active electrode, pacemaker wire, pacemaker tip, right atrial myocardium, body fluids between right atrial myocardium and the

indifferent electrode, indifferent electrode, pacemaker electronics, active electrode. In this geometrically complex circuit the current density is greatest at the pacing electrode tip within the right atrium. It is this differential current density which guarantees that right atrial depolarisation is induced but that chest-wall depolarisation is not. Stimulation and sensing are carried respectively from and to the pacemaker unit via the pacing electrode.

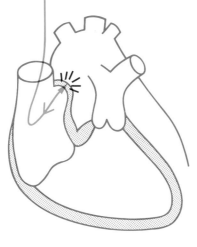

Atrial pacemaker output escape interval (AOEI)

Atrial pacing interval

b) During any rhythm in which P waves are generated and recognised by the pacemaker electronics, the recognition of a P wave induces re-setting of the atrial output escape interval (AOEI). No pacemaker stimulus occurs until one complete AOEI has elapsed following the last recognised P wave. The first five beats in the illustration are sinus beats. The interval between consecutive P waves during this period is less than the AOEI and no pacing stimulus occurs. After the fifth P wave there is a longer pause. When

no P wave is recognised within the defined (for that particular pacemaker) AOEI, the pacemaker unit will deliver a stimulus. This is immediately followed by a pacemaker-induced P wave. Like an atrial ectopic beat, it is abnormally shaped. Since no spontaneous P wave follows the sixth beat within the time interval designated as the automatic pacing interval, a further paced beat occurs. In this case the pacemaker escape interval is longer than the automatic pacing interval. This phenomenon (which is totally

dependent on the form of the pacemaker circuitry or programming) is called "hysteresis". Although it is often possible to programme this property into atrial demand pacemakers it has no obvious advantage (contrast ventricular demand pacing where it helps to maintain atrial transport at slightly lower rates than would otherwise be possible). It is shown only for clarity. Where there is no hysteresis the AOEI and the pacemaker escape interval are identical.

Atrial demand pacing permits only (a) **sensing** atrial activity (sinus-induced P waves, ectopic P waves, retrograde P waves of ventricular depolarisation and (b) **stimulation** of the atrial myocardium if no P wave has been sensed within the atrial output escape interval. Examples of the possible behaviour of such a system are shown in Figure 366.

Figure 366 Atrial demand pacing: some examples of behaviour

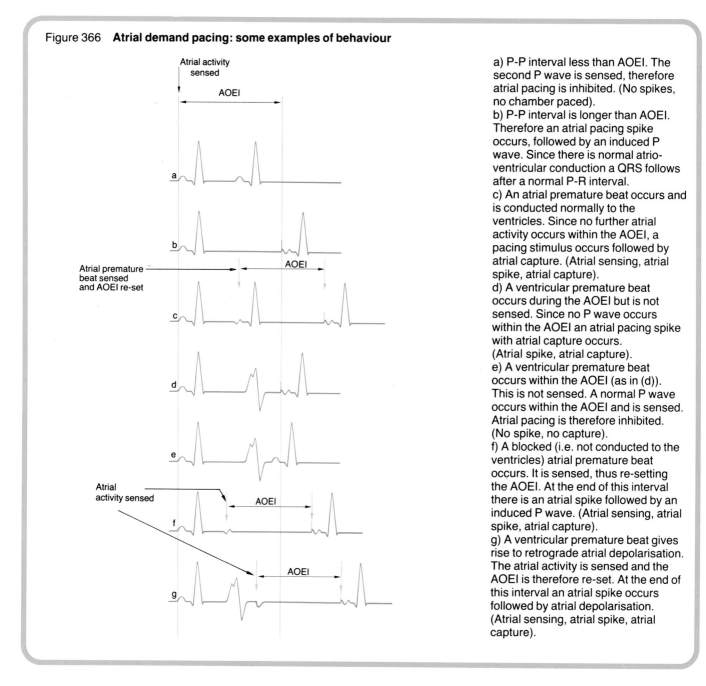

a) P-P interval less than AOEI. The second P wave is sensed, therefore atrial pacing is inhibited. (No spikes, no chamber paced).

b) P-P interval is longer than AOEI. Therefore an atrial pacing spike occurs, followed by an induced P wave. Since there is normal atrio-ventricular conduction a QRS follows after a normal P-R interval.

c) An atrial premature beat occurs and is conducted normally to the ventricles. Since no further atrial activity occurs within the AOEI, a pacing stimulus occurs followed by atrial capture. (Atrial sensing, atrial spike, atrial capture).

d) A ventricular premature beat occurs during the AOEI but is not sensed. Since no P wave occurs within the AOEI an atrial pacing spike with atrial capture occurs. (Atrial spike, atrial capture).

e) A ventricular premature beat occurs within the AOEI (as in (d)). This is not sensed. A normal P wave occurs within the AOEI and is sensed. Atrial pacing is therefore inhibited. (No spike, no capture).

f) A blocked (i.e. not conducted to the ventricles) atrial premature beat occurs. It is sensed, thus re-setting the AOEI. At the end of this interval there is an atrial spike followed by an induced P wave. (Atrial sensing, atrial spike, atrial capture).

g) A ventricular premature beat gives rise to retrograde atrial depolarisation. The atrial activity is sensed and the AOEI is therefore re-set. At the end of this interval an atrial spike occurs followed by atrial depolarisation. (Atrial sensing, atrial spike, atrial capture).

Dual-chamber Pacing Systems

So far, single-chamber pacing of the ventricles or atria (each in the synchronous or asynchronous mode) has been discussed. It is also, of course, possible to pace both atria and ventricles. Such pacing requires two discrete electrodes, one to the right atrium and the other to the right ventricle. Again, fixed rate (asynchronous) atrial and ventricular pacing is possible (with a fixed interval between the atrial and ventricular stimuli) but is very rarely used. Almost without exception, dual-chamber pacing systems involve sensing of ventricular activity, of atrial activity or of both atrial and ventricular activity. The circuitry of the pacing units and the electrocardiographic appearances both become correspondingly more complex.

Figure 367 shows the anatomical situation and one possible set of electrocardiographic appearances in relation to dual-chamber pacing.

Figure 367 Dual-chamber pacing: basic features

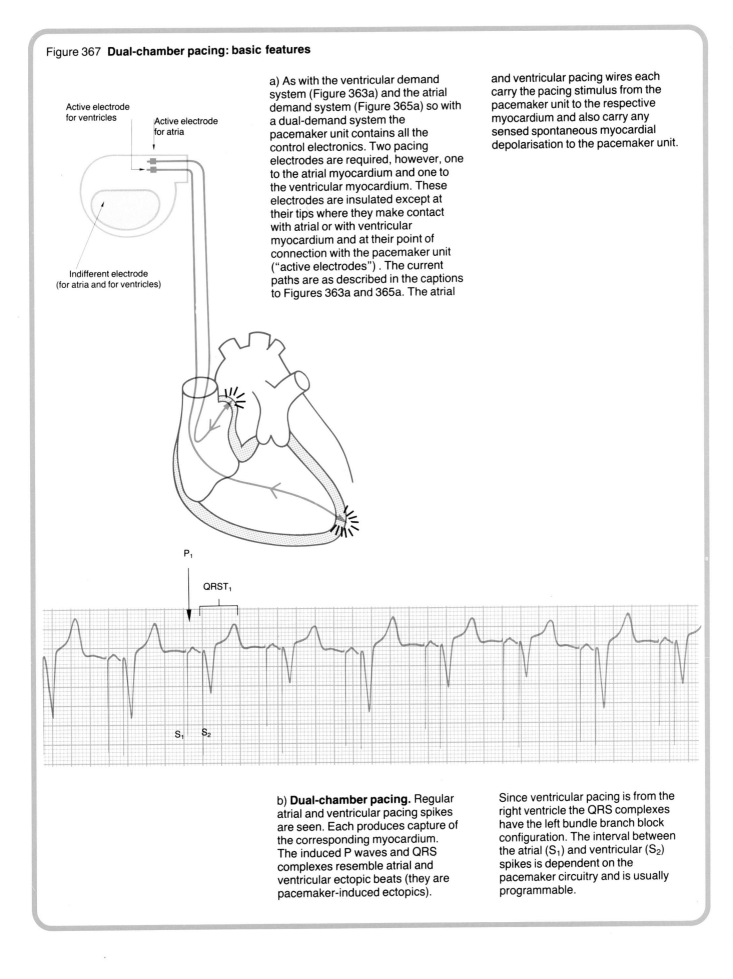

Active electrode for ventricles

Active electrode for atria

Indifferent electrode (for atria and for ventricles)

P₁

QRST₁

S₁ S₂

a) As with the ventricular demand system (Figure 363a) and the atrial demand system (Figure 365a) so with a dual-demand system the pacemaker unit contains all the control electronics. Two pacing electrodes are required, however, one to the atrial myocardium and one to the ventricular myocardium. These electrodes are insulated except at their tips where they make contact with atrial or with ventricular myocardium and at their point of connection with the pacemaker unit ("active electrodes"). The current paths are as described in the captions to Figures 363a and 365a. The atrial and ventricular pacing wires each carry the pacing stimulus from the pacemaker unit to the respective myocardium and also carry any sensed spontaneous myocardial depolarisation to the pacemaker unit.

b) **Dual-chamber pacing.** Regular atrial and ventricular pacing spikes are seen. Each produces capture of the corresponding myocardium. The induced P waves and QRS complexes resemble atrial and ventricular ectopic beats (they are pacemaker-induced ectopics).

Since ventricular pacing is from the right ventricle the QRS complexes have the left bundle branch block configuration. The interval between the atrial (S_1) and ventricular (S_2) spikes is dependent on the pacemaker circuitry and is usually programmable.

The International Pacemaker Code

With the advent of increasingly complex pacemaker systems, the need for an internationally-recognised convention for the abbreviated description of pacing modes became apparent. In response to this need a code of five letters was devised. The fourth and fifth letters refer to the pacemaker's programmability and tachyarrhythmia-inhibiting functions respectively, and these functions are not relevant to this text. This presentation will therefore be confined to the first three letters of the code. This "three-letter" code or "three-position" pacemaker code identifies the major features of the pacemaker function. The first and second letters of the code refer to the chamber(s) paced and the chamber(s) sensed respectively. (A = atrium, V = ventricle, D = double (both), O = neither) and the third letter refers to the mode of response when activity is sensed (I = inhibited, T = triggered, D = atrial-triggered and ventricular-inhibited, O = not applicable). This terminology is presented in Table 41.

Table 41 The three-letter pacemaker code

First letter	Second letter	Third letter
Chamber paced	Chamber sensed	Mode of response
	O = no sensing	O = no response
V = ventricle	V = ventricle	I = inhibited
A = atrium	A = atrium	T = triggered
D = double (atrium and ventricle)	D = double (atrium and ventricle)	D = atrial sensing triggers ventricular stimulation, ventricular sensing inhibits stimulation of atria, ventricles or both

Pacemaker Modalities

The pacemaker code is used to describe the modality (operational characteristics) of the particular pacemaker units. Available modalities are given in Table 42.

Table 42 Modalities of pacemaker function (pacemaker operational characteristics)

Code	Functional description	Common designations
	Atrial Lead Only	
AOO	A 1)* Atrium paced; ventricle not paced O 2)* No sensory function O 3)* No triggering or inhibiting function	"Atrial fixed rate", "Atrial asynchronous"
AAI	A 1)* Atrium paced; ventricle not paced A 2)* Atrium sensed; ventricle not sensed I 3)* Sensed (spontaneous) atrial activity inhibits atrial stimulation	"Atrial inhibited", "P wave inhibited", "Atrial demand"
AAT	A 1)* Atrium paced; ventricle not paced A 2)* Atrium sensed; ventricle not sensed T 3)* Sensed atrial activity triggers atrial stimulation on top of the sensed P wave	"Atrial triggered", "P wave triggered", or "P wave synchronous" **atrial pacing**
	Ventricular Lead Only	
VOO	V 1)* Ventricle paced; atrium not paced O 2)* No sensory function O 3)* No triggering or inhibiting function	"Ventricular fixed rate", "Ventricular asynchronous"
VVI	V 1)* Ventricle paced; atrium not paced V 2)* Ventricle sensed; atrium not sensed I 3)* Sensed (spontaneous) ventricular activity inhibits ventricular stimulation	"Ventricular inhibited", "R wave inhibited", "Ventricular demand"
VVT	V 1)* Ventricle paced; atrium not paced V 2)* Ventricle sensed; atrium not sensed T 3)* Sensed (spontaneous) ventricular activity triggers ventricular stimulation on top of the sensed QRS	"Ventricular triggered", "R wave triggered", "R wave synchronous"
	Atrial and Ventricular Leads	
DOO	D 1)* Atrium paced; ventricle paced O 2)* No sensory function O 3)* No triggering or inhibiting function	"AV sequential fixed rate", "AV sequential asynchronous"
VAT	V 1)* Ventricle paced; atrium not paced A 2)* Atrium sensed; ventricle not sensed T 3)* Sensed (spontaneous) atrial activity triggers ventricular stimulation after suitable (predetermined) delay	"Atrial triggered" "P wave triggered" or "P wave synchronous", **ventricular pacing** Also known as "AV synchronous" pacing
DVI	D 1)* Atrium paced; ventricle paced V 2)* Ventricle sensed; atrium not sensed I 3)* Sensed (spontaneous) ventricular activity inhibits whole unit (i.e. inhibits atrial and ventricular stimulation)	"Atrio-ventricular sequential demand", "Bifocal sequential demand"
VDD	V 1)* Ventricle paced; atrium not paced D 2)* Atrium sensed; ventricle sensed D 3)* Sensed (spontaneous) atrial activity triggers ventricular stimulation after suitable (pre-determined) delay; sensed ventricular activity inhibits (ventricular) stimulation	"P wave synchronous", "Ventricular inhibited"
DDD	D 1)* Atrium paced; ventricle paced D 2)* Atrium sensed, ventricle sensed D 3)* Sensed (spontaneous) atrial activity (a) inhibits ventricular stimulation (b) triggers ventricular stimulation after a suitable (predetermined) delay; sensed (spontaneous) ventricular activity inhibits ventricular stimulation	"Fully automatic", "Optimal sequential", "Universal"

* Numbers refer to position of letter in the code
1) = first letter, 2) = second letter, 3) = third letter.

Electrocardiographic Appearances of Single Function Pacing Modes

No attempt is being made in this section to provide a portfolio of the electrocardiography of normally functioning and malfunctioning pacemakers. The range of possibilities is enormous (especially in relation to DDD pacemakers). In addition, some pacing modes have become obsolete (e.g. VOO) and some have never had any practical value in management (e.g. DOO and AOO). Furthermore pacemaker technology is continually evolving and many currently available pacing modes may not stand the test of time. A few examples, therefore, will serve to illustrate the principles of pacemaker electrocardiography.

AAI Pacing

In relation to this designation the first "A" refers to the ability of the unit to pace the atrium, the second "A" to the ability of the unit to sense any spontaneous atrial activity and the "I" to the ability of the unit to inhibit a pacing output to the atrium whenever spontaneous atrial activity is sensed.

An example is shown in Figure 368.

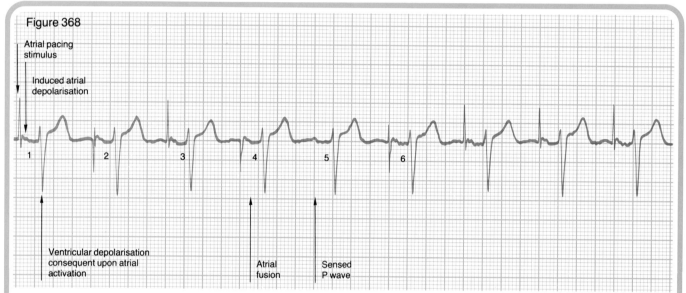

Figure 368

Atrial pacing stimulus

Induced atrial depolarisation

Ventricular depolarisation consequent upon atrial activation

Atrial fusion

Sensed P wave

Chest monitoring lead. AAI pacing.
The first complex shows the atrial pacing stimulus, immediately followed by the induced atrial depolarisation wave (i.e. there is "atrial capture") . The P wave is abnormal in shape since the atrial depolarisation is, in fact, ectopic (induced at an ectopic site by the pacing stimulus). The induced atrial depolarisation wave is followed, after an interval (pacemaker spike to onset of QRS complex) of 0.22 sec, by a normal QRS complex. The depolarisation wave has clearly spread from the atrial myocardium in an entirely normal fashion through the AV node. The true P'-R interval is slightly less than 0.22 sec but one cannot assess this precisely since the moment of onset of atrial myocardial depolarisation cannot be recognised – it must be at some point between the onset of the atrial pacing stimulus and the recognisable onset of the P' wave. Since ventricular myocardial depolarisation is normal (QRS is

normal) ventricular myocardial repolarisation is normal and the S-T segments and T waves are both therefore within normal limits.
The first three beats show exactly the same process (the polarity of the pacing stimulus varies because the axis of the heart and of the pacemaker stimulus vary during the respiratory process). The fourth beat shows atrial fusion. Spontaneous atrial activity presumably begins (but is not seen) just prior to the onset of the pacing stimulus. The atrial myocardium is therefore depolarised by two routes; one initiated at the sino-atrial node and one at the pacemaker electrode. The fusion can only be inferred (not proven). It is inferred because the morphology of the fourth P' wave differs slightly from that of the first three waves and the fourth P' wave is briefer than the other three, suggesting that it began just before or during the onset of the pacing spike. The fifth atrial depolarisation wave is

entirely spontaneous (there is no preceding spike). This P wave is a sinus-initiated beat. The absence of a pacemaker spike indicates that the atrial depolarisation has been sensed. After a normal P-R interval of 0.20 sec a normal QRS and T wave follows. It is possible that the sixth atrial depolarisation is a fusion beat (and it is probable that the second atrial depolarisation was also a fusion beat). All subsequent beats are atrially-paced beats.
In relation to the designation AAI, (1) the second "A" function is demonstrated by the recognition by the pacemaker unit of the fifth atrial activation, (2) the "I" function is indicated by inhibition of the pacemaker spike following this recognition and (3) the first "A" function is indicated by the atrial pacing spike occurring in situations in which no atrial activity is sensed.

AAT and AOO Modes

These are rarely used and will not be discussed here.

VOO Pacing

In relation to this designation, the "V" refers to the ability of the unit to pace the ventricle and the first "O" refers to the fact that no sensing of ventricular activity is possible. The second "O" indicates that no triggering or inhibition occurs but this inevitably follows since there is no sensing function. Although this mode is not used now it is illustrated here because it was the first pacing mode to be developed.

An example is shown in Figure 369.

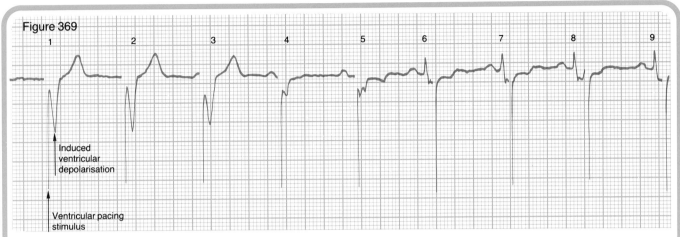

Figure 369

Induced ventricular depolarisation

Ventricular pacing stimulus

Chest monitoring lead. VOO pacing. The first three complexes show the ventricular pacing stimulus immediately followed by the induced ventricular depolarisation (i.e. there is "ventricular capture") . The QRS complex is abnormal in shape and width since the ventricular depolarisation is, in fact, ectopic (induced at an ectopic site by the pacemaker stimulus).

The induced ventricular depolarisation is inevitably followed by an S-T segment and T wave (spontaneous ventricular repolarisation). The sixth, seventh, eighth and ninth ventricular depolarisations are spontaneous, normal QRS complexes, each of which follows the P wave in a completely normal manner. Since the pacemaker has no sensory function (the absence of sensory function is indicated by the first "O" in VOO) a ventricular pacing stimulus occurs exactly on time in relation to these beats (6-9) even though a spontaneous QRS has occurred. Since the pacing stimulus occurs when the ventricular myocardium is still refractory from the spontaneous beats it elicits no response. The fourth and fifth beats show pacing stimuli to the ventricular myocardium occurring after the onset of the spontaneous P wave but before the normal QRS complex. The ventricular depolarisation seen immediately after each of these pacing stimuli is intermediate in shape between that of the spontaneous beats (6-9) and that of the paced beats (1-3). The ventricular depolarisations of these beats 4 and 5 are therefore, in fact, fusion beats with ventricular depolarisation being induced from two sites simultaneously, one from the pacing electrode and one from the normal spread of the sinus-initiated beat via the His bundle.

VVI Pacing

This is an important pacing mode which is still extensively used. In relation to this designation the first "V" refers to the ability of the unit to pace the ventricle, the second "V" refers to the fact that the unit is able to sense spontaneous ventricular activity and the "I" indicates that when the unit recognises spontaneous ventricular activity the pacing output to the ventricle is inhibited. An example of VVI pacing is shown in Figure 370.

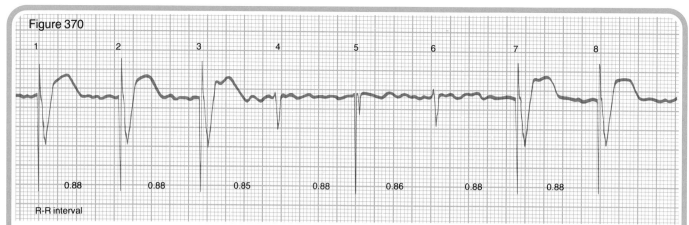

Figure 370

1   2   3   4   5   6   7   8

0.88   0.88   0.85   0.88   0.86   0.88   0.88

R-R interval

In the figure, time intervals are shown in relation to each R-R interval. These are measured from the onset of the pacemaker spike or from the onset of any spontaneous QRS complex which occurs alone or begins sooner.

Chest monitoring lead. VVI pacing.
Atrial fibrillation. The underlying rhythm is atrial fibrillation. No P waves are seen. Irregular fibrillation waves are visible. The first three beats are ventricular paced beats, each one is initiated by a ventricular pacing stimulus and followed by an induced QRS complex ("ventricular capture") which is necessarily abnormally wide and abnormally shaped since the ventricular depolarisation is ectopic. A T wave immediately follows the QRS complex. The pacing rate is 68 beats/min (i.e. the pacing interval is 0.88 sec). The interval between the third pacing spike and the onset of the

fourth QRS complex is 0.85 sec (corresponding to an instantaneous ventricular rate of 70.5 beats/min). Since this pause is less than the ventricular pacemaker escape interval (otherwise known as the ventricular output escape interval or VOEI) a spontaneous QRS complex occurs. The fourth interval is 0.88 sec, exactly the same as the pacemaker escape rate and the pacing stimulus is seen. However, spontaneous ventricular depolarisation must have commenced just before the ventricular depolarisation could be induced by the pacemaker stimulus since the QRS has normal width and an almost normal morphological appearance. The fact that the QRS morphology is slightly different from that of beats four and six suggests that beat five is a fusion beat with a small part of ventricular activity being due to the pacemaker stimulus. Beat 6 follows

beat 5 by an interval of 0.86 sec. This is less than the pacemaker escape interval and this is a spontaneous beat initiated by the atrial fibrillation in the usual way. Beat 7 is a paced beat. No spontaneous QRS has occurred during the pacemaker escape interval of 0.88 sec. The same applies to beat 8. Note that the pacemaker escape interval in this case is the same as the basic pacing interval, i.e. there is no hysteresis (page 512)
In relation to the designation "VVI", (1) the second "V" function is demonstrated by the recognition by the pacemaker of the fourth and sixth ventricular depolarisations, (2) the "I" function is demonstrated by the fact that following this recognition no pacing stimulus occurs until after the next escape interval and (3) the first "V" is indicated by the ventricular pacing spikes demonstrated at beats 1, 2, 3, 5, 7 and 8.

Note that if a VVI unit fails to sense it will become a VOO unit and will give ECG appearances of the type shown in Figure 369. The ECG cannot distinguish between a unit designed to operate in the

VOO mode and one designed to operate as a VVI unit but with failure to sense. An example of a VVI unit failing to sense is shown in Figure 371.

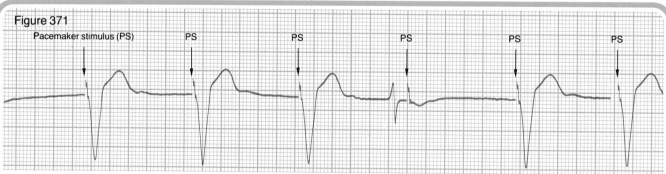

Figure 371

Pacemaker stimulus (PS)   PS   PS   PS   PS   PS

Lead II. VVI pacemaker (failing to sense). The first three beats are ventricular paced beats. After the third paced beat a spontaneous QRS occurs. This is of supraventricular origin (it is narrow). The spontaneous QRS occurs at a shorter time after the third pacing stimulus than the pacemaker escape interval. It should be recognised by the pacemaker and the pacemaker escape interval should then be reset to start again at zero.

That this has not happened is shown by the fact that a pacemaker stimulus occurs just after the spontaneous QRS. This fourth pacemaker stimulus has occurred 0.98 sec after the third pacemaker stimulus – exactly the same gap as that between the first and second and between the second and third and that between the fifth and sixth pacemaker stimuli. The pacemaker has, therefore, failed to sense the spontaneous QRS. In

relation to the designation "VVI", the second "V" (sensing the ventricle) has been inoperative so that the "I" cannot happen (i.e. there cannot be inhibition of the ventricular stimulus). The pacemaker is, therefore, in effect operating in a VOO mode.

An example of a VVI pacemaker
failing to capture the ventricle is
shown in Figure 372.

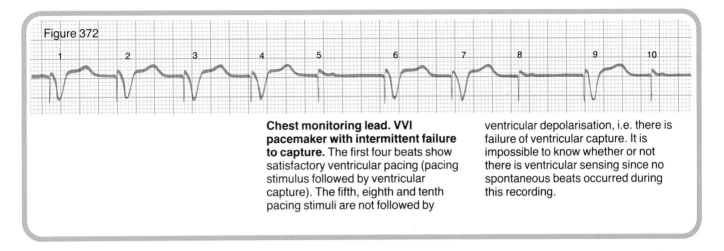

Figure 372

Chest monitoring lead. VVI pacemaker with intermittent failure to capture. The first four beats show satisfactory ventricular pacing (pacing stimulus followed by ventricular capture). The fifth, eighth and tenth pacing stimuli are not followed by ventricular depolarisation, i.e. there is failure of ventricular capture. It is impossible to know whether or not there is ventricular sensing since no spontaneous beats occurred during this recording.

A further example of a VVI pacemaker is shown in Figure 373. Consecutive paced beats show the basic pacing interval. The first paced beats following the last spontaneous beats shows the pacemaker escape interval. Where the latter is greater than the former the pacemaker is said to possess hysteresis (page 512).

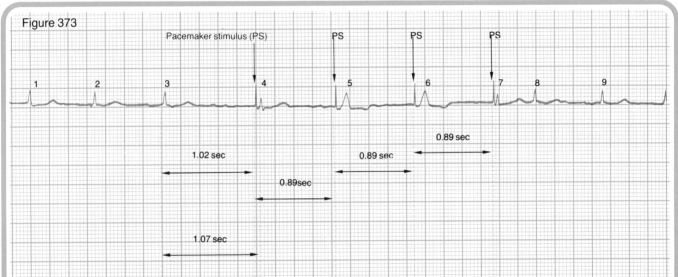

Figure 373

Pacemaker stimulus (PS)   PS   PS   PS

1.02 sec

0.89 sec

0.89sec

0.89 sec

1.07 sec

In this figure, time intervals are shown in relation to some R-R intervals. These are measured from the onset of the pacemaker spike or the onset of any spontaneous QRS complex which occurs alone or begins sooner than a pacemaker spike.

Lead I. VVI pacing. The basic rhythm is atrial fibrillation. The record shows atrial fibrillation throughout. No P waves are seen. The first three QRS complexes are morphologically normal and are conducted beats of supraventricular origin as is usual in atrial fibrillation. The interval between the third and fourth QRS complexes is 1.07 sec, which exceeds the pacemaker escape interval. The interval between the third QRS and the pacing stimulus is 1.02 sec and this gives a direct measure of the **pacemaker escape interval.** The form of the fourth QRS is intermediate between that of the first three QRS complexes and that of the fifth and sixth QRS complexes (these latter two both being preceded by pacing stimuli). Beat 4 is therefore a fusion beat, part of the ventricular activation being initiated via the conduction of the atrial depolarisation through to the His bundle and part being initiated at the ventricular pacing electrode. The fifth and sixth beats are fully paced beats. In each case the interval between the pacing stimulus (4-5 and 5-6) is 0.89 sec, which is the basic **pacing interval** ("pulse interval"). This basic pacing interval (0.89 sec) is less than the pacemaker escape interval (1.02 sec) indicating that the pacemaker shows hysteresis. The seventh beat is a fusion beat. A pacemaker stimulus follows after the basic pacing interval of 0.89 sec but a ventricular depolarisation occurs at the same time as a result of transmission of the stimulus through the His bundle from the fibrillating atria. Beats 8 and 9 are conducted beats from the atrial fibrillation.

VVT Pacing

This is rarely used and will not be discussed.

VAT Pacing

Figure 374 shows the 12-lead ECG appearances in VAT pacing mode. The P waves are normal and spontaneous. In relation to the designation "VAT" the "A" refers to sensing of atrial activity, the "T" to triggering of the ventricular stimulus at a predetermined time interval after the atrial sensing (the pacemaker-controlled P-R interval) and the "V" refers to ventricular pacing.

Figure 374

12-lead ECG. VAT pacing. The P waves are spontaneous. They are recognised by the pacemaker (the "A" in VAT indicates atrial sensing). At a predetermined interval after the P wave (programmable within the pacemaker circuitry) a ventricular pacing stimulus occurs (the "V" refers to ventricular pacing, the "T" refers to triggering of the ventricular pacemaker stimulus after an appropriate delay following sensing recognition of atrial depolarisation). The induced ventricular depolarisation results in an abnormally-wide and abnormally-shaped QRS complex which has the configuration of left bundle branch block (since the depolarisation takes place in the right ventricle – in just the same way as right ventricular ectopic beats give a left bundle branch block configuration (page 414)). The induced QRS complex also shows an abnormal degree of left axis deviation (in this case −75°) since the pacemaker electrode is situated in the apex of the right ventricle and ventricular depolarisation is predominantly from inferior to superior.

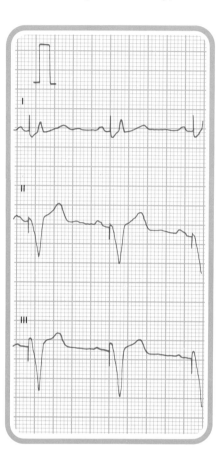

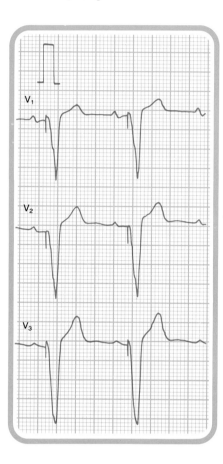

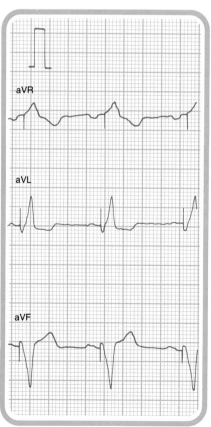

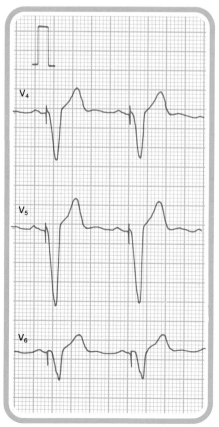

The Electrocardiographic Appearances of Dual or Triple Function Pacing Systems

The more complex pacing systems usually combine together two or more of the functions of the simpler pacing systems and these combinations can be predicted and understood by certain simple rules of arithmetic addition in relation to the pacemaker function.

The Pacemaker Code: Rules of Arithmetic

Since these are "rules of pacemaker addition" they only apply to systems which combine two or more functions. They have no meaning in relation to (a) single-chamber pacing systems (AOO, AAI, AAT, VOO, VVI and VVT (Table 42)) or to (b) VAT pacing which, though it involves two chambers, only has one pacing function (atrial sensing triggers ventricular pacing). Those systems which combine two or more pacing modalities (and which necessarily have both atrial and ventricular leads) can, however, be understood in this way. These systems are DOO, DVI, VDD and DDD. (Note that all have at least one "D" in the code).

The rules of pacemaker arithmetic are as follows:

1. In relation to the first or to the second letter

$$A + A = A$$
$$V + V = V$$
$$O + O = O$$
$$O + V = V$$
$$O + A = A$$
$$A + V = D$$

2. In relation to the third letter

$$O + O = O$$
$$O + I = I$$
$$O + T = T$$
$$T + I = D \text{ (also known as T/I)}$$

Note that the operation of addition is commutative so that $A + V = V + A = D$ i.e. the order of addition is not significant.

Using these rules:

AOO	AVI	VAT	AAI VAT
+ VOO	+ VVI	+ VVI	+ VVI
= DOO	= DVI	= VDD	= DDD

DOO Pacing

This is hardly ever used and will not be discussed further.

VDD Pacing

The VDD pacing mode behaves both like a VAT pacemaker, in that atrial activity is sensed and the recognition of atrial activity results in the triggering of ventricular pacing, and like a VVI pacemaker, in that ventricular pacing is inhibited by the recognition of spontaneous ventricular depolarisation. In relation to the designation "VDD" the first "D" (i.e. "Double") refers to atrial and ventricular sensing, the second "D" ("Double", i.e. both triggering (T) and inhibiting (I) to the fact that pacing of the ventricle is triggered as a result of atrial sensing and inhibited as a result of ventricular sensing, and the "V" refers to ventricular pacing following after a pre-determined delay following the recognition of atrial depolarisation or after a predetermined "output escape interval" if no P wave or QRS complex is sensed. The second "D" is sometimes referred to as "T/I" and the pacing mode may then be referred to as "VDT/I".

The function of the pacemaker in triggering ventricular stimulation following the recognition of spontaneous atrial activity is effectively that of a VAT pacemaker. The function of the pacemaker in inhibiting ventricular stimulation as a result of sensing spontaneous ventricular activity is the same as a VVI pacemaker. A VDD pacemaker therefore, combines the roles of VAT unit and a VVI unit. This may be predicted using the "rules of addition" as they apply to the pacemaker code.

An example of VDD pacing is shown in Figure 375.

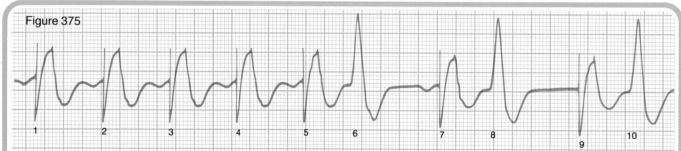

Figure 375

Chest monitoring lead. VDD pacing. The first five beats show spontaneous P waves with ventricular pacing after a predetermined P-pacing interval (VAT pacing). The sixth QRS is a ventricular premature beat. It is recognised by the pacemaker (the "V" part of the first "D") and the pacing output is inhibited. The re-setting of the pacemaker probably occurs early in the QRS complex. About 0.76 sec later a spontaneous P wave occurs. This is sensed (the "A" part of the first "D") and a ventricular pacing stimulus (occurring after the appropriate interval) gives ventricular depolarisation (the seventh QRS complex). The eighth QRS is a ventricular premature beat. 0.96 sec passes after the onset of the eighth (the ectopic) QRS without any P wave or QRS being apparent. This interval equals the pacemaker escape interval and a ventricular paced beat occurs (VVI pacing). The pacemaker has, within this short ECG record, demonstrated its ability to pace the ventricle (the "V" of the first letter), to sense spontaneous activity both in the atrium and in the ventricle (the first "D"), to trigger (T) the ventricle after recognising atrial activity and to inhibit (I) the ventricle after recognising ventricular activity. (The T and I constitute the second "D") . It is thus a VDD pacemaker and has demonstrated both VAT and VVI functions.

DVI Pacing

This form of pacing may be of two types: **"uncommitted"** and **"committed"**. In both cases pacing occurs at atrial and at ventricular level, sensing occurs at ventricular level only and ventricular sensing results in inhibition of both atrial and ventricular stimulation. The difference between the two forms relates to the response of the pacemaker unit when a spontaneous ventricular depolarisation is sensed after the release of an atrial pacing spike. In the committed system a ventricular pacing spike inevitably follows an atrial pacing spike after the appropriate AV interval irrespective of whether or not a spontaneous ventricular depolarisation is recognised within this AV interval. In the uncommitted form the ventricular pacing spike is inhibited if a spontaneous ventricular depolarisation is sensed during the AV interval (i.e. after the release of an atrial pacing spike but before the release of the ventricular pacing spike).

* The duration of the inhibition of the ventricles and of the atria varies. The atrial inhibition (atrial output escape interval (AOEI)) is shorter than the ventricular inhibition (ventricular output escape interval (VOEI)) by an amount which corresponds to the AV interval (equivalent to the P-R interval).

Uncommitted DVI Pacing*

Using the "rules of addition" for the pacemaker code (as described above):

VVI*
+ AVI*
= DVI

In a DVI system, therefore, ventricular activity is sensed and the recognition of ventricular activity inhibits stimulation of the atrium and stimulation of the ventricle.

The possible electrocardiographic appearances of DVI pacing are complex and potentially confusing. Figure 376 demonstrates the principles in relation to the uncommitted form.

Figure 376 **DVI pacing (uncommitted)**

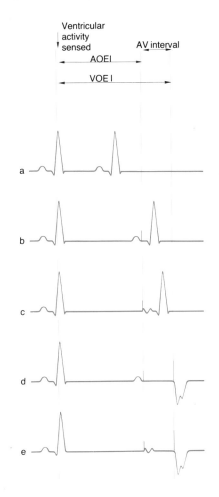

a) The R-R interval is less than AOEI, therefore atrial pacing is inhibited. The R-R interval is also less than VOEI and therefore ventricular pacing is inhibited. (No spikes, no chamber paced).

b) The R-R interval is longer than AOEI, therefore since no R wave is sensed, the atrial pacing stimulus is released (AVI operation). This happens despite the occurrence of the P wave for there is no atrial sensing. The atrial pacing spike follows the P wave and achieves nothing. The R-R interval is less than the VOEI, therefore ventricular pacing is inhibited. (Atrial spike, no ventricular spike, no chamber paced).

c) The R-R interval is longer than the AOEI therefore an atrial pacing spike occurs. Since this has not been preceded by a P wave the atrial pacing spike is followed by an induced P wave. Ventricular depolarisation follows spontaneously (there is atrio-ventricular conduction) so the ventricular pacing spike is inhibited (i.e. the R-R interval is less than VOEI). The fact that a ventricular pacing stimulus is not released at the pre-set AV interval following the atrial pacing spike indicates that the system is "uncommitted". (Atrial pacing spike and atrial capture but no ventricular spike or ventricular capture).

d) The R-R interval is longer than AOEI, therefore an atrial pacing spike occurs. However, a spontaneous P wave develops before the end of the AOEI therefore an ineffective atrial pacing spike follows the spontaneous P wave. No R wave occurs within the VOEI, therefore a ventricular pacing spike occurs with ventricular capture. (Atrial and ventricular spikes, only the ventricle is paced).

e) The R-R interval is greater than AOEI, therefore an atrial pacing spike occurs. Since no P wave has appeared during the AOEI this spike captures the atrium. The R-R interval exceeds VOEI also, so a ventricular pacing spike occurs with ventricular capture. (Atrial and ventricular spikes, atrial and ventricular capture).

Committed DVI Pacing

The form of DVI pacing shown in Figure 376 is referred to as **"uncommitted"** for there is still time to inhibit the ventricular pacing spike after the initiation of an atrial pacing spike should a spontaneous QRS be recognised (as in (b) and (c) of Figure 376). Another form of DVI pacing is the **"committed"** form in which a ventricular output spike is obligatory once an atrial output spike is initiated. Figure 377 demonstrates the principles. Committed DVI systems are becoming less popular and have no advantages over uncommitted systems.

Figure 377 Committed DVI pacing

Ventricular activity sensed

AOEI

VOEI

a) The R-R interval is less than AOEI, therefore atrial pacing is inhibited. The R-R interval is also less than VOEI therefore ventricular pacing is inhibited. (No spikes, no pacing).

b) The R-R interval is longer than AOEI, therefore since no R wave is sensed the atrial pacing stimulus is initiated. This happens despite the occurrence of a P wave, for there is no capability of atrial sensing. The atrial spike follows the P wave and achieves nothing. The R-R interval is less than VOEI but since the system is committed a ventricular pacing stimulus is necessarily emitted at the programmed AV interval after the atrial pacing spike. (Atrial and ventricular spikes, no pacing).

c) The R-R interval is greater than AOEI, therefore an atrial pacing stimulus is released. No spontaneous P wave has preceded the stimulus so atrial pacing occurs. The R-R interval is less than VOEI but a ventricular pacing stimulus still occurs since the system is committed to giving such a stimulus once it has given an atrial stimulus. Since a spontaneous QRS occurs before the ventricular pacing stimulus (normal AV conduction) the ventricular pacing stimulus falls in the refractory period and is ineffective. (Atrial and ventricular spikes, atrial pacing only).

d) The R-R interval exceeds AOEI, therefore an atrial pacing stimulus occurs. A spontaneous P wave has developed prior to the stimulus so the stimulus is ineffective. The R-R interval is greater than the VOEI but a ventricular pacing spike would be delivered irrespective of this since the system is committed to such a spike at the programmed AV interval after the atrial spike. Since no spontaneous QRS precedes this ventricular spike, ventricular capture occurs. (Atrial and ventricular spikes occur, ventricular capture occurs).

e) The R-R interval exceeds AOEI, therefore an atrial pacing spike occurs. No spontaneous P wave precedes the spike so atrial capture is achieved. A ventricular pacing spike inevitably follows at the programmed AV interval after the atrial spike. Since no spontaneous R wave occurs within this interval (i.e. the R-R interval exceeds the VOEI) ventricular capture occurs. (Atrial and ventricular spikes, atrial and ventricular pacing).

Note that one of the risks of committed DVI pacing is that a pacing stimulus can be delivered to the ventricular myocardium during ventricular repolarisation (as in (b) and (c)). This could produce ventricular tachydysrhythmias in the same way as an R-on-T ectopic (Figure 304).

Figure 378 shows an example of uncommitted DVI pacing.

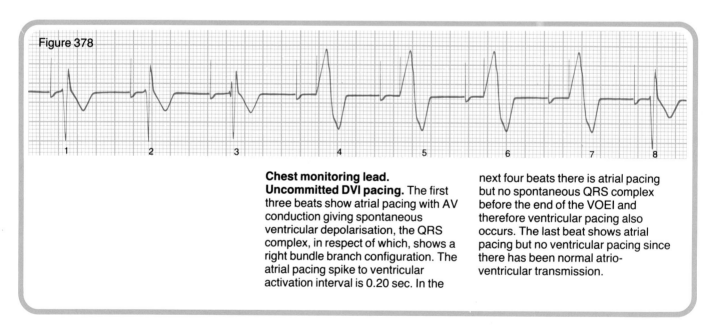

Figure 378

Chest monitoring lead. Uncommitted DVI pacing. The first three beats show atrial pacing with AV conduction giving spontaneous ventricular depolarisation, the QRS complex, in respect of which, shows a right bundle branch configuration. The atrial pacing spike to ventricular activation interval is 0.20 sec. In the next four beats there is atrial pacing but no spontaneous QRS complex before the end of the VOEI and therefore ventricular pacing also occurs. The last beat shows atrial pacing but no ventricular pacing since there has been normal atrio-ventricular transmission.

Figure 379 shows an example of committed DVI pacing.

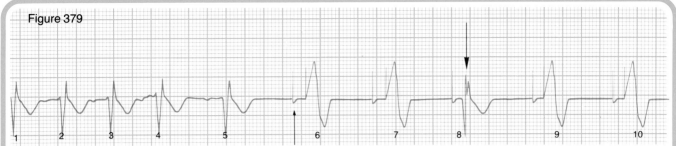

Figure 379

Chest monitoring lead. Committed DVI pacing. Beats 2-4 show sinus rhythm (the first beat is probably also a sinus beat but the record starts during the QRS and one cannot therefore be sure). The fifth beat is also a sinus beat but the sinus rate is slower. These five beats show a right bundle branch block type of QRS configuration. In relation to the sixth beat an atrial pacing spike occurs at 0.78 sec after the onset of the QRS at beat 5. This interval therefore indicates the AOEI. Atrial capture occurs (small inverted P wave indicated by small arrow). After an AV delay of 0.16 sec a ventricular pacing spike occurs with ventricular capture. (Since no spontaneous QRS occurs during the pre-programmed AV delay a ventricular pacing spike would occur whether the system were committed or non-committed). The same sequence of events occurs in beats 7, 9 and 10. **The appearance in beat 8 clearly indicates that the system is committed** for a spontaneous QRS complex (similar to that seen in beats 1-5) begins before the end of the programmed AV delay but despite this a ventricular pacing spike still occurs (large arrow). It produces no effect for it finds the ventricles refractory. (Had the spontaneous QRS occurred fractionally later there might well have been a fusion beat – part of the QRS being initiated spontaneously and part occurring as a result of the ventricular pacing spike). Had the ventricular stimulus occurred later still, i.e. during the ventricular repolarisation period, there would be a risk of inducing ventricular tachydysrhythmias as with R-on-T ectopics (Figure 304).

DDD Pacing

DDD pacing is both versatile and complex. The possible electrocardiographic appearances of normally functioning and of malfunctioning DDD pacemakers are extremely numerous and only the basic principles will be covered here. Basically, the DDD pacemaker has two circuits, one for the atrium (which acts as an AAI pacemaker) and one for the ventricle (acting as a VVI pacemaker). The two circuits are linked so that atrial activity (whether spontaneous and recognised or not spontaneously present and therefore pacemaker-induced) is followed, after a predetermined AV interval, by ventricular activation (if not spontaneous, then pacemaker-induced) i.e. a VAT operation.

Using the "rules of addition" for the pacemaker code:

```
  AAI
  VVI
+ VAT
= DDD
```

Figure 380 shows the principles of DDD pacing.

Figure 380   **DDD pacing**

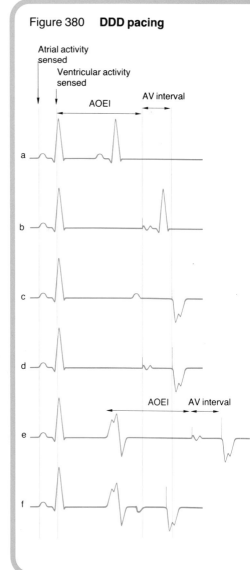

a) Spontaneous atrial rate is faster than the lower tracking rate of the pacemaker (i.e. the P-P interval is less than the AOEI) so no atrial stimulus occurs. The second spontaneous P wave is also sensed and the interval between it and its succeeding R wave is checked by the pacemaker. Since this interval is less than the programmed atrio-ventricular interval, no ventricular stimulus is given. (Atrial and ventricular output inhibited. No pacing).

b) Spontaneous atrial rate is slower than the lower tracking rate of the pacemaker so an atrial stimulus is given and atrial pacing induced. A spontaneous QRS follows the induced atrial activation after a delay which is less than the programmed AV interval so no ventricular stimulus is given. (Atrial spike, no ventricular spike. Atrial pacing only, i.e. AAI behaviour).

c) Spontaneous atrial rate is faster than the lower tracking rate of the pacemaker so no atrial stimulus appears. However, after the second spontaneous P wave there is no spontaneous QRS before the end of the programmed AV interval, so a ventricular stimulus is given and ventricular pacing occurs. (Atrial output inhibited, ventricular spike. Ventricular pacing only, i.e. VDD behaviour*).

d) Spontaneous atrial rate is slower than the lower tracking rate of the pacemaker so an atrial stimulus is given. No spontaneous QRS follows the atrial stimulus within the programmed atrio-ventricular interval so a ventricular stimulus occurs. (Atrial spike, ventricular spike. Atrial and ventricular pacing, i.e. DDD behaviour).

e) Ventricular premature beat occurs during atrial output escape interval. This re-sets the AOEI. Since no P wave is sensed during this re-set AOEI, a pacing spike occurs and atrial capture is induced. Since no spontaneous QRS develops during the AV interval which follows the atrial pacing spike, a ventricular stimulus occurs and ventricular pacing is induced. (Atrial spike, ventricular spike. Atrial and ventricular pacing, i.e. DDD behaviour).

f) Ventricular premature beat (VPB) occurs during the atrial output escape interval. This re-sets the AOEI. However, the VPB is followed by a retrograde P wave. This is sensed and since no further QRS occurs spontaneously within the duration of the programmed atrio-ventricular delay following the retrograde P wave, a ventricular pacing spike is given and ventricular capture occurs. (Ventricular spike only. Ventricular pacing, i.e. VDD behaviour).

* On the electrocardiogram shown this is not distinguishable from VAT behaviour.

Figure 381 shows a 12-lead ECG in a patient with DDD pacing. Note that since no spontaneous P wave and no spontaneous QRS is seen, there is no way of checking the sensing function of the pacemaker from the electrocardiogram. Atria and ventricles are being paced and the system could be DOO, DVI or DDD (i.e.one cannot distinguish these possible pacing modes from the ECG appearances in the context of sustained dual-chamber pacing with no spontaneous P waves or QRS complexes).

Figure 381

12-lead ECG. DDD pacing.
There is regular atrial and ventricular pacing. No spontaneous P waves or QRS complexes are seen so there is no way of knowing if sensing of atrial or ventricular activity is being achieved by the pacemaker. The appearances, therefore, can only be taken to indicate dual chamber pacing which could be DOO, DVI or DDD.

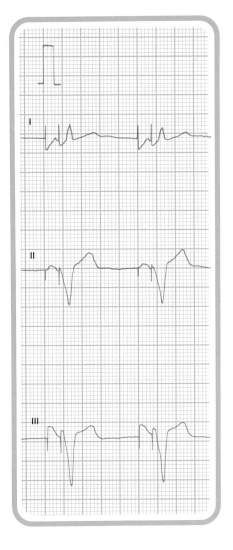

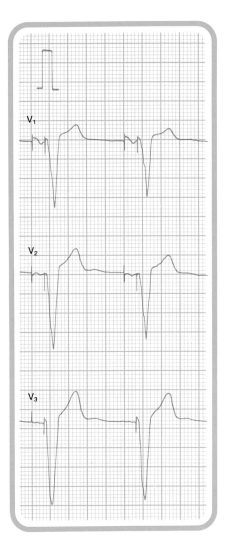

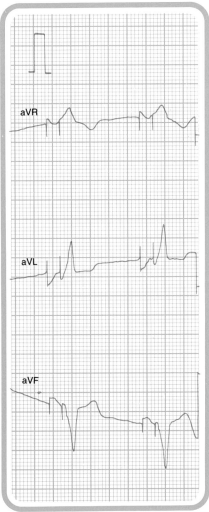

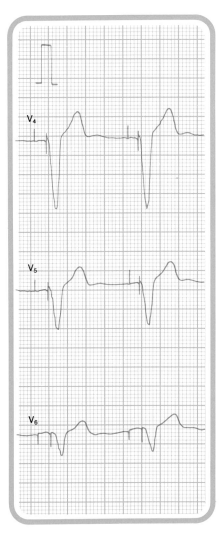

Figure 382 shows a further example of DDD pacing. The record is taken from a chest monitoring lead in the same patient as Figure 381.

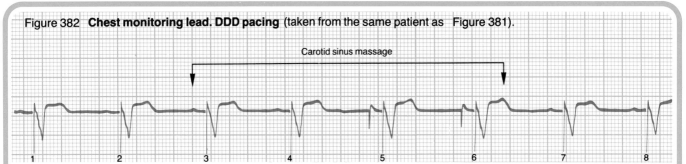

Figure 382 **Chest monitoring lead. DDD pacing** (taken from the same patient as Figure 381).

a) **Effect of brief carotid sinus massage**
The first four complexes show spontaneous P waves with ventricular pacing after an AV interval of 0.16 sec (VAT pacing). Carotid sinus massage is begun within a second or so of the start of the recording and continued only until a change in the pacing mode is seen. The interval between the pacemaker ventricular stimulus and the next spontaneous P wave (in relation to each of the first four beats) is 0.76 sec. Carotid sinus massage slows down the prevailing sinus rate and the interval between the ventricular pacing stimulus of beat 4 and the atrial pacing stimulus of beat 5 is 0.84 sec. This is the atrial output escape interval. Beats 5 and 6 show DDD pacing. Carotid sinus massage is stopped immediately after beat 6. The fact that no atrial spike occurs in relation to beats 1-4 and 7 and 8 (when P waves occur within the atrial output escape interval) demonstrates effective atrial sensing. Beats 1-4 and 7 and 8 show VAT pacing.

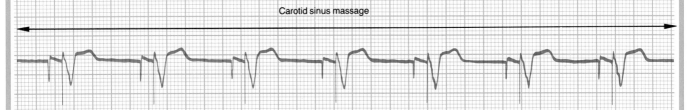

b) **Effect of sustained carotid sinus massage**
Carotid sinus massage is given throughout the recording. The spontaneous atrial rate is depressed and dual chamber pacing occurs throughout.

Figure 383 shows another example of DDD pacing. The versatile behaviour of this pacing mode is illustrated and this example serves to give some idea of the complexity of the electrocardiographic appearances in DDD pacing. This pacemaker is actually functioning normally. When failure of one or more of the functions occurs the electrocardiographic appearances can be even more complex to interpret.

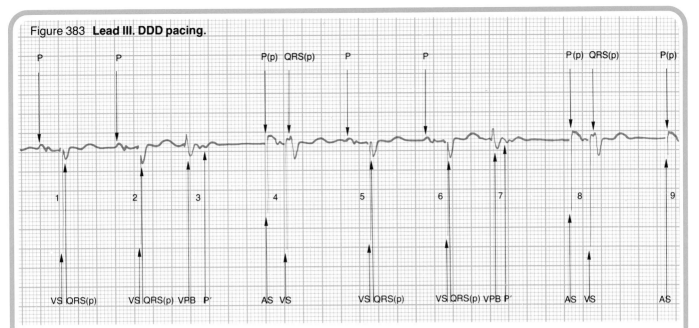

Figure 383 **Lead III. DDD pacing.**

Figure nomenclature:

P = spontaneous P wave
P′ = retrograde conducted P wave
VPB = ventricular premature beat
AS = atrial spike (atrial stimulation)
VS = ventricular spike (ventricular stimulation)
P(p) = pacemaker-induced P wave
QRS(p) = pacemaker-induced QRS

The first two beats show spontaneous P waves. These are recognised by the pacemaker (i.e. there is trial sensing). It is clear that (a) they are recognised and (b) each occurs within the atrial output escape interval of the preceding QRS since no atrial spike occurs. Each of the two spontaneous P waves is followed by a ventricular pacing spike and induced QRS (i.e. VAT pacing). The third beat is a ventricular premature beat (VPB) and it is followed by a P′ wave conducted retrogradely through the atrio-ventricular node. This is not recognised by the pacemaker since it falls during that period after the recognition of the ventricular complex when the atrial sensing function is temporarily blanked out. The atrial output escape interval is re-set by the recognition of the ventricular premature beat and the resulting atrial pacing spike (at 4) follows the ventricular premature beat (3) by an interval of 0.88 sec (the atrial output escape interval). At beat 4, both atrial and ventricular pacing occur. Beats 5 and 6 are like beats 1 and 2. Beat 7 is like beat 3. Beat 8 is like beat 4. This illustration shows examples of (i) atrial sensing (beats 1, 2, 5 and 6), (ii) ventricular sensing (beats 3 and 7), (iii) atrial pacing (beats 4, 8 and 9), (iv) ventricular pacing (beats 1, 2, 4, 5, 6 and 8) and (v) blanking of atrial sensing for a short time after the sensing of ventricular activity (beats 3 and 7).

A further example of DDD pacing is shown in Figure 384.

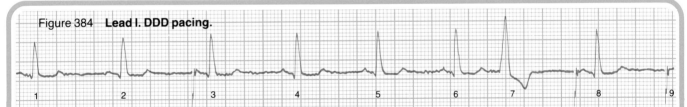

Figure 384 **Lead I. DDD pacing.**

The first two beats are sinus beats. The interval between the onset of the QRS of beat 1 and the onset of the P wave of beat 2 before is 0.83 sec. The interval between the onset of the QRS of beat 2 and the onset of the P wave of beat 3 is also 0.80 sec. This must be very close to the atrial output escape interval for the pacemaker gives an atrial pacing spike indicating either that it has failed to recognise the P wave of beat 3 or (perhaps more likely) that the atrial pacing spike has been released just before the P wave would have been sensed (and that the P wave is therefore a fusion beat). The pacemaker can clearly recognise P waves (since no atrial pacing stimulus occurs at 1 and 2) and can recognise QRS complexes (since no ventricular pacing stimulus occurs at 1 and 2). No ventricular pacing stimulus occurs at 3 since a QRS is recognised at less than the programmed atrio-ventricular interval after the P wave spike. Beats 4, 5 and 6 are sinus beats. Beat 7 is a ventricular premature beat. It is recognised and it therefore re-sets the atrial output escape interval which is 0.83 sec (the same as that between QRS 2 and atrial pacing spike 3). Atrial pacing occurs in beats 8 and 9. No ventricular pacing spike occurs at beat 8 since a spontaneous (conducted) QRS occurs before the end of the programmed atrio-ventricular interval following the atrial spike 8.

It must be emphasised once more that only a tiny proportion of the possible number of electrocardiographic appearances in relation to DDD pacing have been demonstrated.

Combination Arrhythmias

Even within the short time windows provided by conventional 12-lead electrocardiographic recordings, two or more arrhythmias may be apparent, either because two or more arrhythmias are present simultaneously or because two or more arrhythmias are present consecutively within a short time period. Some arrhythmias, of course, preclude the simultaneous (but not the consecutive) presence of other arrhythmias. Thus, for example, the presence of atrial fibrillation precludes the possibility of any form of co-ordinated atrial depolarisation occurring simultaneously but does not prevent co-ordinated atrial depolarisation occurring consecutively. Atrial ectopic beats, atrial tachycardia, sinus rhythm, sinus tachycardia, sinus bradycardia etc cannot occur during atrial fibrillation. Likewise ventricular ectopic beats and ventricular tachycardia cannot occur during ventricular fibrillation.

Arrhythmias are classified (page 375) into the following groups:

1. Disturbances of function at the sino-atrial node

2. Premature ectopic rhythms

3. Escape ectopic rhythms

4. Conduction disturbances

5. Combinations of the above

It is this last group which is now being considered.

Any disturbance of function at the sino-atrial node may be combined simultaneously with (a) either an escape ectopic rhythm or a premature ectopic rhythm, and/or (b) a conduction disturbance. In relation to consecutive arrhythmias any combination is obviously possible. A few examples will serve to illustrate the principles.

1. Sinus tachycardia with first degree heart block

This is a common combination and is illustrated in Figure 385.

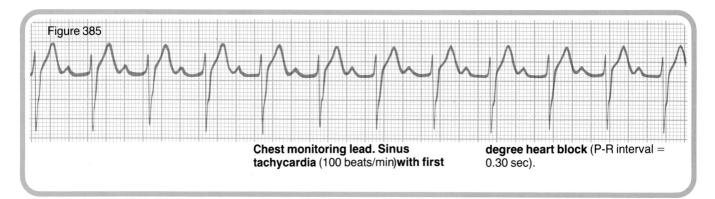

Figure 385

Chest monitoring lead. Sinus tachycardia (100 beats/min)**with first degree heart block** (P-R interval = 0.30 sec).

2. Atrial flutter with complete heart block

This is not a common combination. In most cases of atrial flutter there is 2:1, 3:1, 4:1 or 5:1 atrio-ventricular block with corresponding ventricular rates of 150, 100, 75 or 60 beats/min. Complete heart block can only be diagnosed by the finding of a regular, very slow (usually 50 beats/min or less) ventricular rate in the presence of atrial flutter. Figure 386 shows an example.

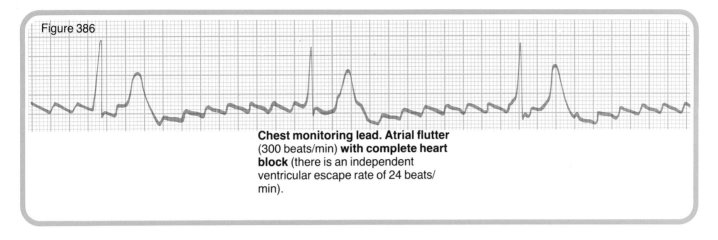

Figure 386

Chest monitoring lead. Atrial flutter (300 beats/min) **with complete heart block** (there is an independent ventricular escape rate of 24 beats/ min).

3. Atrial fibrillation with complete heart block

An example of this relatively uncommon arrhythmia is seen in Figure 387.

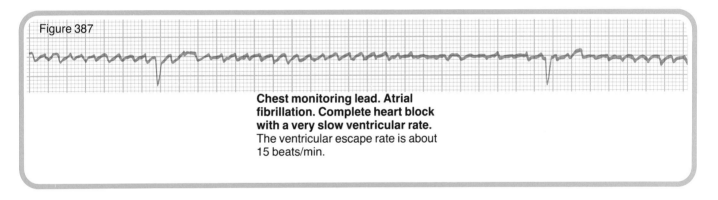

Figure 387

Chest monitoring lead. Atrial fibrillation. Complete heart block with a very slow ventricular rate. The ventricular escape rate is about 15 beats/min.

4. Atrial flutter, VVI pacing and ventricular tachycardia

An example is seen in Figure 388.

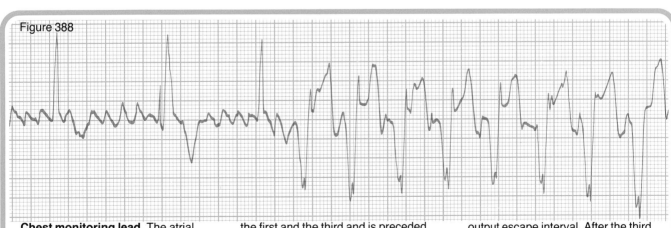

Figure 388

Chest monitoring lead. The atrial rhythm is **atrial flutter.** The first and third QRS complexes are conducted beats. The second QRS is wider than the first and the third and is preceded by a pacing spike. It is an example of **VVI pacing** with the stimulus occurring at the end of the ventricular output escape interval. After the third QRS there is the onset of **ventricular tachycardia.**

5. First degree heart block and ventricular premature beats

This is a common combination and an example is shown in Figure 389.

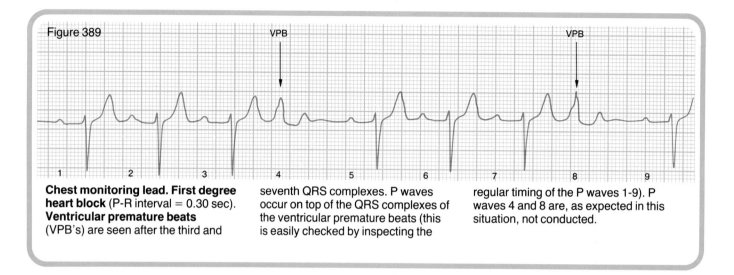

Figure 389

VPB VPB

1 2 3 4 5 6 7 8 9

Chest monitoring lead. First degree heart block (P-R interval = 0.30 sec). **Ventricular premature beats** (VPB's) are seen after the third and seventh QRS complexes. P waves occur on top of the QRS complexes of the ventricular premature beats (this is easily checked by inspecting the regular timing of the P waves 1-9). P waves 4 and 8 are, as expected in this situation, not conducted.

6. 2:1 atrio-ventricular block with unifocal ventricular premature beats

An example of this combination is shown in Figure 390.

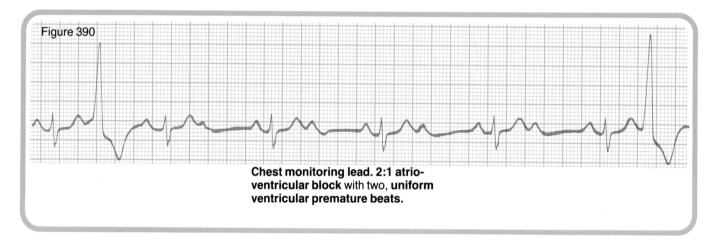

Figure 390

Chest monitoring lead. 2:1 atrio-ventricular block with two, **uniform ventricular premature beats.**

7. Atrial flutter with ventricular premature beats and also bursts of ventricular tachycardia

This combination is shown in Figure 391.

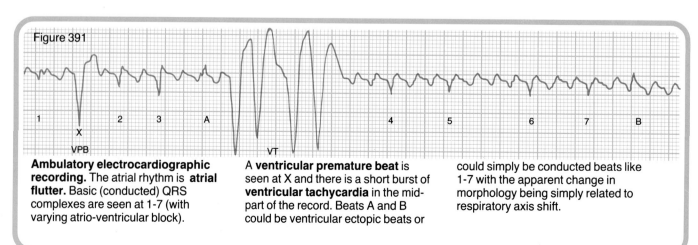

Figure 391

1 X 2 3 A 4 5 6 7 B

VPB VT

Ambulatory electrocardiographic recording. The atrial rhythm is **atrial flutter.** Basic (conducted) QRS complexes are seen at 1-7 (with varying atrio-ventricular block). A **ventricular premature beat** is seen at X and there is a short burst of **ventricular tachycardia** in the mid-part of the record. Beats A and B could be ventricular ectopic beats or could simply be conducted beats like 1-7 with the apparent change in morphology being simply related to respiratory axis shift.

8. Ventricular tachycardia, giving way to atrial fibrillation

This example is shown in Figure 392.

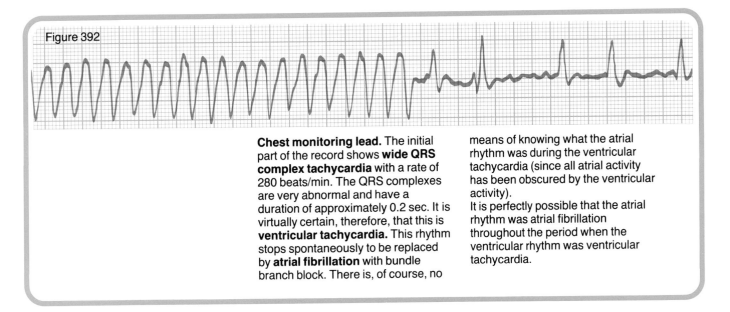

Figure 392

Chest monitoring lead. The initial part of the record shows **wide QRS complex tachycardia** with a rate of 280 beats/min. The QRS complexes are very abnormal and have a duration of approximately 0.2 sec. It is virtually certain, therefore, that this is **ventricular tachycardia.** This rhythm stops spontaneously to be replaced by **atrial fibrillation** with bundle branch block. There is, of course, no means of knowing what the atrial rhythm was during the ventricular tachycardia (since all atrial activity has been obscured by the ventricular activity).

It is perfectly possible that the atrial rhythm was atrial fibrillation throughout the period when the ventricular rhythm was ventricular tachycardia.

9. Sinus rhythm with atrial echo beats, plus atrial tachycardia plus ventricular premature beats

This example is shown in Figure 393.

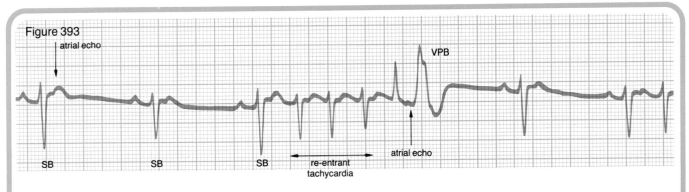

Figure 393
atrial echo
VPB
atrial echo
SB   SB   SB   re-entrant tachycardia

Chest monitoring lead. The first two beats are **sinus beats** (SB). On the upstroke of the T wave following each QRS complex is a perturbation caused by an inverted P wave – an **atrial echo beat.** This does not give rise to a second QRS. However, after the third sinus-initiated QRS (SB) an atrial echo beat again occurs but this time it induces a subsequent QRS and the cycle becomes repeated to give a burst of re-entrant tachycardia. After three beats of the **atrial tachycardia** the QRS axis changes but there is still a re-entrant atrial echo beat. This time, however, the re-entrant tachycardia is not sustained because a **ventricular premature beat** (VPB) happens to depolarise the ventricular myocardium. This probably conducts back into the atrio-ventricular node making it refractory and the re-entrant cycle is therefore broken. Sinus rhythm returns. The next two sinus beats again provoke atrial echoes and the atrial echo after the last sinus beat once more initiates re-entrant tachycardia (only a single beat of this re-entrant tachycardia is shown in the illustration).

10. Atrial tachycardia (from two separate foci) and sinus rhythm

This example is shown in Figure 394.

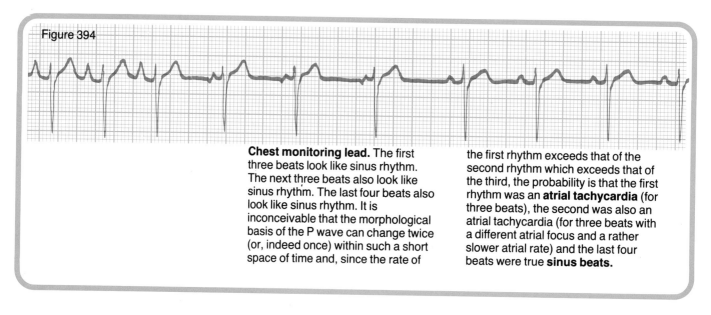

Figure 394

Chest monitoring lead. The first three beats look like sinus rhythm. The next three beats also look like sinus rhythm. The last four beats also look like sinus rhythm. It is inconceivable that the morphological basis of the P wave can change twice (or, indeed once) within such a short space of time and, since the rate of the first rhythm exceeds that of the second rhythm which exceeds that of the third, the probability is that the first rhythm was an **atrial tachycardia** (for three beats), the second was also an atrial tachycardia (for three beats with a different atrial focus and a rather slower atrial rate) and the last four beats were true **sinus beats.**

11. Sinus bradycardia with first degree heart block and a ventricular escape ectopic mechanism

This example is shown in Figure 395. Strictly speaking this shows three rhythm disturbances (sinus bradycardia, first degree heart block, ventricular escape ectopic beats).

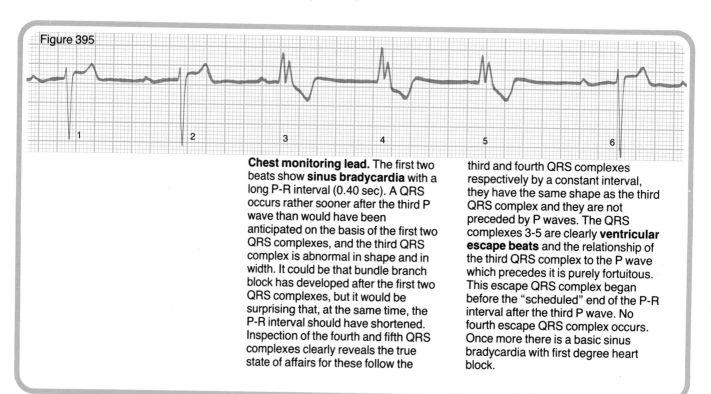

Figure 395

1   2   3   4   5   6

Chest monitoring lead. The first two beats show **sinus bradycardia** with a long P-R interval (0.40 sec). A QRS occurs rather sooner after the third P wave than would have been anticipated on the basis of the first two QRS complexes, and the third QRS complex is abnormal in shape and in width. It could be that bundle branch block has developed after the first two QRS complexes, but it would be surprising that, at the same time, the P-R interval should have shortened. Inspection of the fourth and fifth QRS complexes clearly reveals the true state of affairs for these follow the third and fourth QRS complexes respectively by a constant interval, they have the same shape as the third QRS complex and they are not preceded by P waves. The QRS complexes 3-5 are clearly **ventricular escape beats** and the relationship of the third QRS complex to the P wave which precedes it is purely fortuitous. This escape QRS complex began before the "scheduled" end of the P-R interval after the third P wave. No fourth escape QRS complex occurs. Once more there is a basic sinus bradycardia with first degree heart block.

12. Sinus rhythm with ventricular coupling simulating alternating bundle branch block

This example is shown in Figure 396.

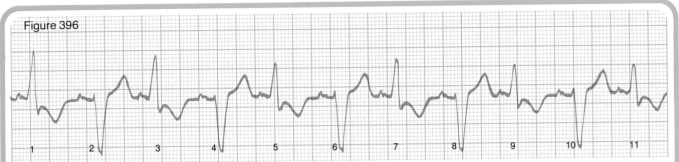

Figure 396

Chest monitoring lead. The rhythm is basically **sinus rhythm with left bundle branch block.** There are **uniform ventricular premature beats** arising in the left ventricle (and having an approximately right bundle branch block configuration) and these beats simulate alternating bundle branch block. The P wave rate is regular and the P wave configuration is constant throughout the record. The even-numbered beats have a left bundle branch block configuration and are associated with an absolutely constant P-R interval of 0.18 sec. At first sight it looks as though the odd-numbered beats are also sinus-initiated but careful inspection shows some variation in the P-R interval. For example the P-R interval of the first beat is 0.10 sec and of the seventh beat is 0.13 sec. A probable mechanism of the odd-numbered beats is a uniform ventricular premature beat mechanism in which the premature beat occurs just before the completion of the P-R interval. If these premature beats had not occurred one would have expected the odd-numbered P waves to be followed by QRS complexes like those of the even-numbered beats.

Pre-excitation and Atrial Fibrillation

Whilst pre-excitation, *per se,* is not arrhythmia and "pre-excitation with atrial fibrillation" is therefore not, strictly speaking, a combination of arrhythmias, it is a combination of electrocardiographic abnormalities and is of great clinical importance. Ventricular pre-excitation of the Wolff-Parkinson-White variety (Section 2, pages 212 to 218) gives rise to a short P-R interval, a delta wave and widening of the QRS complexes (Figures 149 to 151). When atrio-ventricular re-entrant tachycardia (AVRT) develops, atrio-ventricular conduction usually takes place normally down the atrio-ventricular node and His bundle rather than anomalously down the accessory pathway, and the QRS complexes become normal (since antegrade conduction down the normal atrio-ventricular pathway is the usual situation in the presence of AVRT – the ECG evidence of pre-excitation temporarily disappears, i.e. pre-excitation is not actually taking place). Occasionally, during atrial flutter or atrial fibrillation, atrio-ventricular conduction may take place down the bypass tract and, in this situation, the QRS complexes are widened and have an initial delta wave (since there is then ventricular pre-excitation even during the tachycardia).

This is a relatively uncommon occurrence but is very dangerous since extremely high ventricular rates (of 300 beats/min or more) may occur. Figure 397 (a to c) shows examples of ventricular pre-excitation of the Wolff-Parkinson-White type, (a) in sinus rhythm with ventricular pre-excitation, (b) during AVRT without pre-excitation and (c) during atrial fibrillation with ventricular pre-excitation and functional right bundle branch block.

These examples (and Figure 397 (a-c)) are only a small number from the infinite number of possible rhythm combinations and they serve simply to illustrate the concepts of two or more **simultaneous** or **consecutive** disturbances of cardiac rhythm.

Figure 397

ECGs in the Wolff-Parkinson-White syndrome taken from the same patient (a) during sinus rhythm, (b) during atrio-ventricular re-entrant tachycardia (AVRT) and (c) during atrial fibrillation.

(a) Sinus rhythm with ventricular pre-excitation.
Initial slurring of the upstroke of the QRS complexes (the delta wave) can be seen in Leads II, III and aVF and in V_5 and V_6. The total QRS duration is beyond the upper limit of normal (0.13 sec).

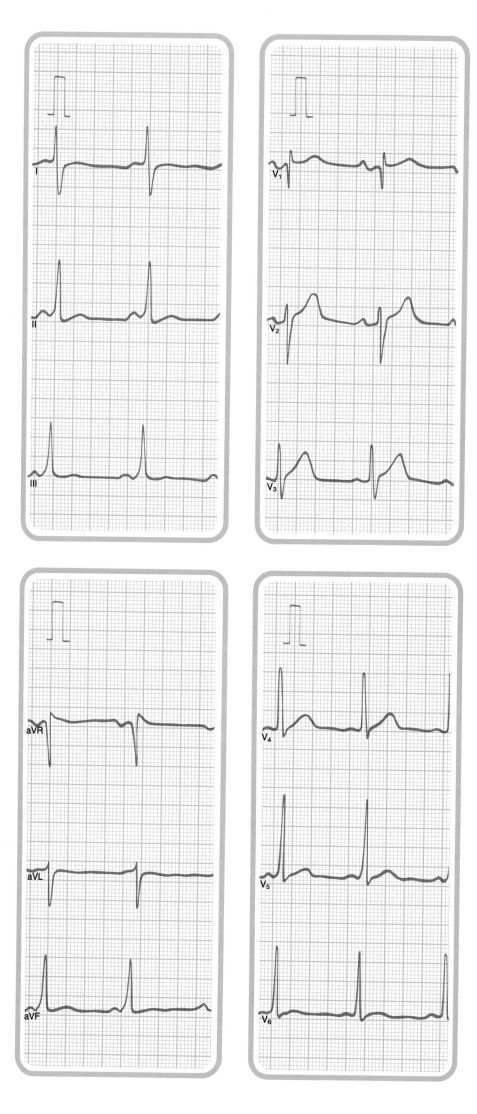

Figure 397

(b) The record taken from the same patient during atrio-ventricular re-entrant tachycardia (AVRT).
The QRS complexes are narrow and have the same overall morphology as those seen in (a) but without the initial delta wave. The total QRS duration is normal. The ventricular rate is regular at 200 beats/min. This is an orthodromic atrio-ventricular re-entrant tachycardia (AVRT) with atrio-ventricular conduction taking place via the AV node and ventriculo-atrial conduction via the anomalous atrio-ventricular pathway.

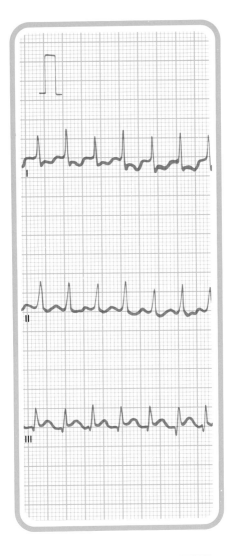

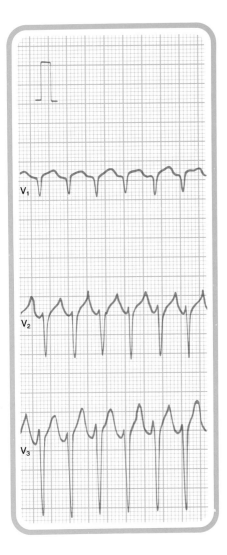

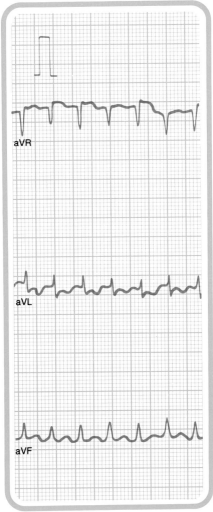

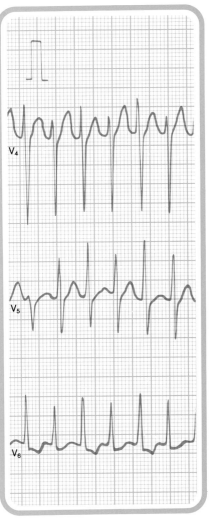

Figure 397

(c) Taken from the same patient during atrial fibrillation.
The ventricular rate is rapid and irregular. The QRS complexes are abnormally wide. There has been a significant shift in the frontal plane QRS axis compared with the records taken during sinus rhythm or during supraventricular tachycardia. The total QRS complex is appreciably widened. This is atrial fibrillation with atrio-ventricular conduction occurring via the anomalous atrio-ventricular pathway. It needs to be distinguished from atrial fibrillation with pre-existing left bundle branch block and from atrial fibrillation with aberrant intraventricular conduction (tachycardia-dependent bundle branch block).

At times it can be difficult to distinguish it from atrial fibrillation with pre-existing left bundle branch block. However, whenever there is atrial fibrillation with abnormally wide QRS complexes and R-R intervals of 0.26 sec or less, it is likely that there is ventricular pre-excitation with atrio-ventricular conduction down the anomalous pathway.

In this case, as is usual, there is no difficulty in distinguishing the rhythm from atrial fibrillation with functional (tachycardia-dependent) bundle branch block, since in this latter rhythm one would expect a more aberrant (wider) QRS complex in a beat which ends a short R-R interval, which was itself preceded by a long R-R interval (e.g. third QRS in V_1, V_2, V_3) and a less aberrant (narrower) QRS complex in a beat which ends a long R-R interval, which was itself preceded by a short R-R interval (e.g. fifth QRS in V_1, V_2, V_3) but this is manifestly **not** the case here.

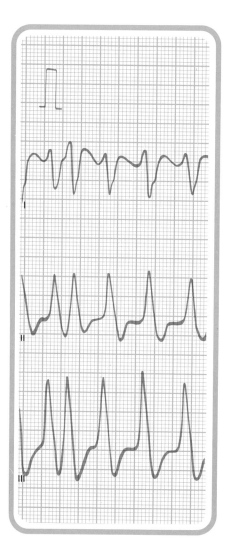
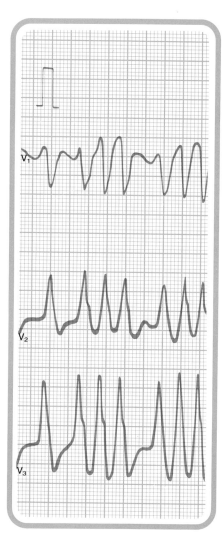
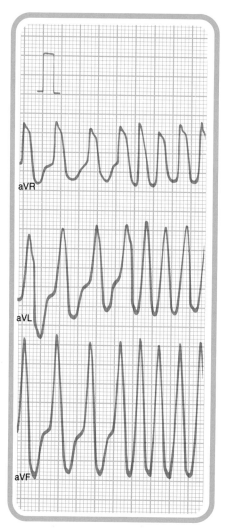
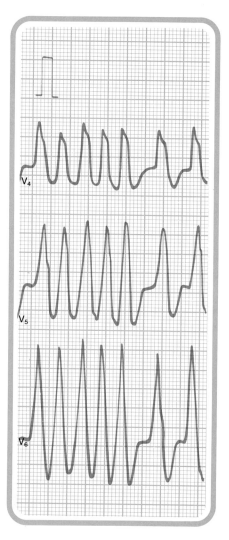

Ambulatory Electrocardiography

The standard 12-lead electrocardiogram displays something of the order of 12 sec of recording when a three-channel machine is used, and 36 sec of recording when a single-channel machine is used. When the cardiac rhythm is "diagnosed" the diagnosis only applies for the duration of the period of observation. The "time window" of the normal 12-lead electrocardiogram is only a tiny proportion of even one day and clearly gives a very inadequate expression of the possible variations in rhythm which might occur over a period of time.

In recognition of the need to create a less inadequate "time window" of observation for rhythm analysis, the technique of ambulatory electrocardiographic monitoring was introduced by Holter in 1961. The terms "ambulatory electrocardiography", "Holter monitoring" and "dynamic electrocardiography" are synonymous and refer to a technique designed to permit relatively long-term electrocardiographic recording in patients going about their normal everyday activities. The technique is most useful in the diagnosis and quantification of arrhythmias, in the evaluation of anti-arrhythmic therapy and for detecting pacemaker malfunction. However, the technique is also applied to the collection of morphological information from the electrocardiogram to investigate intermittent myocardial ischaemia by looking at changes in the configuration of the S-T segments and T waves.

Basic Aspects of Ambulatory Electrocardiography

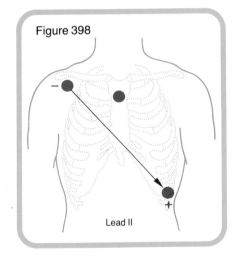

Figure 398

Lead II

Equipment used. Recording and Playback Technique

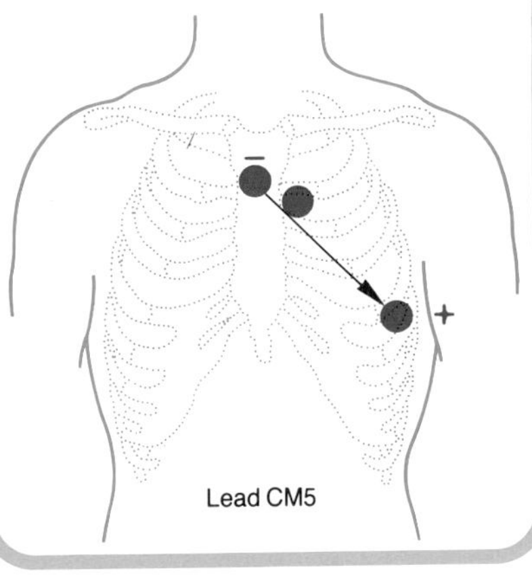

The most commonly used **equipment** is a battery-operated continuous ECG tape-recorder.

The **recording electrodes** are attached to the chest in a manner which is most appropriate to the problem under consideration. In the case of rhythm analysis, for example, the lead chosen is approximately equal to Lead II (negative connection just below the right clavicle, positive connection at the lower anterior left rib margin, indifferent connection in the area of the manubrium sterni, Figure 398) or Lead CM1 (a modified V_1 position in which the positive lead is situated at the fourth right intercostal space adjacent to the sternum, the negative position is on the manubrium sterni and the indifferent position is at the second left intercostal space adjacent to the sternum, Figure 399). However, for the detection of ischaemia, Lead CM5 (a modified V_5 position in which the positive electrode is situated at the fifth left intercostal space in the anterior auxiliary line, the negative electrode is situated over the manubrium and the indifferent electrode at the second left intercostal space adjacent to the sternum, Figure 400) or Lead CC5 (also a modified V_5 position in which the positive electrode is situated at the fifth left intercostal space in the anterior auxiliary line, the negative electrode is situated at the fifth right intercostal space in the anterior auxiliary line and the indifferent electrode is situated at the second left intercostal space adjacent to the sternum, Figure 401) may be used. The Lead II of ambulatory electrocardiography is approximately equivalent to Lead II of the 12-lead ECG (compare Figure 398 with Figure 26 (Section 1, page 21)). Lead CM1 is approximately equivalent to Lead V_1 of the 12-lead ECG (compare Figure 399 with Figures 37 and 36 (Section 1, pages 29 and 28 respectively)). Lead

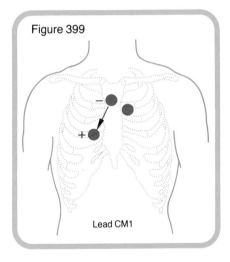

Figure 399

Lead CM1

CM5 is approximately equivalent to Lead V_5 of the 12-lead ECG (compare Figure 400 with Figures 37 and 36 (Section 1, pages 29 and 28 respectively)). Lead CC5 is a less accurate approximation to Lead V_5 of the 12-lead ECG than is Lead CM5.

Figure 400

Lead CM5

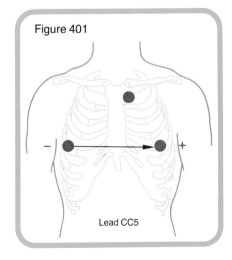

Figure 401

Lead CC5

The **ECG electrodes** are normally connected to the patient via gel-type patch electrodes and the small portable ECG tape-recording box is strapped around the patient's chest and worn under the clothing. Most systems permit the recording of two leads simultaneously as a fail-safe in case one recording lead becomes defective (so that a false arrhythmia diagnosis is less likely to be made). The electrode sitings are chosen to avoid large muscle masses the inclusion of which would result in the intermittent addition of electromyographic signals from active skeletal muscle.

The **play-back system** may provide a full print-out in miniaturised form of 24 hours of recording (on the basis of one sheet of recording per hour or per half hour, Figure 402a) or it may be organised to permit a technician to view the ECG signal on an oscilloscope screen at many times (typically 60–120) the natural speed and subsequently to produce print-outs, at conventional electrocardiographic recording speed, of representative samples of observed arrhythmias (Figure 402b). In the former system the clinician sees the entire recording (although it is in miniaturised form and may be difficult to read in places), whereas in the latter system the clinician is to some extent dependent upon the technician for "reading" of the ambulatory record. The technician using the scanning system will normally, on noticing a deviation from normal, obtain a "natural" speed (i.e. conventional ECG recording speed of 25mm/sec) print-out of the relevant parts of the record. Computer-assisted techniques are becoming available to help to reduce the tedious, time-consuming and error-fraught techniques of analysis.

Figure 402a

30-minute print-out of continuous ambulatory ECG recording

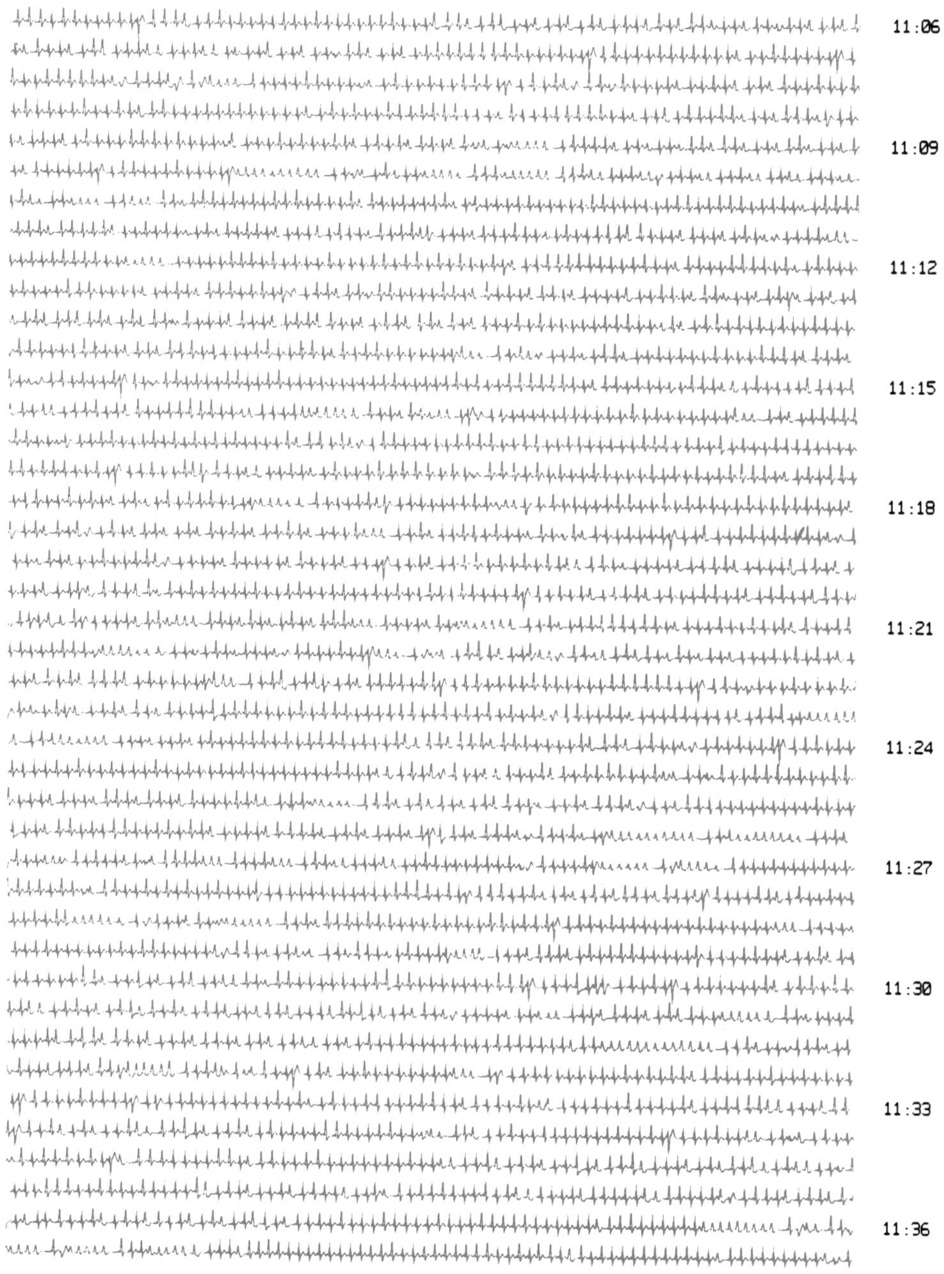

543

Figure 402b

Real-time print-out of technician-selected parts of a 24-hour ambulatory recording of conventional (25mm/sec) recording speed

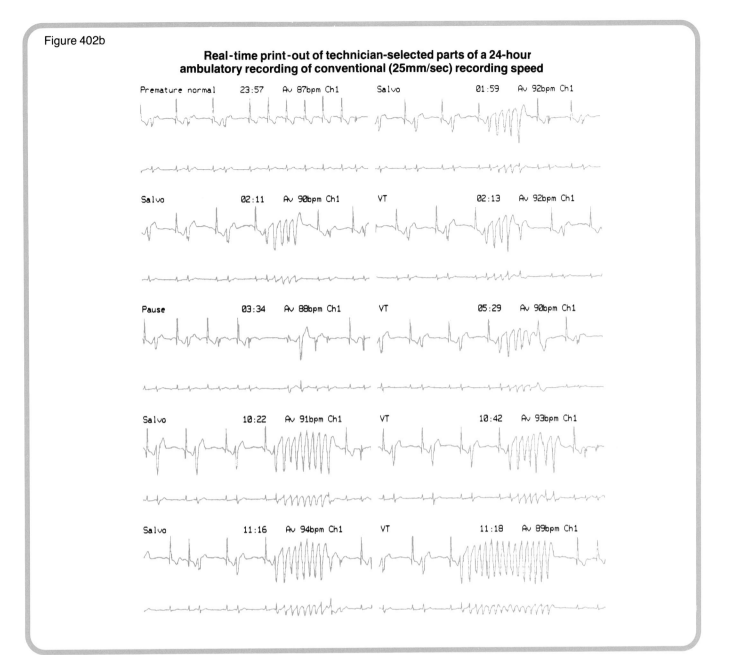

An alternative technique for gaining information about the cardiac rhythm in a real-time situation requires the patient to carry a pocket-sized device which contains a solid-state memory, capable of recording the electrocardiogram for a limited period (typically 30 sec or so). This device has metal contacts which may be applied directly to the bare chest and has a button to activate the recording. The patient is required to open his shirt, place the device on the chest with the electrodes touching his skin and then press the button. The recording then take place automatically. The memory is non-volatile although it can be overridden if required by a further push on the button. The contents of the memory may be unloaded by taking the equipment to the recording centre or by a telephone transmission where the appropriate facilities are available.

Intermittent recording devices of this type are clearly useful when there are symptoms suggestive of a dysrhythmic event (particularly palpitations or dizziness) but are not useful when the presenting symptom is syncope.

Patient Diary

Patients undergoing ambulatory electrocardiography are required to keep a log during the day of all relevant activities and symptoms and of the times when various medications (especially anti-arrhythmic drugs) are taken. This diary forms a very important part of ambulatory monitoring for it demonstrates the correlation (or lack of it) between the observed changes in the electrocardiogram and the symptoms which are being investigated. Most recorders are equipped with an event marker which permits the patient to identify the precise timing of relevant events with respect to the ECG recordings. The use of this event marker in conjunction with the patient diary helps also to establish a clear frame of reference for time.

544

24-hour Rhythm Analysis in Normal Subjects: The Normal Database

With the increasing use of ambulatory monitoring it soon became apparent that the ECG in the normal subject varied much more than had formerly been realised. Variations in heart rate and rhythm were found to be common.

Heart Rate

In normal subjects the heart rate may vary widely during a 24-hour period of day and night. A variation can clearly be recognised. In the absence of sufficient physical activity to disturb the heart rate, the minimal heart rate usually occurs between 3 and 5 am and the maximal heart rate between late morning and noon. Taking into account the normal everyday activities of healthy subjects variations in rate between 35 and 190 beats/min may be seen in the absence of heart disease. Women tend to have a faster heart rate than men and it is clear that the heart rate in normal subjects increases appreciably, not only with physical exercise, but also as a result of mental stress. Substantial changes in heart rate have been observed to occur in relation to driving. In athletes the heart rate during sleep may be as low as 24 beats/min.

Sinus Arrhythmia

Sinus arrhythmia is found to be extremely common in healthy subjects and R-R intervals may vary between 0.8 and 2.0 sec at rest within seconds.

Ectopic Beats

Occasional asymptomatic supraventricular (atrial or junctional) ectopic beats are observed in more than half of the normal population. However, although it is very common to find these beats in a 24-hour recording, it is not usual for large numbers of beats to be found during a 24-hour period.
The majority of healthy subjects will have no more than 10 or 20 of these beats and only a tiny proportion of the healthy population will have more than 100 of these beats within a 24-hour period.
The situation with respect to ventricular ectopic beats is very similar. Again more than half the population will have some ventricular ectopic beats during a 24-hour period, but in most cases the numbers will be small (again typically 10 or 20 per 24 hours). Only a tiny minority of the normal population will have more than 100 ventricular ectopic beats in a 24-hour period. More complex forms of ventricular ectopic activity (ventricular coupling, multi-form ventricular ectopic beats, R-on-T ectopics, couplets and more than 30 ventricular ectopics per hour) are relatively less frequently found in normal subjects, but are found with increasing frequency the older the age of the population studied.

Brady-arrhythmias

As indicated above, marked sinus bradycardia is common in the normal ambulatory electrocardiographic recording and is almost universally present during sleep in the early hours of the morning. At this stage the bradycardia can be associated with a junctional escape rhythm and this may be found in up to 20 percent of healthy subjects. Sinus arrest for periods of half to one sec and sino-atrial block for a single beat at a time may be seen in up to one-third of normal subjects. First degree heart block and type I second degree atrio-ventricular block may be found in normal subjects. These findings are most common in those with high levels of physical activity either in their occupation or as a hobby, and may be most noticeable at the end of such activity or during sleep.

Tachy-arrhythmias

Short episodes of atrial tachycardia (typically lasting for 2 or 3 sec) may be seen in about two percent of young adults as with the ventricular ectopic beats. This finding tends to be commoner in older members of the population.

Junctional and ventricular tachycardias are rarely found in healthy subjects who do not have symptoms of tachy-dysrhythmia.

Arrhythmias not found in Healthy Subjects

Type II second degree atrio-ventricular block, complete heart block and sustained ventricular tachycardia are not found in the ambulatory electrocardiogram of normal subjects.

Indications for Ambulatory Electrocardiographic Recording

The most common indication for ambulatory electrocardiographic recording is the presence of symptoms which might have a cardiac arrhythmic cause. This group obviously includes palpitations but also, very importantly, includes dizziness and/or syncope. The ambulatory electrocardiogram may also be used to help to monitor the effects of anti-arrhythmic therapy in patients known to have cardiac arrhythmias and may be used to look for the presence of arrhythmias in patients with heart disease where arrhythmias are known to carry prognostic significance (even if they are not symptomatic). The technique may be used in the assessment of pacemaker function or malfunction and also to detect occult myocardial ischaemia. If it is used for the latter purpose it is of the greatest importance to establish that the physical characteristics of the equipment are adequate for the purpose. In particular the low-frequency response of the recording system must be completely reliable.

Ambulatory Monitoring for Palpitations

"Palpitations" (or the unusual awareness of the cardiac action) frequently disturb patients and often constitute an indication for ambulatory monitoring in the hope that an electrocardiographic explanation of the symptoms will become apparent and that suitable treatment will then be possible. Examples of rhythm strips obtained from 24-hour ambulatory records used in this way are shown in Figures 403 to 408.

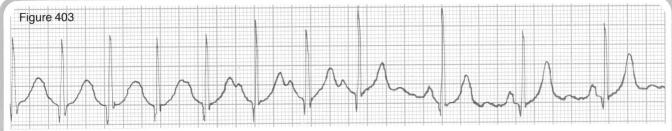

Figure 403

Ambulatory electrocardiographic recording. Varying sinus rate. The first four complexes show a very rapid sinus rate (approximately 115 beats/min) with each P wave superimposed on the preceding T wave. The sinus rate then slows spontaneously and rapidly and within two sec is down to about 80 beats/min.

This patient was complaining of intermittent pounding of the heart. Treatment with a beta-blocking drug suppressed the symptoms.

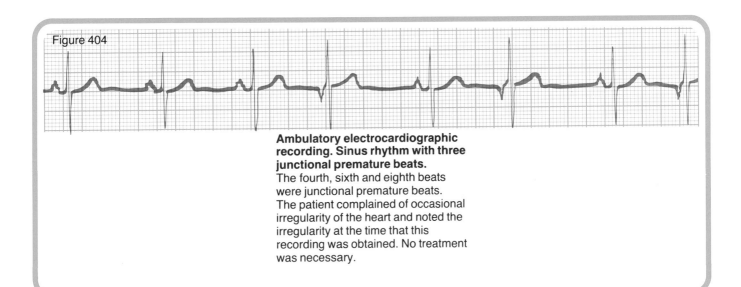

Figure 404

Ambulatory electrocardiographic recording. Sinus rhythm with three junctional premature beats. The fourth, sixth and eighth beats were junctional premature beats. The patient complained of occasional irregularity of the heart and noted the irregularity at the time that this recording was obtained. No treatment was necessary.

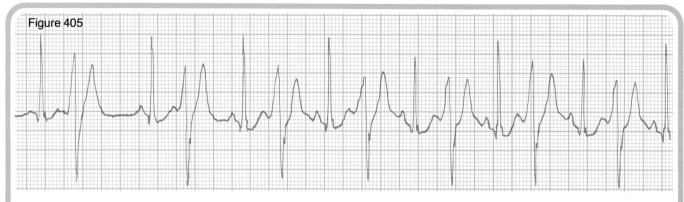

Figure 405

Ambulatory electrocardiographic recording. Sinus rhythm with uniform, coupled, interpolated ventricular premature (ectopic) beats. Such an arrhythmia will frequently give rise to symptoms. The possible role of hypokalaemia and of digitalis should be considered.

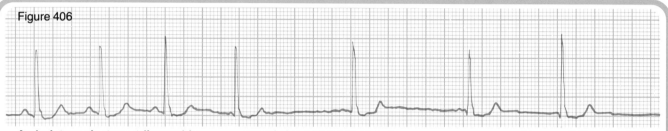

Figure 406

Ambulatory electrocardiographic recording. The onset of atrial fibrillation. The first three beats are sinus beats. The remainder of the strip shows atrial fibrillation with a slow ventricular rate. The patient complained of irregularity of the heart and occasional episodes of dizziness. No symptoms were noted in association with the rhythm change shown.

Findings of this type raise the possibility that other findings of more obvious haemodynamic significance (such as episodes of rapid atrial fibrillation or substantially slower ventricular rates) might occur at other times and treatment might well be necessary. The possibility of the Sick Sinus Syndrome should be considered. Further arrhythmia monitoring is likely to be necessary for the use of anti-arrhythmic drugs might result in aggravation of bradycardia with possible increase in the symptoms. Cardiac pacing might need to be considered.

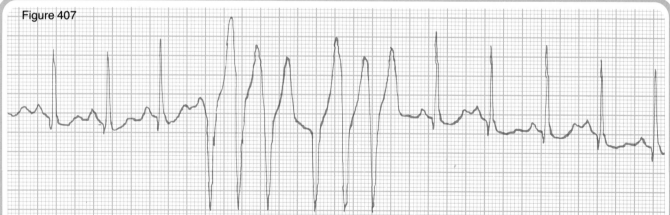

Figure 407

Ambulatory electrocardiographic recording. Sinus rhythm with a run of wide QRS complex tachycardia. The tachycardia may well be a short burst of ventricular tachycardia but it is difficult to be certain of this. It looks as though the P wave rhythm is probably undisturbed during the burst of wide QRS complex tachycardia (if the timing of the P waves in relation to the first three beats is traced throughout the record, they match up perfectly with the timing of the P waves following the burst of tachycardia) and this supports the suggestion that the arrhythmia is ventricular tachycardia (since the P waves have presumably continued at an unchanged rate during the tachycardia, i.e. there has been atrio-ventricular dissociation). However, the ventricular rate is strikingly irregular during the tachycardia. Although irregularity of the heart rate is recognised in association with ventricular tachycardia, the variation is usually minimal and this raises the possibility that the rhythm is a short burst of rapid atrial fibrillation with aberrant intraventricular conduction.

However, this explanation is relatively unlikely since the long R-R interval occurring in the middle of the tachycardia is not followed by a more normal QRS.

This example illustrates the difficulty of interpretation often found in association with ambulatory records (or with any rhythm analysis for that matter). The correct diagnosis in this case is probably ventricular tachycardia (possibly with two short bursts of three beats each and a gap in between).

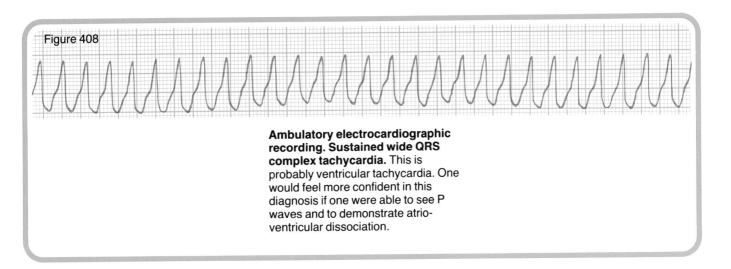

Figure 408

Ambulatory electrocardiographic recording. Sustained wide QRS complex tachycardia. This is probably ventricular tachycardia. One would feel more confident in this diagnosis if one were able to see P waves and to demonstrate atrio-ventricular dissociation.

Ambulatory Monitoring for Dizziness or Syncope

Dizziness and syncope are clearly potentially very important symptoms. They can be indicative of serious or life-threatening arrhythmias and the transient impairment of consciousness may itself, in appropriate situations, pose a major danger to the subject. Such symptoms may have cardiac or extra cardiac causes. Even when the cause is cardiac, routine clinical, electrocardiographic, radiographic and echocardiographic assessment may not reveal any abnormality. The use of short-term, patient-initiated, solid state memory devices is clearly inappropriate for this kind of problem but 24-hour Holter monitoring may yield very useful information. The ambulatory electrocardiogram may be helpful in one of two ways. First of all, when the patient develops a rhythm disturbance of a type which is capable of giving rise to profound haemodynamic disturbance and simultaneously experiences dizziness, the likelihood that the arrhythmia is the cause of the symptomatic problem is extremely high. By the same token when a patient experiences a rhythm disturbance and is unaware of any symptoms it may reasonably be concluded that the symptoms are not related to the demonstrated rhythm changes (although, of course, the possibility that other rhythm changes occur at times when the recording is not being made needs to be considered) and when the patient has a typical episode of syncope or dizziness at a time when the cardiac rhythm is unchanged, that particular episode (at least) could not have been due to a cardiac arrhythmia. Some rhythm changes, of course, are inevitably associated with loss of consciousness (such as ventricular fibrillation or asystole persisting for 15 sec or longer). Some arrhythmias might give rise to symptomatic disturbances in some situations but not in others. These would include rapid ventricular tachycardia or profound bradycardia. Young subjects with relatively healthy hearts and relatively normal cerebral circulations might well tolerate these arrhythmias much better than those with impaired myocardial function, valve disease or cerebrovascular disease. Unfortunately, there will be many situations when the electrocardiographic recording will not permit the confident diagnosis or exclusion of a cardiac cause for the symptoms. For example, when the record shows atrial fibrillation with a rapid ventricular rate, short bursts of supraventricular or ventricular tachycardia or pauses of two or three seconds between consecutive QRS complexes it may not be possible to reach a definitive conclusion about the role of the rhythm in producing symptoms. Such transient arrhythmias **may** but **do not necessarily** cause impairment of consciousness. Further periods of ambulatory monitoring may be indicated.

Although a 24-hour ambulatory record represents a considerable advance in the magnitude of data collection compared with a 12-lead ECG (typically a 24-hour record involves about 85,000 cardiac cycles and a 12-lead ECG fewer than 50) it still represents an extremely small time window and has, for example, only a 1 in 30 chance of catching an event which occurs monthly.

Examples of records obtained in the investigation of patients complaining of dizziness or syncope are shown in Figures 409 to 412.

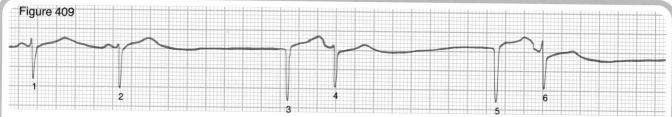

Ambulatory electrocardiographic recording. Sick sinus syndrome.

The first two beats (1 and 2) are sinus beats. There is then a long pause without atrial activity (sinus arrest). This pause is ended by a junctional escape beat (3). This beat is followed by what is either an atrial echo beat or an atrial ectopic (premature) beat which conducts to the ventricle to give a normal QRS (beat 4). There is then a period of sinus arrest which ends with a junctional escape beat (5) and a further atrial echo beat or atrial ectopic premature beat (6). Although the pauses here are not sufficient to guarantee that dizziness or syncope will result the record leaves little doubt that the sino-atrial and atrio-ventricular nodes are diseased. The patient had the Sick Sinus Syndrome and was disturbed by symptoms of dizziness. A pacemaker was inserted with relief of the symptoms.

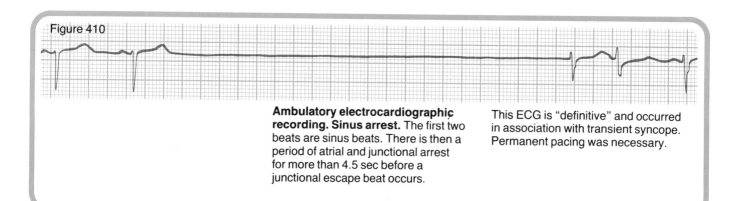

Ambulatory electrocardiographic recording. Sinus arrest.

The first two beats are sinus beats. There is then a period of atrial and junctional arrest for more than 4.5 sec before a junctional escape beat occurs. This ECG is "definitive" and occurred in association with transient syncope. Permanent pacing was necessary.

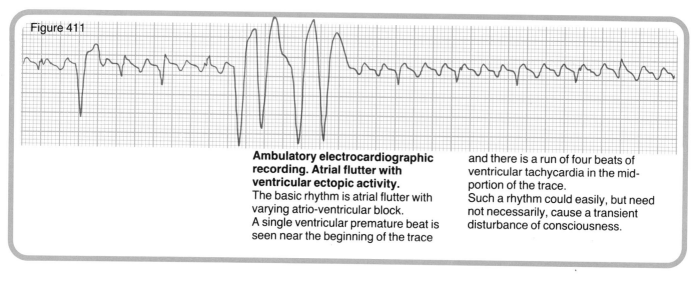

Ambulatory electrocardiographic recording. Atrial flutter with ventricular ectopic activity.

The basic rhythm is atrial flutter with varying atrio-ventricular block. A single ventricular premature beat is seen near the beginning of the trace and there is a run of four beats of ventricular tachycardia in the mid-portion of the trace.

Such a rhythm could easily, but need not necessarily, cause a transient disturbance of consciousness.

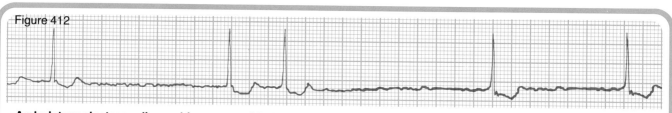

Ambulatory electrocardiographic recording. Atrial fibrillation with a slow mean ventricular rate.

Two pauses of 2 sec each are seen in a short segment of trace. The mean ventricular rate was very slow. The cardiac action could certainly be inefficient at such a rate and it is possible that consciousness might be impaired. On the other hand it is equally possible that the patient could tolerate this kind of heart rate without any symptoms. The finding of such a slow rate, however, would suggest that drugs which increase the refractory period of the atrio-ventricular node (digitalis preparations, beta-blocking drugs, verapamil and similar calcium antagonists) should be withdrawn or withheld. Permanent pacing might be necessary if symptomatic bradycardia persisted after these drugs had been withdrawn.

Innocent Arrhythmias Recorded by Ambulatory Monitoring

As explained earlier, studies of ambulatory electrocardiographic recordings from subjects with no overt evidence of ischaemic heart disease have demonstrated that a wide variety of arrhythmias (which in some cases at least had formerly been considered to have prognostic importance) may occur. Thus occasional (but not very frequent) atrial and ventricular premature beats are found in a significant proportion of young subjects and in higher proportions of older subjects. Profound sinus bradycardia (Figure 413) is common during sleep and transient type I second degree atrio-ventricular block (Figure 414) occurs in a few percent of healthy subjects, particularly those who are regularly involved in vigorous physical activity. In these subjects it is most likely to occur at the completion of such activity or during sleep. Normally if there is a sufficiently slow sinus rate there will be a junctional escape mechanism. An example is shown in Figure 415.

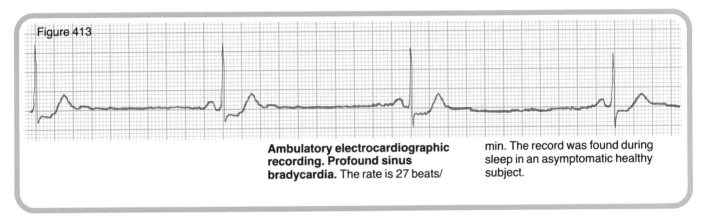

Figure 413

Ambulatory electrocardiographic recording. Profound sinus bradycardia. The rate is 27 beats/min. The record was found during sleep in an asymptomatic healthy subject.

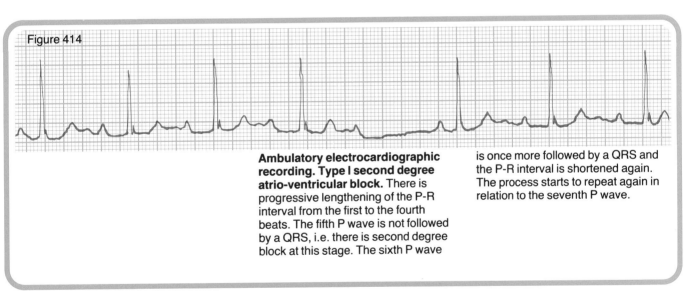

Figure 414

Ambulatory electrocardiographic recording. Type I second degree atrio-ventricular block. There is progressive lengthening of the P-R interval from the first to the fourth beats. The fifth P wave is not followed by a QRS, i.e. there is second degree block at this stage. The sixth P wave is once more followed by a QRS and the P-R interval is shortened again. The process starts to repeat again in relation to the seventh P wave.

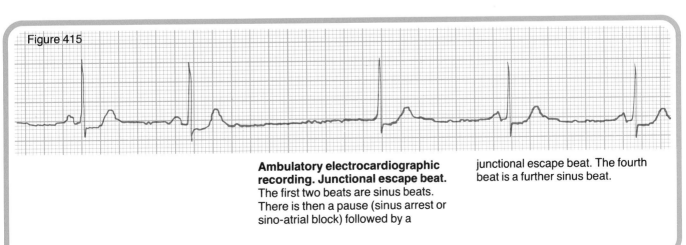

Figure 415

Ambulatory electrocardiographic recording. Junctional escape beat. The first two beats are sinus beats. There is then a pause (sinus arrest or sino-atrial block) followed by a junctional escape beat. The fourth beat is a further sinus beat.

When there is a sinus pause without a junctional escape beat the implication is that the junctional area is depressed as well as the sinus node. An example is shown in Figure 416.

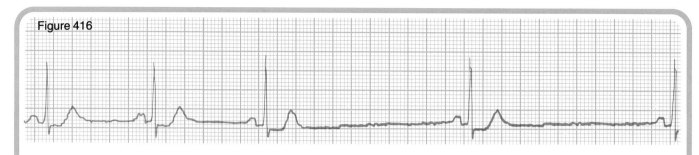

Figure 416

Ambulatory electrocardiographic recording. Sinus arrest. The first three beats are sinus beats. There is then a sudden drop in the sinus rate. Since the R-R interval between the third and fourth beats is not exactly twice the control (preceding) R-R interval, the suggestion is that the mechanism is sinus arrest rather than sino-atrial block. The period of sinus arrest is ended not by a junctional escape beat (which would be expected after a pause of almost 2.3 sec) but by a further sinus beat. The implication is that the atrio-ventricular node is depressed as well as the sinus node.

Ambulatory Monitoring in Ischaemic Heart Disease

Ambulatory electrocardiographic monitoring may reveal changes in the S-T segments and T waves occurring in the absence of any primary disturbance of rate or rhythm. Such changes are often thought to be associated with coronary artery spasm. The changes may consist of S-T segment depression or T wave inversion or, less frequently, of S-T segment elevation. An example is shown in Figure 417.

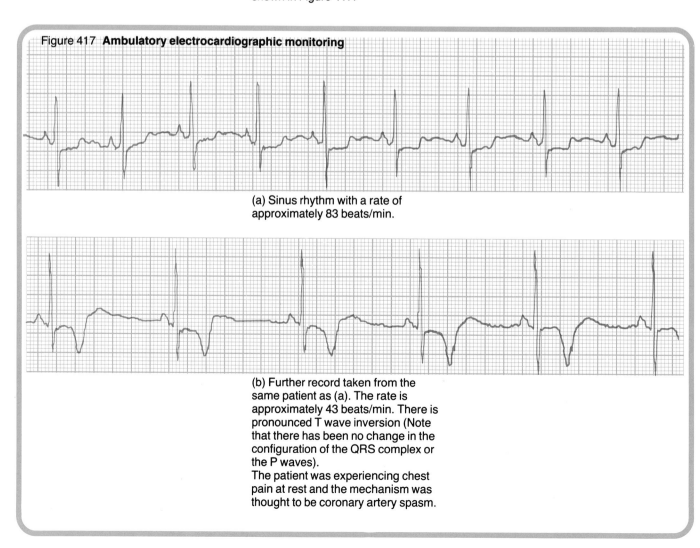

Figure 417 **Ambulatory electrocardiographic monitoring**

(a) Sinus rhythm with a rate of approximately 83 beats/min.

(b) Further record taken from the same patient as (a). The rate is approximately 43 beats/min. There is pronounced T wave inversion (Note that there has been no change in the configuration of the QRS complex or the P waves).
The patient was experiencing chest pain at rest and the mechanism was thought to be coronary artery spasm.

Great caution should be exercised in the interpretation of S-T segment depression and T wave inversion recorded during ambulatory electrocardiography. The first problem which may arise is a technical one. For adequate recording of the information contained in the T waves and S-T segments the frequency response of the recorder and play-back system must extend down to 0.5 cycles per sec or better. The second problem concerns the currently very inadequate database for the normal dynamic electrocardiogram. All electrocardiographic interpretation is empirical and only when an extensive database of dynamic electrocardiographic recording has been obtained both in healthy and in defined disease states, will reasonably confident prediction of the significance of S-T segment and T wave changes observed during such recordings become possible. It is already apparent that all subjects (100%) show variation in T wave amplitude and morphology (including the development of T wave inversion) within a 24-hour period. The vast majority of these changes are innocent and they are more commonly seen in association with (i) changes in body positions (ii) eating (iii) anything which induces substantial changes in the heart rate. S-T segment depression is less commonly seen than T wave change but seems to occur in about 30 percent of normal subjects. It also occurs without associated symptoms in about 70 percent of subjects with proven ischaemic heart disease.

Ambulatory Monitoring in Pacemaker Patients

Pacemaker malfunction may be intermittent and in cases of suspected intermittent pacemaker malfunction, ambulatory monitoring is sometimes of value, for example, in demonstrating the intermittent failure of a pacing stimulus to "capture" the myocardium or the intermittent failure of the pacemaker system to sense a spontaneous myocardial depolarisation. The ambulatory electrocardiogram can also, of course, be useful in showing the absence of pacing malfunction at a time when the patient experiences symptoms.

Clearly it is perfectly possible for any of the cardiac arrhythmias to be demonstrated during the course of an ambulatory electrocardiographic recording. No attempt has been made in this chapter to provide a comprehensive demonstration of rhythms which can be recorded by ambulatory techniques. Some of the most helpful varieties have been shown.

Inter-relationship of Morphological Changes and Arrhythmias

"Morphological analysis" relates to the electrocardiographic evaluation (a) of P waves to gain useful information concerning the atria (atrial hypertrophy, atrial infarction, atrial ischaemia) and, more particularly, (b) of QRS complexes, S-T segments and T waves to give useful information concerning the ventricles (hypertrophy of left or right ventricles, intraventricular conduction disturbances (left or right bundle branch block, left anterior hemiblock, left posterior hemiblock, combinations of these)), myocardial infarction, myocardial ischaemia etc. This morphological assessment depends upon the recognition of deviations from the normal appearances of the P waves, QRS complexes, S-T segments and T waves (as described in Sections 1 and 2). Ectopic arrhythmias necessarily interfere with this process to some extent since supraventricular ectopic arrhythmias involve abnormal pathways of atrial myocardial depolarisation and therefore are associated with abnormal shape and/or polarity of the P waves and since ventricular arrhythmias involve abnormal pathways of ventricular myocardial depolarisation with abnormal shape and/or polarity of the QRS complexes. In the case of the ventricles, the abnormal depolarisation process (giving abnormal QRS complexes) results in abnormal repolarisation also and this is usually apparent as abnormalities of shape of the S-T segments and T waves (Atrial repolarisation is similarly abnormal in supraventricular arrhythmias but since the Ta wave is only occasionally visible in the normal ECG (page 166) changes in atrial repolarisation occurring in association with atrial arrhythmias are only very rarely apparent). Since no database can readily be available for the "normal" P wave associated with a given supraventricular arrhythmia or for the "normal" QRS, S-T or T of the ventricular arrhythmias, **it is not possible for a reliable morphological assessment of the atria to be made during a period of supraventricular arrhythmia or of the ventricles during a period of ventricular arrhythmia.**

Theoretically, it should be possible to make a morphological assessement of the atria in the presence of ventricular arrhythmias (provided there is no retrograde conduction to the atria (i.e there is ventriculo-atrial dissociation) but in practice this is impossible since the P waves are usually barely detectable because of the large QRS (and possibly the large T) deflections (e.g. see Figure 308, page 466). It often is possible, however, to make a morphological assessment of the ventricles during a supraventricular arrhythmia. This is not possible if, during the period of the supraventricular arrhythmia, there is pre-existing ventricular pre-excitation or bundle branch block and it is not easily possible if, during the period of the supraventricular arrhythmia, there is aberrant intraventricular conduction.

Table 43 shows the effect of arrhythmias on the possibility of morphological assessment of the electrocardiogram.

Table 43 Ability to make a morphological assessment of the electrocardiogram during an ectopic arrhythmia

Cardiac rhythm	Possibility of morphological assessment of P waves	Possibility of morphological assessment of QRS complexes, S–T segments and T waves
Sinus rhythm	Possible	Possible
Sinus tachycardia	Possible	Possible
Sinus bradycardia	Possible	Possible
Sinus arrest	No P wave at time of sinus arrest	Possible if junctional escape Not possible if ventricular escape
Atrial ectopic beats	Not possible. P wave distorted	Possible unless aberrant intraventricular conduction, bundle branch block or pre-excitation
Atrial tachycardia	Not possible. P wave distorted	
Atrial flutter	Not possible. Flutter waves not P waves	
Atrial fibrillation	Not possible. Fibrillation waves not P waves	
Junctional premature beats	Not possible. Polarity reversed	
Junctional tachycardia	Not possible. Polarity reversed	
AV nodal re-entrant tachycardia	Not possible. Polarity reversed and P wave usually hidden in QRS	
Re-entrant tachycardia with anomalous pathway	Not possible. Polarity reversed	Possible if anterograde path is via the AV node Impossible if anterograde path is via anomalous pathway
Ventricular tachycardia with ventriculo-atrial conduction	Not possible. Polarity reversed	Not possible
Ventricular tachycardia with no ventriculo-atrial conduction	Not possible. Morphology unchanged but obscured	Not possible
Ventricular fibrillation	Not possible. Morphology unchanged but obscured	Not possible
First degree atrio-ventricular block	Possible	Possible
Second degree type I atrio-ventricular block	Possible	Possible
Second degree type II atrio-ventricular block	Possible	Possible
Third degree atrio-ventricular block	Possible	Possible if His bundle escape rhythm Impossible if ventricular escape rhythm

Influence of Morphological Changes on Rhythm Analysis

The essence of the influence of morphological changes on rhythm analysis in the electrocardiogram is contained in the phrase (used very frequently in the section on Ectopic Arrhythmias) that the P wave or QRS complex is "normal for the subject at the time". Thus, for example, an ectopic P wave has a morphology different from that of a sinus-initiated P wave. But patients with morphological abnormalities of the atria (hypertrophy, infarction etc) also have morphologically abnormal P waves and the P wave of atrial hypertrophy can be very similar to or identical to that of an atrial ectopic beat. The distinction between abnormal P waves due to morphological abnormality of the atria and abnormal P waves due to the site of initiation of atrial depolarisation is indicated by the timing and morphology of adjacent complexes (Figure 418).

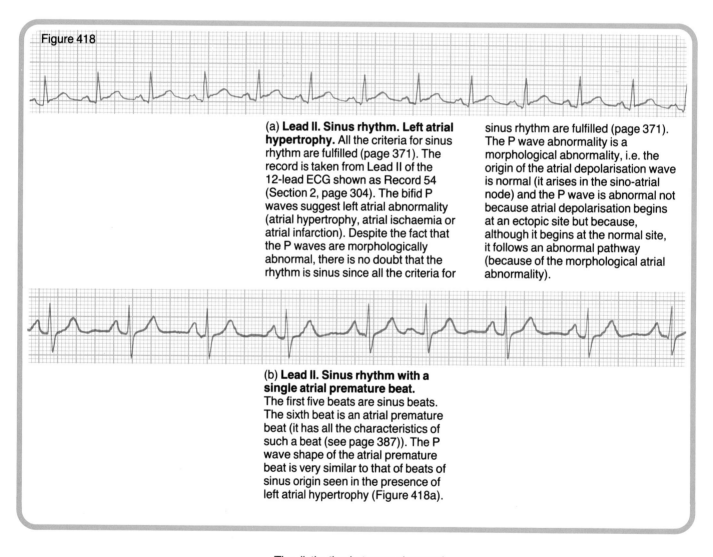

Figure 418

(a) **Lead II. Sinus rhythm. Left atrial hypertrophy.** All the criteria for sinus rhythm are fulfilled (page 371). The record is taken from Lead II of the 12-lead ECG shown as Record 54 (Section 2, page 304). The bifid P waves suggest left atrial abnormality (atrial hypertrophy, atrial ischaemia or atrial infarction). Despite the fact that the P waves are morphologically abnormal, there is no doubt that the rhythm is sinus since all the criteria for sinus rhythm are fulfilled (page 371). The P wave abnormality is a morphological abnormality, i.e. the origin of the atrial depolarisation wave is normal (it arises in the sino-atrial node) and the P wave is abnormal not because atrial depolarisation begins at an ectopic site but because, although it begins at the normal site, it follows an abnormal pathway (because of the morphological atrial abnormality).

(b) **Lead II. Sinus rhythm with a single atrial premature beat.** The first five beats are sinus beats. The sixth beat is an atrial premature beat (it has all the characteristics of such a beat (see page 387)). The P wave shape of the atrial premature beat is very similar to that of beats of sinus origin seen in the presence of left atrial hypertrophy (Figure 418a).

The distinction between abnormal QRS complexes due to morphological abnormality of the ventricles and abnormal QRS complexes indicative of ventricular ectopic beats is indicated by the timing and morphology of adjacent complexes (Figure 419).

Figure 419

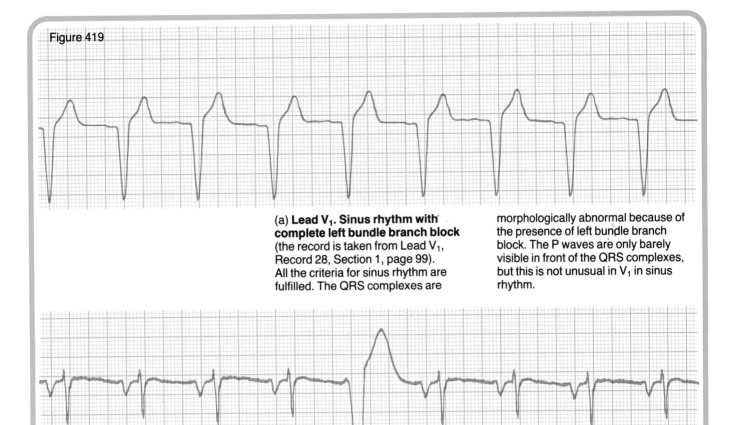

(a) **Lead V₁. Sinus rhythm with complete left bundle branch block** (the record is taken from Lead V₁, Record 28, Section 1, page 99). All the criteria for sinus rhythm are fulfilled. The QRS complexes are morphologically abnormal because of the presence of left bundle branch block. The P waves are only barely visible in front of the QRS complexes, but this is not unusual in V₁ in sinus rhythm.

(b) **Lead V₁.** The basic rhythm is sinus. There is a strong negative component to the P wave in this lead suggesting the presence of left atrial hypertrophy (see Section 2, pages 162 to 165). A single ventricular ectopic beat is seen. This ectopic QRS complex has the configuration of left bundle branch block and is therefore arising in the right ventricle (page 413). The form of the QRS complex in relation to the ectopic beat in this recording is virtually indistinguishable from the QRS complexes in association with left bundle branch block in Figure 419a.

Thus the potentially confusing impact of morphological abnormalities on the analysis of the cardiac rhythm is minimised or abolished by referring to the P wave or QRS appearances which are "usual for the subject at the time" (rather than to P wave or QRS complexes which are "normal") in the criteria for a given rhythm. It follows that if the P waves or QRS complexes are morphologically abnormal (i.e. are abnormal during sinus rhythm) an ectopic atrial or ventricular beat may actually present with a P wave or QRS (respectively) which is closer to **normal** than is the corresponding appearance during sinus rhythm in that subject with that morphological abnormality. It also follows that an abnormal P wave may be due to a morphological abnormality of the atrial myocardium or to an ectopic atrial depolarisation and that an abnormal QRS complex may be due to a morphological abnormality of the ventricular myocardium or to an ectopic ventricular depolarisation. In each case the distinction is made by assessing what happens before and after the deflection in question.

Cardiac Rhythm Assessment

It will be apparent from the foregoing sections that the cardiac rhythms are numerous and that many are complex. No truly systematic approach to rhythm analysis has yet been devised and all attempts to do so inevitably come up against the conflict between simplicity and comprehensiveness. This conflict was acknowledged earlier (pages 359 to 370), when a simple approach to rhythm analysis was initiated. Now that the individual arrhythmias have been covered it is possible to produce a more complex (but still by no means comprehensive) approach.

The Record: Single or Multiple Lead Analyses

The cardiac rhythm is often interpreted from a single lead of the ECG. In most cases a single lead is adequate, provided the lead has been optimally chosen. **Rhythm analysis requires elucidation of the QRS complexes, the P waves and the relationship between them.** Almost any lead will show the QRS complexes so it follows that for effective rhythm analysis, if a single lead is used, it should be chosen as a lead which best shows the P waves. Leads II and V_1 are probably the best individual leads for this purpose (Section 2, page 158). However, if more than one lead is available, the process of rhythm analysis may be made much simpler since

a) the greater the number of leads available the greater is the likelihood of being able to recognise P waves, and

b) the greater the number of leads available, the more likely one is to be able to make conclusions about the direction (and hence by inference the site of initiation) of depolarisation of the atria and of the ventricles.

These are powerful factors in rhythm analysis.

Figure 420 shows an example of a situation in which **the availability of more than one lead helps rhythm analysis.**

It is an illustration of Leads I, II and III from an ECG showing atrial flutter. The flutter waves are readily apparent in Leads II and III but are barely detectable in Lead I. The latter feature simply indicates that the vector of the flutter wave was approximately at right angles to Lead I and emphasises the need to find a lead which shows atrial activity (P waves, P' (ectopic P) waves, F (flutter waves) etc).

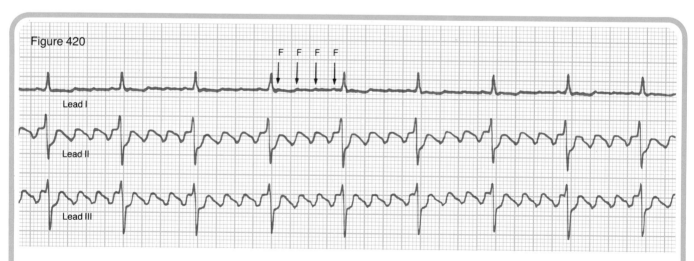

Figure 420

F F F F

Lead I

Lead II

Lead III

Atrial flutter. Leads I, II and III simultaneously recorded. There is atrial flutter with 4:1 atrio-ventricular block. The atrial rate is 300 beats/min and the ventricular rate is 75 beats/min. Flutter waves are easily seen in Leads II and III but are difficult to see in Lead I. Careful analysis of Lead I reveals the flutter waves (arrowed). If Lead I alone were used the flutter waves could easily be missed. The usefulness of inspecting several leads during rhythm analysis is apparent.

Figure 421 shows an example of how **the knowledge of the location of a lead influences the conclusions about the rhythm.** In this lead the QRS complexes are upright in each beat (indicating that the ventricular depolarisation vector travels towards the lead in each of these beats). The P waves are upright in all beats but one, indicating that in most beats the P wave vector also travels towards that lead but that in one it travels away from that lead.

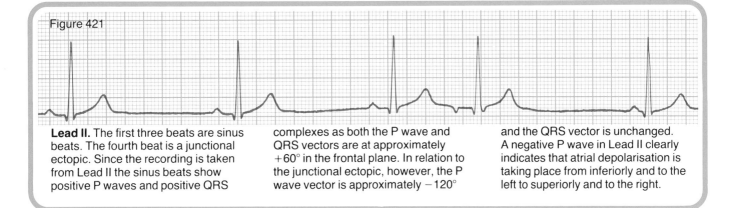

Figure 421

Lead II. The first three beats are sinus beats. The fourth beat is a junctional ectopic. Since the recording is taken from Lead II the sinus beats show positive P waves and positive QRS complexes as both the P wave and QRS vectors are at approximately +60° in the frontal plane. In relation to the junctional ectopic, however, the P wave vector is approximately −120° and the QRS vector is unchanged. A negative P wave in Lead II clearly indicates that atrial depolarisation is taking place from inferiorly and to the left to superiorly and to the right.

The Initial Approach

The initial approach to rhythm analysis is important in obtaining maximal information.

1. Choose the Time Window

It has to be remembered that the rhythm of the heart is, like Easter, a variable feast and that any description of cardiac rhythm is only valid in respect of that time during which the rhythm analysis is being made. When choosing such a time window it is helpful not only to attempt to analyse the ECG during a period when the appearances are constant, but also to make a careful inspection of a time window at any time when the rhythm appears to change (e.g. Figure 266, page 430). For example, consider the appearances in Figure 266: Inspection of the time window involving beats 1-5 or 6-11 reveals a rapid regular heart rate with narrow QRS complexes, i.e. a supraventricular tachycardia. P or P′ waves cannot be recognised with confidence. However, during the time interval between beat 5 and beat 6 and during the time interval between beat 11 and beat 12 P′ waves are recognisable and are seen to be occurring regularly. Their timing can be extrapolated in both directions throughout the record (see caption to Figure 266). **It is frequently very rewarding to analyse the rhythm at times of apparent change.**

2. Choose the ECG Lead

Every effort must be made to choose a lead which either (a) **actually** shows P or P′ waves or (if no P or P′ waves can be recognised with confidence), (b) **usually** shows P or P′ waves. The leads most likely to be helpful in this respect are Leads II and V_1.

3. If possible use Multiple Leads to assess the QRS Duration

If the morphology of the QRS complex is constant throughout the period for which the rhythm is to be analysed, assess the QRS duration as the greatest QRS duration seen in any of the leads, for it is perfectly possible for a QRS complex to look narrower in one lead than another if the vector of the initial or terminal part of the QRS is at right angles to that lead. Figure 422 shows an example of this.

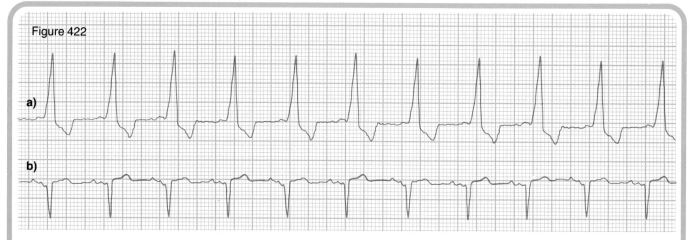

Figure 422

This figure shows Leads I (a) and V$_1$ (b) from the same patient as Record 70, page 320. Inspection of Lead V$_1$ would suggest that the QRS complex is of normal duration (0.08 sec). Inspection of **simultaneously-recorded** Lead I shows that the QRS is actually abnormally wide at 0.14 sec. This patient had ventricular pre-excitation and the delta wave is well seen in Lead I but is approximately at right angles to V$_1$ and is therefore not seen in this latter lead. Ventricular activation actually begins before it is apparent in V$_1$ (of course it is also possible that the **very** earliest or latest part or both of the ventricular activation vectors is at right angles to Lead I and that the QRS is actually **longer** than 0.14 sec). All that can be concluded is that **provided the QRS morphology does not change between the recording of one lead and another** (manifestly impossible when the leads in question are recorded simultaneously) the widest QRS seen most closely approximates to the actual duration of ventricular depolarisation. In this respect it is worthwhile also to compare the varying appearances of atrial activity in the different leads of Figure 420. The duration of the flutter waves is apparently very short in Lead I but clearly much longer in Leads II and III.

4. Carotid Sinus Massage

The value of carotid sinus massage in providing additional electrocardiogaphic data which contribute to the diagnostic information relating to supraventricular tachycardia should not be underestimated. A few examples may serve to illustrate this.

Sinus tachycardia is a supraventricular tachycardia and one cannot always be absolutely certain that the rhythm is sinus since, if the rate is sufficiently rapid, the P wave of a given beat may be buried in the T wave of the preceding beat or it may be suspected that an additional P wave may be present, perhaps obscured by the QRS complex. In either case, carotid sinus massage may reveal the true situation (Figure 423 a-e).

Figure 423

The value of carotid sinus massage in the elucidation of the cardiac rhythm. Carotid sinus massage may (i) transiently slow down the prevailing sinus rate, (ii) prolong atrio-ventricular conduction time or produce an increase in atrio-ventricular block (e.g. during atrial tachycardia or during atrial flutter) or (iii) may both slow the sino-atrial discharge frequency and also prolong AV conduction time.

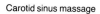

Carotid sinus massage

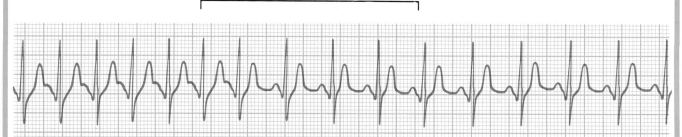

a) **Lead II. Sinus tachycardia.** During the first part of the trace there is sinus tachycardia at the rate of 150 per min. Carotid sinus massage temporarily slows down the sinus rate revealing clearly that the underlying rhythm is sinus enabling one to be reasonably confident that the earlier part of the record did not contain additional P waves obscured by the QRS complexes (i.e. that the rhythm had not previously been atrial tachycardia with 2:1 atrio-ventricular block).

Figure 423 (continued)

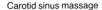
Carotid sinus massage

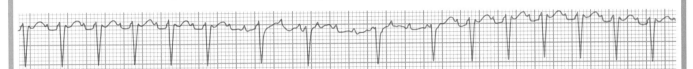

b) **Lead V₁. Atrial tachycardia.**
The first six beats show a regular supraventricular tachycardia and the appearances suggest sinus tachycardia. Carotid sinus massage produces a greater degree of atrio-ventricular block and reveals that the true rhythm is atrial tachycardia. The ectopic atrial rate remains constant throughout. In the initial and terminal parts of the record there is atrial tachycardia with 2:1 AV block (alternate P′ waves being hidden in the terminal part of the QRS complexes).

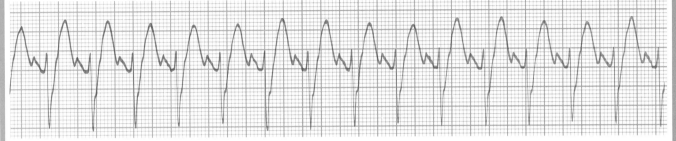

c) **Lead II. Sinus tachycardia.**
The rhythm seems clearly to be sinus tachycardia but one might wonder about the possibility that there could be twice as many P waves as initially seems apparent, i.e. that there could be atrial tachycardia with 2:1 AV block and alternate P waves buried in the QRS. Carotid sinus massage (d) slows the sinus rate and indicates that the rhythm simply is sinus tachycardia. QRS complexes are wide since there is a pre-existing left bundle branch block.

Carotid sinus massage

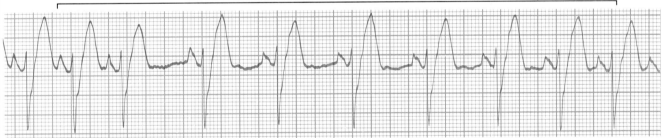

d) The record is taken from the same patient as Figure 423c. Carotid sinus massage transiently slows the sinus rate.

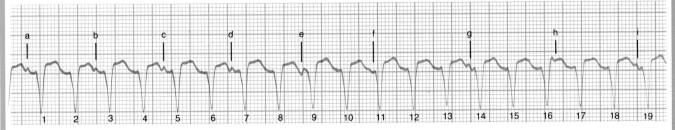

e) **Chest monitoring lead. Ventricular tachycardia.**
There is a tachycardia with wide QRS complexes (0.11 sec). The ventricular rate is 168 beats/min. P waves can be seen at a, b, c and d. They are regular and are at half the ventricular rate. The rhythm is, therefore, clearly ventricular tachycardia with ventriculo-atrial conduction every second beat (i.e. 2:1 ventriculo-atrial block). At beat 7 carotid sinus massage is commenced. There is no change in the ventricular rate but the atrial rate falls (intervals d-e, e-f, f-g, g-h and h-i are all longer than intervals a-b, b-c and c-d (these three all being the same)). Clearly carotid sinus massage has influenced the atrial rate without affecting the ventricular rate (a clear demonstration of the ventricular nature of the tachycardia). Either this was initially ventricular tachycardia with retrograde AV block (i.e. VA block) and with an independent sinus mechanism at exactly half the ventricular rate (statistically unlikely) in which case carotid sinus massage reduced the sinus rate, or there was originally ventricular tachycardia with 2:1 ventriculo-atrial block (every alternate ventricular activation being transmitted back through the AV node to the atria) in which case, carotid sinus massage increased the ventriculo-atrial activation time.

Caution must be exercised in relation to carotid sinus massage. In sensitive subjects asystole may be produced and carotid massage must never be undertaken without simultaneous observation of a real-time ECG display or at least continuous simultaneous, auscultation of the heart (Figures 424 and 425). Carotid sinus massage must be discontinued immediately ventricular slowing is apparent.

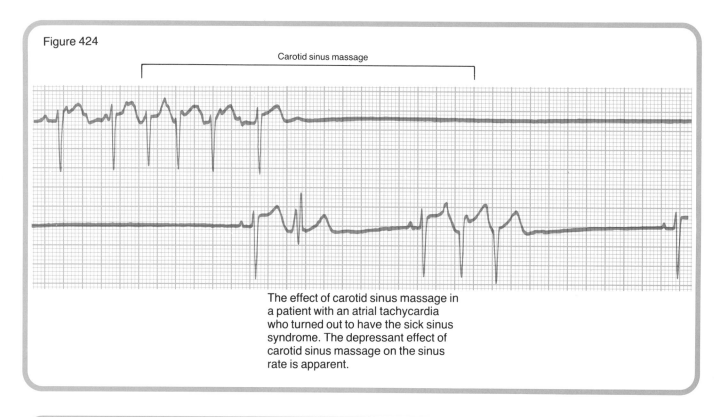

Figure 424

Carotid sinus massage

The effect of carotid sinus massage in a patient with an atrial tachycardia who turned out to have the sick sinus syndrome. The depressant effect of carotid sinus massage on the sinus rate is apparent.

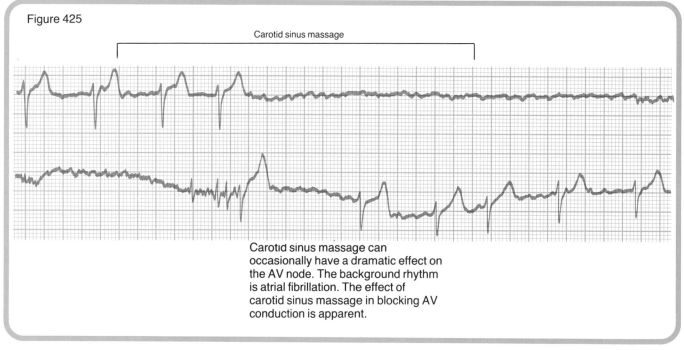

Figure 425

Carotid sinus massage

Carotid sinus massage can occasionally have a dramatic effect on the AV node. The background rhythm is atrial fibrillation. The effect of carotid sinus massage in blocking AV conduction is apparent.

From this point onwards a decision-making tree is inevitably followed, whether intuitively or knowingly, or whether haphazardly or systematically. It clearly makes manifest good sense that it should be both knowingly and systematically and therefore an attempt at a systematic approach is given here. It must, however, be conceded at the outset that no comprehensive, systematic approach has yet been devised which results in the successful delineation of every cardiac rhythm and that even if such an approach were available it would still fail to elucidate some cardiac rhythms from the 12-lead ECG or from a single-lead rhythm strip simply because some of the required ECG data may be obscured (e.g. P waves may be present but may always be obscured by QRS complexes). The following systematic approach should therefore be seen in the light of this limitation. Sometimes it is not possible to be sure what the cardiac rhythm is.

Ventricular fibrillation, when present, must be recognised immediately (pages 473 to 475). The scheme which follows assumes that ventricular fibrillation is not present.

The Systematic Approach to ECG Rhythm Interpretation

Having chosen a suitable lead and an appropriate time zone, as indicated above, the systematic analysis may begin.

These questions should be answered systematically (with respect to the chosen time zone) and Tables 44 to 50 referred to as indicated.

1. Is the QRS rate (frequency) regular?
2. Is the rate rapid (>100 beats/min), **slow** (<60 beats/min) **or "normal"** (60<rate<100)?
3. Is the QRS width normal (<0.12 sec) **or wide** (≥0.12 sec)?

At this stage (Table 44) the rhythm can be categorised as:
a) bradycardia (ventricular rate<60 beats/min)
b) normal rate (ventricular rate between 60-100 beats/min)
c) tachycardia (ventricular rate >100 beats/min)
d) intermittent, short R-R intervals (early beats)
e) intermittent, long R-R intervals (pauses)
f) cyclical variation in R-R interval
g) no recognisable pattern of R-R interval

In turn the tachycardias can be sub-divided into:
i) **a narrow QRS complex tachycardia** (ventricular rate >100 beats/min; QRS width normal)
ii) **wide QRS complex tachycardia** (ventricular rate >100 beats/min; QRS width > 0.12 sec)
iii) **irregular QRS rate tachycardia** (mean ventricular rate >100 beats/min, R-R interval very variable).

Flow Chart of Systematic Rhythm Analysis

Table 44 shows a diagnostic flow chart covering the more common cardiac rhythms.

Table 44 Rhythm Analysis

Is the QRS rate regular?

YES

NO

What is the QRS rate?
(tachycardia?, normal rate?, bradycardia?)

What is the QRS rate pattern?

† If there is a previous electrocardiogram showing wide QRS complexes (bundle branch block or intraventricular block) and the present record shows identical QRS morphology, proceed as if the QRS were of normal width.

‡ Use multiple leads. Assuming that no change occurs in the QRS during the 12-lead recording the widest QRS complex seen given that estimate of QRS width which is closest to the truth.

* Digitalis compounds, beta-blocking drugs, calcium antagonists of the verapamil type.

** These obvious possibilities should always be considered first in each respective heart-rate group. Any of these sinus mechanisms (sinus tachycardia, sinus rhythm, sinus bradycardia) may be accompanied by a long P-R interval (i.e. first degree heart block).

EARLY R WAVES   NO

YES

INTERMITTENT SHORT R-R INTERVALS   **D**

Sinus premature beats
Atrial premature beats   } conducted to the   { Occurring on the
Junctional premature beats   ventricles   { background of a
                                                   { regular rhythm as
                                                   { listed in A, B or C
Atrial parasystole
Junctional parasystole

Capture beats

Improvement in AV conduction during a supraventricular tachycardia with 2:1 or greater AV block

Ventricular premature beats occurring on a background of a regular rhythm as listed in A, B or C

Ventricular parasystole

Refer to Table 49 and Figure 428

Is the QRS abnormally†‡ wide
(>0.12 sec)?

YES†

NO

There are four possibilities

The rhythm is supraventricular with pre-existing bundle branch block   **1**

Supraventricular rhythms listed above are shown in red boxes

The rhythm is supraventricular
Supraventricular rhythms listed
above are shown in red boxes

The rhythm is supraventricular with functional (rate-related) bundle branch   **2**
block (i.e. with aberrant intraventricular conduction)

Supraventricular rhythms listed above are shown in red boxes

The rhythm is supraventricular with antegrade conduction down an   **3**
anomalous pathway

Supraventricular rhythms are shown in red boxes

For tachycardias with narrow QRS complexes refer to Table 45.
For bradycardias with narrow QRS complexes refer to Figure 426.
For intermittent pauses with narrow QRS complexes refer to Table 48 and Figure 427.

The rhythm is ventricular   **4**

Ventricular rhythms listed above are shown in purple boxes

RAPID (> 100 beats/min) ➤ NO ➤ "NORMAL" (60-100 beats/min) ➤ NO ➤ SLOW (< 60 beats/min)

YES   YES

TACHYCARDIA   **A**
(> 100 BEATS/MIN) : REGULAR

Sinus tachycardia**
Atrial tachycardia (1:1 or 2:1 AV conduction)
Atrio-ventricular nodal re-entrant tachycardia (AVNRT)
Atrial flutter (1:1 or 2:1 AV conduction)
Atrio-ventricular re-entrant tachycardia with bypass tract (AVRT)

Any of the above rhythms with additional bundle branch block, acceleration-dependent aberrancy or ventricular pre-excitation

Ventricular tachycardia

NORMAL RATE   **B**
(60-100 BEATS/MIN) : REGULAR

Sinus rhythm**
Sinus tachycardia with 2:1 AV block
Atrial tachycardia with 2:1 AV block
Atrial flutter with 3:1 or 4:1 AV block
Non-paroxysmal junctional tachycardia

Any of the above rhythms with additional bundle branch block, acceleration-dependent aberrancy or ventricular pre-excitation

Idioventricular rhythm (slow VT)
Ventricular tachycardia with 2:1 exit block

BRADYCARDIA   **C**
(< 60 BEATS/MIN : REGULAR)

Sinus bradycardia**
2:1 sino-atrial block
Coupled, blocked atrial premature beats
Coupled, blocked junctional premature beats
Sinus rhythm with high grade AV block
Sinus rhythm with 2:1 AV block
Sinus rhythm with complete heart block

Atrial fibrillation
Atrial tachycardia   } with complete heart block
Junctional tachycardia
Atrial flutter

Junctional escape rhythm

Any of the above rhythms with additional bundle branch block, deceleration-dependent aberrancy or ventricular pre-excitation

Idioventricular escape rhythm

PAUSES

YES

**INTERMITTENT LONG
R-R INTERVALS**   **E**
Intermittent increase in AV block during { Sinus tachycardia / Atrial tachycardia / Atrial flutter

Intermittent, non-conducted atrial extrasystoles

Pauses following premature beats (sinus, atrial, junctional, ventricular)

Sinus rhythm with Type I second degree AV block

Sinus rhythm with Type II second degree AV block

Concealed conduction

Concealed supraventricular extrasystoles

Repeated long R-R intervals suggest atrial fibrillation treated by drugs*

Any of the above rhythms with additional bundle branch block, deceleration-dependent aberrancy or ventricular pre-excitation

Concealed ventricular extrasystoles

Refer to Table 47 and Figure 426

CYCLICAL VARIATION ➤ NO ➤

YES

**"CONCERTINA"
R-R INTERVALS**   **F**
Sinus rhythm with Type I second degree AV block
Sinus arrhythmia

Any of the above rhythms with additional bundle branch block, rate – (acceleration – or deceleration –) dependent aberrancy or ventricular pre-excitation

Refer to Table 48 and Figure 427

**NO RECOGNISABLE
R-R INTERVAL PATTERN**   **G**

Atrial fibrillation
Atrial flutter with varying AV conduction
Multifocal atrial ectopic beats
Any of the above rhythms with additional bundle branch block, rate – (acceleration – or deceleration –) dependent aberrancy or ventricular pre-excitation

Multifocal ventricular ectopic beats
Ventricular parasystole

Combinations of the above

These three possibilities consist of supraventricular rhythms and can only be distinguished if (a) a pre-existing record shows bundle branch block(1) or pre-excitation(3) at a time when there is no disturbance of rate and the QRS duration and morphology is identical to that of the rhythm being considered, in which case supraventricular rhythm with pre-existing bundle branch block or supraventricular rhythm with antegrade conduction down an anomalous pathway (respectively) may be diagnosed or if (b) the rate became more normal (usually less rapid (of a tachycardia) but occasionally less slow (of a bradycardia)) and the QRS shape and duration simultaneously became less abnormal in which case supraventricular rhythm with rate-related bundle branch block can be diagnosed

These are all supraventricular rhythms with abnormal intraventricular conduction

The distinction between supraventricular rhythm with abnormal intraventricular conduction and ventricular rhythm is particularly important if there is also a tachycardia

Ventricular rhythm

Wide QRS rhythm

For wide QRS complex tachycardias refer to Table 46

Flow Chart for the Diagnosis of Narrow QRS Complex Tachycardia

Narrow QRS complex tachycardias are, almost without exception, supraventricular. (The only exception is fascicular tachycardia which is a very high ventricular tachycardia arising close to the His bundle). Re-entrant tachycardias associated with an anomalous pathway are regarded as supraventricular although strictly speaking the term is inaccurate since part of the re-entrant pathway is ventricular (page 452).

Once sinus tachycardia has been excluded as the mechanism of a narrow QRS complex tachycardia, the important diagnostic possibilities are atrial flutter, atrial fibrillation, atrial tachycardia, junctional tachycardia and anomalous pathway re-entrant tachycardia.

A schematic approach to the differential diagnosis of narrow QRS complex tachycardias is shown in Table 45.

The use of this table depends upon the assumption that sinus tachycardia has already been excluded as the cause of the supraventricular tachycardia.

Flow Chart for the Diagnosis of Wide QRS Complex Tachycardia

This is the single most important diagnostic sub-group of the tachycardias. The distinction between supraventricular and ventricular tachycardia is important in relation to diagnosis, prognosis and therapy. Whilst knowledge of the clinical background (e.g. young and otherwise fit patients with repeated episodes of paroxysmal tachycardia are likely to have supraventricular tachycardia whereas patients with multiple myocardial infarction are more likely to have ventricular tachycardia*) may help in relation to **clinical** diagnosis such concepts are irrelevant to this text which is concerned with the **electrocardiographic** diagnosis of the rhythm.

Rarely, one or more of four features may be found which permit of a confident diagnosis of ventricular tachycardia (Table 46 a-d). If **fusion beats** or **capture beats** can be seen or if the **QRS rate is demonstrably consistently greater than the P wave rate** or if the **QRS duration is 0.16 sec or more** in a subject known to have normal width ($\not> 0.10$ sec) QRS complexes when in sinus rhythm then the ventricular origin of the underlying rhythm is established (Table 46, pages 567 and 568). The first two features are rarely seen and the third only occasionally, so that whilst these features are invaluable when present their relative infrequency makes them of limited usefulness in the general approach.

Occasionally a previous ECG may be available to provide a clue to the current rhythm (Table 46 (e and f)).

More commonly none of the above features is present and the rhythm may be diagnosed with a varying degree of confidence depending on other features (Table 46 (1-6)).

*A common clinical misconception is that the onset of ventricular tachycardia is inevitably associated with appreciable haemodynamic deterioration whereas the onset of supraventricular tachycardia is not. This is a completely unreliable method of assessing the problem. The most important aspect of an arrhythmia in relation to its haemodynamic consequences is the ventricular rate.

Table 45 Narrow QRS complex tachycardia (rate > 100 beats/min, QRS complexes 0.10 sec or less in width)‡

1. The commonest supraventricular tachycardia is sinus tachycardia

2. Are flutter waves visible?

YES

NO

Atrial flutter

3. Is the ventricular rate irregular* and is there absence of consistently recognisable P waves?

YES

NO

Atrial fibrillation

4. Is there a regular atrial rate in the range of 180-240 beats/min with twice as many P waves as QRS complexes (2:1 AV block)?

YES

NO

Atrial tachycardia with 2:1 AV block

5. Is there a regular ventricular rate within the range 180-240 beats/min with no P waves visible?

YES

NO

The rhythm is probably AV nodal re-entrant tachycardia of the common "slow-fast" type

6. Is there a regular ventricular rate within the range 180-240 beats/min with one P wave to each QRS. If so, is the R-P′ interval equal to, greater than or less than the P′-R interval?

R-P′ < P′-R

R-P′ > P′-R

R-P′ = P′-R†

The rhythm is probably AV re-entrant tachycardia involving an AV bypass tract (AVRT) but could also be AV nodal re-entrant tachycardia (AVNRT) with slight delay in ventriculo-atrial conduction

The rhythm is probably AV nodal re-entrant tachycardia (AVNRT) of the uncommon "fast-slow" type (this configuration may also occasionally be seen, however, in re-entrant tachycardia using an anomalous pathway (antegrade through the AV node) when the anomalous pathway conducts slowly in a retrograde direction)

The rhythm may well be atrial tachycardia with 2:1 AV block (alternate P waves being in the QRS)†

* Random variation in R-R interval between the maximum and minimum values seen in the given time zone.

† Consider carefully the possibility that the additional P′ wave may be hidden in the QRS complex (whenever a P wave is seen half-way between QRS complexes such a possibility must be considered).

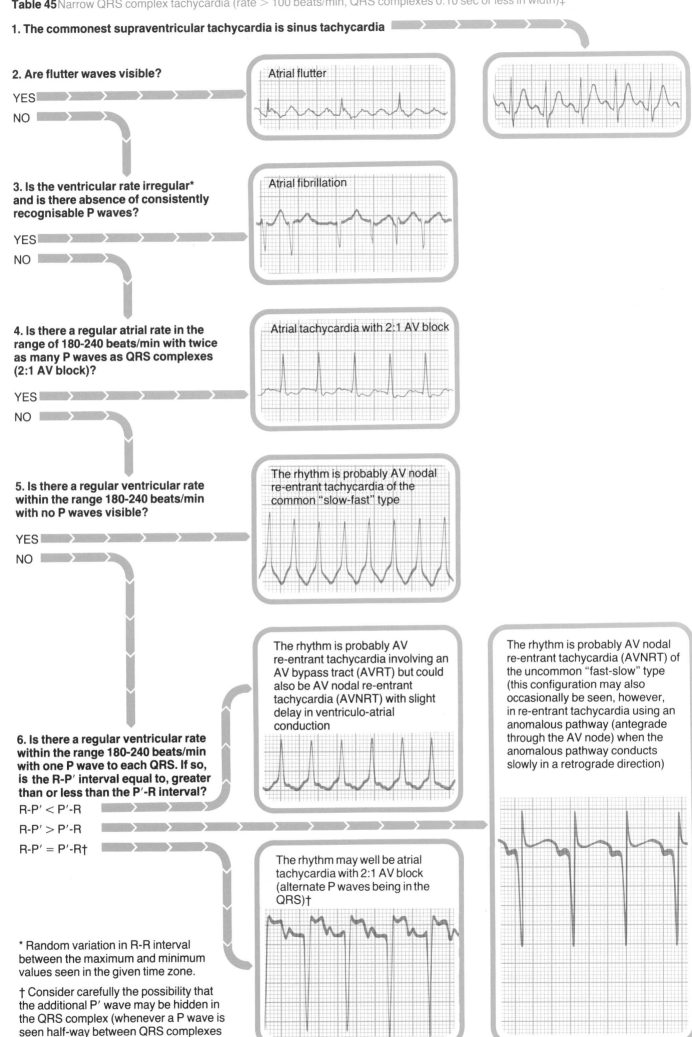

Table 46 Wide QRS complex tachycardia†

Rarely one of the following features may be observed. If any is present the tachycardia is definitely ventricular in origin.

(a) If capture beats can be seen the underlying rhythm is ▶▶▶▶ | VENTRICULAR TACHYCARDIA |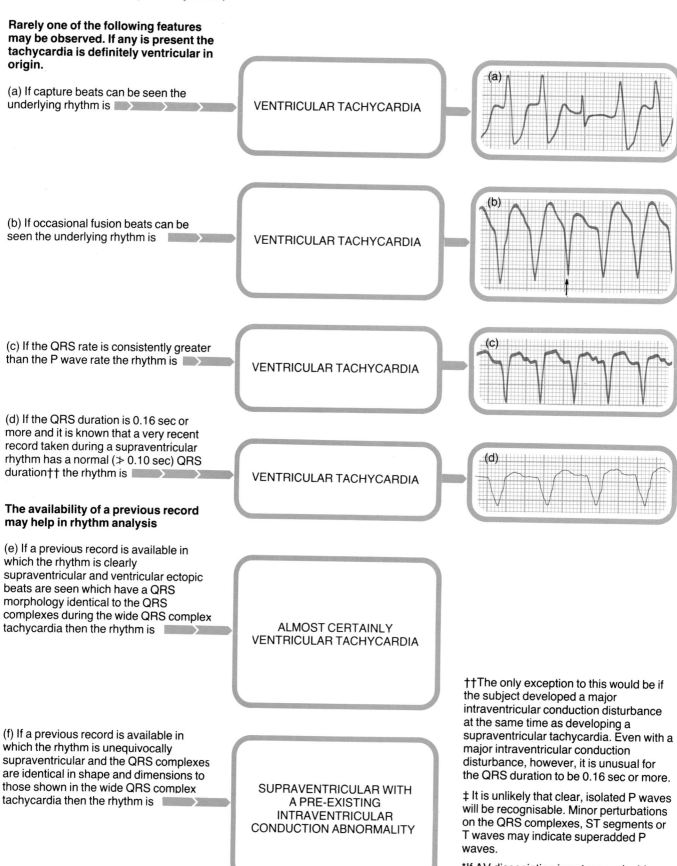

(a)

(b) If occasional fusion beats can be seen the underlying rhythm is ▶▶ | VENTRICULAR TACHYCARDIA |

(b)

(c) If the QRS rate is consistently greater than the P wave rate the rhythm is ▶▶ | VENTRICULAR TACHYCARDIA |

(c)

(d) If the QRS duration is 0.16 sec or more and it is known that a very recent record taken during a supraventricular rhythm has a normal (≯ 0.10 sec) QRS duration†† the rhythm is ▶▶ | VENTRICULAR TACHYCARDIA |

(d)

The availability of a previous record may help in rhythm analysis

(e) If a previous record is available in which the rhythm is clearly supraventricular and ventricular ectopic beats are seen which have a QRS morphology identical to the QRS complexes during the wide QRS complex tachycardia then the rhythm is ▶ | ALMOST CERTAINLY VENTRICULAR TACHYCARDIA |

(f) If a previous record is available in which the rhythm is unequivocally supraventricular and the QRS complexes are identical in shape and dimensions to those shown in the wide QRS complex tachycardia then the rhythm is ▶ | SUPRAVENTRICULAR WITH A PRE-EXISTING INTRAVENTRICULAR CONDUCTION ABNORMALITY |

††The only exception to this would be if the subject developed a major intraventricular conduction disturbance at the same time as developing a supraventricular tachycardia. Even with a major intraventricular conduction disturbance, however, it is unusual for the QRS duration to be 0.16 sec or more.

‡ It is unlikely that clear, isolated P waves will be recognisable. Minor perturbations on the QRS complexes, ST segments or T waves may indicate superadded P waves.

*If AV dissociation is not recognisable this may mean that (i) the P waves are absent or obscured (very common), (ii) that there is AV association with a supraventricular rhythm (very common) or (iii) that there is ventriculo-atrial association with the ventricular rhythm (less common, not rare). Inspect multiple leads to have the best chance of recognising the presence of P waves. If P waves are recognised and do not bear a constant relationship to adjacent QRS complexes, there is atrio-ventricular dissociation.

†The QRS complexes are regular (i.e. no irregularity is detectable. Effectively this means less than 10 percent variation in R-R interval – the largest compared with the shortest.) have a QRS duration of 0.12 sec or more (Use multiple leads. Assuming that no change occurs in the QRS during the 12-lead recording the widest QRS complex seen given that estimate of QRS width which is closest to the truth.) and a rate of more than 100 beats/min (These can either be ventricular tachycardia or supraventricular tachycardia with pre-existing bundle branch block or with aberrant intraventricular conduction. Rarely they might be supraventricular tachycardia with antegrade conduction down an anomalous pathway)

More commonly the above features are not present. In that event it is more difficult to be certain of the ventricular origin of a tachycardia with wide QRS complexes but the following features are the most helpful ones.

1. Can P waves be recognised?‡

NO ▷▷▷▷▷▷ Does not help to distinguish ventricular from supraventricular tachycardia.

YES ▷▷

Is atrio-ventricular dissociation recognisable?* ▷▷▷▷▷▷▷

2. Is the QRS duration > 0.14 sec? ▷▷▷

3. Is the frontal plane QRS axis within the range −30° to −120° (travelling anticlockwise, i.e. superior axis)? ▷▷▷

4. Is the shape of the QRS in V₁: ▷▷

5. Is the shape of the QRS in V₆: ▷▷

(i.e. r/s ratio <1)

(QS)

(R)

(RS)

(QS)

(QR)

(Rr)

6. If previous records available, is R (tachycardia) >r (sinus rhythm)? ▷▷

NO	YES
TO SOME EXTENT FAVOURS SUPRA-VENTRICULAR TACHYCARDIA with bundle branch block aberration	STRONGLY FAVOURS VENTRICULAR TACHYCARDIA

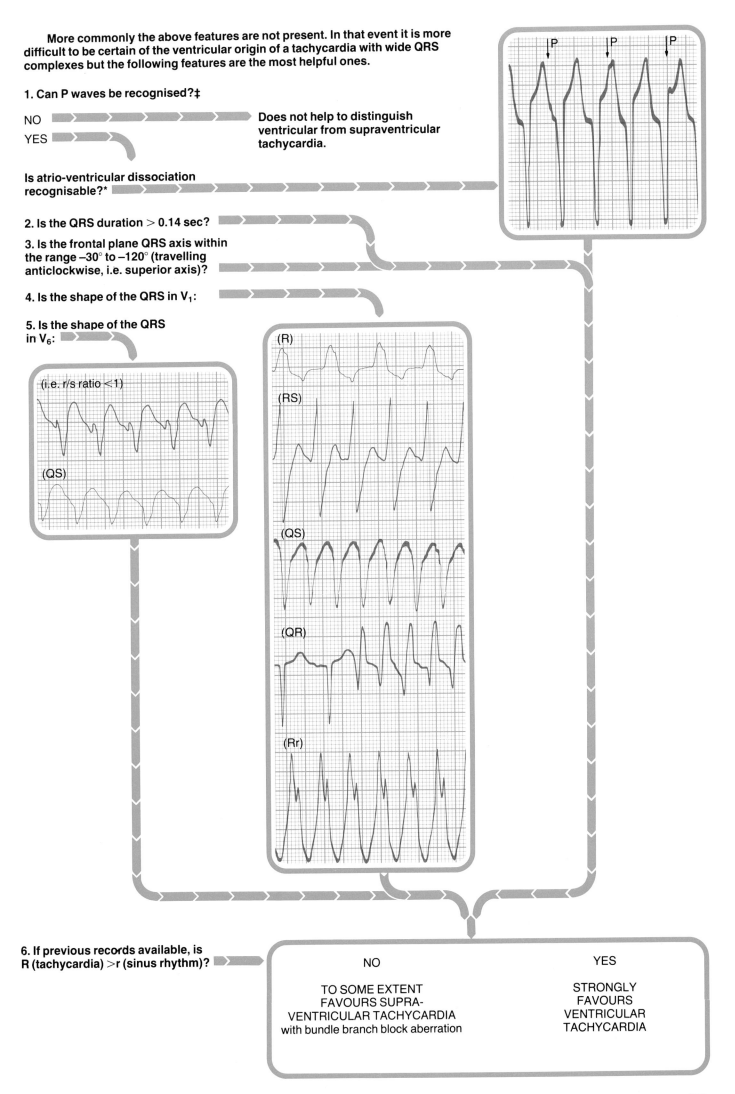

Tachycardias with Irregular Ventricular Rate (Irregular QRS Rate Tachycardias)

The commonest cause of a tachycardia with irregular rate* is atrial fibrillation. This is the only tachycardia in which there is no predictable relationship between one R-R interval and the next (in any given time window there will be a maximum and a minimum R-R interval but between these limits the R-R interval will not be predictable). The QRS duration is usually normal in atrial fibrillation (Figure 281) except for those beats associated with aberrant intraventricular conduction (Figure 285) or unless there is pre-existing bundle branch block or ventricular pre-excitation (Figure 301).

Bradycardias

The diagnosis of bradycardias does not, in general, present the same difficulty as the diagnosis of tachycardia. Nevertheless it is worth viewing the common causes (Table 47).

Table 47   Common Causes of Bradycardia

Sinus bradycardia

Junctional escape rhythm (with underlying (occult) sinus bradycardia**)

Ventricular escape rhythm (with underlying (occult) sinus bradycardia**)

Coupled, blocked (non-conducting) atrial premature beats

Third degree atrio-ventricular block, "complete atrio-ventricular block"; "complete heart block". (The atrial rhythm may be sinus rhythm, atrial tachycardia, atrial flutter, atrial fibrillation).

Second degree atrio-ventricular block with frequent failure of conduction (e.g. 2:1 atrio-ventricular block)

Examples of the common causes of bradycardias are given in Figure 426.

*This excludes tachycardias with **transient** irregularities such as those produced by capture beats, fusion beats, occasional ectopic beats or changes in the mechanism of the rhythm.

** The implication is that the sinus rate is slower than the junctional escape rate. In the presence of a continuous escape rhythm background sinus bradycardia cannot be distinguished from background sinus arrest.

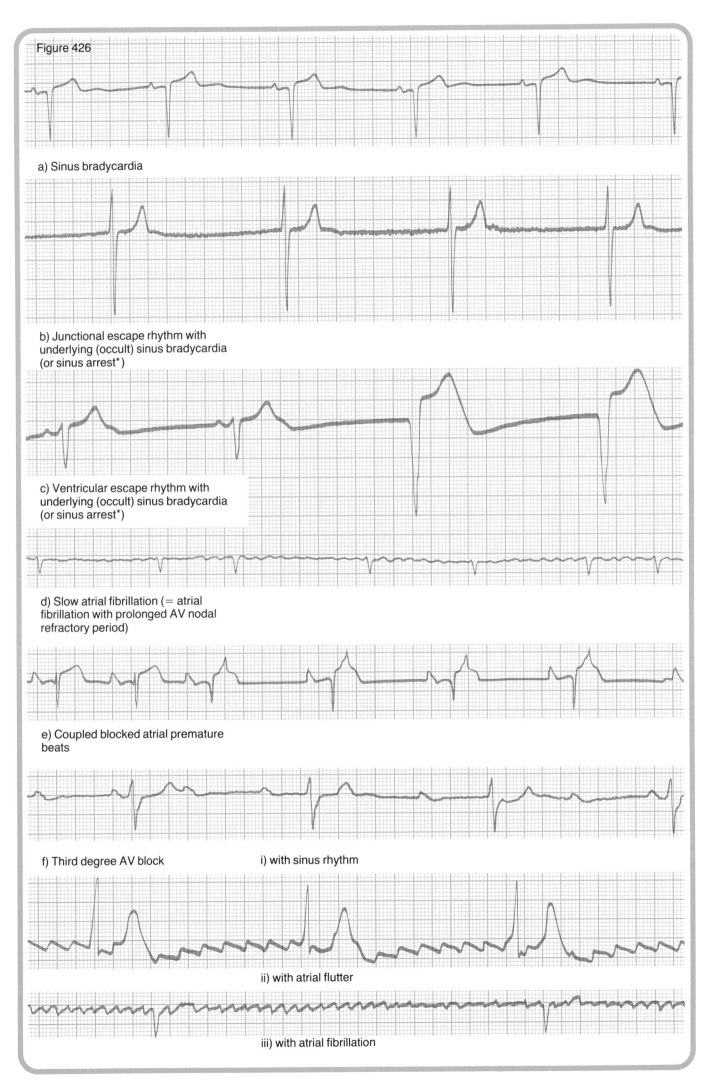

Figure 426

a) Sinus bradycardia

b) Junctional escape rhythm with underlying (occult) sinus bradycardia (or sinus arrest*)

c) Ventricular escape rhythm with underlying (occult) sinus bradycardia (or sinus arrest*)

d) Slow atrial fibrillation (= atrial fibrillation with prolonged AV nodal refractory period)

e) Coupled blocked atrial premature beats

f) Third degree AV block   i) with sinus rhythm

ii) with atrial flutter

iii) with atrial fibrillation

570

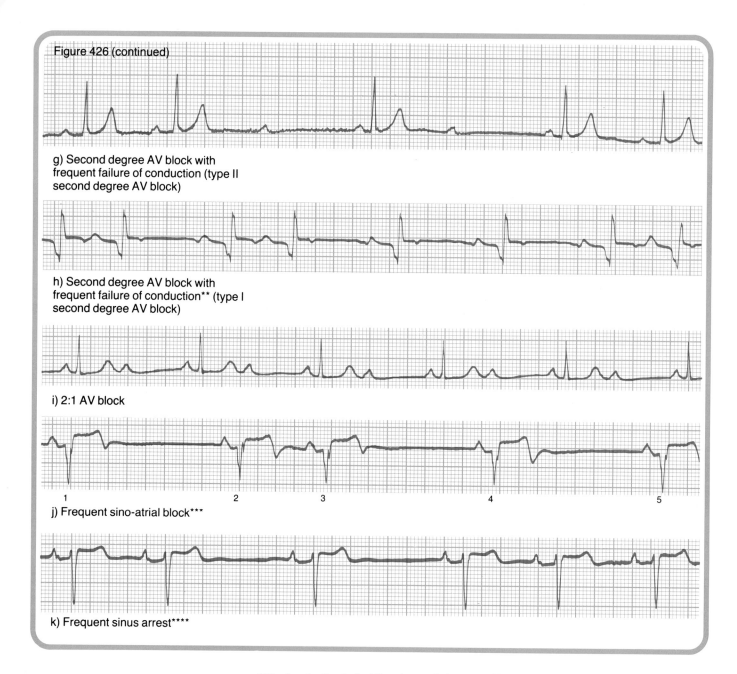

Figure 426 (continued)

g) Second degree AV block with frequent failure of conduction (type II second degree AV block)

h) Second degree AV block with frequent failure of conduction** (type I second degree AV block)

i) 2:1 AV block

j) Frequent sino-atrial block***

k) Frequent sinus arrest****

* The implication is that the sinus rate is slower than the junctional escape rate. In the presence of a continuous escape rhythm background sinus bradycardia cannot be distinguished from background sinus arrest.

** Lead V$_1$ after acute anteroseptal infarction. There is right bundle branch block and anterior infarction (compare the QRS complexes in Lead V$_1$, Figure 169, page 254). There is type I second degree AV block. In parts of the record there is 2:1 AV block. This can either be type I or II (pages 496 to 498) but since two consecutive conducted beats can be seen (on three occasions) with the second P-R interval longer than the first and each time preceding a blocked (non-conducted P wave the thythm is clearly type I second degree AV block.

*** The basic sinus rate is probably similar to that of interval 2-3. Intervals 1-2, 3-4 and 4-5 are almost exactly twice this interval, therefore the rhythm is probably sinus (cf. 2-3) with sino-atrial block after 1, after 3 and after 4. (Intervals 1-2, 3-4 and 4-5 are not exactly twice interval 2-3, probably because the sinus rate varies slightly).

**** The appearances are similar (as far as the rhythm is concerned) to j but the pauses are less than twice the normal sinus interval. Therefore the rhythm is likely to be sinus rhythm with transient sinus arrest after the second and third beats. If the sinus arrest occurs frequently, a bradycardia results. If it is occasional a pause occurs.

Pauses

Intermittent pauses seen on the electrocardiogram often reveal very useful information about the mechanism of the cardiac rhythm. The main causes of intermittent pauses are given in Table 48.

Table 48	Common Causes of Pauses
Non-conducted atrial premature beats	
Second degree AV block type I	
Second degree AV block type II	
Intermittent sino-atrial block	
Intermittent sinus arrest	
Concealed conduction*	

Examples of the common pauses are given in Figure 427.

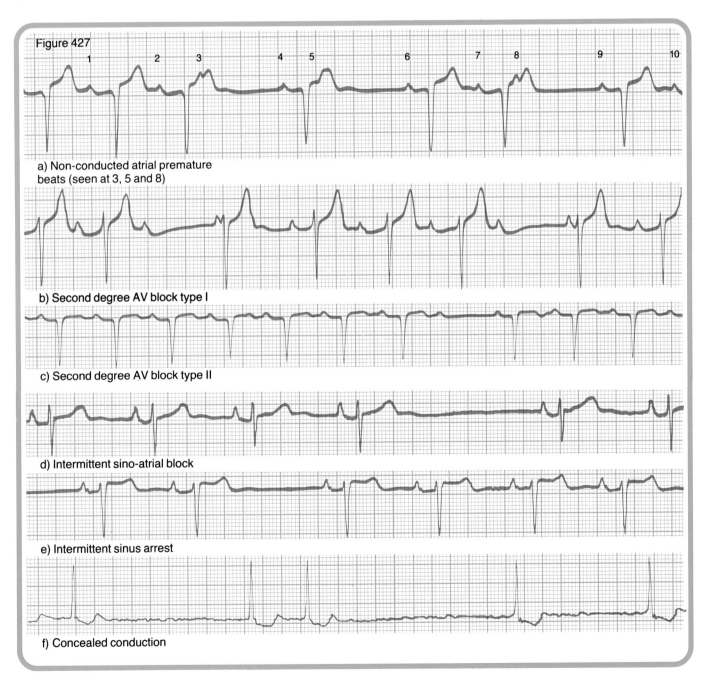

Figure 427

a) Non-conducted atrial premature beats (seen at 3, 5 and 8)

b) Second degree AV block type I

c) Second degree AV block type II

d) Intermittent sino-atrial block

e) Intermittent sinus arrest

f) Concealed conduction

*The commonest example of concealed conduction is the intermittent very long ventricular pause in atrial fibrillation which indicates concealed conduction through the AV node.

Intermittently Short R-R Intervals

Common causes are given in Table 49.

Table 49 Common Causes of Intermittently Short R-R Intervals
Atrial premature beats
Ventricular premature beats
Junctional premature beats
Parasystolic rhythm
Capture beats
Echo beats
A rhythm change involving improvement in a previously appreciable degree of AV conduction block
A rhythm change involving the onset of a significantly greater ventricular rate than that of the previously prevailing rhythm

Examples of the common causes of intermittently short R-R intervals are given in Figure 428.

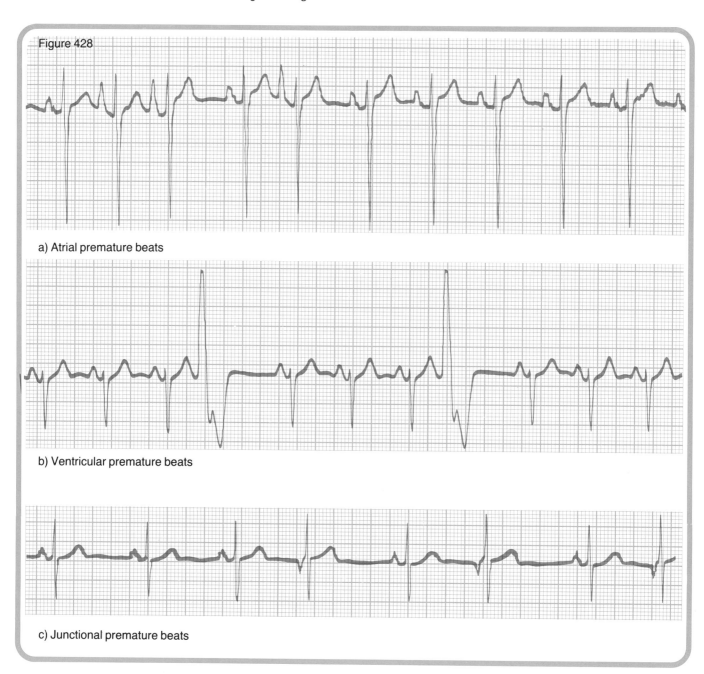

Figure 428

a) Atrial premature beats

b) Ventricular premature beats

c) Junctional premature beats

Figure 428 (continued)

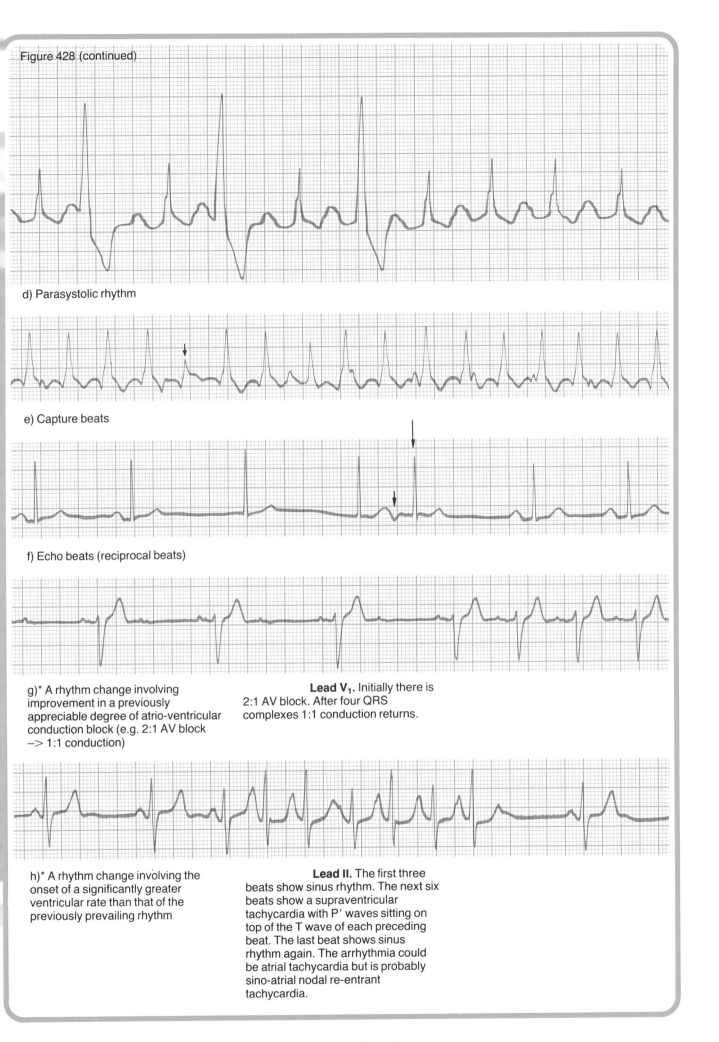

d) Parasystolic rhythm

e) Capture beats

f) Echo beats (reciprocal beats)

g)* A rhythm change involving improvement in a previously appreciable degree of atrio-ventricular conduction block (e.g. 2:1 AV block —> 1:1 conduction)

Lead V$_1$. Initially there is 2:1 AV block. After four QRS complexes 1:1 conduction returns.

h)* A rhythm change involving the onset of a significantly greater ventricular rate than that of the previously prevailing rhythm

Lead II. The first three beats show sinus rhythm. The next six beats show a supraventricular tachycardia with P′ waves sitting on top of the T wave of each preceding beat. The last beat shows sinus rhythm again. The arrhythmia could be atrial tachycardia but is probably sino-atrial nodal re-entrant tachycardia.

* In this situation the "early beat" occurs only at the onset of the rhythm change.

Clues to the Diagnosis of the Main Groups of Arrhythmias

It must be emphasised that it is not **always** possible confidently to assign a given tachycardia to one of the following types on the basis of the conventional 12-lead ECG recording alone (though electrophysiological studies can make the distinctions). But there are **often** sufficient clues in the recording to make the distinctions possible and for the vast majority of practising cardiologists the 12-lead electrocardiogram is the only diagnostic investigation likely to help them in rhythm analysis. Some useful clues in the various categories are presented here.

Clues to the Differential Diagnosis of Narrow QRS Complex Regular Tachycardias

Sinus Tachycardia

This rhythm will usually present no problem. The rate will typically be between 100-150 beats/min for the resting subject, although it may lie in the range of 100-190 beats/min in relation to exercise. The P waves will have a normal shape and axis (they will be upright in Leads II, III and the foot lead) and they will usually be readily visible. They may, however, be slightly taller than usual in association with tachycardia and, if the rate is approximately 150 beats/min, the P waves may well be superimposed on the preceding T waves. The P-R interval will be normal. It is most unusual for aberrant intraventricular conduction to occur with sinus tachycardia so the QRS complexes will be of the usual form for that subject (and typically will be normal). When the ventricular rate is around 150 beats/min and no clear P waves are seen, it is worth trying carotid sinus massage which may transiently slow the rate and in so doing may separate the P waves from the preceding T waves.

Atrial Flutter

Atrial flutter may or may not be associated with a regular ventricular rate (though usually the rate is regular over a relatively short time span) but the diagnosis is usually straightforward, especially if multiple ECG leads are inspected. With the use of multiple leads the chances are very high that one will be able to see the saw-tooth pattern of atrial activity (Figure 267).

Atrial Fibrillation

Atrial fibrillation is almost always associated with an irregular ventricular rate, but if the rate is very rapid the degree of irregularity may not be striking unless looked for carefully in the manner described in relation to Figure 201.

Other Narrow QRS Complex Tachycardias

The following rhythms may be less easy to diagnose with confidence:
Sino-atrial nodal re-entry
Paroxysmal (re-entrant) atrial tachycardia
Non-paroxysmal (enhanced automaticity) atrial tachycardia
Paroxysmal junctional tachycardia (AV nodal re-entrant tachycardia (AVNRT)) of the common "slow- fast" type
Paroxysmal junctional tachycardia (AV nodal re-entrant tachycardia (AVNRT)) of the uncommon "fast- slow" type
Paroxysmal (re-entrant) arrhythmias associated with anomalous pathways (Paroxysmal Atrio-ventricular Re-entrant Tachycardia (AVRT)).

Sino-atrial Nodal Re-entrant Tachycardia

The appearances in this rhythm will be very similar to those in sinus tachycardia except that the P-R interval tends to be short and the R-R interval long. However, this is unlikely to provide a clear distinction between the two possibilities since the P-R interval may be entirely within the normal range. It may be quite impossible to distinguish this from sinus tachycardia except that sino-atrial nodal re-entrant tachycardia will either be unaffected by carotid sinus massage or will be abruptly stopped by it (with the restoration of sinus rhythm at a normal rate). If one is fortunate enough to see the onset of the arrhythmia or the offset of the arrhythmia (compare Figure 264) then the sudden change from the abnormal re-entrant rhythm to normal sinus rhythm or sinus tachycardia will be apparent.

Paroxysmal Re-entrant Atrial Tachycardia

The atrial rate is typically in the range of 160-250 beats/min and there is often 2:1 atrio-ventricular block. In the presence of 2:1 block it may be very difficult to recognise the P waves during tachycardia. Any part of the record in which the ventricular rate transiently slows should be inspected carefully (compare Figure 266, page 430). Such a transient increase in the degree of AV block may reveal P waves which were previously obscured. It is also worth remembering that if a P wave appears to sit equally spaced between adjacent QRS complexes (i.e. when the P-R interval is approximately equal to the R-P interval) there is a high probability that another P wave will be occurring at the same time as the QRS, i.e. that there is 2:1 atrio-ventricular block (Figure 266, page 430). The P waves will be abnormally shaped but their morphological difference from the sinus P waves may be slight. Carotid sinus massage may (i) have no affect on the arrhythmia, (ii) cause a transient increase in the degree of AV block, (iii) (rarely) stop the arrhythmia and permit the restoration of sinus rhythm.

Non-paroxysmal Atrial Tachycardia

This is less common than the re-entrant (paroxysmal) variety. The atrial rate tends to be slower but unless the gradual onset and offset (of the non-paroxysmal type) is actually witnessed, it can be impossible to distinguish from the paroxysmal variety.

AV Nodal Re-entrant Tachycardia (AVNRT) of the (common) "Slow-fast" Type

This most typically shows either (a) rapid, narrow QRS complexes with no P′ waves visible (Figure 290) or (b) rapid, narrow QRS complexes with inverted (negative in II, III and aVF, positive in aVR etc) P′ waves occurring immediately (typically 0.06 sec or less) after the QRS (Figure 291).

AV Nodal Re-entrant Tachycardia (AVNRT) of the (less common) "Fast-slow" Type

This is a rare rhythm. It looks similar to the usual slow-fast type except that the inverted P waves tend to occur much later after the QRS so that the P′-R interval is less than the R-P′ interval and the P′ wave precedes the QRS (see Table 45).

Arrhythmias Associated with Accessory Atrio-ventricular Pathways

This group contains numerous possibilities including the following:

a) Sinus rhythm with conduction down the anomalous pathway.

b) Sinus rhythm with conduction through the AV node (i.e. anomalous pathway concealed).

c) Reciprocating tachycardia down the AV node (i.e. orthodromic) and back up the bypass tract. (The common paroxysmal tachydysrhythmia in patients with pre-excitation).

d) Reciprocating tachycardia with bundle branch block (i.e. antegrade depolarisation through the AV node (orthodromic) and back up the bypass tract but with bundle branch block).

e) Orthodromic tachycardia with slow retrograde conduction through the accessory pathway (resulting in a very long R-P′ interval).

f) Antidromic tachycardia in which the depolarisation spreads down the accessory pathway and back up the AV node.

g) Atrial fibrillation with conduction down the AV node. (The bypass tract is thus "concealed" and the ECG is the same as in any case of atrial fibrillation).

h) Atrial fibrillation with conduction down the accessory pathway. (This may give rise to an extremely rapid (e.g. 300 beats/min) ventricular rate).

i) Atrial flutter with conduction down the normal pathway. (The re-entrant pathway is therefore concealed and the ECG appearances are the same as in any case of atrial flutter).

j) Atrial flutter with conduction down the accessory pathway. (This may give rise to an extremely rapid (typically 300 beats/ min) ventricular rate).

Paroxysmal Atrio-ventricular Re-entrant Tachycardia (AVRT)

This is the common tachycardia associated with an anomalous atrio-ventricular pathway. In its common form atrio-ventricular conduction occurs through the AV node (orthodromic).

Appearances in this rhythm will be of rapid, regular QRS complexes having the duration and shape usual for the subject at the time (and most commonly, therefore, narrow) with a rate typically in the region of 150-250 beats/min. If an ECG is available during sinus rhythm this will most commonly show a short P-R interval, delta wave and wide QRS complex of the Wolff-Parkinson-White syndrome (pages 212-220) but not infrequently the record may be normal even when the subject is in sinus rhythm. This is because the accessory pathway may fail to conduct from atrium to ventricle (during sinus rhythm) but may conduct from ventricle to atrium (during tachycardia). Thus it is possible to have a re-entrant bypass tract tachycardia without any evidence of re-entry during sinus rhythm. There is then said to be re-entry over a "concealed" (i.e. not apparent during sinus rhythm and, of course, not apparent during the tachycardia). One may get a clue to the presence of this conduction pathway if retrograde P waves (i.e. inverted P waves in Leads II, III and the footlead or upright P waves in aVR) are seen during the tachycardia and if those P waves are well clear of the QRS complex (i.e. seen in the S-T segment or in the early part of the T wave). The situation in this respect is not very dissimilar from the uncommon form of AV nodal re-entrant tachycardia ("fast-slow") and not all that different from the common form of AV nodal re-entrant tachycardia ("slow-fast") in those cases when there is also some delay in retrograde conduction. However, subjects with a reciprocating tachycardia due to an accessory atrio-ventricular pathway in general have an R-P′ interval in excess of 0.07 sec whereas the majority of patients with AV nodal re-entrant tachycardia of the common "slow-fast" variety usually have an R-P′ interval of less than 0.07 sec and those with AVNRT of the very rare "fast-slow" variety have very long QRS-P′ intervals with the P′ wave just in front of the next QRS. In addition, although both groups have, of course, rapid ventricular rates the patients with anomalous pathways during episodes of tachycardia tend to have higher ventricular rates than the patients with intra AV nodal re-entrant tachycardias.

Clues to the Differential Diagnosis of Wide QRS Complex Tachycardias

A most important question in relation to wide QRS complex tachycardias is whether the tachycardia is ventricular in origin or whether it is a supraventricular tachycardia associated with

a) pre-existing bundle branch block

b) functional (tachycardia-dependent) bundle branch block or

c) atrio-ventricular conduction down an anomalous pathway.

Distinction between tachycardias of ventricular and of supraventricular origin is of far more practical importance than the distinction between the various kinds of supraventricular tachycardias. (Probably the most important aspect of the distinction between the supraventricular tachycardias is the recognition of the existence of an accessory pathway for such a pathway may give rise to extremely rapid ventricular rates in the presence of a supraventricular tachycardia).

From a clinical point of view more harm is done by wrongly concluding that ventricular tachycardia is supraventricular than by wrongly concluding that a supraventricular tachycardia is ventricular.

It is a prerequisite to this discussion that the QRS complexes are regular, i.e. no irregularity is detectable, which effectively means that there is less than 10 percent variation in the R-R intervals, the longest being compared with the shortest, and that the QRS complexes have a duration of 0.12 sec or more* and a rate of more than 100 beats/min. When these criteria are fulfilled, questions outlined in Table 46 should be followed.

It will be noted that the comments made in Table 46 indicate that certain appearances "favour ventricular tachycardia" or "favour supraventricular tachycardia". As indicated in the table it is only in certain special situations that one can be **absolutely confident** of the distinction.

Ventricular Tachycardia

1. If one is fortunate enough to have a 12-lead ECG taken prior to the onset of the tachycardia and if the QRS complexes during the tachycardia are identical with those during sinus rhythm, then the rhythm is supraventricular in type and (by inference) there is an intraventricular conduction abnormality during sinus rhythm.

2. If the QRS during the tachycardia is identical with the QRS of ventricular ectopic beats seen in the same lead during a recent recording in sinus rhythm, then the probability is that the record is one of ventricular tachycardia.

3. If there is atrio-ventricular dissociation (no consistent time relationship between P waves (probably seen intermittently)) and QRS complexes, then the rhythm is ventricular tachycardia.

4. If there is a consistent relationship between the P waves and the QRS complexes then either the rhythm is supraventricular tachycardia or the rhythm is ventricular tachycardia with retrograde (VA) conduction.

5. If the total QRS duration is equal to or greater than 0.14 sec, then the probability is high that the rhythm is ventricular.

6. If the frontal plane QRS axis during the tachycardia is superiorly orientated in the range of −30° to −120° then the rhythm is likely to be ventricular.

It should be noted that the above are only clues. The systematic approach of Table 46 should be followed.

General Electrocardiographic Features of Tachycardias

Finally, it might be helpful if some of the general electrocardiographic features to be found in a variety of tachycardias are compared. These are therefore listed in Table 50.

* Use multiple leads. Assuming that no change occurs in the QRS during the 12-lead recording the widest QRS complex seen gives that estimate of QRS width which is closest to the truth.

Table 50 ECG Appearances of Tachycardias (+ implies possible appearance)

| | QRS COMPLEXES | | | | | | | ATRIO-VENTRICULAR (OR VENTRICULO-ATRIAL†) ASSOCIATION OR DISSOCIATION | | | ATRIO-VENTRICULAR RATE RELATIONSHIPS | | |
| | DURATION | | | AXIS¹ | | | | | | | | | |
	<0.10	≥0.12 <0.16	>0.16	N	Slight shift to the right	Slight shift to the left	Very abnormal	Association	Complete dissociation	Partial dissociation	A>V	A=V	V>A
Supraventricular tachycardia*	+	−	−	+	−	−	−	+	−	−	+	+	−
Supraventricular tachycardia* with pre-existing bundle branch block	−	+	−	+	+‡	+‡	−	+	−	−	+	+	−
Supraventricular tachycardia* with aberrant intraventricular conduction	−	+	−	+	+‡	+‡	−	+	−	−	+	+	−
Supraventricular tachycardia* with accessory AV conduction pathway	+	−	−	+	+	+	+	+	−	−	+	−	−
Supraventricular tachycardia* with accessory AV conduction pathway and with superadded aberrant intra-ventricular conduction	−	+	−	+	+	+	+	+	−	−	+	−	−
Ventricular tachycardia	−	+	+**	−	−	−	+²	(+)***	+	+***	−	+⁴	+
Polymorphic ventricular tachycardia (Torsade de pointes)	−	+	+**	−	−	−	+²	3	3	3	3	3	3

† A more appropriate term if the origin of the arrhythmia is ventricular.

‡ With pre-existing or functional right bundle branch block a slight shift to the right may occur. With pre-existing or functional left bundle branch block a slight shift to the left may occur.

* Sinus tachycardia, junctional tachycardia, atrial tachycardia, atrial flutter, atrial fibrillation, fascicular tachycardia (The latter is not strictly supraventricular but has essentially the same electrocardiographic appearances).

** When the QRS duration is 0.16 sec or a more ventricular origin for the rhythm is highly likely.

*** In the majority of cases of ventricular tachycardia there is ventriculo-atrial dissociation

¹ Assuming no abnormal axis prior to onset of tachycardia.

² The QRS axis is nearly always grossly abnormal in ventricular tachycardia.

³ P waves usually obscured.

⁴ In most cases V>A.

Rhythm Abnormalities

This final chapter will review a series of 94 demonstrations of cardiac arrhythmias each consisting of a single lead rhythm strip. A similar approach was used at the end of Sections 1 and 2 where Records 1-30 and 31-70 were presented.

The records in this section will be numbered 71-164 to prevent confusion with the earlier records and with the illustrations. The first 20 records (i.e. 71-90) will be presented with the rhythm diagnosis and with a brief explanation of the factors which led to the diagnostic conclusion. The diagnostic process in relation to these first 20 records will, in general, follow the scheme used in the preceding section ("Cardiac rhythm assessment", pages 557-579). In each case the "time window" (page 558) and the electrocardiographic lead(s) (page 558) have already been chosen prior to the presentation of the recording. The approach therefore follows that in pages 562-574 and uses Tables 44-46 and Figures 426-428.

Record 71

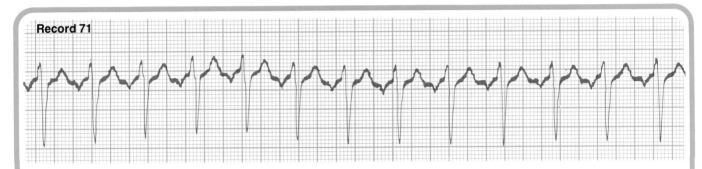

Sinus tachycardia

The lead in question is V_1. The QRS rate is regular and rapid (page 562) and we are therefore dealing with a tachycardia (Box A, Table 44, page 564). The QRS duration is normal (page 562) and we are therefore dealing with a supraventricular tachycardia (red boxes, Table 44). The rhythm fulfils all the criteria for sinus tachycardia (page 378) and does not show features diagnostic of other supraventricular tachycardias (Table 45).

Record 72

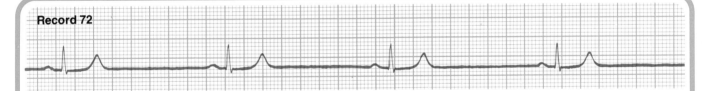

Sinus bradycardia

The QRS rate is regular and slow (page 562) and we are therefore dealing with a bradycardia (Box C, Table 44). The QRS duration is normal (page 562) and we are therefore dealing with the upper (red) part of Box C. The record fulfils all the criteria for sinus bradycardia (page 377) and does not show features diagnostic of other bradycardias (Figure 426).

Record 73

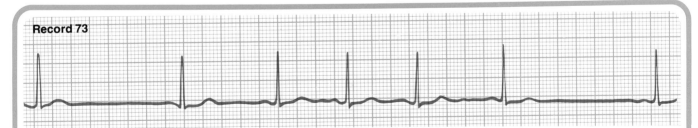

Sinus arrhythmia

The QRS rate is irregular and there is a cyclical variation in the rate with "concertina" R-R intervals (Box F, Table 44). There is no evidence of atrio-ventricular conduction disturbance (every P wave is followed by a QRS complex after a constant P-R interval) and the criteria for sinus arrhythmia are fulfilled (page 379). Note that there is a small U wave following each T wave and the U wave bears a constant relationship to the preceding T wave. This U wave should not be confused with additional P waves.

Record 74

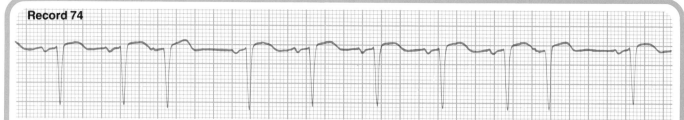

Sinus rhythm with atrial premature ectopic beats

The basic QRS rate is regular but there are intermittent short R-R intervals (early beats). The basic rhythm is clearly sinus rhythm and the appearances fulfil all the criteria for this rhythm (page 371) except in respect of the third and ninth beats.

These are the beats associated with intermittent short R-R intervals (Box D, Table 44). Since the QRS complexes of these beats are morphologically the same as the QRS complexes of the sinus beats the beats are clearly supraventricular

premature beats. They are preceded by abnormally-shaped P waves and are atrial premature ectopic beats (Table 49 and Figure 428a). All the criteria for atrial premature ectopic beats (page 388) are fulfilled.

Record 75

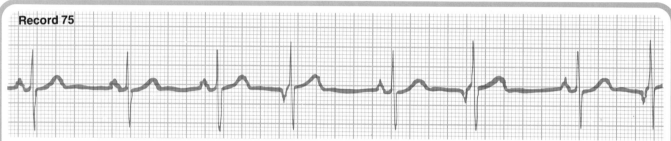

Sinus rhythm with junctional premature ectopic beats

The rhythm is clearly sinus except in relation to the fourth beat. The basic QRS rate is regular but there is one short R-R interval (early beat). The basic rhythm is clearly sinus rhythm and the appearances fulfil all the criteria for this rhythm (page 371) except in respect of the fourth beat. This is the beat associated with a short preceding R-R interval (Box D, Table 44). Since the QRS complex of this beat is morphologically the same

as the QRS complexes of the sinus beats the beat is clearly a supraventricular beat. The QRS of this fourth beat is preceded by an abnormally-shaped P wave. It is clear from the fact that the P waves have a polarity opposite that of normal that atrial depolarisation is proceeding in a direction opposite from normal and since the QRS complexes are the same as those in the sinus beats ventricular depolarisation is

proceeding in a normal direction. Beat 4 is clearly an example of an intermittent short R-R interval (Box D, Table 44) and in view of the morphology of the P'waves and QRS complexes it is clearly a junctional premature ectopic beat (Table 49, Figure 428c). All the criteria for junctional premature ectopic beats are fulfilled (page 395).

Record 76

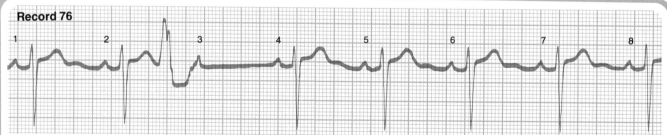

Ventricular premature ectopic beats

The basic rhythm is clearly sinus (there are prominent, but not abnormal, U waves following each T wave). The third QRS is clearly a premature QRS and this is an example of an intermittent short R-R interval (Box D, Table 44). The QRS in question is abnormally wide and could be a ventricular premature ectopic beat (purple part of Box D,

Table 44) or a supraventricular premature ectopic beat with aberrant intraventricular conduction (red part of Box D, Table 44 and pages 403-407). Since the P wave rate remains completely undisturbed (i.e. intervals 1-2, 2-3, 3-4, 4-5 etc are constant) and since the extra beat in question is followed by a compensatory pause so that the time interval between the

second and fourth QRS complexes is exactly the same as twice the time interval between the first and second QRS complexes the extra beat is clearly a ventricular premature beat (Table 49, Figure 428b). The criteria for ventricular premature ectopic beats (page 392) are completely fulfilled.

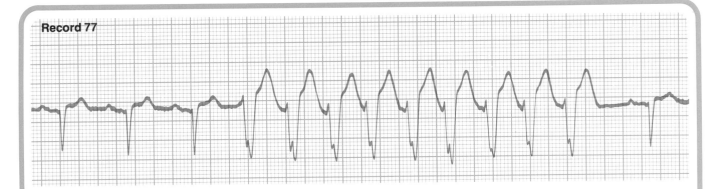

Record 77

Sinus rhythm with transient, self-limiting ventricular tachycardia

The first three beats show sinus rhythm with first degree heart block (there is a constant prolonged (0.24 sec) P-R interval). The fourth QRS is premature (in relation to the timing anticipated from inspection of the first three QRS complexes) and is abnormally wide and abnormally shaped. This abnormally wide premature QRS complex is followed by eight further virtually identical QRS complexes occurring at a constant rate. It is clear that a tachydysrhythmia interrupts the basic sinus rhythm and the tachycardia is associated with wide QRS complexes. This could be ventricular tachycardia or supraventricular tachycardia with rate-related bundle

branch block (Box 2, Table 44) or supraventricular tachycardia and antegrade conduction down an anomalous pathway (Box 3, Table 44). Of these, supraventricular tachycardia with antegrade conduction down an anomalous atrio-ventricular pathway is a very unlikely possibility. There is no possibility that the rhythm is supraventricular with pre-existing bundle branch block (Box 1, Table 44) since there was no pre-existing bundle branch block when the rhythm was clearly sinus. In the vast majority of cases in which there is ventricular pre-excitation the anomalous atrio-ventricular pathway conducts antegrade during sinus rhythm and retrograde during an

episode of tachycardia (pages 449-453). Since the first beat of the tachycardia is clearly a ventricular premature ectopic beat (there is no atrial or junctional P wave seen in front of the abnormal QRS and in fact the beginning of a normal (in timing and morphology) P wave is just seen immediately prior to the initial upstroke of the first abnormally wide QRS) one can conclude that the rhythm is initiated by a ventricular ectopic premature beat and since the morphology of the QRS complexes during the period of sustained tachycardia is the same as that of the ventricular premature ectopic beat the rhythm is almost certainly ventricular tachycardia (Table 46).

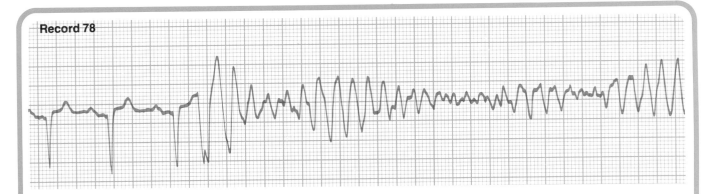

Record 78

Sinus rhythm with an R-on-T ventricular ectopic beat giving rise to ventricular fibrillation

The first three beats are sinus beats. The fourth QRS is abnormally wide and begins on the peak of the T wave of the preceding QRS. This premature ventricular ectopic beat immediately initiates ventricular fibrillation (this record is taken from the same patient as that of Record 77). The P-R interval in this case is 0.21 sec. The forms of the P waves and of the QRS complexes of the sinus beats are similar to those in Record 77. The initial ventricular ectopic beat in this record is virtually identical with that in Record 77 except that in this record the beat is clearly R-on-T.

Record 79

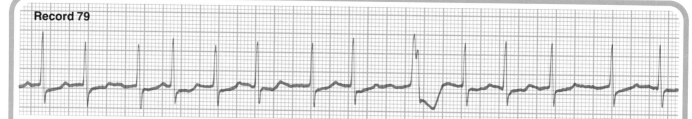

Atrial fibrillation with a single broad QRS complex

The ventricular rate is irregular, and with the exception of one beat, the QRS complexes are of normal width (page 562). It is clear that the single wide QRS complex is a manifestation of a different form of rhythm from that of the "background" rhythm. The background rhythm will be discussed first. This background rhythm has no recognisable R-R interval pattern (Box G, Table 44). The QRS complexes of the background rhythm are of normal width and they are therefore supraventricular in origin (red part of Box G, Table 44). No flutter waves can be seen and there is no evidence of any co-ordinated atrial

activity. The basic rhythm is therefore clearly atrial fibrillation and the background rhythm satisfies all the criteria for atrial fibrillation (page 440). The main problem in the analysis of this rhythm strip is to identify the nature of the wide (ninth) QRS complex. The most obvious possibility is to suggest that this is a ventricular ectopic premature beat but the beat is manifestly not premature. It is separated from the preceding beat by the longest R-R interval seen in the rhythm strip. It could, therefore, be a ventricular ectopic escape beat (page 392). This is one real possibility. Another possible explanation is that

the broad QRS complex might be an example of deceleration-dependent aberrancy (page 406) but, as indicated earlier (page 406) one can only be sure that there is deceleration-dependent aberrancy when two or more consecutive aberrant QRS complexes are each preceded by the same P-R interval and, since the "background" rhythm in this case is atrial fibrillation there can be no P-R interval. The data obtainable from this electrocardiogram do not permit one to distinguish between these two possible explanations for the wide QRS complex.

Record 80

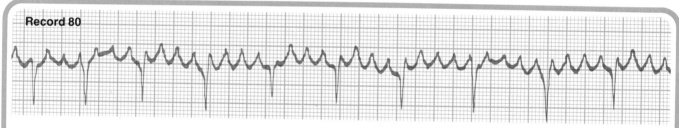

Atrial flutter with varying AV block

The QRS rate is irregular (page 562) and there is no clearly recognisable pattern in the R-R interval (Box G, Table 44). The QRS complexes are narrow and the rhythm is clearly supraventricular (red part of Box G, Table 44). Flutter waves are clearly recognisable (Table 45) and it is

obvious that the rhythm is atrial flutter. The degree of AV block varies. The situation is probably a little more complicated still since the relationship between the QRS complexes and the preceding flutter waves is not constant. This suggests that there is Wenckebach AV conduction

(compare Figure 266, page 430 and contrast this with the more usual finding in atrial flutter where there is a constant relationship between the QRS complexes and the immediate antecedent flutter wave as in Figure 269, page 432).

Record 81

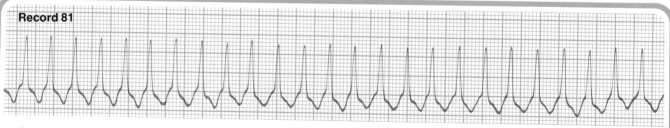

AV nodal re-entrant tachycardia

The QRS rate is regular and rapid (page 562) and there is clearly a tachycardia (Box A, Table 44). The QRS width is normal (page 562) and the rhythm is therefore clearly supraventricular (red part of Box A,

Table 44). As indicated in Table 44 reference should be made at this point to Table 45 which shows the narrow QRS complex tachycardias. Since this particular record shows a regular ventricular rate within the range 180 to

240 beats/min and with no P waves visible the rhythm is probably AV nodal re-entrant tachycardia of the common "slow-fast" type.

Record 82

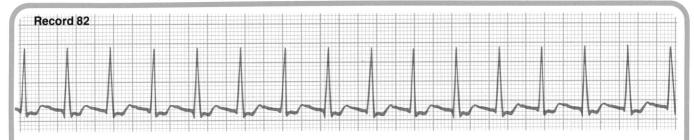

AV re-entrant tachycardia

The QRS rate is regular and rapid (page 562) and the rhythm is therefore a tachycardia (Box A, Table 44). The QRS width is normal (page 562) and the rhythm is therefore one of those listed in the red part of Box A,

Table 44. Table 44 in this situation refers us to Table 45, which shows the important supraventricular tachydysrhythmias. P waves are seen after the QRS (arrows). Since (Question 5, Table 45) the R-P'

interval is less than the P'-R interval the rhythm is probably atrio-ventricular re-entrant tachycardia involving an atrio-ventricular bypass tract (i.e. it is AVRT).

Record 83

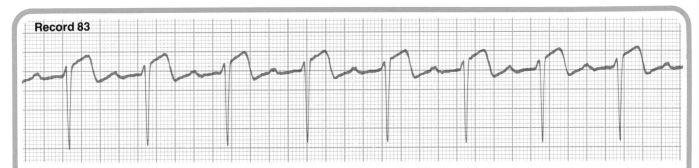

Sinus rhythm with first degree heart block

The QRS rate is regular and "normal" (page 562) and it is therefore a "normal rate" rhythm (Box B, Table 44). The QRS complexes are narrow and this is therefore one of the

rhythms listed in the red part of Box B, Table 44. All the criteria for sinus rhythm (page 371) are fulfilled except that the P-R interval is abnormal (0.36 sec). The record clearly shows a

constant, prolonged P-R interval and the rhythm is therefore sinus rhythm with first degree heart block. All the criteria for first degree heart block are fulfilled (page 488).

Record 84

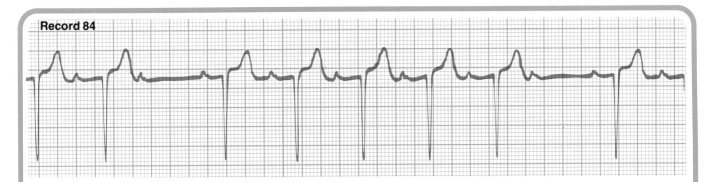

Sinus rhythm with type I second degree atrio-ventricular block

The QRS rate is irregular and there are occasional pauses (Box E, Table 44). The QRS complexes are narrow and the rhythm is therefore included in the red part of Box E, Table 44. There is clearly one P wave to each QRS complex except in relation to the pauses where there are two P waves. A close inspection of the P-R intervals in the beats preceding the pause shows that there is progressive prolongation of the P-R interval before

the transient failure of atrio-ventricular conduction and the rhythm is therefore type I second degree atrio-ventricular block (pages 489-492). However, this is not an entirely complete explanation since the R-R intervals preceding the block do not behave precisely as anticipated in type I second degree block (Figure 340, page 490). One normally expects a progressive shortening of the R-R intervals (accompanying the

progressive prolongation of the P-R intervals – see Figure 340, page 490) before the transient failure of atrio-ventricular conduction. This pattern is not seen in this particular case since the P-P interval is not constant. The rhythm is sinus rhythm with type I second degree atrio-ventricular block with some additional variation in the sinus rate. The criteria for type I second degree atrio-ventricular block (page 492) are fulfilled.

Record 85

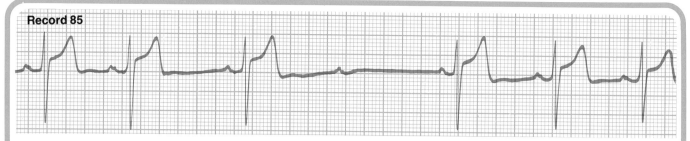

Type II second degree atrio-ventricular block

The QRS rate is irregular and there is one pause (Box E, Table 44). The QRS complexes are narrow (red part of Box E, Table 44). There is one P wave to each QRS complex except after the third QRS complex when there are two P waves, the first one of which is not followed by a QRS complex. This is clearly an example of second degree atrio-ventricular block. Since there is no prolongation of the P-R interval before the transient failure of atrio-ventricular conduction it is clearly type II second degree atrio-ventricular block. The issue is complicated slightly by the fact that the basic sinus rate is not precisely constant, the second P-P interval being longer than the first P-P interval. Nevertheless, all the criteria for type II second degree atrio-ventricular block (page 495) are fulfilled.

Record 86

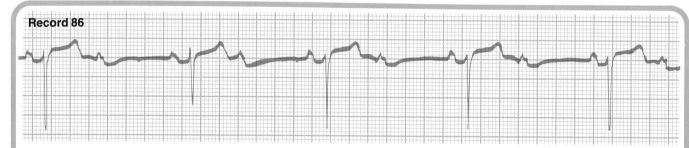

Sinus rhythm with 2:1 atrio-ventricular block

The QRS rate is regular and slow (page 562) the rhythm is therefore a bradycardia (Box C, Table 44). The QRS complexes are narrow (page 562) and the rhythm is therefore supraventricular (red part of Box C, Table 44). The P wave rate is regular and the P waves have a constant morphology so this rules out coupled, blocked atrial premature beats and coupled, blocked junctional premature beats. Since the P wave rate is constant, the P-R interval (in relation to those P waves followed by QRS complexes) is constant and there are two P waves to each QRS complex, the rhythm is clearly 2:1 atrio-ventricular block (page 496).

Record 87

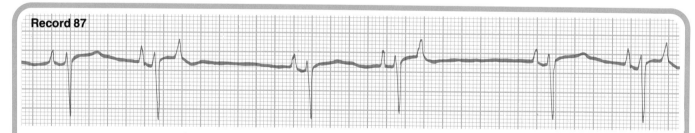

Sinus rhythm with blocked atrial premature beats

The QRS rate is not regular, it is "normal" (page 562).Clearly we are dealing with a situation in which the rate is basically regular but in which there are pauses (Box E, Table 44). Those cardiac cycles which have QRS complexes fulfil all the criteria for sinus rhythm (page 371) but premature P waves are seen after the second, fourth and sixth QRS complexes. Although the P wave morphology of these additional atrial beats is **similar** to that of the sinus beats it is not exactly the same (the premature beats have P waves which are taller and broader than the sinus P waves) so it is clear that the premature beats are ectopic as well as premature, i.e. they are atrial premature ectopic beats and not sinus premature beats. The atrial ectopic beats occur during the S-T segment which follows the preceding QRS complex and they are not followed by their own QRS complex, indicating that some part of the conducting tissue (AV node, bundle of His, or right and left bundle branches simultaneously) is refractory when the premature beats reach that point. We are therefore dealing with intermittent, non-conducted (i.e. blocked) atrial premature ectopic beats. (Note the occurrence of blocked atrial premature beats substantially reduces the effective ventricular rate and that if there were alternate blocked atrial premature beats (i.e. coupled but blocked atrial premature beats) the appearances would be very similar to those in Record 86. Coupled blocked atrial premature beats are an important cause of bradycardia. An example is shown in Figure 426e).

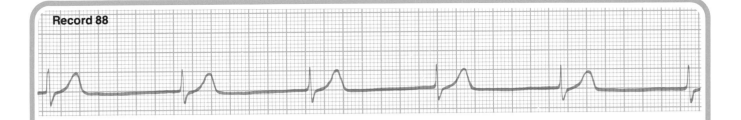

Record 88

Junctional escape rhythm ("nodal rhythm")

The QRS rate is regular and slow (less than 60 beats/min, page 562). The rhythm is therefore a bradycardia (Box C, Table 44). The QRS width is normal (page 562) and this directs us to the red part of Box C, Table 44. No P waves are seen. The rhythm is not therefore sinus bradycardia, 2:1 sino-atrial block, coupled blocked atrial premature beats, coupled blocked junctional premature beats, sinus rhythm with high-grade AV block, sinus rhythm with 2:1 AV block or sinus rhythm with complete heart block. The base-line is absolutely flat and there is no evidence of atrial tachycardia, atrial fibrillation, junctional tachycardia or atrial flutter. The rhythm is clearly a junctional escape rhythm. Since there are no P waves visible it follows that either the retrograde (reverse polarity) P waves are hidden in the QRS complexes (which seems unlikely since the QRS complexes in this case are so "clean") or, much more likely in this case, there is blocked retrograde conduction of the P waves (page 479 and Figure 328a). All the criteria for junctional escape rhythm are fulfilled (page 480).

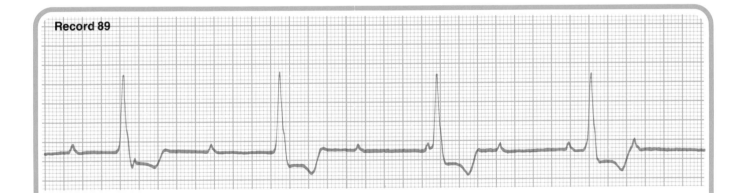

Record 89

Sinus rhythm with complete heart block

The QRS rate is regular and slow (page 562) and the rhythm is therefore a bradycardia (Box C, Table 44). The QRS complexes are abnormally wide (page 562) and we are therefore dealing with the rhythms from the purple part of Box C, Table 44. Inspection of the individual P wave and QRS complex rates clearly indicates that each is regular and that the two are independent of one another and there is no doubt at all that this is complete heart block. The ventricular rhythm is an idioventricular escape rhythm as is usual in complete heart block. All the criteria for complete heart block (page 504) are fulfilled and the criteria for ventricular escape rhythms (page 481) are fulfilled.

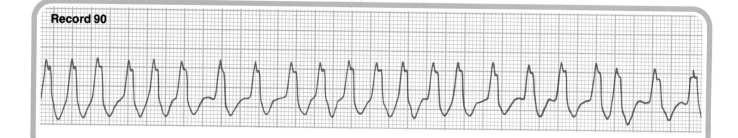

Atrial fibrillation with ventricular pre-excitation

The QRS rate is irregular and the rate is rapid (page 562). There is no recognisable pattern to the R wave frequency (Box G, Table 44). The QRS complexes are abnormally wide (page 562). We are therefore dealing with one of the rhythms listed in the purple section of Box G, Table 44. All the QRS complexes have the same morphology so the rhythm is not multifocal ventricular ectopic beats. There is no background regular rhythm with intermittent variation in the R-R interval so the rhythm is not background regular rhythm with ventricular parasystole. The behaviour of the R-R intervals is absolutely typical of atrial fibrillation in that there is no means of predicting what the next R-R interval will be having seen several previous R-R intervals (although one will, of course, be able to predict the likely maximum and minimum R-R intervals from preceding R-R intervals) (pages 436-440) and all the criteria for atrial fibrillation are fulfilled (page 440). Since the QRS complexes are abnormally wide there must either be additional bundle branch block (probably left bundle branch block), ventricular pre-excitation or rate-related aberrancy. The latter is very unlikely since the QRS complexes have the same morphology irrespective of the preceding R-R interval. We are therefore left with two possibilities, namely (i) that this is atrial fibrillation with additional (and probably pre-existing) left bundle branch block or (ii) that this is atrial fibrillation with additional (pre-existing) ventricular pre-excitation. It is not possible with absolute confidence to distinguish between these two possibilities but, in general, whenever the minimum R-R interval is 260 milliseconds or less (i.e. 0.26 seconds, i.e. one large square plus one and a half small squares on the ECG graticule) it is extremely unlikely that atrio-ventricular conduction is taking place through the AV node since such an R-R interval corresponds to an instantaneous ventricular rate of 230 beats/min which, in the absence of vagal blockade and intense sympathetic drive is most unlikely to be achieved by atrio-ventricular nodal conduction. The third from last R-R interval in this record measures 0.22 seconds (one large ECG square plus half a small square) and this corresponds to an instantaneous R-R interval of 273 beats/min. It is virtually certain, therefore, that this is atrial fibrillation with ventricular pre-excitation. **Whenever, in atrial fibrillation, the QRS complexes have a bundle branch block configuration and R-R intervals of 0.26 seconds or less and are seen without any simultaneous change in the QRS morphology, it is likely that there is atrial fibrillation with ventricular pre-excitation** (page 541, Figure 397). **Whenever the R-R interval is equal to or less than 205 milliseconds during atrial fibrillation with ventricular pre-excitation the development of ventricular fibrillation becomes a real possibility.**

Following is a selection of examples of various cardiac rhythms. Unless indicated to the contrary, each rhythm strip is taken from a chest monitoring lead. No description is given with the record. The rhythm diagnoses are listed on pages 599 and 600. Following this (pages 601 to 606) a brief description of the most important aspects of the analysis of each rhythm strip is given. All the rhythms shown in this section are abnormal in some way(s). In general, the rhythm analyses follow the guidelines provided in pages 562 to 579.

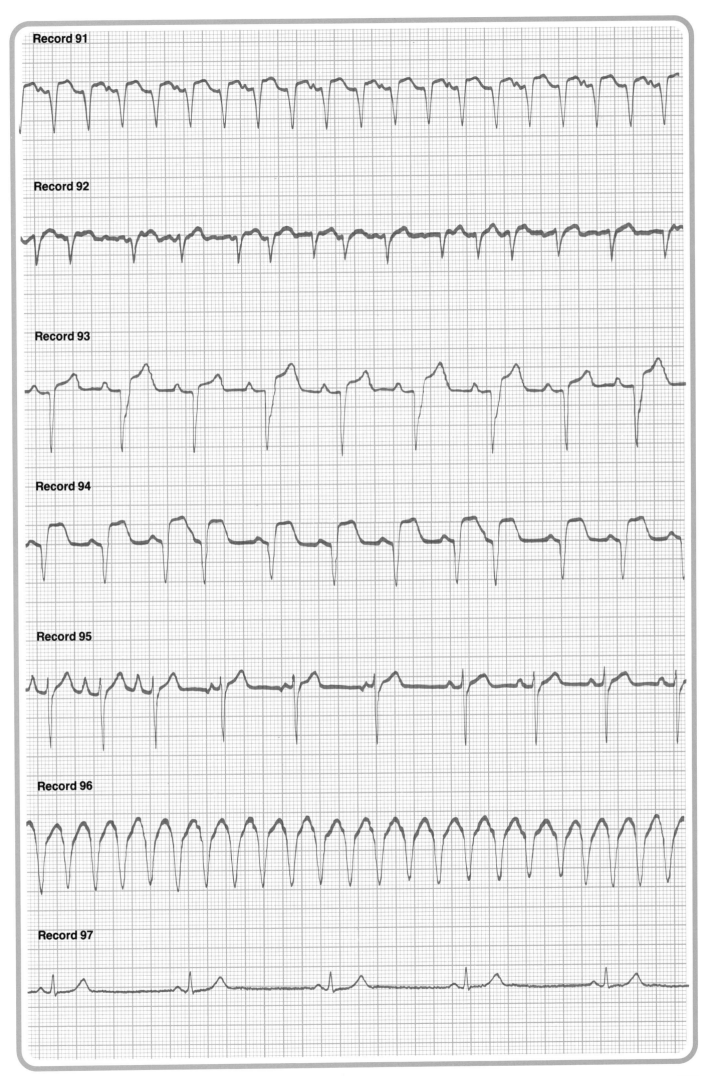

588

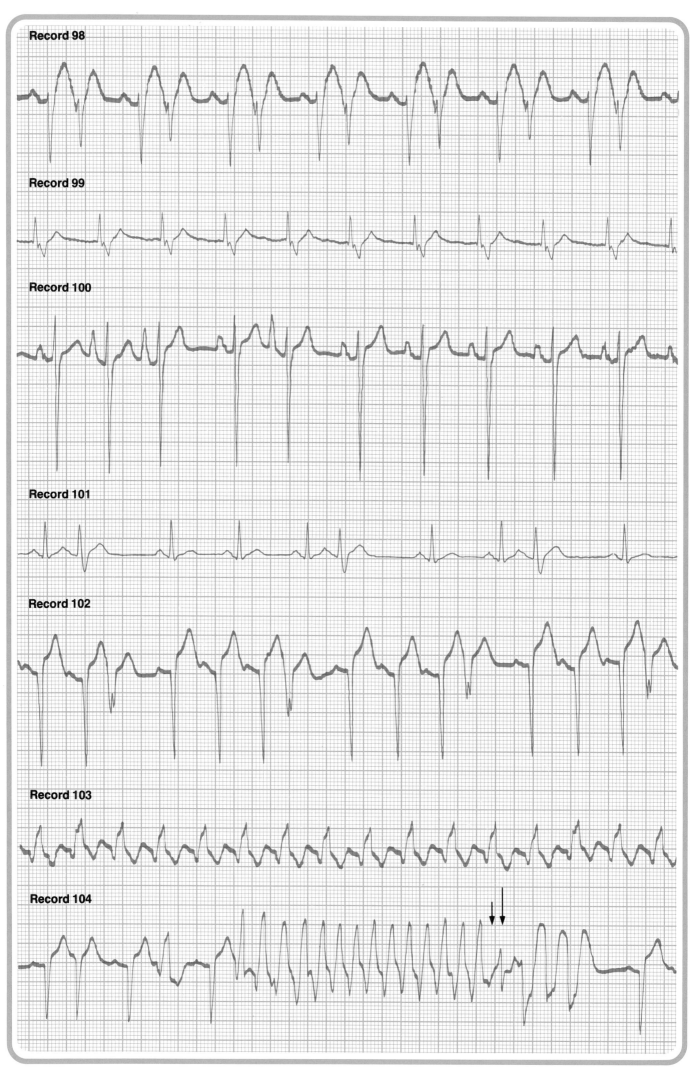

Record 98

Record 99

Record 100

Record 101

Record 102

Record 103

Record 104

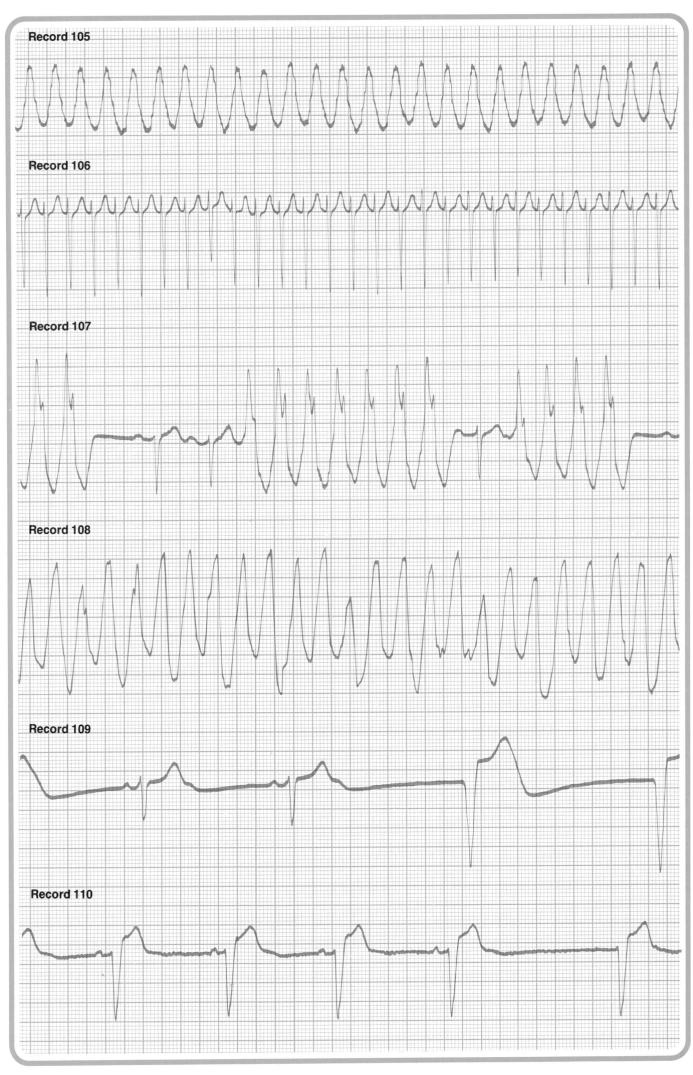

Record 105

Record 106

Record 107

Record 108

Record 109

Record 110

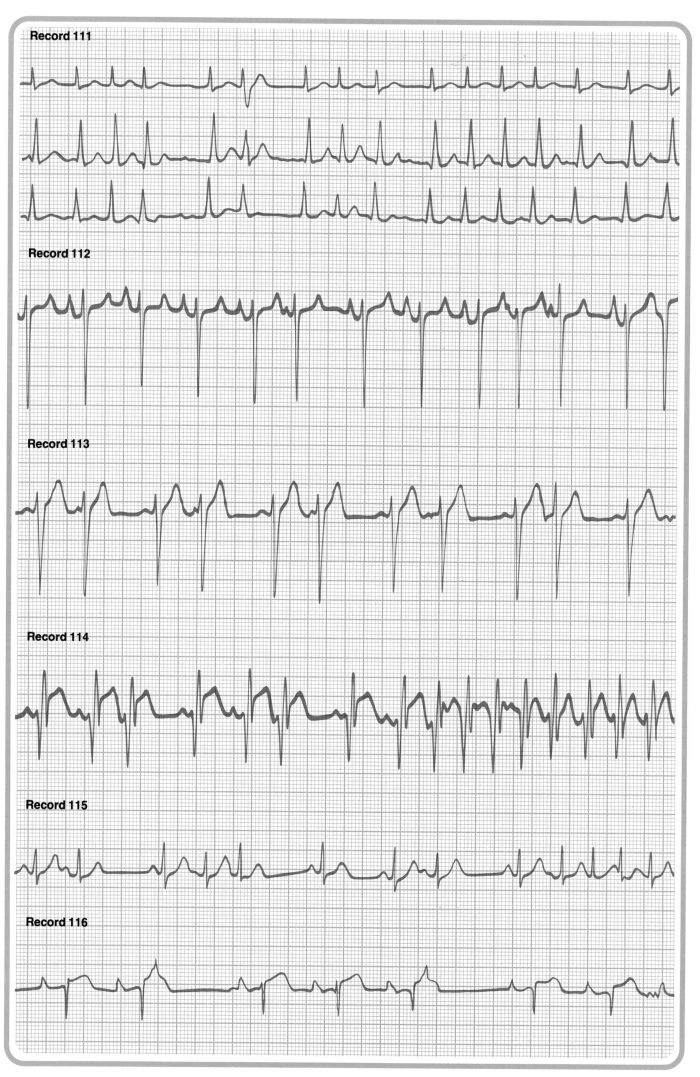

Record 111

Record 112

Record 113

Record 114

Record 115

Record 116

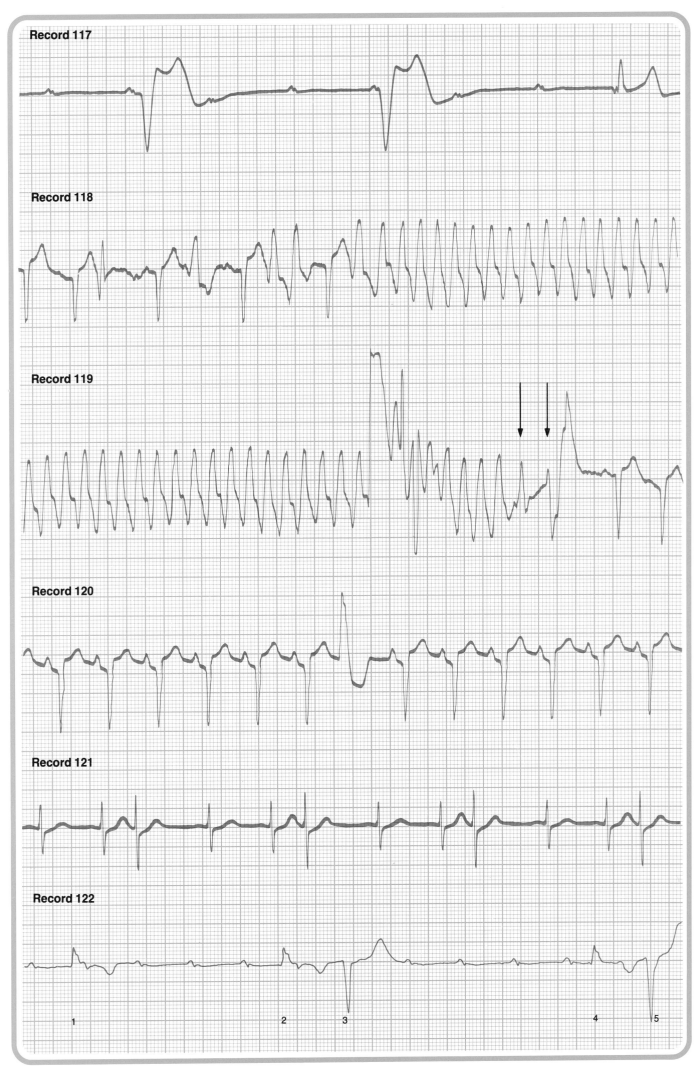

Record 117

Record 118

Record 119

Record 120

Record 121

Record 122

1   2   3   4   5

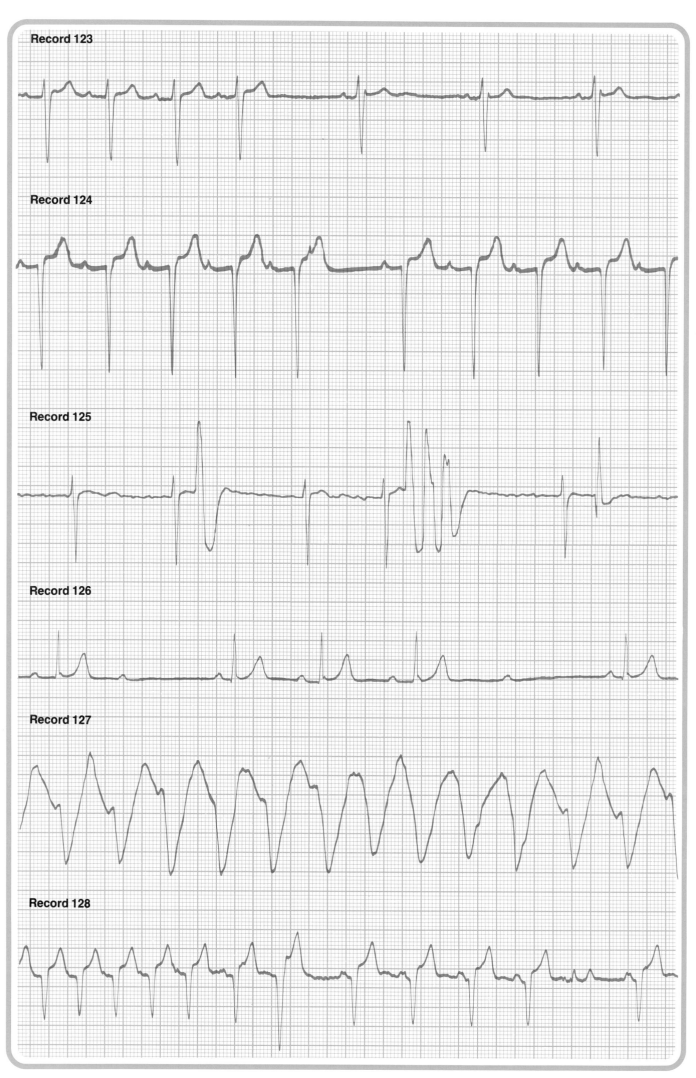

Record 123

Record 124

Record 125

Record 126

Record 127

Record 128

593

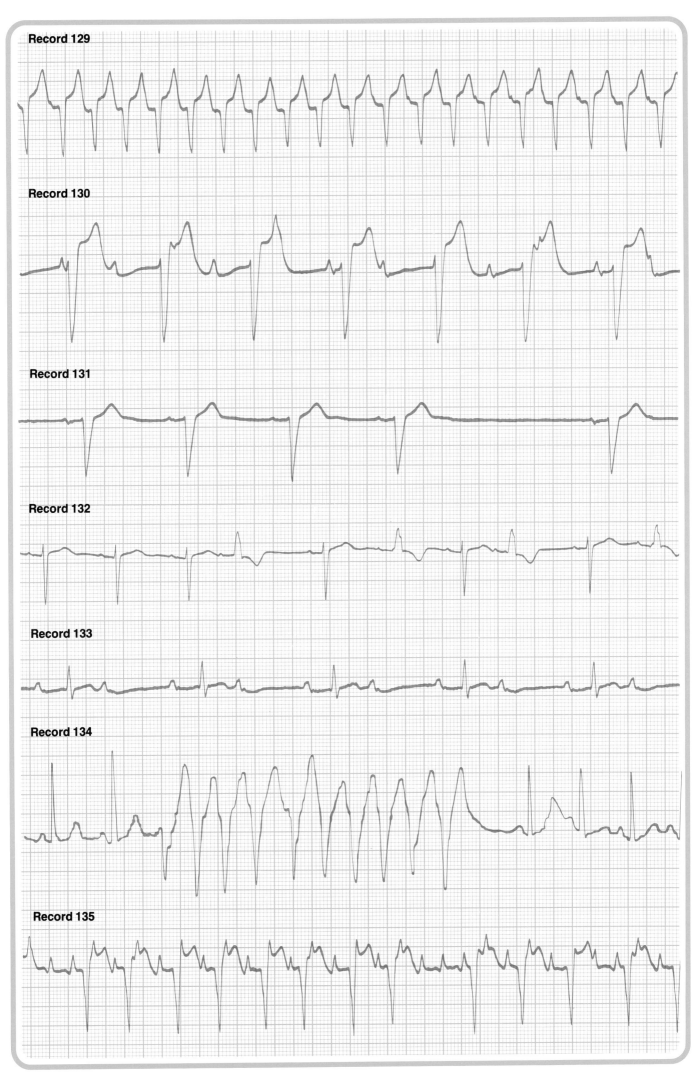

Record 129

Record 130

Record 131

Record 132

Record 133

Record 134

Record 135

594

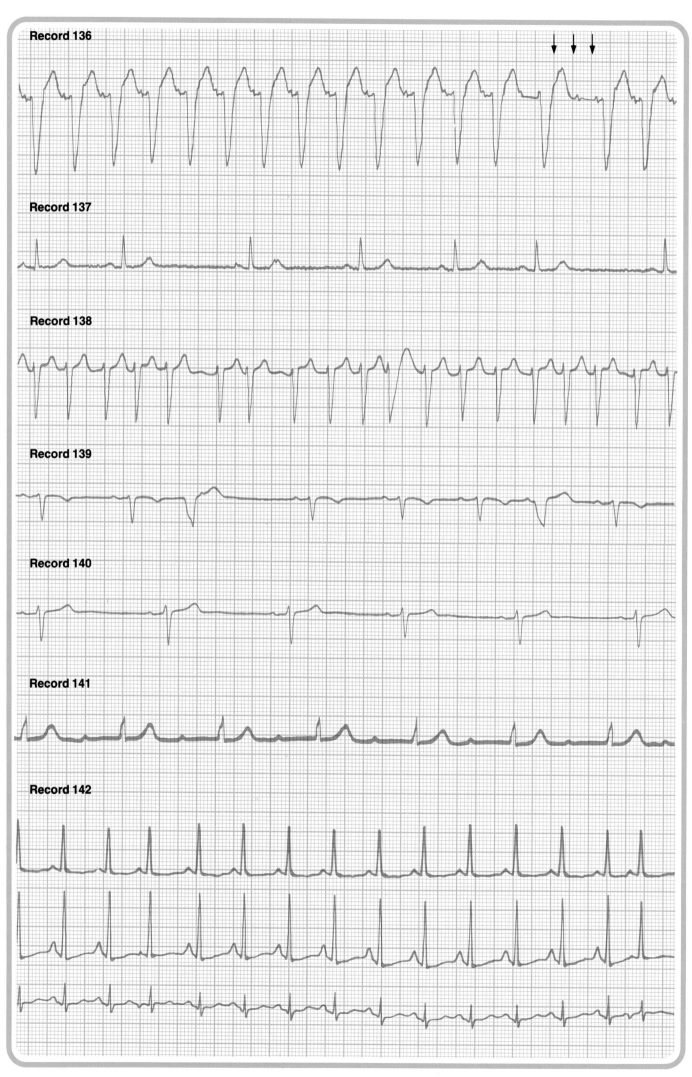

Record 136

Record 137

Record 138

Record 139

Record 140

Record 141

Record 142

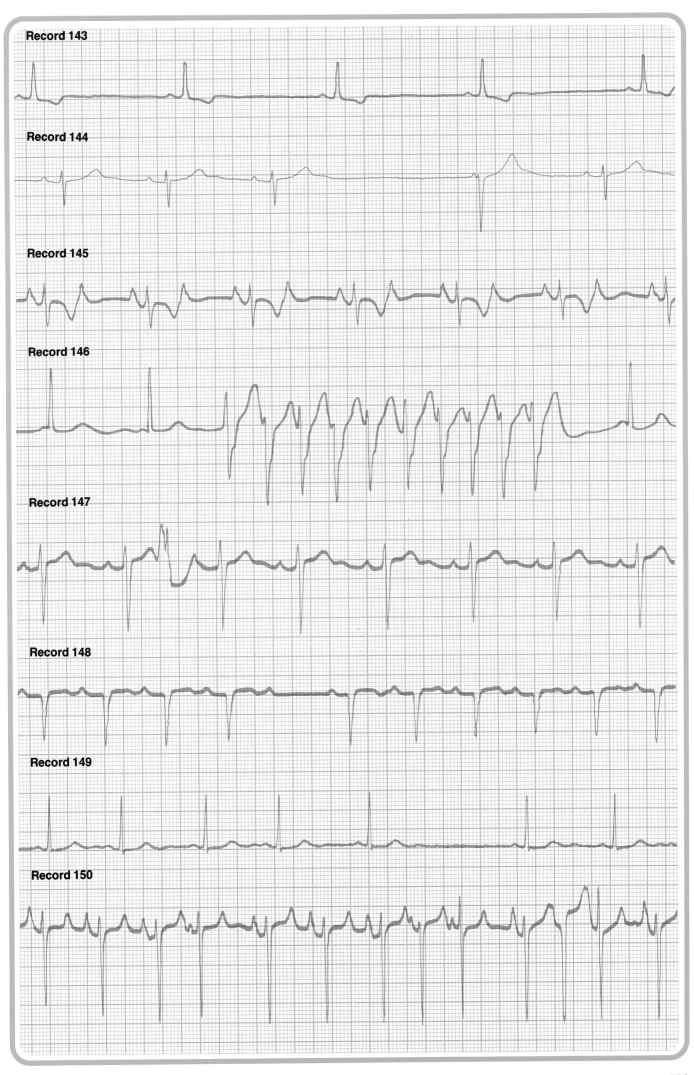

Record 143

Record 144

Record 145

Record 146

Record 147

Record 148

Record 149

Record 150

596

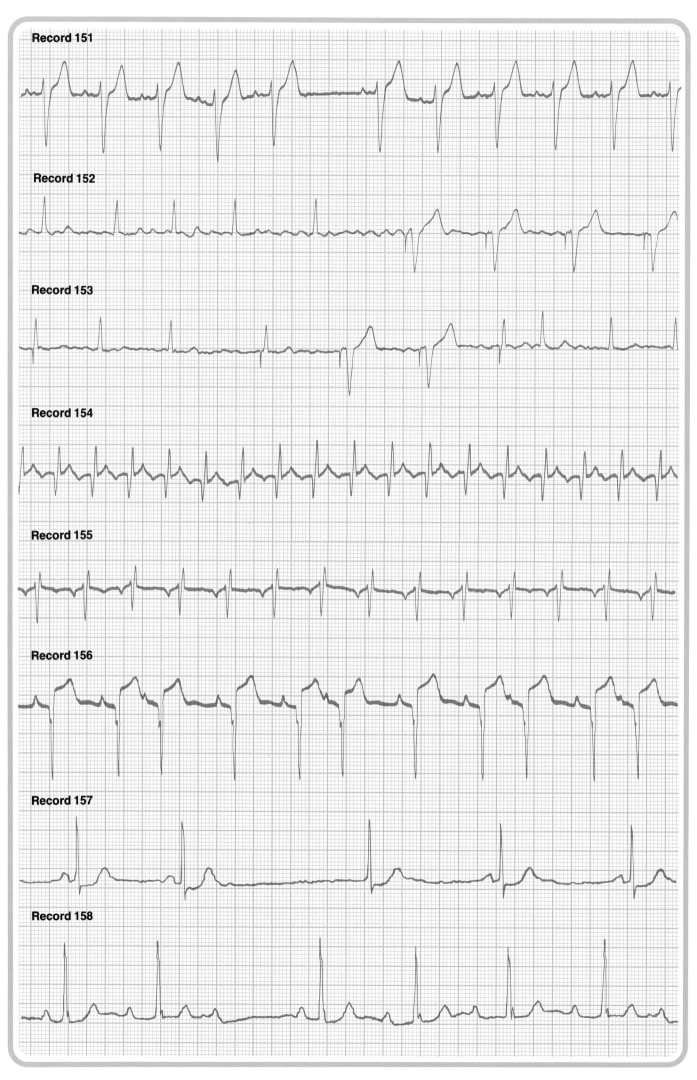

Record 151

Record 152

Record 153

Record 154

Record 155

Record 156

Record 157

Record 158

597

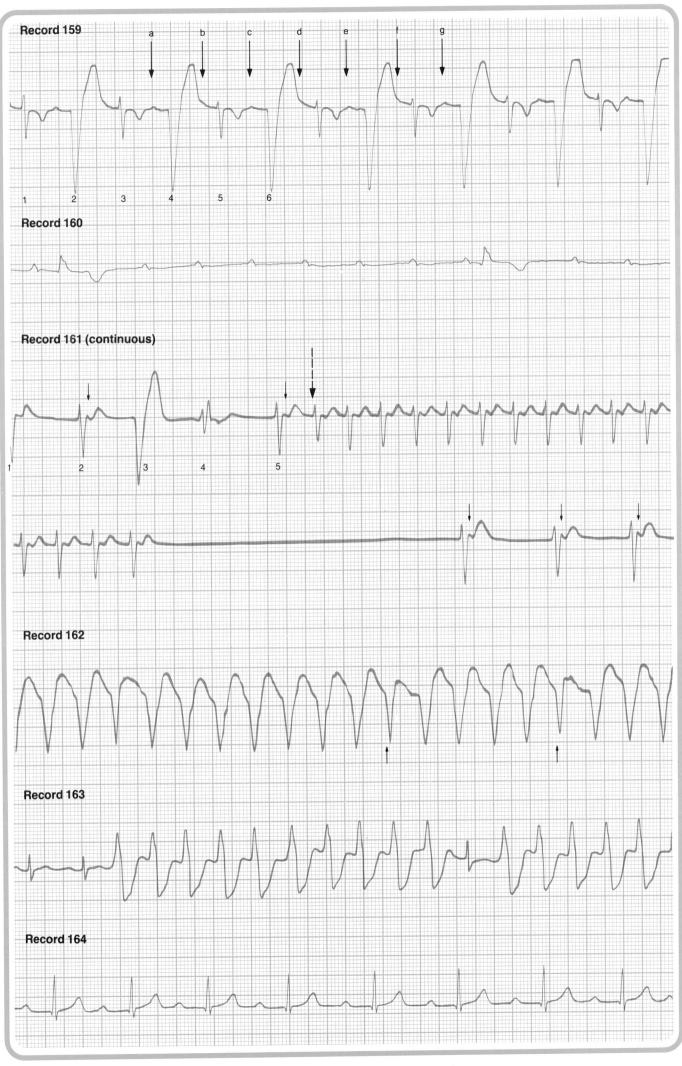

598

Records 91 to 164

Record 91
Ventricular tachycardia with 2:1 ventriculo-atrial block.

Record 92
Atrial fibrillation.

Record 93
Sinus rhythm with intermittent left bundle branch block. Recent myocardial infarction.

Record 94
Sinus rhythm with atrial premature ectopic beats. Recent myocardial infarction.

Record 95
Varying atrial rhythm – three independent atrial pacemakers, one of which could be sino-atrial.

Record 96
Ventricular tachycardia.

Record 97
Sinus bradycardia.

Record 98
Sinus rhythm with coupled ventricular ectopic premature beats.

Record 99
Non-paroxysmal junctional tachycardia.

Record 100
Sinus rhythm with atrial premature ectopic beats.

Record 101
Sinus rhythm. Atrial premature beats with aberrant intraventricular conduction.

Record 102
Sinus rhythm with ventricular ectopic premature beats of the R-on-T type.

Record 103
Atrial flutter with 2:1 atrio-ventricular block and bundle branch block.

Record 104
Sinus rhythm. Atrial premature ectopic beats. Ventricular premature ectopic beat. Ventricular premature ectopic beat of R-on-T type initiating ventricular tachycardia. Capture beat.

Record 105
Ventricular flutter.

Record 106
Atrio-ventricular nodal re-entrant tachycardia (AVNRT) or atrial flutter with 1:1 conduction via an anomalous atrio-ventricular pathway.

Record 107
Sinus rhythm with repetitive short bursts of ventricular tachycardia.

Record 108
Ventricular flutter.

Record 109
Sinus bradycardia with ventricular escape rhythm.

Record 110
Sinus bradycardia with a junctional escape beat.

Record 111
Atrial fibrillation with a single example of aberrant intraventricular conduction.

Record 112
Sinus rhythm with atrial premature ectopic beats.

Record 113
Sinus rhythm with complete atrial premature ectopic beats ("atrial coupling").

Record 114
Sinus rhythm with frequent atrial premature ectopic beats, one of which initiates atrial fibrillation. Complete right bundle branch block and recent myocardial infarction.

Record 115
Sinus rhythm with multiform atrial premature ectopic beats, one of which initiates re-entrant atrial tachycardia.

Record 116
Sinus rhythm with blocked atrial premature ectopic beats.

Record 117
Complete heart block. Ventricular escape rhythm from two foci.

Record 118
Sinus rhythm with frequent ventricular premature ectopic beats, one of which initiates ventricular tachycardia.

Record 119
Ventricular tachycardia ended by a ventricular premature beat interrupting the re-entrant pathway.

Record 120
Sinus tachycardia with a single ventricular premature beat.

Record 121
Sinus rhythm with frequent, uniform (unifocal) atrial premature beats, each of which is associated with aberrant intraventricular conduction.

Record 122
Complete heart block, with two independent ventricular escape foci.

Record 123
SA nodal re-entrant tachycardia, giving way to sinus rhythm.

Record 124
Sinus rhythm with type I second degree atrio-ventricular block (the Wenckebach phenomenon).

Record 125
Atrial fibrillation, R-on-T ventricular ectopics with a short burst of ventricular tachycardia.

Record 126
Sinus rhythm with type I second degree atrio-ventricular block (the Wenckebach phenomenon).

Record 127
Ventricular tachycardia.

Record 128
Varying rhythm. Atrial tachycardia, ventricular ectopic beat, sinus rhythm, blocked atrial premature ectopic beats.

Record 129
Atrial fibrillation.

Record 130
Sinus rhythm with complete heart block and a high ventricular escape rhythm.

Record 131
Sinus rhythm with transient sino-atrial block. Bundle branch block.

Record 132
Sinus rhythm with atrial premature beats associated with aberrant intraventricular conduction.

Record 133
Sinus rhythm with complete heart block and ventriculo-phasic sinus arrhythmia.

Record 134
Sinus rhythm with a short burst of ventricular tachycardia.

Record 135
Atrial tachycardia with varying, but predominantly 2:1 atrio-ventricular block.

Record 136
Atrial tachycardia with 2:1 atrio-ventricular block and bundle branch block. There is a single instance of 3:1 atrio-ventricular block.

Record 137
Sinus rhythm with type I sino-atrial block.

Record 138
Atrial fibrillation with a single example of aberrant intraventricular conduction.

Record 139
Sinus rhythm with two uniform premature ventricular ectopic beats.

Record 140
Sinus bradycardia.

Record 141
Sinus rhythm with first degree heart block.

Record 142
Sinus rhythm with atrial premature ectopic beats.

Record 143
Sinus bradycardia. Non-specific S-T, T changes.

Record 144
Sinus rhythm, sinus arrest and a high ventricular escape beat.

Record 145
Sinus tachycardia with 2:1 atrio-ventricular block.

Record 146
Sinus rhythm with a short burst of ventricular tachycardia.

Record 147
Sinus rhythm with a single interpolated premature ectopic ventricular beat with concealed retrograde conduction into the atrio-ventricular node.

Record 148
Sinus rhythm with first degree atrio-ventricular block (first degree heart block) and a single example of type II second degree atrio-ventricular block.

Record 149
Sinus arrhythmia.

Record 150
Sinus rhythm with atrial premature ectopic beats.

Record 151
Sinus rhythm with transient sinus arrest.

Record 152
Atrial fibrillation. Normally functioning VVI pacemaker with hysteresis.

Record 153
Atrial fibrillation.
Normally functioning VVI pacemaker.
Fusion beat. Pacemaker hysteresis.

Record 154
Sinus tachycardia. Right bundle branch block.

Record 155
Sinus tachycardia. Right bundle branch block.

Record 156
Sinus rhythm with atrial premature ectopic beats. Recent myocardial infarction.

Record 157
Sinus rhythm with transient sinus arrest and junctional escape.

Record 158
Sinus rhythm with type I second degree atrio-ventricular block (the Wenckebach phenomenon).

Record 159
Sinus rhythm with alternating left bundle branch block and normal intraventricular conduction.

Record 160
Complete heart block. Low ventricular escape rhythm.

Record 161
Sick sinus syndrome. Sinus arrest. Ventricular escape beats. Echo beat. Re-entrant junctional tachycardia. Asystole. Ventricular escape rhythm.

Record 162
Ventricular tachycardia. Fusion beats.

Record 163
Ventricular tachycardia. Capture beat.

Record 164
Sinus rhythm with first degree atrio-ventricular block.

Record 91

There is a tachycardia (approximate rate 165 beats/min). The rate is regular. The QRS complexes are abnormally wide (0.13 sec). On the basis of these findings the rhythm could be i) ventricular tachycardia or ii) supraventricular tachycardia with pre-existing bundle branch block, aberrant intraventricular conduction or with atrio-ventricular conduction down an anomalous pathway.

Examination of the electrocardiogram for P waves shows that P waves are visible in relation to every alternate QRS complex. This is an unusual finding, since the ventricular rate is twice the atrial rate. Clearly, therefore, the rhythm cannot be a supraventricular tachycardia. It must be ventricular tachycardia although it looks as though the P waves are upright and in front of the QRS complex to which they are related, since the rhythm is obviously ventricular tachycardia, the P waves can only either be independent or related to the ventricular tachycardia by retrograde conduction to the atria. The P waves are clearly not independent since their time relation to the QRS complexes is constant in relation to each alternate beat. The true explanation is that this is ventricular tachycardia with alternating ventriculo-atrial conduction, i.e. 2:1 ventriculo-atrial block. Each alternate ventricular activation is conducted backwards to the atria.

Record 92

There is a rapid heart rate. The heart rate is irregular. The QRS complexes are of normal width. No P waves are seen. There is irregularity of the baseline. The appearances are those of atrial fibrillation.

Record 93

Sinus rhythm with intermittent left bundle branch block. The first, third, fifth and eighth beats do not show an intraventricular conduction problem but the remaining beats show left bundle branch block. The record was taken from a patient with acute myocardial infarction and the beats which do not show left bundle branch block are consistent with this in that there are abnormally deep QS complexes and S-T segment elevation, but since one cannot be confident of the positioning of the lead with respect to the heart (it is a chest monitoring lead) one could not make a confident morphological diagnosis of myocardial infarction on the basis of this record alone. In relation to those beats showing left bundle branch block the morphological diagnosis of myocardial infarction could not be made with confidence in any event (page 268).

Record 94

Chest monitoring lead. The record was taken from a patient with acute myocardial infarction. There is sinus rhythm with atrial premature beats. The fourth and ninth beats are atrial premature beats. In each case the ectopic P wave can be seen slightly deforming the down-slope of the T wave (the T wave is merged into the elevated S-T segment). The QRS complexes following these premature P waves have the usual form for the subject at that time (as evidenced by the fact that they are the same as the QRS complexes in relation to the sinus beats).

Record 95

Three separate atrial rhythms are visible here. The first three beats show one atrial focus, the next three show a second atrial focus and the last four show a third atrial focus. It is possible that all three atrial foci are ectopic and that none of the beats shown is a sinus beat but it is more likely that either the first three or the last four beats are sinus beats. Beats 4-6 have abnormal looking P waves and probably initiate an ectopic atrial focus. The P waves of beats 1-3 and beats 7-10 are consistent with their having a sinus origin but both groups cannot be sinus. Since the P waves of the last group (7-10) look more normal and have a slower rate they are probably the sinus beats. Note that each atrial focus (whether it be three separate ectopic atrial foci or one sino-atrial nodal discharge and two ectopic atrial foci) has not only its own P wave morphology (indicating its own anatomical location within the atrial myocardium) but also its own intrinsic discharge rate. Note also that all the QRS complexes are identical irrespective of the atrial ectopic focus.

Record 96

There is a regular tachycardia at a rate of approximately 185 beats/min. The QRS complexes are abnormally wide (0.13 sec). There are occasional perturbations of the wave-form which might indicate the presence of a P wave but these cannot be recognised with absolute confidence. The rhythm could be a supraventricular tachycardia with pre-existing bundle branch block or a supraventricular tachycardia with aberrant intraventricular conduction or a supraventricular tachycardia with conduction down an accessory pathway or ventricular tachycardia. It is impossible, with absolute confidence, to distinguish between these rhythms. Independent P waves cannot be recognised with absolute confidence, there are no fusion beats, there are no capture beats.

No electrocardiographic data concerning the appearances when the subject was in sinus rhythm are available. This is a not-uncommon clinical situation. The **electrocardiographic** probability is that this is ventricular tachycardia.

Record 97

Sinus bradycardia.

Record 98

The record is taken from a patient with recent myocardial infarction. There is sinus rhythm with coupled ventricular premature ectopic beats of the R-on-T type. Each sinus beat is followed by a ventricular ectopic. The QRS complex of the ectopic beat is abnormally wide. No P wave is seen in relation to the premature beats. The down-slope of the T wave following the sinus beat merges straight into the beginning of the QRS complex of the premature beat. However this is only just "R-on-T" and is therefore unlikely to promote ventricualr tachycardia or fibrillation since it is probably outside the vulnerable period.

Record 99

Non-paroxysmal junctional tachycardia. The ventricular rate is regular at 90 beats/min. Although such a rate does not constitute a "tachycardia" in the general sense, such a rate is considered to be a tachycardia in relation to intrinsic rhythmicity of the AV node. The QRS complexes are normal. Inverted P waves are seen following each QRS complex.

Record 100

Sinus rhythm with atrial premature beats. The second, third and fifth beats are atrial premature beats. The remainder of the record shows sinus rhythm. The atrial premature beats are premature, abnormally (i.e. different from the usual one for that subject) shaped P waves with normal QRS complexes.

Record 101

Sinus rhythm with atrial premature beats associated with aberrant intraventricular conduction. The second, sixth and ninth beats are clearly premature. The remainder of the record shows sinus rhythm. These premature beats have abnormally-shaped, abnormally-wide QRS complexes and might initially, therefore, be thought to be ventricular premature beats. However, careful inspection of the T waves of the sinus beats immediately preceding the premature QRS complexes shows that they are slightly deformed (pointed) compared with the two "control" T waves which are clearly seen in relation to the third and fourth beats. The premature and ectopic P waves are present superimposed on top of the T waves of the first and fifth beats and they are followed by premature QRS complexes which are conducted as a result of the atrial premature beats. The QRS complexes of the premature beats show the right bundle branch block configuration and there is no reasonable doubt that this is an example of atrial premature beats with aberrant intraventricular conduction.

Record 102

Sinus tachycardia with ventricular premature beats of the R-on-T type occurring after every three sinus beats.

Record 103

There is a tachycardia at a rate of 136 beats/min. The QRS complexes are abnormally wide. The rate is regular. This could either be a supraventricular tachycardia with pre-existing bundle branch block, functional bundle branch block or atrio-ventricular conduction down an accessory pathway or it could be ventricular tachycardia.

The probability is that this is atrial flutter with 2:1 block and bundle branch block. Carotid sinus massage might confirm this if a transient increase in the degree of AV block could be induced.

Record 104
Sinus rhythm with atrial and ventricular premature beats and two short bursts of ventricular tachycardia. The first beat is a sinus beat. This is followed by a premature, normal QRS complex. The P wave in relation to this beat cannot be clearly seen but the beat is probably an atrial or junctional premature beat. The third beat is a sinus beat and following this there is an abnormally-shaped and premature QRS complex, i.e. a ventricular premature beat. The fifth QRS complex occurs as a result of a sinus-initiated beat. Towards the end of the down-slope of the T wave following this fifth QRS complex there is a ventricular premature beat of the R-on-T type and this initiates a burst of ventricular tachycardia which continues for approximately three seconds.

The ventricular tachycardia is disturbed when an atrial beat (small arrow) is transmitted to the ventricles to give a capture beat (large arrow). Although three ventricular ectopic beats are seen following this the re-entrant cycle has been disturbed and sinus rhythm ultimately returns.

Record 105
Ventricular flutter. There is a rapid regular heart rate of 210 beats/min with abnormally-wide QRS complexes. This could conceivably be supraventricular tachycardia with pre-existing bundle branch block, supraventricular tachycardia with aberrant intraventricular conduction or supraventricular tachycardia with conduction down an anomalous pathway. It could also be ventricular tachycardia. P waves cannot be seen with confidence and there are no examples of capture beats or fusion beats. The very wide QRS complexes powerfully suggest that the rhythm is ventricular and the symmetry of the QRS complexes suggests that the rhythm is ventricular flutter.

Record 106
This is clearly a supraventricular tachycardia. The QRS complexes are of normal width and the rate is regular and very rapid at approximately 250 beats/ min. Such a rapid rate occurring in association with what is very clearly a supraventricular tachycardia raises the possibility of atrial flutter with 1:1 conduction down an anomalous atrio-ventricular pathway. The rhythm could also be atrio-ventricular nodal re-entrant tachycardia.

Record 107
Sinus rhythm with repetitive short bursts of ventricular tachycardia.

Record 108
Ventricular flutter.

Record 109
Sinus bradycardia with ventricular escape. The first two beats are sinus beats. The sinus rate is slow (38 beats/ min). No P wave is seen after the second QRS complex and two consecutive ventricular escape beats are then seen. These are late ventricular ectopic beats.

Record 110
Sinus rhythm with a junctional escape beat. The first four beats are sinus beats. The QRS complex in relation to these beats is abnormally wide suggesting the presence of bundle branch block (this diagnosis cannot be made with certainty from this single lead). After the fourth beat there is a long pause (sinus arrest) followed by a junctional escape beat. The QRS complex of this escape beat is abnormally wide but it does in fact have exactly the same morphology as the QRS complexes of the conducted beats and in this way can be recognised to be a junctional escape beat rather than a ventricular escape beat (i.e. it has the morphology which is usual for that subject).

Record 111
Leads I, II and III. Atrial fibrillation with a single example of aberrant intraventricular conduction.

The rhythm is clearly atrial fibrillation. No P waves are seen. The QRS complexes (with one exception) are of normal width and the rhythm is clearly supraventricular. The QRS complexes are irregular with no organised pattern to the R-R intervals. The obvious feature for comment is the sixth QRS complex which is clearly different from the others. It could be a ventricular premature ectopic beat but the fact that it follows the preceding QRS complex after a short R-R interval and the fact that the preceding QRS complex itself followed the one before that by a long R-R interval, makes it very likely that the unusually shaped QRS complex is an example of aberrant intraventricular conduction. Aberrant intraventricular conduction is most likely to occur in a beat which ends a short R-R interval immediately following a long R-R interval (page 403).

Record 112
Sinus tachycardia with frequent atrial premature beats. The rhythm is clearly sinus tachycardia. The sixth QRS complex follows an ectopic premature P wave. The tenth, eleventh, and thirteenth QRS complexes likewise follow premature ectopic P waves. The QRS morphology is effectively constant throughout.

Record 113
Sinus rhythm with coupled atrial premature ectopic beats. The first beat is a sinus beat and this is followed by an atrial premature ectopic beat. This pattern continues throughout the recording but the morphology of the ectopic P waves varies indicating that the site of origin of the ectopic focus is not constant.

Record 114
Sinus rhythm with frequent atrial premature beats, one of which precipitates a run of sustained atrial fibrillation. There is complete right bundle branch block and evidence of recent infarction.

The lead in question is a chest monitoring lead. The QRS complexes are abnormally wide and are of the RSR′ type. In those beats of sinus origin this clearly indicates that there is complete right bundle branch block. There is S-T segment elevation and the record is taken from a patient with recent myocardial infarction. The third, sixth and ninth beats are atrial premature ectopic beats in which the ectopic P wave can be seen deforming the T wave of the preceding beat. The ninth atrial premature beat is followed by what superficially looks like a sustained burst of atrial tachycardia. The QRS complexes have the same morphology as those in the sinus beats and they are therefore "usual for that patient" The rhythm is therefore clearly supraventricular. The R-R intervals are, however, quite variable and the rhythm is therefore almost certainly atrial fibrillation.

Record 115
Sinus rhythm with frequent atrial premature ectopic beats and a short run of atrial tachycardia. The second, fourth and fifth beats are premature atrial ectopic beats. These beats have different P wave morphologies from each other and are arising from different foci in the atrial myocardium. The eighth beat is also an atrial premature beat. The tenth beat is an atrial premature beat and this then initiates a re-entrant atrial tachycardia which is seen to continue for four beats before the rhythm strip ends.

Record 116
Sinus rhythm with first degree heart block and frequent blocked atrial premature beats. The first two beats are sinus beats with a long P-R interval (0.26 sec). Following the second QRS complex there is a premature, abnormally-shaped P wave seen superimposed on the S-T segment. This P wave is not conducted to the ventricles but the sino-atrial node is re-set and, as is usual with atrial premature beats, the interval between the P′ wave and the next P wave is slightly greater than the interval between two consecutive P waves. The interval between the QRS immediately preceding the atrial ectopic beat and the QRS following the next sinus beat is very significantly prolonged since this interval

is the sum of the P'-P interval, the P-R interval of the beat following the atrial ectopic and the time interval between the QRS preceding the atrial ectopic and the atrial ectopic beat. Blocked atrial premature beats are a common cause of abnormal pauses between R waves.

Record 117
Complete heart block. The atrial rate is regular at 69 beats/min. Three ventricular escape beats are seen. The first two have identical morphology with very wide QRS complexes and an escape rate (R-R interval) of 24 beats/min. The third QRS has a different morphology indicating that the escape beat has occurred from a different focus within the ventricle. The escape rate is still of a similar order of magnitude at about 23 beats/min (interval between the second and the third QRS complexes).

Record 118
Sinus rhythm with frequent R-on-T ectopic beats, one of which is followed by ventricular tachycardia. The first two beats are sinus beats, the third beat is an R-on-T ectopic. Just after the down-slope of the T wave of the fourth beat there is a P wave which is probably an atrial premature beat. This is followed by an abnormally-wide, abnormally-shaped QRS complex. This could be aberrant intraventricular conduction resulting from the atrial premature beat or it could be an ectopic premature ventricular beat arising before conduction of the P wave to the ventricles can occur. The sixth beat is a sinus beat and this is followed by an R-on-T ectopic which is followed immediately by a second ectopic beat. The second ectopic probably occurred on a re-entry basis following the first ectopic. After these two consecutive ventricular ectopic beats, there is a further sinus beat followed by an R-on-T ectopic which gives rise to a sustained burst of ventricular tachycardia.

Record 119
This record is continuous with that demonstrated in Record 118. There is a period of sustained ventricular tachycardia. An artefact appears just to the right of centre of the illustration when a blow was applied to the subject's lower sternum as part of the resuscitating manoeuvres. This produces no immediate detectable effect in the rhythm but after a further two seconds of ventricular tachycardia there is a QRS complex with a different morphology (arrowed). This appears to be an ectopic beat from a different focus and it may well have resulted in depolarisation of part of the re-entrant pathway thus breaking the re-entrant cycle.
This ectopic beat is followed by a further QRS with abnormal morphology (second arrow). It is difficult to tell where this QRS complex ends and part of the subsequent upward deviation may be a further artefact due to a second sternal blow. Following this sinus rhythm is restored. This record is an example of a ventricular

ectopic beat from a site other than the area of the re-entry mechanism, giving rise to depolarisation in the area of the re-entry and thereby interrupting the re-entrant tachycardia.

Record 120
Sinus tachycardia with a single ventricular premature beat. The pause following the premature beat is precisely compensatory. If the P wave timing is traced through the record it can be seen that the P wave which follows the onset of the ventricular premature beat would be expected to occur at about the mid-portion of the QRS complex. The timing corresponds to the slight irregularity in the down-slope of the QRS at the ectopic beat just after its peak. This irregularity could be produced by the P wave but equally could simply be related to the pathway of intraventricular conduction during the ectopic beat.

Record 121
Sinus rhythm with frequent, uniform (unifocal) atrial premature beats each of which is associated with aberrant intraventricular conduction. The first two beats are sinus beats. The third beat is premature. The T wave of the second beat is taller than that of the first beat and this difference represents superimposition of the P wave of the atrial premature beat on top of the T wave of the preceding beat. The third QRS, whilst narrow, is morphologically slightly different from the first two and this represents a minor degree of aberrant intraventricular conduction (not complete bundle branch block). The cycle is then repeated, every third beat being an atrial ectopic with aberrant intraventricular conduction. When every third beat is an atrial ectopic the word "trigeminy" may be used.

Record 122
Lead III. Complete heart block.
The record is taken from the same subject as Record 160. During the trace two separate ventricular escape foci are seen (beats 1, 2 and 4 arising from one focus and beats 3 and 5 from a different focus).

Record 123
Chest monitoring lead. Sino-atrial nodal re-entrant tachycardia, followed by sinus bradycardia. The first four beats look exactly like sinus rhythm (and indeed in so far as sinus rhythm is considered to be that rhythm in which myocardial depolarisation is initiated at the sino-atrial node it **is** "sinus rhythm"). After the fourth beat there is a sudden dramatic fall in the sinus rate and sinus bradycardia follows. This is not sinus arrhythmia since the rate change is abrupt and sustained. It is likely that there has been a sino-atrial nodal re-entrant tachycardia which has stopped spontaneously. No change occurs in the morphology of the P waves or of the QRS complexes. The first four beats satisfy the criteria for sinus rhythm at a rate of about 86 beats/min and the last three satisfy the

criteria for sinus bradycardia at a rate of about 47 beats/min. The record shows sinus rhythm throughout but the abrupt rate change suggests that the initial rhythm was SA nodal re-entrant tachycardia.

Record 124
Chest monitoring lead. AV nodal Wenckebach (Type I second degree AV block). The first P-R interval is normal. The first five beats are followed by QRS complexes with progressively lengthening P-R intervals. The sixth P wave (seen disturbing the upstroke of the T wave of the preceding beat) is not followed by a QRS. Measurement of the P-P interval indicates that the P wave is premature. Not surprisingly (since (a) it is premature and (b) there is already evidence of a progressively lengthening P-R interval) it fails to conduct. Because of the presence of the premature P wave it cannot be said that AV nodal Wenckebach has occurred but since (a) the P-R interval "starts again" at a normal value after the ensuing sinus P wave and progressively lengthens in successive beats (b) the R-R interval shortens progressively during the first five beats, it is very likely that type I block is occurring (see Record 84).

Record 125
Chest monitoring lead. The basic rhythm is atrial fibrillation. (No P waves are seen, there is irregularity in the baseline consistent with chaotic atrial activity). Five QRS complexes of normal morphology are seen and this clearly indicates the usual ventricular response in atrial fibrillation. The third QRS is abnormally wide and abnormally shaped. It represents a premature ectopic ventricular beat of the R-on-T type (it begins before the anticipated completion of the T wave following the second QRS. Although the T wave cannot be seen its timing can be predicted since the (slow) ventricular rate of the underlying atrial fibrillation means that one would expect a Q-T interval of the order of 0.40 sec and the approximate timing of the end of the T wave can therefore be predicted). A further (similarly shaped) R-on-T ectopic occurs after the fourth beat and this gives rise to three more ventricular ectopics in quick succession. This is technically a short burst of ventricular tachycardia. The tachycardia is not sustained. After the fifth normal QRS a further abnormally shaped QRS occurs. This has the right bundle branch block configuration. It could either be a ventricular ectopic beat arising at the left ventricle or an example of aberrant intraventricular conduction.

Record 126
Lead II. Second degree atrio-ventricular block type I. The second and sixth P waves are not followed by QRS complexes. The remainder of the P waves are followed by QRS complexes. This is second degree atrio-ventricular block. The first P-R interval is long. In relation to the first and second P

waves, therefore, one cannot be certain whether the fact that no QRS has followed the second P wave is due to type I or type II second degree block but the third to sixth P waves are followed by QRS complexes with gradually increasing P-R intervals before the failure of conduction occurs indicating clearly that the conduction disturbance of the atrio-ventricular node is of the type I variety.

Record 127
Chest monitoring lead. Ventricular tachycardia. Very wide, bizarre QRS complexes occur. The shape is so bizarre that one cannot tell where the QRS ends and the S-T segment begins. Although this is technically classified as a "wide QRS complex tachycardia" the QRS complexes are well in excess of 0.16 sec in duration. This rules out any possibility of aberrant intraventricular conduction.

Record 128
Chest monitoring lead. Variable rhythm. The first four beats show a regular supraventricular tachycardia. On the basis of the appearance of these beats alone the rhythm could conceivably be sinus tachycardia. After the fifth beat there is a longer pause followed by what also looks like a sinus beat but has a P wave morphology different from the earlier beats. The probability at this stage is that the first five beats represent atrial tachycardia and the sixth beat is the sinus beat. There is then a ventricular ectopic premature beat followed by a pause. In view of the irregularity of the rate preceding this beat it is not possible to say whether or not the pause is "compensatory". There are then four beats of what is clearly sinus rhythm and this reinforces the view that the first four beats represented atrial tachycardia. After four consecutive sinus beats there are two atrial ectopic beats occurring in quick succession, neither of which is conducted to the ventricles. This is surprising in view of the time interval between the first of these atrial ectopic beats and the preceding sinus beat and this failure to conduct after such a time interval suggests that there is depression of atrio-ventricular nodal function. The final beat is the sinus beat.

Record 129
Chest monitoring lead. Atrial fibrillation. The total QRS duration is at the upper end of the normal range. The rhythm is therefore supraventricular. A casual inspection might suggest that this is a regular supraventricular tachycardia but more careful examination of the R-R intervals indicates that these vary considerably. The rhythm is atrial fibrillation.

Record 130
Chest monitoring lead. Complete heart block. The basic sinus rate can clearly be recognised. The sinus rate is not absolutely constant but is approximately

so and the basic sinus mechanism can be "traced through" the record. The basic QRS rate is a constant ventricular rate of approximately 50 beats/min. The QRS complexes are abnormally wide. The ventricular rhythm is a relatively high ventricular escape rhythm.

Record 131
Chest monitoring lead. Basic sinus rhythm with transient sino-atrial block. The first four beats show sinus rhythm at a relatively slow rate. The interval between the fourth and fifth P waves is almost exactly twice the interval between consecutive P waves prior to this and the probability, therefore, is that there has been sino-atrial block causing the beat. The QRS complexes are abnormally wide indicating bundle branch block (they are clearly conducted beats of supraventricular origin since the P-R intervals are constant).

Record 132
Chest monitoring lead. Sinus rhythm with atrial premature beats associated with aberrant intraventricular conduction. The underlying rhythm is sinus rhythm but three premature P waves are seen, each followed by a QRS complex which is abnormally wide and has a configuration suggesting delay in conduction in the right bundle branch system. These are examples of atrial premature beats associated with aberrant intraventricular conduction. It is a manifestation of acceleration-dependent aberrancy in the intraventricular conducting tissue.

Record 133
At first sight this looks like 2:1 atrio-ventricular block. In fact the P-R interval in relation to those P waves immediately followed by a QRS complex is slightly variable and the probability is that this is complete heart block. Careful inspection reveals that those P-P intervals which "contain" a QRS complex are shorter than those P-P intervals which do not contain a QRS complex. This is an example of complete heart block with ventriculo-phasic sinus arrhythmia.

Record 134
Ambulatory ECG recording. The first two beats show sinus rhythm . The second T wave is followed by a premature, abnormally shaped QRS complex which is not of the R-on-T type. This is followed by repeated consecutive ventricular ectopic beats with a slightly irregular rate. This is a short burst of ventricular tachycardia. Following the cessation of the tachycardia there is a pause before the next sinus beat.

Record 135
Paroxysmal atrial tachycardia with varying AV block. In most of the record there is 2:1 atrio-ventricular block. Two pauses are seen, one right at the beginning of the record and the other between the eighth and ninth beats. It is

always worth carefully inspecting such pauses. In both these pauses the true atrial ectopic rate can be seen and the atrial activity can be recognised in other parts of the record by extrapolation forwards and backwards as indicated in Figure 266. In this way it can be seen that in most of the record there is 2:1 atrio-ventricular block and that during the pauses there is 4:1 atrio-ventricular block.

Record 136
Atrial tachycardia with predominantly 2:1 atrio-ventricular block. There is a tachycardia with a rate of 150 beats/min. The QRS complexes are abnormally wide. On the basis of the rapid, regular QRS rate and wide QRS complexes the rhythm could be i) a supraventricular tachycardia with pre-existing bundle branch block, ii) a supraventricular tachycardia with functional bundle branch block, or iii) a supraventricular tachycardia with conduction down an anomalous pathway, or iv) ventricular tachycardia. For most of the record the appearances look to be consistent with sinus tachycardia and left bundle branch block, but a longer than usual pause is seen towards the end of the rhythm strip. It is always worthwhile looking carefully at such pauses.
In relation to that pause three P waves can be seen (arrowed). The clear state of affairs is revealed. The rhythm is actually atrial tachycardia and there is bundle -branch block. In most of the recording the degree of atrio-ventricular block is 2:1, but for one interval the block is 3:1. The P-R interval in relation to the beat at the beginning of this pause is slightly prolonged indicating that some increase in the degree of atrio-ventricular block is already beginning.
The fact that the QRS complex following the pause is identical with all previous QRS complexes effectively rules out acceleration – dependent aberrancy as a cause of the abnormal QRS complexes. The clear record of atrial tachycardia during the pause rules out atrio-ventricular tachycardia using an anomalous pathway. The fact that there are more P waves than QRS complexes (seen during the pause) rules out ventricular tachycardia.

Record 137
The basic rhythm is clearly of sinus origin. All the P waves have a consistent morphology and the P-R interval is constant. There is variation in the P wave rate (and therefore in the QRS rate) and superficially the appearances resemble sinus arrhythmia. However, it can be seen that there is progressive shortening of the P-P interval (and therefore in the R-R interval) before a sudden increase in the P-P (and therefore in the R-R interval). The appearances are probably those of type I **sino-atrial** block. This diagnosis can only be inferred. The behaviour of the P waves in type I second degree sino-atrial block is similar to the behaviour of the QRS complexes in type I second degree atrio-ventricular block, i.e. in both cases there is progressive

shortening of the interval between (either the P waves or the QRS complexes) until there is a sudden lengthening of the interval for one beat followed by progressive shortening once more.

Record 138
Atrial fibrillation with a single example of aberrant intraventricular conduction. QRS complexes have a duration within normal limits. No consistent P waves are seen. The R-R interval is irregular. Just past the mid-point of the record there is a single QRS complex which is abnormally wide. The interval between the preceding R wave and this R wave is less than all the other intervals and this is an example of acceleration-dependent aberrant intraventricular conduction.

Record 139
Sinus rhythm with two uniform ventricular premature beats. The first two beats are clearly sinus beats. The third beat has an abnormally-wide, abnormally-shaped QRS complex and it occurs without any preceding P waves. A normally timed P wave can, in fact, be seen disturbing the upstroke of the S-T segment of the ectopic beat. The pause following the ectopic beat is fully compensatory. There is no doubt that this is a ventricular premature ectopic beat. The penultimate beat has a QRS, S-T and T morphology identical with that of the ventricular premature ectopic beats which occurred earlier. The penultimate QRS does have a P wave in front of it with a short P-R interval but the probability is that this is also a ventricular ectopic beat arising from the same focus as the earlier ectopic and occurring just before the completion of the P-R interval (i.e. just before conduction of the P wave to the ventricles).

Record 140
Sinus bradycardia.

Record 141
Sinus rhythm with first degree heart block.

Record 142
Leads I, II and III. Sinus rhythm with atrial premature beats. The fourth QRS complex occurs as a result of conduction of an atrial premature beat to the ventricles. The P wave preceding this QRS is clearly abnormal in morphology and is premature. The final beat is also an atrial premature beat. The P-R interval of the first atrial premature beat appears slightly less than that of the sinus beats, and that of the final atrial premature beat appears slightly longer than that of the sinus beats. The abnormality of morphology of the ectopic P waves is difficult to see in Lead I but is easily appreciated in Leads II and III, emphasising the value of multiple leads in rhythm analysis.

Record 143
Sinus bradycardia with non-specific S-T, T changes.

Record 144
Sinus rhythm, followed by a period of sinus arrest with a high ventricular escape beat. The fourth QRS complex does follow a P wave but after a very short P-R interval it is likely that this fourth QRS is entirely independent of the P wave which precedes it. After the first three P waves there is a long pause before the next P wave indicating there has been a period of sinus arrest. The fourth QRS has a morphology different from that of the three preceding QRS complexes so the probability is that this is a ventricular escape beat but the QRS is still narrow indicating that the escape focus is situated high in the ventricles, probably high up in the interventricular septum. The time interval between the third and fourth P waves is not an integral multiple of the time interval between the first and second or second and third P waves so the sinus mechanism is sinus arrest and not sino-atrial block.

Record 145
Sinus tachycardia with 2:1 atrio-ventricular block. There is clearly a P wave in front of each QRS complex. There is clearly also an identically shaped P wave "attached" to the terminal part of the inverted T wave. The interval between the P wave preceding and the P wave following a QRS complex is the same as the interval between the P wave following one QRS complex and the P wave preceding the next one. Because of this we can be sure the rhythm is sinus rhythm with 2:1 atrio-ventricular block and is not the result of blocked atrial premature beats. In the case of 2:1 atrio-ventricular block it is not possible to tell whether this is of type I or type II.

Record 146
Ambulatory recording. Two sinus beats followed by a short burst of what is probably ventricular tachycardia.
The burst of tachycardia is initiated by what is clearly a ventricular ectopic beat. It is not of the R-on-T type.
The tachycardia subsequently has a rapid regular rate with abnormally wide QRS complexes.

Record 147
Sinus rhythm with a single interpolated ventricular premature beat. After the first two sinus beats there is a premature, abnormally-shaped, abnormally-wide QRS complex. This is clearly a ventricular ectopic premature beat. The P-R interval following this beat is abnormally long indicating that the depolarisation from the ventricular premature beat has spread backwards into the atrio-ventricular node resulting in subsequent delay in conduction through the node. This is an example of concealed retrograde conduction of a ventricular premature beat.

Record 148
Sinus rhythm with first degree atrio-ventricular block (the P-R interval is 0.24

sec). There is transient type II second degree atrio-ventricular block. The first four beats are sinus beats. There is then a P wave with normal timing and normal configuration. This P wave is not followed by a QRS. Sinus rhythm returns immediately afterwards. This is an example of type II second degree atrio-ventricular block.

Record 149
Sinus arrhythmia. The criteria for sinus rhythm are fulfilled but the rate is irregular. The pattern does not follow a gradual "compression" of the R-R interval until a sudden large R-R interval occurs but rather involves a waxing and waning of the R-R interval. Small U waves are seen consistently.

Record 150
Sinus rhythm with atrial premature ectopic beats. The fourth, eighth, ninth, eleventh and twelfth beats are atrial premature ectopic beats.

Record 151
Sinus rhythm with a single episode of sinus arrest. The record shows sinus rhythm, a pause and then the restoration of sinus rhythm. The pause is not an integral multiple of the normal P-P interval and the probability is that there has been a period of sinus arrest.

Record 152
Atrial fibrillation with a normally functioning VVI pacemaker. The pause after the fifth spontaneous QRS complex is followed by a pacing spike and an induced QRS. Subsequently there is regular ventricular pacing. The time interval between the fifth spontaneous QRS and the first pacing spike is greater than that between consecutive pacing spikes indicating that the pacemaker shows hysteresis.

Record 153
Atrial fibrillation with a VVI pacemaker and fusion beats. The first complex shows a pacing spike followed by a QRS. This QRS has a normal morphology and duration indicating that it is a supraventricularly-initiated beat resulting from the spread of a depolarisation from the fibrillating atria travelling through the atrio-ventricular node. The second and third QRS complexes are likewise those associated with atrial fibrillation. Following the third QRS complex there is a long pause which is ended by a pacing spike and a QRS which is slightly different in form from the basic QRS complexes and is probably a fusion beat. The fifth and sixth QRS complexes are paced beats with the pacing stimulus clearly visible. The seventh complex is a fusion beat which has a pacing stimulus at the beginning of it. The final three complexes are related simply to the atrial fibrillation.
The pause between the third QRS and the pacing spike in front of the fourth QRS is greater than that between the consecutive pacing spike seen in relation

to the fourth and seventh beats, indicating that the pacemaker shows hysteresis.

Record 154
Sinus tachycardia (the patient also had right bundle branch block). Because of the possibility that an additional P wave might be hidden in the QRS complex, S-T segment or T wave, carotid sinus massage was undertaken (see Record 155).

Record 155
Sinus tachycardia (the patient having complete right bundle branch block). The record is taken from the same patient as that in Record 154 but is recorded during carotid sinus massage.

Record 156
Sinus rhythm with atrial premature beats. The third, sixth, ninth and eleventh beats are atrial premature ectopic beats. The patient had recently sustained a myocardial infarction.

Record 157
Sinus rhythm followed by sinus arrest and junctional escape. The first two beats are sinus beats. Following the second beat there is a pause of approximately 2 sec. This pause is ended by a QRS complex which is not preceded by a P wave. This is a junctional escape beat. The next two beats are sinus beats.

Record 158
Sinus rhythm with Wenckebach block (Möbitz Type I second degree atrio-ventricular block). The first P-R interval is normal, the second P-R interval is prolonged and the third P wave is not followed by a QRS complex. The fourth P wave is followed by a QRS complex with a P-R interval at the upper end of the normal range and there is progressive prolongation of the P-R interval in relation to the next two P waves.

Record 159
Chest monitoring lead. At first sight the appearances suggest coupled ventricular premature beats. Alternate R-R intervals (1-2, 3-4,5-6 etc) are terminated by abnormally-wide, abnormally-shaped QRS complexes. Close inspection, however, reveals the seemingly anomalous situation that the abnormal QRS complexes consistently follow P waves after a normal P-R interval and that the normal QRS complexes do not seem to be preceded by P waves. If the P waves preceding beats 4 and 6 are marked by arrows (a) and (c) and a mark is then made exactly half way between (a) and (c), at (b), a P wave can be recognised deforming the terminal part of the T wave of beat 4. The interval a-b, b-c can be extrapolated as e-f etc. Thus it can be seen that the rhythm is sinus throughout with a constant sinus rate and P-R interval and with alternating left bundle

branch block. This illustration is taken from the same patient as that shown in Figure 245b(i), page 405.

Record 160
Lead III. Complete heart block. The sinus rate is 101 beats/min. The ventricular rate is 13 beats/min.*

* This is a truly extraordinary situation. One would expect partial or complete loss of consciousness. The record was actually taken from a 64-year-old lady who attended the cardiology clinic saying that she had felt tired and slightly light-headed for about a year. She had never lost consciousness.

Record 161(continuous).
Sick sinus syndrome. The first QRS complex is incompletely seen. The second QRS complex is abnormally wide and is a ventricular escape beat. It is virtually identical in shape and dimensions to the last three QRS complexes seen (on the second row) which are also ventricular escape beats. These ventricular escape beats are occurring on the background of sinus arrest. Careful inspection of the S-T segment in relation to the second and last three QRS complexes shows what appears to be retrograde P waves (arrowed). It seems likely that the ventricular escape rhythm is giving rise to depolarisation of the atria via retrograde transmission through the atrio-ventricular node. QRS complexes 3 and 4 are also abnormally wide and abnormally shaped and these are also likely to be ventricular ectopic escape beats. The only alternative explanation is that they are ventricular ectopic premature beats. In this case the distinction is largely a semantic one since QRS complexes 3 and 4 as well as QRS complex 2 and the last three QRS complexes are all occurring on the background of sinus arrest and complexes 3 and 4 are only marginally "premature" in relation to the ventricular escape interval demonstrated by the last three QRS complexes. Complexes 3 and 4 may therefore be "premature" only in the sense that the escape focus represented by these two beats transiently has a shorter escape interval than the dominant ventricular escape rhythm. The matter is of no consequence. QRS complex 5 is also a ventricular escape beat similar to the second and last three QRS complexes. It likewise is followed by a retrograde P wave (arrowed) but this retrograde atrial depolarisation is able to gain access again via the atrio-ventricular node to the ventricles producing an echo beat (dashed arrow). The mechanism of this echo beat is as described on page 481 and is shown in Figure 330. In this particular case, however, the process is self-perpetuating and a burst of atrial tachycardia occurs for a period of approximately 4 sec. This atrial tachycardia stops when, following the last QRS in the tachycardia series the retrograde P wave does not gain access once more to the ventricles to initiate

ventricular depolarisation. Note that during the period of atrial tachycardia the QRS configuration is entirely normal, clearly showing that this is not a ventricular escape rhythm at this time but is a supraventricular rhythm. Following the end of the reciprocal ("echo") rhythm there is a period of complete asystole for almost 4 seconds followed by a ventricular escape mechanism once more.
This combination of marked depression of sino-atrial nodal function giving rise to periods of slow idioventricular escape rhythm and of asystole together with episodes of supraventricular tachycardia is typical of the sick sinus syndrome.

Record 162
There is a tachycardia with a regular rate and a constant QRS morphology except in relation to the two QRS complexes arrowed which occur marginally closer to the preceding QRS complexes and are followed by a marginally longer gap before the next QRS complex. All the QRS complexes are abnormally wide but the two QRS complexes arrowed are fractionally narrower than the majority. These arrowed QRS complexes give a clear clue to the nature of the rhythm disturbance. They are similar to the predominant form of QRS in their shape but they are significantly narrower and are almost certainly fusion beats. This means that these beats are partly initiated from the ventricular ectopic focus and partly from the results of supraventricular depolarisation and they clearly indicate that the underlying rhythm is ventricular tachycardia (see Table 46b).

Record 163
Sinus rhythm giving way to ventricular tachycardia. The first two beats are sinus beats with a P-R interval at the upper end of the normal range. The third QRS is clearly premature, abnormally wide and abnormally shaped and is a ventricular premature ectopic beat. This ventricular premature ectopic beat is followed by nine further identical QRS complexes with constant morphology and an almost constant rate. This is clearly a short burst of ventricular tachycardia. It is interrupted by a single QRS complex which has a morphology identical with that of the first two sinus beats and then the ventricular tachycardia resumes. The QRS complex seen in the middle of the burst of ventricular tachycardia is clearly a capture beat. This demonstrates the ventricular origin of the wide QRS complex tachycardia (Table 46a).

Record 164
Sinus rhythm with first degree heart block. All the criteria for sinus rhythm (page 371) are fulfilled except one. The one exception is that the P-R interval is abnormal and 0.34 sec. The P-R interval is constant. Since there is a constant, prolonged P-R interval the criteria for first degree heart block are fulfilled (page 488).

Glossary

Aberration, aberrant intraventricular conduction

Transient abnormality of the pathway of intraventricular conduction following a supraventricular impulse and occurring as a result of a change in the R-R interval. This response most commonly occurs in association with transient shortening of the R-R interval (i.e. a transient increase in the ventricular rate) in which case it is sometimes known as acceleration-dependent aberrancy. Sometimes the aberration occurs in association with transient slowing of the rate (i.e. a transient increase in the R-R interval (in which case it is known as 'deceleration-dependent aberrancy')).

Acceleration-dependent aberrancy
see Aberration

Accelerated idio-nodal rhythm

Enhanced activity of the atrio-ventricular nodal (junctional) area, giving rise to a junctional rhythm at a rate greater than the normal junctional escape rate and usually lying between 60-100 beats/min.

Accelerated idio-ventricular rhythm

An increase in the highest intrinsic ventricular depolarisation rate, giving rise to an ectopic ventricular rhythm occurring at a rate greater than the usual ventricular escape rate and typically at between 50-100 beats/min.

Antegrade

Conduction of the depolarisation impulse in the normal (forward) direction. The term is usually used in respect of conduction through the atrio-ventricular junctional area.

Anterograde

Sometimes used in place of "antegrade".

Antidromic

A term used in respect of circus movement tachycardias occurring in association with accessory pathways and referring to the fact that the circus pathway is the reverse of the normal direction and goes from atrium via accessory pathway to interventricular septum and back through the AV node to the atrial myocardium. The reverse pathway is called "orthodromic".

Arrhythmia

Any cardiac rhythm (transient or sustained) other than sinus rhythm with a regular rate in the range of 60-100 beats/min.

Asynchronous

This term (in respect of artificial pacemakers) refers to the regular stimulation of myocardium by a pacemaker unit without any reference to the spontaneous electrical activity of that unit, i.e. a fixed-rate pacing system.

Atrial capture

Retrograde conduction of the depolarisation impulse to the atria from the atrio-ventricular junctional area or from the ventricles occurring on the background of a period of atrio-ventricular dissociation. The term is also used in respect of depolarisation of the atrial myocardium by an artificial atrial pacing stimulus.

Atrial fibrillation

Irregular unco-ordinated activity of the atria. This is usually associated with irregular transmission of the impulse to the ventricles.

Atrial flutter

Rapid, regular atrial depolarisation, usually at approximately 300 beats/min occurring from an atrial pacemaker site.

Atrial premature beat (atrial premature contraction)

A depolarisation initiated within the atrial myocardium occurring earlier in the cardiac cycle than would be anticipated on inspection of the preceding cycles and resulting in re-setting of the sinus node pacemaker.

Atrial tachycardia

Regular, rapid depolarisation from an ectopic focus in the atrial myocardium. Only occasionally associated with 1:1 atrio-ventricular conduction and more often associated with 2:1, 3:1 or 4:1 conduction. The atrial rate is usually significantly less than that of atrial flutter and there is usually time for an iso-electric interval in the electrocardiogram between adjacent manifestations of atrial depolarisation.

Atrio-ventricular block

Impairment of conduction in the atrio-ventricular node (atrio-ventricular junctional area) or in the His bundle or simultaneously in the proximal part of the right and left bundles. First degree atrio-ventricular block implies conduction of every beat from atria to ventricles but implies also a longer than normal atrio-ventricular conduction time (P-R interval). Second degree atrio-ventricular block indicates intermittent failure of conduction of impulses from the atria to the ventricles. Type I second degree atrio-ventricular block implies a progressive prolongation of the P-R interval before transient failure of conduction. Type II second degree atrio-ventricular block implies a constant P-R interval before the intermittent failure to conduct. In this situation the P-R interval may be normal or prolonged. Third degree atrio-ventricular block (synonymous with complete heart block) indicates complete failure of atrio-ventricular conduction of all atrially-initiated impulses. Retrograde atrio-ventricular block indicates failure of impulses originating within the ventricular myocardium to pass backwards through the atrio-ventricular conduction area.

Automaticity

The inherent rhythmic spontaneous depolarisation of pacemaker tissue.

Atrio-ventricular dissociation

Independent depolarisation of the atria and of the ventricles. This can occur when the atrial rate is more rapid than the ventricular rate and there is failure of antegrade conduction (complete heart block) or when the ventricular rate is more rapid than the atrial rate and there is failure of retrograde conduction (ventricular tachycardia).

Bigeminy

Alternating foci of depolarisation. This implies that there are two separate cardiac pacemakers. The most common examples are provided by sinus rhythm with alternating atrial, nodal or ventricular premature beats giving respectively atrial, nodal (junctional) and ventricular bigeminy.

Bradycardia

A heart rate below the arbitrary lower limit of normal of 60 beats/min.

Capture

This term in general refers to depolarisation of a cardiac chamber in response to a stimulus. It tends to be used only when it is an intermittent phenomenon or when reference is being made to response of the myocardium to an artificial pacemaker. In respect to the latter the atrial pacing spike may be said to give rise to atrial capture and the ventricular pacing spike to ventricular capture. In relation to the former, see 'Capture beat'.

Capture beat

A conducted beat occurring at a time when the rhythm immediately preceding the beat is showing atrio-ventricular dissociation. This may therefore occur during complete heart block when, transiently, a P wave is seen to give rise to conduction through the atrio-ventricular junctional area into the ventricles or in association with ventricular tachycardia when, transiently, a P wave may succeed in passing through the junctional area and produce a ventricular capture with a normal QRS or when, consistently, on a 2:1, 3:1 or 4:1 basis, activation passes retrogradely through the AV node and produces atrial capture.

Circus movement tachycardia

A tachycardia occurring on the basis of a re-entrant mechanism (within the sinus node, atrial myocardium, AV node or ventricular myocardium or involving both the AV node and an anomalous pathway).

Compensatory pause

The increment in the time-interval between a ventricular premature beat and the subsequent, sinus-initiated, ventricular depolarisation which is just sufficient to offset the shorter interval between the preceding sinus-initiated QRS and the ventricular premature beat so that the total time-interval between the preceding and succeeding QRS complexes is exactly twice the normal R-R interval.

Complete atrio-ventricular block

Complete heart block. Third degree heart block. (See Atrio-ventricular block).

Concealed conduction

This refers to situations in which conduction of an impulse from one part to another of the pacemaker and conducting tissue cannot be seen directly but can only be inferred by its effect on the subsequent cycle time or depolarisation route.

Concealed pre-excitation

That situation in which an anomalous atrio-ventricular pathway exists but can only conduct in a reverse (ventriculo-atrial) direction. During sinus (or any supraventricular) rhythm there will be no electrocardiographic evidence of pre-excitation. Any re-entrant tachycardia involving the accessory pathway will be orthodromic and again there will be no electrocardiographic evidence of pre-excitation. The diagnosis can only be confirmed by electrophysiological studies.

Coupling interval

The interval between a premature or ectopic beat and the beat preceding it (normally measured from the beginning of the preceding QRS to the beginning of the ectopic or premature QRS or from the beginning of the preceding P wave to the origin of the ectopic or premature P wave).

Deceleration-dependent aberrancy
see Aberration

Delta wave

Deformity of the initial part of the QRS complex giving rise to slurring of the initial QRS deflection. This is most commonly associated with a short P-R interval and is seen in pre-excitation syndromes.

Demand mode pacemaker

A mode of artificial pacing in which, whether or not pacing is activated, depends on the current spontaneous depolarisation. Atrial or ventricular stimulation in such systems is initiated only when spontaneous activation does not occur within a predetermined interval.

Dissociation

Separation of depolarisation processes which are normally inter-related. This term is usually applied in respect of atrio-ventricular inter-relationships.

Dysrhythmia

Synonymous with arrhythmia.

Ectopic

Arising at any site in the cardiac tissue other than the sino-atrial node.

Entrance block

The phenomenon by which part of the myocardium fails to be activated by an oncoming depolarisation wave-front even though that part of the myocardium is no longer refractory. The term is most commonly used in association with ectopic sites giving rise to parasystolic rhythms.

Escape beat

A depolarisation arising at a site other than the sino-atrial node but not occurring prematurely. These beats only occur as a result of the (usually temporary) suppression of a pacemaker which would normally have an intrinsically higher discharge rate.

Extrasystole

A premature ectopic beat.

Exit block

Failure of conduction of a depolarisation process from its site of origin to adjacent tissue (e.g. sino-atrial block).

Fascicular block

Conduction failure is one or more of the three fascicles which normally transmit supraventricularly-initiated beats from the distal end of the His bundle to the ventricular myocardium. (The three "fascicles" are (i) the right bundle, (ii) the antero-superior division of the left bundle branch and (iii) the postero-inferior division of the left bundle branch).

Fibrillation

Chaotic, disorganised, electrical depolarisation of myocardium (may refer to the atria or to the ventricles).

Flutter

Very rapid co-ordinated atrial depolarisation of a cardiac chamber, usually with a rate of 300 beats/min. The term is most often applied to atrial depolarisation but has, in the past, been equally applied to ventricular depolarisation.

Fusion beat

A depolarisation produced by two independent and merging depolarisation waves, each arising from a separate site. The term may be used in respect of depolarisation within the atria (atrial fusion beats) or more commonly within the ventricles (ventricular fusion beats).

Idio-nodal rhythm

Rhythm initiated by regular depolarisation at the atrio-ventricular nodal (junctional) area. This differs from accelerated idio-nodal rhythm in that it can only be revealed if the higher rate pacemaker (principally the sinus node) is suppressed, i.e. it is an escape rhythm.

Idio-ventricular rhythm

Rhythm initiated by regular depolarisation within the ventricular myocardium. This is an escape rhythm which can only be revealed if the higher rate pacemakers (principally the sinus node and the AV node) are suppressed.

Interference dissociation

A form of atrio-ventricular dissociation which occurs when an accelerated ventricular rhythm is partially conducted backwards through the atrio-ventricular node rendering it refractory to simultaneously-occurring supraventricular depolarisations.

Interpolated

Ectopic premature depolarisations which do not interfere with the subsequent, anticipated normal depolarisation. Such beats are ectopic and premature but they occur in between the normally-initiated beats giving rise to an additional beat within the given time zone.

Junctional

Referring to that zone in the region of the atrio-ventricular node and the common bundle where automatic depolarisation is possible and where such depolarisation usually gives rise to

ventricular activation with normal QRS morphology and to atrial depolarisation with reversal of the normal P wave direction. The term is synonymous with "atrio-ventricular junctional".

Möbitz block

That form of second degree atrio-ventricular block in which intermittent failure of atrio-ventricular conduction occurs without any preceding increase in the P-R interval. This is also known as type II second degree atrio-ventricular block. This can occur at sites other than the atrio-ventricular node but it is most commonly recognised at the AV node.

Multifocal (usually applied in relation to ectopic beats)

Arising from several different anatomical sites.

Nodal rhythm, idio-nodal rhythm, atrio-ventricular junctional rhythm

These terms are synonymous and refer to the regular initiation of depolarisation at the AV nodal junctional area with antegrade spread to the ventricles and sometimes with retrograde spread to the atria. The ventricular rate is typically in the range of 40-60 beats/min. The rhythm is an escape rhythm and occurs when sinus nodal activity is depressed.

Nodal tachycardia

A rhythm originating at the atrio-ventricular junctional area. This differs from nodal rhythm in not being an escape rhythm but in being a sustained repetitive depolarisation arising in the AV junctional area at a rate higher than the prevailing sinus rate.

Orthodromic

A term used in respect of circus movement tachycardias occurring in association with accessory pathways and referring to the fact that the circus pathway is in the usual direction – atrial myocardium, via AV node to interventricular septum and back via the accessory pathway to the atrial myocardium.

Parasystole

An automatic ectopic (atrial, junctional or ventricular but most commonly recognised in relation to the ventricles) rhythm in which the ectopic pacemaker site is protected (by entrance block) from being prematurely discharged by other spontaneous impulses which reach the ectopic pacemaker site. Because of the entrance block the ectopic pacemaker site maintains its own regular automatic spontaneous discharge rate. It will give rise to myocardial depolarisation (and thus to a QRS complex if one is referring, for example, to ventricular parasystole) when and only when adjacent myocardium has not been made refractory as a result of depolarisation spreading from another site. It follows that the interval between consecutive depolarisations initiated by the parasystolic mechanism will be an integral multiple (one or more) of the basic interval between the parasystolic depolarisations.

Paroxysmal

This term is used to refer to episodic tachy-dysrhythmias which have a sudden onset and offset.

Pre-excitation

Activation of the ventricular myocardium earlier than would be expected by supraventricularly-initiated beats which travel by the normal atrio-ventricular conduction pathways. The presence of ventricular pre-excitation reveals the existence of an anomalous, fast-conducting, atrio-ventricular pathway.

Premature beat

A beat occurring earlier than would be anticipated as a result of inspection of preceding beats.

Re-entry phenomenon

A phenomenon in which a repetitive cyclical passage of the depolarisation wave within a segment of myocardium is made possible because the depolarising wave-front enters an inhomogeneous zone of myocardium in which different areas have different conduction velocities and different refractory periods. Because of these differences the depolarisation wave-front is able to travel along that part of the pathway which is not refractory and out into the distant myocardium, but is also able to return, retrogradely, through the inhomogeneous myocardium as a result of there having been sufficient time during its antegrade passage through that myocardium for recovery of the formerly refractory part of that inhomogeneous zone. If the circuit length, conduction velocities and refractory periods are appropriate, then the retrogradely-returning activation wave may once more find its initial antegrade pathway sufficiently recovered to permit a return in the antegrade fashion. In this way a cyclical movement within the inhomogeneous zone occurs and each time the depolarisation circuit passes the distal end of the zone transmission to the adjacent myocardium occurs. The re-entry phenomenon is the electrophysiological basis for the vast majority of ectopic tachy-dysrhythmias.

Re-entrant tachycardia

A tachycardia occurring on the basis of a re-entrant mechanism (synonomous with "circus movement tachycardia").

Refractory period

That interval immediately following depolarisation of myocardium during which the sensitivity of the myocardium to a subsequent depolarisation is markedly diminished. The refractoriness may be **absolute** (so that no stimulus, however powerful, can be effective) or may be **relative** (so that a normal stimulus will be ineffective but a more powerful stimulus than normal might initiate a further response).

Retrograde

Backward conduction of the depolarisation process, i.e. depolarisation taking place in a direction the opposite of normal. This term is usually applied to the atrio-ventricular node.

Sino-atrial block

Exit block at the sino-atrial node. This implies that the depolarisation process takes place normally within the SA nodal tissue but does not spread to the adjacent atrial myocardium.

Sinus arrest

A (usually transient) cessation of automaticity in the sino-atrial node.

Sinus arrhythmia

An exaggeration of the normal (though often only found on careful inspection) phasic variation in the rate of discharge from the sino-atrial node.

Sinus bradycardia

Sinus rhythm with a rate below 60 beats/min.

Sinus pause

Transient cessation of automaticity in the sino-atrial node. Effectively synonymous with sinus arrest except that "sinus pause" clearly indicates that the cessation of activity is transient, whereas "sinus arrest" could, strictly speaking, be applied to a transient or sustained cessation of sinus activity.

Sinus tachycardia

Sinus rhythm with a rate above 100 beats/min.

Supraventricular

This refers to a site of initiation of a depolarisation event or rhythm as being above (proximal to in electrophysiological terms) the ventricles. This description includes the sinus node, the atrial myocardium, the AV node (junctional area) and the His bundle, i.e. all electrical sites within the heart proximal to the bifurcation of the His bundle.

Synchronous pacemaker

A system of artificial pacemaking in which ventricular activation is controlled by and related to a spontaneous atrial activity. In the **atrial synchronous ventricular pacemaker** (VAT pacing) ventricular pacing occurs at a pre-determined interval following the recognition of a P wave. In **atrial synchronous ventricular inhibited pacing** (VDD pacing) ventricular pacing follows the recognition of a spontaneous P wave provided no spontaneous ventricular depolarisation occurs within the programmed atrio-ventricular delay.

Tachycardia

A heart rate (ventricular rate) above 100 beats/min.

Tachy-dysrhythmia

A rhythm in which the ventricular rate is more than 100 beats/min and the initiation of atrial and/or ventricular myocardial depolarisation is ectopic. A tachy-dysrhythmia is synonymous with tachy-arrhythmia.

Threshold

That intensity of stimulation which is just sufficient to cause a response in electrically-responsive tissue.

Trigeminy

A pattern of electrical activity in which, within each group of three beats, the first two are normal sinus beats and the third is an ectopic beat. Thus in atrial trigeminy the first two beats are sinus beats and the third beat is an atrial premature beat. Likewise for nodal and ventricular trigeminy. (Note. This is a rather loose term, the use of which is best avoided. Texts can be found in which it is defined as the recurring pattern of normal sinus beats followed by two unifocal ventricular ectopic beats).

Ventricular aberration

Aberrant intraventricular conduction.

Ventricular capture

Conduction to the ventricles of a depolarisation process initiated at supraventricular level occurring on the background of pre-existing atrio-ventricular dissociation (i.e. in the presence of complete heart block or during ventricular tachycardia).

Ventricular tachycardia

An abnormal ectopic rhythm resulting from rapid repetitive depolarisation being initiated at a site within the ventricular myocardium. Although the normal idio-ventricular rate is 50 beats/min or less and any discharge rate in excess of this could be considered to be a ventricular tachycardia, it is only when the rate begins to exceed approximately 130 beats/min that the term is used in general and in most cases of ventricular tachycardia the QRS rate is 180 or more, although "accelerated idio-ventricular rhythm" or "slow ventricular tachycardia" may be used when the ventricular rate is in the region of 70-130 beats/min.

Vulnerable period

That time-interval during the later part of the repolarisation process in which the tissue is unusually sensitive to stimulation and in which a less than normally adequate stimulus may initiate a depolarisation. It is also an interval during which a normally adequate (supra-threshold) stimulus may initiate local re-entry circuits which might result in an abnormal rhythm (e.g. ventricular tachycardia or ventricular fibrillation).

Wenckebach phenomenon

That form of second degree atrio-ventricular block in which failure of atrio-ventricular conduction is preceded by a progressive lengthening of the P-R interval. Although this definition is given in respect of conduction at the atrio-ventricular node, a similar phenomenon can occur at other sites in the conducting tissue. The Wenckebach phenomenon is also known as "type I block" or (when it is specifically referring to atrio-ventricular conduction problems) to "type I second degree atrio-ventricular block".

Wolff-Parkinson-White syndrome

This "syndrome" consists of a combination of ventricular pre-excitation (apparent from the electrocardiogram) together with clinical episodes of paroxysmal tachycardia. Electrocardiographic features consist of a shortened P-R interval, a widened QRS complex and slurring of the initial part of the QRS to give a delta wave.

Index

Bold numbers (e.g. **598**, **299** etc.) in this index refer to annotated electro-cardiogram records.

A

action potential, 347
  pacemaker cell, 349
  propagated, 347
activation, electrical
  definition, 8
  initiation and spread, 6
  magnitude and direction, 7
  vectors *see* vectors
ambulatory electrocardiography, 542
  arrhythmias, 546
    normal subjects, 545, 550
  dizziness, 548–9
  equipment, 542–4
  indications, 546–9
  ischaemic heart disease, 551–2
  pacemaker patients, 552
  palpitations, 546–8
  patient diary, 544
  syncope, 548–98
amiodarone, 224
amyloidosis, 242
aneurysm
  dissecting, 244
  ventricular, 199
angina, Prinzmetal (variant), 187
antidepressants, tricyclic, 223
aorta, coarctation, 244
apridine, 223
arrhythmias
  associated with atrio-ventricular
    pathways, 577
  classification, 375–6
  combination, 533–41
  definition, 61
  diagnosis, 575
  digitalis toxicity, 222
  ectopic, 385
  and hypokalaemia, 227
  and infarction, 197
  influence on morphological analysis,
    553–4
  mechanisms, 358
  normal subjects, 545, 550
  supraventricular, effect on P waves,
    269
  ventricular, effect on QRS complexes,
    269
  see also specific arrhythmias
Ashman phenomenon, 399
asystole, **598**
  ventricular, 475–6
ataxia, Friedreich's, 241
atelectasis, pulmonary, 244
atrial
  abnormality, left, **299**, **303**, **315**
  activation, 6

beats
  non-premature (escape), 387, 389
  premature, **594**
  premature blocked, **585**
  premature ectopic, 386–7, 388, 396,
    397–402, **581**, **588**, **589**, **591**, **593**,
    595, **596**, **597**
  depolarisation, 43, 59, 158, 386
  fibrillation, 436, **583**, **589**, **591**, **593**,
    594, **595**, **597**
    in combination with other
      arrhythmias, 534, 536
    criteria, 440
    diagnostic clues, 575
    ECG features, 436–40
    and ventricular pre-excitation, 454,
      538, 541, **587**
  flutter, 431, **583**, **589**, **590**
    in combination with other
      arrhythmias, 534, 535
    criteria, 435
    diagnostic clues, 575
    ECG features, 431–5
  hypertrophy, 158, 159
    bi-atrial, 165
    clinical significance, 162, 165
    congenital heart disease, 244
    criteria, 165, 269
    left, 162–5, 244, 250, 269, **292**, **293**,
      310
    right, 159–62, 167, 244, 250, 269,
      313, **318**
  infarction, 199
  repolarisation, 166–7
  rhythm, varying, **588**
  septal defect, 244
  tachycardia, 229–40, 402, 420–4,
    593, **594**, **595**
    in combination with other
      arrhythmias, 536, 537
    non-paroxysmal, 576
    normal subjects, 545
    paroxysmal re-entrant, 576
    re-entrant, **591**
atrio-ventricular (AV)
  block *see* heart block
  conduction
    accelerated *see* ventricular pre-
      excitation
    antidromic, 451
    normal, 111, 213–15
    orthodromic, 451
  dissociation, 369, 462
    causes, 370
  junctional area, 342
    see also junctional …
  node, 6, 11
    activation, 6
    anatomy, 342–4
    decremental conduction and
      concealed conduction at, 437
    refractory period, 420
    in supraventricular tachycardia, 420
    see also tachycardia, atrio-ventricular
      nodal re-entrant; tachycardia, atrio-
      ventricular re-entrant
axis, electrical *see* electrical axis

B

Bachmann's bundle, 343
baseline drift, 62
beats
  capture, 477, 565, **589**, **598**
  echo (reciprocal), 481, 536, **598**
  fusion, 386, 476–7, 565, **597**, **598**
  premature, 352, 376
  supraventricular, 396, 424–6
  see also atrial beats; ectopic beats;
    escape beats; junctional beats;
    ventricular beats
beta-blockers, 223
bifascicular blocks, 129, 139–42
  clinical significance, 143
bradycardia, 362
  causes, 363, 569
  diagnosis, 569–71
  sinus, **580**, **588**, **590**, **595**, **596**
    causes, 383
    in combination with other
      arrhythmias, 537
    diagnostic criteria, 377
    normal 545
bundle
  Bachmann's, 343
  branches
    anatomy, 343–4
    left, 6, 111, 343
    right, 6, 111, 343
  common (bundle of His), 6, 111, 342
    anatomy, 344
    electrocardiography, 486
bundle branch block, **589**, **594**
  functional *see* conduction,
    intraventricular aberrant
  left, 120–3, 198, **303**, **312**, **598**
    clinical significance, 129
    diagnostic criteria, 124–5, 213–15,
      268
    hemiblocks, 129–38
    incomplete, 126
    intermittent, 127–8, **598**
    with myocardial infarction, 250–1
  rate-related *see* conduction,
    intraventricular aberrant
  right, 114–17, **298**, **309**, **591**, **597**
    with anterior myocardial infarction,
      250–2
    clinical significance, 120
    congenital heart disease, 244
    diagnostic criteria, 118, 268
    incomplete, 119
    intermittent, 120
    with left anterior hemiblock, 139–40,
      143, 250
    with left posterior hemiblock, 141–3
  and Wolff–Parkinson–White
    syndrome, 454–5

C

calcium, serum levels, 229
calibration signal checking, 64–5
camel hump sign, 236
capture beats, 477, 565, **589**, **598**

Notes

Notes

Notes

Notes

Notes

Notes